Advance Praise for *Empowerment of Women for Promoting Global Health and Quality of Life*

"There is a growing consensus about the importance of women's empowerment both as a means for development and as an end in itself. The book on this topic by Snehendu B. Kar, focused on health promotion and quality of life, is a major achievement. It not only reviews the models dealing with empowerment and the most relevant literature on this topic, but also analyses a large number of case studies that clearly illustrate the way in which ordinary women empower themselves and, by doing so, improve the health and quality of life of their families and communities."

Julio Frenk, MD, MPH, PhD, President, University of Miami; Former Dean of the Faculty, Harvard T.H. Chan School of Public Health and Harvard John F. Kennedy School of Government, Cambridge and Boston

"I am aware of no other publications for this topic that begin to equal Kar's broad scope and depth of analysis, greatly benefited by the use of meta-analysis to draw general conclusions from diverse data. I am confident it will receive much attention and likely generate additional important research and publications. Those favoring women's empowerment for promoting health and quality of life will find it an excellent resource."

Bertram Raven, PhD, Professor Emeritus of Psychology and Founding Director of Health Psychology, UCLA

"It is rare to find a book that integrates theory, research, and practice and provides the compelling, credible support for the results of this integration. The author of this book does it brilliantly while highlighting the lived experience narrative of global ordinary (who are extraordinary) women who organized movements to deal with threats to themselves and their families. There are many books written about women and their health, yet this book stands out as it highlights the empowerment (not the vulnerability) of women. It is a must for reading and studying as a resource in the classroom, in practice, in legislative sessions, and by those who want to advocate for women. It provides a rich and in-depth analysis of women globally and the context within which they can develop and practice their empowerment."

Afaf I. Meleis, PhD, DrPS (hon), FAAN, Professor of Nursing and Sociology and Margaret Bond Simon Dean Emerita, University of Pennsylvania School of Nursing

T0177925

"At the heart of this impressive book is a meta-analysis of eighty cases of women's self-organized empowerment movements—both in low and high income countries. Dr. Kar found that each movement sprang from real threats to women's basic survival or safety, not from desires for personal growth or status. Small initial gains from the grassroots brought vital external support, which propelled movements forward and led to demonstrable impact. He also discovered a unifying theme: women often mobilized to prevent harm to the next generation. His meta-analysis yielded valuable insights into the strategies used by successful women-led movements and the specific barriers they face. This book will definitely be a welcome addition to anyone seeking greater understanding of the mechanics of women's empowerment globally."

Paula Tavrow, PhD, Co-Director, Center of Expertise on Women's Health and Empowerment, University of California Global Health Institute

"This is an incredibly invaluable resource for those interested in the potential of socially and economically disadvantaged women to improve the well-being of their communities, thus closing the health gap from the grassroots. Professor Kar builds on his extensive community-based experiences in Southern California by conducting a highly insightful meta-analysis of case studies from throughout the world, from rich to poor nations. The combination of theoretical concepts and extensive evidence from grounded collective action yields critical lessons for activists, scholars and policy makers."

Paul Ong, PhD, Professor and Director, Center for the Study of Inequality, UCLA Luskin School of Public Affairs

"This fascinating account of what empowerment means to women in most arduous situations and how empowerment translates into improving health and well-being is a must-read for both scholars and development practitioners alike. All those struggling to understand 'how to' empower women must learn from women how they empower themselves in most difficult situations. This volume comprehensively reviews empowerment theories followed by eighty in-depth case studies from across the globe of how ordinary women empower themselves when faced with great barriers and threats. The meticulous analysis presented in this book provides critical insights bridging theory and facts."

Ravi Verma, PhD, Regional Director, International Center for Research on Women (ICRW), Asia

"*Empowerment of Women for Promoting Global Health and Quality of Life* is a must-read for public health students and professionals interested in making a difference in the health of communities through empowerment.

Using the EMPOWER model, Dr. Kar reports on a meta-analysis of 86 real world cases in which women are empowered to change their communities. These cases of real women and real solutions is inspiring and uplifting—making it possible to believe that indeed, empowered women can change the world."

Theresa Byrd, DrPH, Associate Dean and Chair, Department of Public Health, University of Texas Health Science Center at Houston School of Public Health (UTSPH)

"This book is an invaluable addition in our understanding of issues related to empowerment of women for promoting global health and quality of life. Professor Kar's work is current, contextual, and addresses a felt-need for scholarly work on this topic. This work will be useful for both students and researchers across the developed and developing world."

Prof. Sanjay Zodpey, MD, PhD, Director, Indian Institute of Public Health, Delhi; Academic Vice-President and Director, Public Health Education, Public Health Foundation of India, New Delhi

"This book could not be more timely as women's empowerment, once again, takes center stage in health and development efforts with the World Bank, Gates Foundation, and others, prioritizing women's empowerment in their efforts. Dr. Kar grounds women's empowerment in a rich history of public health and development efforts, while highlighting their deep roots at the intersection of East and West, North and South, ancient and modern. Kar then elaborates empowerment theory at multiple domains, stages, strategies and dimensions, but most importantly, grounds this work in an extensive evidence-base of over 80 case studies of women-led, grassroots, empowerment projects from around the world working for human rights, equal rights, and health promotion and disease prevention. Students, scholars, researchers, and program designers alike will find this book to be an invaluable resource."

Dallas Swendeman, PhD, MPH, Co-Director, University of California, Global Health Institute, Center of Expertise on Women's Health and Empowerment

"This book is timely and makes several original and innovative contributions in global health and empowerment research. It contains many theoretical and empirical discussions, with special emphasis on women's empowerment as it relates to Global Public Health and the UN's Human Development Approach. I recommend it highly."

Abdelmonem A. Afifi, PhD, Dean Emeritus, UCLA Fielding School of Public Health

Empowerment of Women for Promoting Global Health and Quality of Life

Empowerment of Women for Promoting Global Health and Quality of Life

Snehendu B. Kar

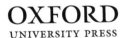

OXFORD
UNIVERSITY PRESS

Oxford University Press is a department of the University of Oxford. It furthers
the University's objective of excellence in research, scholarship, and education
by publishing worldwide. Oxford is a registered trade mark of Oxford University
Press in the UK and certain other countries.

Published in the United States of America by Oxford University Press
198 Madison Avenue, New York, NY 10016, United States of America.

Author's manuscript submitted in Fall, 2014

CIP data is on file at the Library of Congress
ISBN 978-0-19-938466-2

9 8 7 6 5 4 3 2 1

Printed by Edwards Brothers Malloy, United States of America

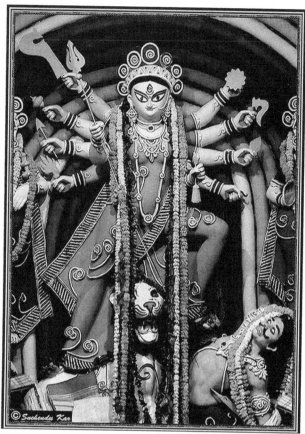

PHOTO 1 Durga Slaying Mahishasur. An idol of the goddess Durga
slaying the vicious demon Mahishasur to save the world from destruction.
The Bengalees worship Durga as the most powerful goddess.
Photo by Snehendu Kar.

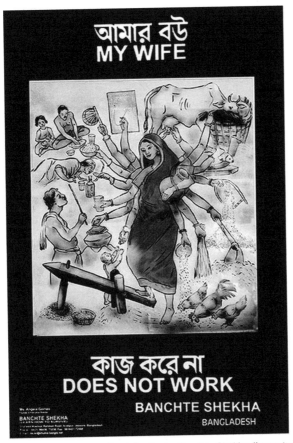

PHOTO 2 Women's Hard Work Undervalued. Poster by Banchte Shekha (Learn to Live).

With permission from Ms. Angela Gomes, the Founder and Executive Director of "Banchte Shekha" (a women's empowerment organization), Bangladesh.

Photo by Snehendu Kar.

These are the two common stereotypes of women in India. One is Durga, the supreme goddess of power, slaying an evil demon (Mahishasur) to save the world from disaster. The Hindu goddess Durga represents the power of the Supreme God and is the cosmic mother who protects and takes care of everyone. Durga Puja (worship) is the biggest religious ceremony and festival in West Bengal and several other states of India; it lasts for five days each year. Hundreds of "Durga Protima" (idols) are made and worshiped in the city of Kolkata alone; countless across the state and the nation. Durga Protimas are immersed in the Ganges or the nearest rivers after the five-day festival is over. There are other incarnations of Durga (Dussehra) worshipped in the rest of India. The second illustration is a rural Bengali housewife who, with her 16 hands (i.e., more than Durga's 10 hands), is a multitasking woman. She is overwhelmed by her daily chores, yet her husband says "My wife does not work"; he means she is unemployed. Her work is not valued, and she does not get paid.

Shabala

(*Sha* meaning "self"; *bal* meaning "power" or "strength")

Rabindranath Tagore

(Translation by Snehendu Kar)

Dear Lord, tell me why
a woman is denied
the right to seek her own fortune
with the power of her own?

Why must I forever await
by the wayside,
with my head bent,
and with weary expectation,
for the day when destiny may
let me find my own way.

Why must I keep gazing
at the empty horizon,
and not look for the way
to my own emancipation?

Why not let me harness
my fearless stallions
and race my sturdy chariot
with brave anticipation
on the way to my liberation?

Sanchayita (Mahua), pp. 631–632.

CONTENTS

LIST OF BOXES, FIGURES, AND TABLES

Boxes

Figures

Tables

ACKNOWLEDGMENTS

The seed of the tree that has produced this fruit was planted more than five decades ago when I was first appointed as a social scientist by the visionary leader of Indian Public Health Education, Dr. Venkata Ramakrishna, the founding director of the Central Health Education Bureau (CHEB) at the Ministry of Health and Family Planning in India. His trust and confidence in me surprised and energized me. Like most public health professionals at that time, I had no idea what "public health" was. Later, at the University of California–Berkeley, my mentors, including professors William Griffiths and Dorothy Nyswander, encouraged and supported me beyond my expectations. Without them, I would not be in public health today. The profound imaginings and writings of Rabindranath Tagore, the pioneering work of Amartya Sen on human development, the lyrics of the spiritual Baul music of rural Bengal, and the extraordinary courage and grace my mother showed as she took care of our family when we became refugees twice and I was still a child, inspired me to study women as a powerful force for combating the sufferings of the powerless and poor. From the hundreds of case studies reviewed for this project, I have discovered that powerless women are not a burden on society; they are the unselfish caregivers and the vastly unappreciated social and cultural capital in our unequal and unjust societies. It would be impossible for me to thank them personally.

Several research grants and awards over the past three decades enabled me to carry on my work, which served as the foundation of this book. In 1983, the World Health Organization (WHO), Geneva, awarded me a grant to develop a simplified consensus method (based on the Delphi technique) to identify meaningful and feasible indicators of primary health care (PHC). Public Health Experts from 42 countries identified and ranked the PHC indicators they considered most important. The results showed that women were major actors in effective global PHC, child health, and family planning initiatives. In 1984, the Centers for Disease Control and Prevention (CDC) awarded me a second grant to focus on the development of health promotion (HP) indicators in developed nations by US experts. Once again, families and women emerged as key forces of program effectiveness. I received a third grant from the Kellogg International Fellowship Program in Health (KIFP/H: 1986–1989) which was designed to bring together 27 senior fellows from across the world for a three-year period; each fellow worked on a project of her or his choice, and all helped one another. My project was on leadership in public health innovations; in addition to quantitative indicators of leadership, I began to collect case studies of effective movements (e.g., Mothers Against Drunk Driving [MADD], International Planned Parenthood Federation [IPPF], Madres de Playa Mayor). These case studies showed that poor and ordinary women across the world were taking the lead in designing and implementing innovative empowerment movements; social scientists in the health field were not writing about them, nor about empowerment for HP.

In the 1990s through 2010, a series of grants and awards allowed me to explore multicultural dimensions of health and HP that are a central focus of this book. The first was a four-year grant from the University of California's Pacific Rim Research Project that allowed me to study the influence of acculturation on quality of life among Asian American immigrants and compare them with US-born Whites, African Americans, and Hispanics. My colleagues and I have published several papers in peer-reviewed journals. The second opportunity was a series of training and program grants from the Health Resources and Services Administration (HRSA) of US Public Health Services (PHS), which focused on demonstrating excellence in HP practices in multicultural communities (MCC; defined as communities where people of different ethnic and national origins reside and no one group has the absolute majority). They supported our foundational work on women's empowerment projects for several years. These projects led to our national award-winning Rescatando Salud (Rescuing Health) project and the first meta-analysis work that led to the EMPOWER model (described in Chapters 5 & 6). Subsequent grants, contracts, and awards that supported our empowerment projects included: a Fulbright scholarship, multiyear grants and contracts from the State of California Department of Health, and the financial and staff support from the Office of Public Health Practice at the University of California–Los Angeles (UCLA). We are deeply indebted to these sources for supporting our work on empowerment of women for HP.

I must thank Cherri Todoroff, MPH (then-director of the L.A. County Immunization Program); Nancy H. Ibrahim, MPH (then–executive director of La Esperanza Community Housing Corporation); and John Kotick, JD (executive director of the LA South Central Community Health Center)—we served as the four co-directors of the Rescatando Salud project. Three former students and research associates who closely worked on our empowerment meta-analysis and Rescatando Salud projects at various stages are: Kirstin Chickering, MPH, who ably served as the project manager and supported me in all aspects of the Public Health Practice Office at UCLA; Catherine Pascual, MPH, served as the key research associate and assisted me with the meta-analysis and case studies; and Laticia Ibarra, MPH, who directed all field operations and outreach work by the *promotoras* for the Rescatando

Salud project. Without their talents and commitment, we could not have accomplished the meta-analysis and the Rescatando Salud project. Over the past 15 years, numerous graduate students have worked on various projects mentioned above. They include Felicia Ze, Sangeeta Gupta, Jasmeet Gill, Shaha Alex, John Talbot, Wendy Coleman, Armando Jimenez, Kevin Campbell, Nancy Hazelton, and Mary Schmitz. They have worked very hard, often beyond the call of their duties, and contributed immensely. I wish to thank Professor William Cumberland for his continued guidance of the statistical analyses in these projects.

Countless colleagues, both in the United States and abroad, have continued to support and inspire me. They include the eminent UCLA psychologist Bertram Raven (of Raven and French's "Six Bases of Social Power" fame), who has graciously shared his ideas on social power and has enhanced my work with his thoughtful comments for more than three decades; A. A. Afifi, Dean Emeritus of UCLA Fielding School of Public Health, a close friend and a fellow foreign-born eminent scholar, who fully supported my every initiative at UCLA; Rina Alcalay, professor and an eminent cross-cultural communication scholar, who has worked closely with me as we co-edited a volume on multicultural health communication and who introduced me to subtle cross-cultural issues, especially in Latin cultures in the United States and South America; Scott K. Simonds, the former head of the Health Education Program, and Leslie Corsa, Jr., the former head of the Population Planning Program, both at the University of Michigan (UM), Ann Arbor. Scott and Les offered me my first faculty position at UM and mentored me during my early career in the United States.

Prominent among my overseas colleagues, who continue to serve as my lifelines to global cultures and health, are Nelly Candeias, former professor and head of Health Education at the University of Sao Paulo, Brazil; Dr. H. S. Dhillon, the former director of Health Information, Education and Communication (IEC) at WHO, Geneva (he and I co-founded the first Research and Evaluation Division at the CHEB in India); and the eminent psychologist, prolific author, poet, and musician Jagadindra Mondal, former professor and Chair of Applied Psychology and former Dean of Sciences at the University of Kolkata, India. I am immensely fortunate to have them enrich my life and work. Most recently, Adam Grotsky, the Executive Director of the United States-India Educational Foundation (USIEF) in India, and the senior leaders of the Fulbright Commission, both in the United States and in India, were immensely helpful in my research activities for my Fulbright-Nehru Distinguished Chair award which allowed me rare opportunities to interview over fifty authors and innovators of several case studies included in this volume.

I am most grateful to Dana Bliss, senior editor, and Brianna Marron, assistant editor, at Oxford University Press (OUP). Dana's reassuring encouragement and Brianna's highly efficient, prompt, and substantive help during the entire process of writing this book are deeply appreciated. When Brianna assumed a deservedly higher position at OUP, Andrew Dominello seamlessly took over her role and helped me through the completion of this book. I am also thankful to Devi Vaidyanathan, the project manager, and Gail Cooper, the copy editor, and Shanmuga Priya for their patience and valuable support as we completed the manuscript. This book would not be possible without the invaluable support from OUP under Dana's leadership.

My immediate family members have been supportive of me beyond the bounds of reason; I am deeply indebted to them. My younger son Sanjib has given up making any demands on my time and has quietly abandoned many fun projects we normally enjoyed together. My older son Robin Kar, a full professor of philosophy and law, has been my strongest argumentative comrade. His deep and thoughtful comments on key issues have sharpened my ideas, and his substantive suggestions have encouraged my frequent journeys into literatures that extend beyond my area of expertise. My wife, Barbara, played a very important role; she patiently reread multiple versions of each chapter, line by line. Her two graduate degrees (an MPH and an MA in Romance Languages) and more than four decades of professional experience as a director of health education, made her eminently qualified to critique my text from a professional's perspective and to make valuable suggestions. I believe that the book is richer because of Robin's and Barbara's substantive contributions.

I wish to dedicate this book to all women who enrich and empower others' lives and to those who help them.

ABOUT THE AUTHOR

Snehendu B. Kar, Dr. P.H., MPH, M.Sc., is a Fulbright-Nehru Distinguished Chair, Professor Emeritus of Public Health and Asian American Studies, and the Founding Director of the MPH for Health Professionals Program in Community Health Sciences at the Fielding School of Public Health (FSPH), University of California at Los Angeles (UCLA). As the Associate Dean and Chair of the then single department FSPH, he led all academic programs of that school. Kar's other fulltime positions include: Distinguished Professor and Academic Advisor at the Public Health Foundation of India (New Delhi), a full-professor at UCLA for nearly four decades, and tenured professorships at the Public Health School of the University of Michigan. Before coming to the US, Kar served as an Assistant Director General of Health Services at the Indian Ministry of Health and Family Welfare, New Delhi. His research and teaching have focused on social determinants of health, health education and promotion, population planning, health communication, global health, and women's empowerment for human development. He has served as a consultant in many countries and has directed several multi-national collaborative research projects sponsored by organizations including the: WHO, UNDP, UNICEF, UNESCO, CDC, USAID, Fulbright Commission, UC Pacific-Rim Research Program, and Kellogg and Ford Foundations. His honors include elected fellowships of the Delta Omega Honor Society, American Psychological Association, SPSSI, Kellogg International Fellowship Program/Health, US-India Education Foundation, Public Health Leadership Institute (UC Berkeley & CDC), and invited keynote addresses at several international conferences. He has authored six books and more than 125 peer-reviewed research papers, book chapters, monographs, and technical reports. Kar's latest book, *Coming and Going: Poems and Songs of Rabindranath Tagore* (2015; the Bee Books, Kolkata), presents his translations of the Nobel Laureate poet's spiritual poems illustrated by his award-winning photos.

Email contact: kar@ucla.edu
Website: http://ph.ucla.edu/faculty/kar

ABBREVIATIONS

APA	American Psychological Association
APHA	American Public Health Association
ASPPH	Association of Schools and Programs of Public Health (formerly: ASPH)
BOL	Bottom of the Ladder
BOP	Bottom of the Pyramid
CDC	Centers for Disease Control and Prevention
CEDAW	Commission on Elimination of Discrimination Against Women
GEE	Gender Equity and Empowerment
GEM	Gender Equality Measures
GDI	Gender Development Index
DPHP	Disease Prevention and Health Promotion (sometimes: Health Promotion and Disease Prevention—HPDP)
EMPOWER	Empowerment model/methods
EOW	Empowerment of Women
EURO	European Regional Office (WHO)
FGM/C	Female Genital Mutilation/Cutting
GPH	Global Public Health
HDA	Human Development Approach
HDI	Human Development Index
HDR	Human Development Report (of UNDP)
HEP	Health Education and Promotion
HHS	Health and Human Services
HPDP	Health Promotion and Disease Prevention
HRQOL	Health-Related Quality of Life
IEC	Information, Education, and Communication
IMF	International Monetary Fund
IOM	Institutes of Medicine
NIH	National Institutes of Health
MLI	Multi-Level Intervention
MDGs	Millennium Development Goals
OECD	Organization for Economic Co-Operation and Development
PAHO	Pan American Health Organization
PHC	Primary Health Care

PHS	Public Health Service
PHN	Public Health Nursing
QOL	Quality of Life
SDG	Sustainable Development Goals (UNDP)
SEARO	South East Asian Regional Office
SOPHE	Society for Public Health Education
SOWEM	Self-Organized Women's Empowerment Movement
SG	Surgeon General (US SG)
SSR	System Sciences Research
WHO	World Health Organization
UCLA	University of California, Los Angeles
UN	United Nations
UNDP	United Nations Development Program
UNW	United Nations Women
USIEF	US-India Educational Foundation
US PHS	US Public Health Service
WPRO	Western Pacific Regional Office (WHO)
WAM	Women and Mothers

Introduction

The primary aim of this book is to critically review selected theories and literature on empowerment, with special emphasis on women's empowerment, as a major strategic option for promoting global public health (GPH) in rapidly globalized and multicultural communities. This book presents a balanced perspective of theoretical and empirical literature on empowerment in general and on women's empowerment in particular, and a meta-analysis of 80 case studies of self-organized empowerment movements by ordinary women that promote the health and well-being of their families and communities. Women are conceptualized as agents for positive change rather than as passive beneficiaries of welfare programs.

The book is organized as follows. Chapters 1 through 4 provide a critical review of the major theoretical literature on empowerment in general and on women's empowerment in particular for promoting GPH and health-related quality of life (HRQOL) in communities. Included is the evolution of GPH and the role of women's empowerment as a powerful component of GPH in a multicultural context. Chapters 5 and 6 present our theoretical framework, methodology including the EMPOWER model, and the key findings from a major meta-analysis of 80 successful case studies of self-organized women-led grassroots empowerment movements that significantly enhanced the health-related quality of life (HRQOL) of their families and communities in both rich and poorer nations across the world. The meta-analysis is based on our ongoing research on women's empowerment for health promotion that began over a 15-year period (Kar, 2000b; Kar et al., 1999). The 80 case studies were selected from empowerment movements in four domains of life: human rights, equal rights, health, and economic well-being; Chapters 7 through 10 include a two to three-page summary of each case study to give the readers a direct glimpse of each empowerment process and reference(s) for further study of these movements. Chapter 11 summarizes the issues and implications of this book including areas for future research and actions for empowerment of women for GPH promotion and HRQOL.

The intended audiences for this book include researchers, educators, students, and policy makers in several health and human services fields (e.g., GPH, Public Health, Gender Studies, Health Psychology, Community Health Sciences, Social Welfare/Work, Community Nursing, and Human Development).

Rationale and Significance of Empowerment: The Third Path

Powerlessness and poverty are two major threats to our HRQOL. Consequently, the United Nations (UN) has emphasized women's empowerment and poverty reduction as two of its eight current Sustainable Development Goals (SDGs) (UN, 2000). On aggregate indicators, our world has made major progress in several areas over the past few decades. For instance, people now live longer, there are fewer world wars comparable to World War I or World War II, major infectious diseases that killed or disabled millions annually (e.g., small pox, malaria, polio, cholera) have been either eradicated or controlled; literacy has risen; more countries live in democracies; and millions have risen above poverty. But these and other aggregate indicators hide serious failures and persistent inequalities have worsened HRQOL in vulnerable sections of populations in both rich and poorer nations (UNDP, 2015).

There are *three paths* or options for promoting HRQOL for poor and disadvantaged populations. The *first path* involves offering developmental aids, including grants and charitable contributions, to poorer nations and poor communities. However, giving foreign aid to poor countries which has been the standard economic development model of past decades has failed to narrow the gaps between the rich and the poor nations and between the rich and the poor people within all nations. Worldwide gender and health inequalities are still unacceptably high. For example, about 2.2 billion people in the world are under or near the poverty line (UNDP, 2015); more than 70% of the people under the poverty line worldwide are women; there is a poor gender ratio in many countries; 60% of infants born in the poorest countries do not survive their first year of life; and the prevalence of child labor, child marriages, and trafficking of women and children for forced labor or prostitution are unacceptably high. Clearly, the standard economic development model does not solve the increasing problem of powerlessness and income disparities between the poor and the rich.

The *second path* to enhance health and well-being uses increased efforts by local/national governments to promote economic growth. The claim of this approach is that when countries become richer, they will have more money to invest in the human development of their poor. Again, available records of the past decades show that this second path mostly befits the rich and the middle classes; growth in national wealth does not reduce income disparities, poverty, and powerlessness of the people at the bottom of the economic pyramid. In recognition of this problem, the world communities, under the leadership of the United Nations Development Programme (UNDP) and other multinational development agencies (e.g., World Bank, International Monetary Fund [IMF]), have adopted the human development approach (HDA) that focuses on the enhancement of human capabilities through increased participatory governance, freedom, education, health, equalities, and opportunities as well as economic growth for a better life for all.

However, in numerous countries and in poor communities there is a strong disagreement between the proponents of the "economic growth" and the "human development" approaches. Advocates of the "economic growth" approach argue that the poor countries must first enlarge the overall size of their economic pie before they will have the funds needed to invest in "human development" (e.g., health, education, and employment). Advocates of the HDA, including the UN/UNDP, the World Bank, and the IMF, argue that a poor country cannot become economically self-reliant unless it has a healthy and literate workforce; besides, a healthy life is a basic right and necessity (Piketty, 2014; UNDP, 2015). We need effective alternative models, or a third path, to empower the poor and the powerless for better HRQOL in addition to the conventional economic growth that tends to bypass the poor.

The third path advocates focusing on the empowerment of the poor and powerless to enhance their capabilities and quality of life with effective structural support from communities and human service agencies. Some argue that the third path (community empowerment including microfinance initiatives) at best tends to have limited and local impact. This may be true, but the critics should recognize the two antitheses to their argument. First, the other two alternative paths are not helping the poorest and powerless; so why dismiss the third path that has demonstrated proven success (e.g., Grameen Bank, Self-Employed Women's Association in India [SEWA]) just because it may have a small local impact. Second, when used effectively, the Third Path has the potential for large effects. The records of the Grameen Bank in Bangladesh and the SEWA movement in India have demonstrated dramatic successes. Our response to those who argue that women's empowerment is not a viable policy option because this method is ineffective or has a small local impact, we offer these justifications. First, as this volume shows, empowerment movements by ordinary women often have huge global and national impacts; we have presented more than 80 examples of successful self-organized women's movements even when these women faced serious adversities. Many of these movements have received prestigious national and international recognitions including the Nobel prize. Second, if indeed women's movements have small local impacts, then the logical option would be to support a much larger number of women's movements so that more people would benefit from the cumulative impacts the larger number of movements. Finally, we are not proposing women's empowerment as an exclusive but a complementary and third option. Also, these three paths need not be mutually exclusive; indeed, they may complement one another and generate significant synergy.

Finally, there are serious problems rooted in our social and cultural systems that cannot be resolved by an exclusive focus on economic growth; violence against powerless and vulnerable groups including women and stigmatized racial groups are examples of such situations. Wealth does not protect affluent women from gender prejudice and domestic violence; nor does having money shield a member of a stigmatized minority from exclusion and abuse (e.g., the first fatal victim of racial hatred after the 9/11 tragedy in the United States was a Sikh male from India who was wrongly perceived by his murderer as a Muslim because the Sikh religion requires men to wear a turban and prohibits shaving of facial hair). Racial, gender based, and other forms of discrimination hurt billions (not millions) of women and other vulnerable groups. The latest UNDP Human Development Report (HDR) (UNDP, 2015) released on July 24, 2014, estimates that our world now has 2.2 billion poor and near poor people (UNDP, 2015); meanwhile, the rich are becoming richer. This HDR report concludes that while the world has made substantial gains on several aggregate measures, these improvements cannot be sustained unless the poor and vulnerable groups are protected from unacceptable levels of poverty, discrimination, and human abuse.

The third path or, empowerment of women, especially in poor and vulnerable communities, has a significant role to play in averting major global miseries and disasters. In recognition of this imperative, the world as a whole under the auspices of the UN, adopted eight millennium development goals (MDGs) for the year 2015; two of these were aimed at gender development (including gender equality and gender empowerment, MDG number 3) and elimination of extreme poverty and hunger (UN, 2000–2009). A new emphasis for the years beyond the 2015 MDGs is on "sustainable progress" that must include reducing "vulnerabilities" and building "resilience" among the poor and powerless. Women's empowerment for human development subsumes both reduction of vulnerabilities and increase of resilience in communities. The main goal of this book is to study how powerless women empower themselves, to learn from their movements, and to make that knowledge widely available.

EMPOWERMENT PHILOSOPHY

The empowerment philosophy of this book is informed not only by the author's formal education and decades of multicultural research and teaching experience, but also from studying numerous innovations in social action in poor and disadvantaged communities. These innovations grew out of a desperate need in a resource-deprived community and the genuine concerns of innovative professionals who cared and tried to find inexpensive solutions through collective group-work for empowerment. A few examples include: Uri Triesman's "Merit Immersion for Students and Teachers" (MIST) which demonstrated that promoting "collaborative learning" and group problem-solving assignments, supported by competent mentors, while de-emphasizing lectures by teachers and tests, dramatically improves math and science performance of minority students (Triesman, 2007). Sugata Mitra's "Hole in the Wall" projects (Mitra, 1982) that won the one-million dollar TED prize, showed that poor slum children in Delhi and elsewhere can, through group work, can learn computer competencies without having teachers in classrooms, or owning personal computers. Salman Khan's "Khan Academy" has shown that children and adults alike can learn math, science, and other technical subjects, without a teacher in the classroom, from free online lessons that Khan initially designed for his cousin and later made available online free of cost to everyone (Khan Academy, 2015). The Forbes Magazine summed up the success story of the Khan Academy in an article entitled: "One Man, One Computer, 10 Million Students: How Khan Academy is Reinventing Education" (Khan Academy, 2015). Rabindranath Tagore, the pioneer of the "microcredit" project in rural India, Ela Bhatt (of SEWA) in urban slums also in India, and Muhammad Yunus (of the Grameen Bank) in Bangladesh and in numerous nations, have shown that small microcredit loans, combined with small working-groups as co-operatives of peers, with support of benevolent mentors, can significantly enhance income and quality of life (QOL) for the poorest farmers, laborers, and powerless women; but investing hundreds of billions of dollars of foreign aid per year over the last several decades failed to benefit the poorest and poor countries; the poorest became poorer. Jody Heymann (2010) has shown that investments at the "bottom of the ladder" of employees that promote their health and working conditions increases economic benefits to all employees and the company. Business scholar C. K. Prahalad's research (2006) has demonstrated innovative methods for partnering with poor consumers (as business partners) that benefit both the business entrepreneurs and their participating poor partners; it happens because it creates a win–win arrangement in which poor clients are treated as empowered business partners, not as poor and passive consumers.

These and other innovations show the inherent power of "self-organized" and "collaborative groups" when learning is supported by competent mentors and trusted professionals; but above all these succeed when peer groups work together to maximize synergy and mutual support. Vicarious learning from these and similar movements is a rich source of learning how the poor and powerless women empower themselves. Teaching is learning; it empowers the teacher as well as the learner.

Finally, three thinkers who have influenced this author's philosophy of empowerment are Paulo Freire, Amartya Sen, and Rabindranath Tagore.

Freire's axiomatic book titles emphasize the importance of *Education for Critical Consciousness* (Freire, 1973, 1974). In his books, Freire emphasizes the value of a "praxis" or a two-way learning through a collaboration between the teacher and the learner through which both learn. He holds that it is not enough for people to gain knowledge about their social reality; they must work together to critically reflect upon their reality and transform it through collective and action (Freire, 2015, p. 1). Sen, in his book *The Argumentative Indian* has argued that the argumentative nature of Indians has enriched their ancient culture and served them very well (Sen, 2006a). As an educator, I am not satisfied if I do not learn something new from teaching a graduate-level course or working with the powerless in poor communities. Finally, the philosopher-poet Rabindranath Tagore nearly a century ago prophesized: "When races come together, as in the present age, it should not be merely the gathering of a crowd; there must be a bond of relation, or they will collide with each other" (Tagore, "On Education," 1925). As our communities are becoming multicultural, professionals working in these communities must learn what divides or unites people from different cultures, and how some communities effectively cope with the problems unique to multicultural communities. These lessons cannot be learned from scholarly literature alone. This book is guided by the philosophy of self-organization, vicarious learning, and critical analysis of exemplary case studies as important sources of learning about empowerment. The meta-analysis of 80 women-led empowerment case studies (Chapter 6) and the summaries of these movements presented in this book (Chapters 7–10) have shown that poor and ordinary women across the world can and do lead self-organized movements that fundamentally transform them and promote HRQOL for their families and communities. These case studies demonstrate how these women succeeded with a little help from dedicated professionals; they teach us how professionals have helped these movements.

Finally, in examining the evolution of GPH, this book looks beyond modern western medicine and public health both geographically and historically. The two most cited books on the history of public health by Rosen (1993) and Porter (1999) focus on historic developments from the Euro-American (European and North-American) perspectives; Rosen primarily focuses on North America and Porter on Britain. Other systems of health care (e.g., Chinese medicine, Indian Ayurveda) are mostly neglected. This omission is not an isolated event among the Western scholars who tend to be preoccupied with the Euro-American heritage (both in time and space); this leads to an incomplete history of human civilization. R. B. Kar (2012a) observed that Western scholars who search for the origins of Western Civilizations, tend to trace back their roots to ancient Abrahamic religions and civilizations in Greece, Rome, and ancient Israel. Writing on the origins of Western Civilization, he states:

Although the so-called "Indus Valley" civilization (a.k.a. the "Harappan" or "Sindhu-Sarasvati" civilization) represents one of the very first such successful transformations in our natural history as a species, and although the Indus Valley civilization long predates similar developments in ancient Greece, Rome or Israel, most scholars deem these early developments irrelevant to Western prehistory because of a specific linguistic proposition: they believe that the Indus Valley civilization spoke a non-Indo-European language and that its traditions are therefore phylogenetically unrelated to the larger family of Indo-European civilizations that show up in the subsequent historical record (first in ancient Persia, Greece, Rome and India—and then much later in Western Europe and Russia). If this traditional linguistic assumption is wrong, however, then many of our modern attempts to understand the basic causes and conditions of Western development are being shaped by a fundamental misunderstanding—and often to their detriment.

After triangulating more recent archeological, linguistic, and genomic evidence, R. B. Kar (2012a) concludes that based on this entire combined body of evidence, we now have compelling reasons to think that the Indus Valley civilization spoke dialects of Proto-Indo-European language.

This means that the roots of western civilization extend far beyond the Abrahamic civilizations. R. B. Kar (2012a) cautions that if we begin the origin of western civilization with Greece, Rome, and Israel, and go no further in time and geographic space, then our history of western civilization will remain incomplete; like beginning to tell a story at the middle, we will not know what happened before and how the past affected subsequent developments. This is especially true for the history of GPH. While this book is not on the history of public health, it goes back to developments that predate the discovery of "germ theory" and the modern western biomedical model of health research and care. It includes evidence from both western and non-western cultures that led to GPH and the HDA approach led by the UN. It extends beyond primary health care and preventive medicine, and extends to sociocultural realities that affect human health and well-being (e.g., freedom, equality, and empowerment).

SELF-ORGANIZED WOMEN'S EMPOWERMENT MOVEMENTS (SOWEM)

A recent Google Scholar search using the key words "Empowerment Books" generated over 3,420,000 results (accessed February 20, 2018). A closer examination shows that the largest categories of these results deal with self-help/care, personal skill-development (e.g., resistance and negotiation skills), personal growth including the New-Age movements for health and spiritual growth (e.g., Yoga, Transcendental Meditation [TM], nutrition, and complementary and alternative medicine [CAM]). In addition, many items have multiple listings. Public health, by definition, deals with health promotion and disease prevention (HPDP) of the public or defined groups of people; its unit of analysis and intervention is not the individual patients, but the community or groups of people. Once the items that do not directly deal with the Public health model or population-based interventions for clinical care (e.g., patient care, clinical care) are excluded, the number of books on empowerment drops significantly. We could not identify any books that exclusively deal with meta-analysis of women's empowerment movements organized and led by women.

Some of the most cited publications on empowerment theory and research are journal articles or chapters in books edited by scholar(s) who are not directly involved in public health. For instance, in social psychology, one of the most cited theories of power is the "Six Social Bases of Power" by Raven (Raven, 2012); this is an expansion of the original French & Raven's "Five Bases of Social Power." Raven added a sixth power base, "information," to their original theory. Information as a base of power could be either negative (e.g., false information about weapons of mass destruction used to justify the US-led invasion of Iraq) or positive in nature such as a sound justification and facts in support of a preventive health practice (danger of tobacco smoking and lung cancer). The information source may also be direct (interpersonal) or impersonal (ubiquitous social media or traditional media). The Raven–French theory of "Six Bases of Power" has had a major impact on health psychology.

Other major social psychological and behavioral theories that deal directly or indirectly with empowerment and human motivation include Lewin et al.'s theory of "Level of Aspirations" (1944); Cantril's "Self-Anchoring Striving" and scale (1967); Maslow's theory of "Hierarchy of Needs" (1962); McClelland's theory of "Need for Achievement" (1953 and 1961) which identifies three major human motivations for action (needs for: achievement, affiliation, and power); Zimbardo's theory on the role of value expectancy and situation, as expounded in his volume entitled *The Lucifer Effect* (2007); the "social cognitive theories" of Bandura (1986) and Vroom (1964); Kahneman's theory of two systems (fast and slow) of human decision (Kahneman (2011); and recent theories by "behavioral economists" [Piketty (2014) and Acemoglu and Robinson (2012)]. In addition there is a recent explosion of literature on over-simplified "self-help" books that try to motivate others and management gurus who claim that what works for successful corporations also works for marginalized and powerless communities; they often forget that corporations are the causes rather than the solutions of many problems in our increasingly globalized economies. These theories and related issues are discussed in greater details in Chapters 4 and 5. The common denominators of these theories are that they do not theorize gender and culture as determinants of empowerment; nor do they explain or predict how gender and culture affect empowerment. Several prolific scholars involved in empowerment research in public health have been inexplicably silent on women's empowerment for health promotion and human development.

This book combines both deductive and inductive methods; in the first five chapters it reviews important literature on empowerment in general and women's empowerment issues using the perspective of the social planners and scholars ("top-down") and in the remaining chapters it uses an inductive approach (meta-analysis of case studies) and focuses on the issues and problems faced by women and how they empowered themselves. The meta-analysis includes a large number of cases ($n = 80$) to observe common trends and differences between empowerment movements across the world in four domains of life and by rich and poor nations. The four domains of empowerment are: human rights, equal rights, health, and economics.

There are three important differences between this book and other books on empowerment for better health and HRQOL. First, the other books are generally gender- and color-blind in their treatment of empowerment. They deal with empowerment at the aggregate level as if gender and ethnic differences do not matter. The major global consensuses that have evolved under the leaderships of the UN, the UNDP, UNICEF, and the World Health Organization (WHO) have repeatedly cautioned the world that persistent gender inequalities and disparities in health, education, and income are serious threats to our collective well-being. Consequently, the UNDP's current Millennium Development Goals (MDGs) specifically emphasize women's empowerment and the reduction/elimination of extreme poverty and hunger. Empirical data from 75 nations support the utilitarian contention that gender empowerment strongly correlates with several health and human development indicators. In a recent global study, Varkey, Kureshi, and Lesnick (2010) state:

> We used the gender empowerment measure (GEM), a composite index measuring gender inequality in economic participation and decision making, political participation and decision making, and power over economic resources. All 75 countries with GEM values in the 2006 Human Development Report (HDR) were included in the study. (p. 71)

This study concluded that

> After adjusting for GDP, GEM was significantly associated with low birth weight, fertility rate, infant mortality, and age ≤ 5 mortality; the strongest correlation was found to be between GEM and infant mortality ($R^2 = 0.601$) ... The results of this study suggest that the empowerment of women is associated with several key health indicators at a national level. (p. 71)

While a correlation does not prove a causality, it does provide a strong justification for further testing a proposed causal hypothesis while experimentally or statistically controlling for spurious relationships and external causal factors.

Second, some volumes focus on women exclusively, but they are descriptive case studies and deal with a small number of cases. There is a big difference between encouraging people to participate in programs designed by someone else (as is the case with community development and organization) and people's self-organized movements that empower them. Unfortunately there are no in-depth meta-analyses of large numbers of cases that examine whether there are common trends, similarities, or differences in women's empowerment movements in diverse situations dealing with different problems and cultures. This book includes a meta-analysis that uses a common analytical framework (using comparable data on six research questions from all case studies and the proposed EMPOWER model to guide data extraction and analysis) and a large number of case studies from diverse societies in richer and poorer nations.

Third, evidence from recent innovative educational programs emphasize the power of "self-organized learning" (SOL) through group problem-solving assignments (discussed before). This book includes 80 self-organized group-based problem-solving processes. It is not suggested that self-organized women's empowerment movements do not need or seek help from outside; indeed one of our six research questions is about who support and oppose these movements and how. The central point is that powerless women can and do organize and lead movements and in that process they need and obtain support from outside allies (including professionals); but these women initiate and remain in charge of their movements. Among the 80 case studies, all except one, the Grameen Bank project, were organized and led by women who were themselves victims. Even in the case of the Grameen Bank, the collateral-free loans were given to groups of powerless women and these women worked in stable groups and reinforced one another in their collective efforts. We have not seen another volume that systematically examines such a large number of self-organized women's empowerment movements in different domains from across the world.

In response to the global consensus, demands from students, and recognition of needs, during the last three decades, the numbers of Gender Studies, Public Health, Social Work/Welfare and Allied Health Sciences degree programs have expanded exponentially. In addition, hundreds of online Master of Public Health (MPH), Master of Social Work (MSW), and related degree programs have sprung up nationally and globally while the available literature has not kept up with the needs of these educational programs. This book would be an important resource for these and related educational programs as well as for others interested in GPH and the Human Development Approach.

Organization of The Book and Scope of the Chapters

Unlike a textbook, this book is not a summary of major theories and research in social and behavioral sciences. This book focuses on women's empowerment as it relates to GPH as one of the three important paths to better health for all. The book has 11 chapters that deal with four theoretical and empirical content areas; First: sociocultural foundations of GPH (Chapters 1–3); second: women's empowerment for better health and human development in multicultural contexts (Chapters 4 and 5); third: a meta-analysis of 80 self-organized women's movements using the EMPOWER model designed to extract data on seven dimensions or methods of empowerment used in the meta-analysis (Chapter 6); and fourth: summaries of the case studies in four domains of empowerment: human rights, equal rights, economics, and health. These case studies constitute the original sources of learning how powerless women self-organized movements that enhanced the HRQOL of their families and communities (Chapters 7–10). The concluding chapter (Chapter 11) includes: (a) a critical review of key issues in empowerment and the implications for the human development approach (HDA) that emerged from all previous chapters, (b) an application of the EMPOWER model for the "Rescatando Salud" (Save Health) project designed to promote childhood immunization coverage by empowering Latina women, as *promotoras* in underserved communities in Los Angeles, and (c) the implications of the content of the entire volume for women's empowerment theory, research, and action.

I hope that the substantive analyses of the topics, the meta-analysis methodology and the key results, and the summaries of the case studies presented in this volume would better inform and inspire us to serve our collective self-interest in empowering women for better health and quality of life for all.

1

Empowerment of Women for Health Promotion

Many of the laws and social regulations guiding the relationships of men and women are relics of a barbaric age, when the brutal pride of an exclusive possession had its dominance in human relations, such as those of parents and children, husbands and wives, masters and servants, teachers and disciples. The vulgarity of it still persists in the social bond between the sexes because of the economic helplessness of women. Nothing makes us so stupidly mean as the sense of superiority which the power of the purse confers upon us.

—Rabindranath Tagore, Nobel laureate, Indian poet, philosopher, and educator, in *Woman and Home*, 1905–1910

Justifications

The aim of this chapter is to present an analytical discussion of social determinants of health related quality of life (HRQOL) in general, and justifications for women's empowerment as a strategy for promoting HRQOL for their families and communities. To that end, the chapter reviews several models dealing with empowerment from different perspectives, ranging from the Human Development Approach (HDA) used by the United Nations, and the United Nations Development Programme's (UNDP) Human Development Index (HDI) (UNDP, 1999, 2014) ranking nations on measures of human development and freedom, using individual or psychological perspectives of empowerment used by social and community psychologists who focus on individual empowerment, self-efficacy, and personal growth as legitimate indicators of empowerment (e.g., French & Raven, 1959; Kar, 2000b; Kar et al., 1999; Maslow, 1962; McClelland, 1961; Perkins & Zimmerman, 1995; Rappaport, 1984, 1987; Raven, 1992; Zimmerman, 1992, 1995). In their seminal paper, French and Raven (1959) proposed a theory of five bases of social power. Social power is defined by them as a person's ability to influence opinion and/or action of other people and thus constitute a measure of social influence. The five bases are (a) reward power, based on P's perception that O has the ability to mediate rewards for him/her; (b) coercive power, based on P's perception that O has the ability to mediate punishments for him/her; (c) legitimate power, based on the perception by P that O has a legitimate right to prescribe behavior for him/her; (d) referent power, based on P's identification with O; (e) expert power, based on the perception that O has some special knowledge or expertness (French & Raven, 1959). Raven (1992) added "information" as the sixth independent base of French and Raven's Social Power Theory expanding it to a theory of "six bases." We will focus on empowerment movements led and organized by the powerless and poor women, who are usually neglected by the standard economic development model/paradigm.

In this book, we place greater emphasis on the empowerment of women for better HRQOL for several reasons. First, women are the primary caregivers in most societies; at the same time they have less power than men in making decisions that affect the HRQOL of their families and communities. Second, empirical evidence shows that investment in the health and education of women produces better health outcomes for the family as a whole than does making the same investment in men (Boserup, 1970/2007; Sen, 1990, 1999). Third, women spend their discretionary money and time differently than men do; women spend their time and money in ways that are more likely to directly benefit their children and families. Consequently, empowered women make greater contributions to the HRQOL of their children, families, and communities. Fourth, one theory suggests that women have a higher tolerance for distress or have a higher family "breakdown point" that leads to divorces; furthermore, women's definition of self-interest is more inclusive of their children and families (see Sen, 1990, *Theory of Cooperative Conflict*). Consequently, even when they are in serious conflict with their spouses or partners, women continue to take care of the children.

Available (vast) literature on empowerment theories and models tends to be theoretical, context-independent, and deductive. For instance, these theories and models do not deal with gender disparity and ethnic factors that disempower people; the UN and the World Health Organization (WHO) consider that, at the macro level of analyses, gender, poverty, and ethnic/racial disparities are primary causes of powerlessness, poor health, and quality of life. The study by the WHO Commission of Social Determinants of Health (WHO, 2008) reported the powerful effects of social determinants or social gradients of health and mortality. In 2000, the UN adopted eight MDGs to be achieved by 2015; women's empowerment and poverty-elimination are two of these

MDGs. A report by the UN Secretary-General Ban Ki-moon confirmed that the MDG on women's empowerment (MDG No. 3) remains mostly unfulfilled, and income disparities between rich and poor nations and between the poor and rich people within each country are steadily increasing (UNDP MDG Report, 2014). Paul Collier, the former director of development research at the World Bank, in his book *The Bottom Billion*, concludes: "The real challenge of development is that there is a group of countries at the bottom that are falling behind, and often falling apart" (Collier, 2007, p. 3). More than a billion people fall in that category, as the title of the book connotes. The same is true for the poorest segment of the populations of most countries, including the world's richest nation, the United States of America (USA).

Our review of literature discussed in this book identifies two basic processes of community empowerment: (a) the top-down (or induced) approach promoted by external agencies, including national governments and international donors; and (b) the bottom-up (or self-organized) movements by the powerless victims themselves. Examples of the bottom-up approach include various liberation and freedom movements, such as the Gandhian nonviolent civil disobedience movement for India's freedom that has been adopted by others, including Lech Walesa in Poland, Vaclav Havel in the Czech Republic, Nelson Mandela in South Africa; Martin Luther King, Jr.'s civil rights movement in the USA; Madam Aung San Suu Kyi in Myanmar (formerly Burma); and the women's liberation/equality movements globally.

One does not master surgery by reading textbooks; one must also observe how best surgeons perform surgery and then use "dedicated practice" (the 10,000 hours rule by Malcolm Gladwell) to master surgery. Most scholars are stronger in theories and research; they are less effective as professionals in real life where contextual factors and forces often determine the outcomes. The empowerment literature is theory-rich and weak in practice. One reason is that people who are engaged in bottom-up empowerment movements are not scholars; they are preoccupied with actions to make things better for themselves and writing is not their top priority. And scholars hardly work at the grass-roots level. Learning how to empower people requires learning "what works." Our understanding of empowerment will be incomplete if we do not study and learn how ordinary people and women empower themselves in real life. One empowerment scholar Julian Rappaport once stated, Those who are engaged in empowerment research have two important obligations. First they must study how people empower themselves; and second, pass on that knowledge to others. (J. Rappaport, September 22, 2014, personal communication)

This book does precisely that. After the first five substantive chapters deal with the conceptual and theoretical issues of empowerment, the rest of the volume analyzes 80 case studies of how ordinary women empower themselves, their children, and their families (Chapters 7–10 present summaries of all cases). Chapter 11 presents a critical discussion about the implications of the key findings for policy, research, and action. The meta-analysis examines 80 "successful" cases of self-organized empowerment movements by women from across the world to answer six specific research questions that emerged from an extensive literature review in preparation for this book (the details are given in Chapter 6). The focus of the literature review is on key issues and processes of empowerment from women's perspectives, and the implications of the findings for future research and action.

This chapter is not intended to be an exhaustive summary of relevant empowerment literature; however, many of the excellent studies and reports on human development, women's empowerment, and health promotion are highly relevant and are cited in this chapter. There are three paths to empowerment and social progress; these are

1. multinational collaborative initiatives (e.g., UN, World Bank, the International Monetary Fund [IMF]);
2. economic growth and human development initiatives by national and local governments and community-based organizations (CBOs); and
3. self-organized empowerment movements by marginalized and powerless people who are confronting existential challenges that are often ignored by those engaged in economic development and social planning.

Although in an ideal world these three paths would work together for maximum effect, that does not happen often. The literature reviews for this book include all three categories of initiatives: the meta-analysis focuses on case studies of self-organized empowerment movements, or the *third path,* as it works in actual contexts. The two objectives of this chapter are to identify major factors and forces affecting health and empowerment and to present exemplary case-study analyses for understanding how powerless women across the world organize to empower themselves (the third path). It is important to note that the UN has several ongoing global empowerment initiatives that are designed to enhance women's status. These global initiatives include the establishment of the UN Development Fund for Women (UNIFEM), the UN Commission on Elimination of Discrimination Against Women (CEDAW), the UN Commission on Status of Women (UNCSW), the Beijing Declaration of 1995, the adoption of the UNDP's HDA that includes several indicators of gender equality and women's empowerment, the UN Assembly Special Session (UNGASS) for the Beijing Plus Five review, and setting the MDGs in June 2000. Several perspectives of empowerment theories and practices are reviewed briefly in this chapter.

The Human Development Approach (HDA): The Multinational Initiatives

FREEDOM AND DEMOCRACY AS MEANS AND ENDS
OF EMPOWERMENT

The Nobel Laureate developmental economist Amartya Sen and his colleague Mahbub ul Haq have been major intellectual forces that guided the HDA used by the UN for promoting the freedom and well-being of UN member nations. Based upon Sen's (1999) pioneering research presented in his book *Development as Freedom*, Dr. Mahbub ul Haq, then director of the UNDP, took the lead that evolved into the current UN system for ranking nations on their human development. Sen speaks for many when he advocates an empowerment approach:

> Focusing on human freedoms contrasts with narrower views of development, such as identifying development with the growth of gross national products, or with the rise in personal incomes, or with industrialization, or with technological advance, or with social modernization. (Sen, 1999, p. 3)

Sen sums up his thesis on development by the title of his book, *Development as Freedom*. According to Sen's analysis, "Expansion of freedom is viewed, in this approach, both as the primary end and as the principal means for development" (Sen, 1999, p. xii).

Initially, the UN HDR used a composite HDI to rank nations on levels of human development. It combines average life expectancy at birth (as a proxy measure of health), educational attainment (adult literacy and combined school enrollment ratio as a measure of human capacities), and standard of living (adjusted per capita income as a measure of economic progress). It soon became clear that these three aggregate measures do not capture the level of pain and suffering that a large segment of people endure in both rich and poor nations alike, even when nations as a whole show remarkable progress on these three aggregate measures. Gender- and race-based discrimination and poverty can seriously disempower people and diminish their quality of life. In recognition of this problem, the current HDI includes two additional indicators—gender equality or gender empowerment measures and human poverty level—which have been included for assessing overall quality of life

(QOL) or well-being of nations.[1] The central focus of the UN approach is on enhanced freedom and equity; both are essential requirements for empowered peoples.

Freedom and democracy may be looked at as two sides of the same coin. Development is incomplete if individual freedom is diminished or does not exist. Indeed, increased freedom, political participation, economic advancement, and social progress, including equity and better health, are all integral parts of development and empowerment; they all interact. Democracy is justified on both moral (deontological) and practical (utilitarian) grounds. This book does not permit a detailed discourse on the moral basis for the justification of democracy. However, we present two empirical studies as utilitarian justification of why democracy is good for QOL.

Sen reports that, contrary to popular wisdom, life expectancy in England and Wales during the first and second world wars actually increased (Sen, 1999, pp. 49–51; Table 2.2). Between 1901 and 1911, in the decade preceding World War I, life expectancy increased by only four years. In comparison, between 1911 and 1921, or during the decade of WWI, life expectancy improved by 6.5 years. Similarly, between 1931 and 1940, the decade preceding World War II, life expectancy improved by only 1.4 years; while during 1940 through 1951, during the decade of World War II, life expectancy improved by nearly five times, or by 6.8 years (the data sets for England and Wales were used for these comparisons because reliable data were available for these populations for those years).

Logic would drive us to conclude that life expectancy would fall during wars. Sen's earlier studies concluded that famines in poor nations are not caused by food shortages per se, but by the inability of the poor to buy food in the open market (when many unscrupulous sellers increase the price). But fortunately, in the case of England and Wales during the two world wars, they had a democratically elected government that was responsible for the safety of their populations. They also had a free press that informed the public on government initiatives or inaction. In crises like these, a responsible government steps in and rations basic food supply. Sen concludes:

> During the second world war also, unusually supportive and shared social arrangements developed, related to the psychology of sharing in beleaguered Britain, which made these radical public arrangements for distribution of food and health care acceptable and effective. Even the National Health Service was born during those war years. (Sen, 1999, p. 50)

---

[1] For more information on the Human Development Index (HDI), Gender Development Index (GDI), Gender Empowerment Measures (GEM), and Human Poverty Index (HPI 1 & 2), see UNDP (2013).

During World War II, food prices in Britain were not driven by the profit motives of greedy sellers (Sen, 1999), and the amount of food distributed to a family was determined by the need (size) of the family rather than how much money the family/buyers could spend. The democratic and responsible government also started relief services that fed those who could not buy food or pay for medical care of the sick. Consequently, the poor people had more food and medical care during these two wars. But this only happens, Sen explains, with a democratic government that is responsive and answerable to the public and a free press. India, which used to have famines routinely during the British Raj, has not had a famine since 1947 when the country became independent. Communist China, on the other hand, had a massive famine in the mid-1960s, during which an estimated 30 million people died. Thus, Sen concludes that a well-functioning democracy with a free press saves lives, and in our modern history, no democratic country has had a famine.

In a meticulous study presented in their book *Why Nations Fail*, Daron Acemoglu and James Robinson (2012) demonstrate that the nature of social institutions or the governance system is the primary cause of the success or failure of nations. There are several dominant theories of why societies and civilizations rise or fall: initial advantages (natural resources), good communication systems (including access to river systems), favorable climate and geography, gene pool, culture, social organization, and demographic pressures have been suggested as key causes for the rise and fall of nations. Acemoglu and Robinson studied societies that shared major sociocultural and ecological attributes equally, and yet one segment failed while the other prospered. For example, the city of Nogales is cut in half by a fence: the northern half is in Arizona (USA), and the southern part, just a few feet away, is in Sonora (Mexico). They both share the same culture, language, geography, ecology, etc. Yet Nogales, Arizona, is prosperous, and "democracy is second nature to them" (Acemoglu & Robinson, 2012, pp. 7–8). Nogales in Sonora, Mexico, is a different story. The population has significantly lower literacy rates, income, and life expectancy (all HDI measurers); they also have higher infant mortality, crimes, and corruption. It does not have a functional democracy. The authors of that study asked: how could the two halves of what is essentially the same city be so different? Their answer is: "They live in a different world shaped by different institutions. These different institutions create very disparate incentives for the inhabitants of the two Nogaleses and for the entrepreneurs and businesses willing to invest there" (Acemoglu & Robinson, 2012, p. 9). The authors conclude that nations that succeed have "inclusive" social institutions of governance that promote human development, innovation, freedom, and social participation by all people; the nations that fail have an "extracting" type of institution of governance that exploits their people, neglects investments in human development, abuses national resources, and robs the people's motivation and opportunities to succeed. We saw the same types of differences on several occasions. For instance, East and West Germany during the Cold War and before the Berlin Wall was torn down could not have been more different. Communist-ruled East Germany was like a ghost town: stores with empty shelves, empty streets without cars, poverty and squalor were ubiquitous, and people were shot when they tried to escape. Within decades after the Berlin Wall fell and the two Germanys were unified, the differences almost disappeared in today's unified Germany. We saw the same situation between North and South Vietnam; in today's unified Vietnam we do not see such differences. But the North and South Koreans, who were divided by the Korean War, live in two different worlds.

The findings by Acemoglu and Robinson provide a strong endorsement of Sen's thesis that freedom and inclusive institutions promoting sustainable human development opportunities empower people and promote QOL. It is important to remember that the UN's HDA uses nations as the unit of analysis and action. Local institutions and individuals do not have direct control over their national institutions to effect change. However, the five indicators they use to develop the composite HDI are equally relevant for planning and evaluating changes at the local level.

Equity and Empowerment

The poor and the powerless deserve more investment and support than the rich and the powerful. Unfortunately, our collective experience of human development initiatives in the past decades shows that we are moving in the wrong direction; the poor are becoming poorer and the rich are becoming richer. This persistent inequality is a major cause of social distress and poor HRQOL. For these reasons, women's empowerment for health promotion has emerged as a major policy priority. In spite of major economic and human development gains, the latest UN HDR (2015) concludes that:

> Human development has been uneven among regions, across countries and within countries. In 2014 Latin America and the Caribbean's HDI value was 0.748, compared with 0.686 in the Arab States. And the maternal mortality ratio was only 21 per 100,000 live births in Organisation for Economic Co-operation and Development countries, compared with 183 in South Asia. (UNDP 2015, p. 5)

Specific to the challenges we still face in the 21st Century, the report says that:

> Globally women earn 24 percent less than men and hold only 25 percent of administrative and managerial positions in the business world—while 32 percent of businesses have no women in senior management positions. Women still hold only 22 percent of seats in single or lower houses of national parliament. (UNDP2015, p. 5)

A recent study by UNICEF concludes that:

> Using different estimation models, we find a world in which the top 20 percent of the population enjoys more than 70 percent of total income, contrasted by two paltry percentage points for those in the bottom quintile in 2007 under Purchase Power Parity [PPP]-adjusted exchange rates; using market exchange rates, the richest population quintile gets 83 percent of global income with just a single percentage point for those in the poorest quintile. While there is evidence of progress, it is too slow; we estimate that it would take more than 800 years for the bottom billion to achieve ten percent of global income under the current rate of change. Also disturbing is the prevalence of children and youth among the poorest income quintiles, as approximately 50 percent are below the $2/day international poverty line. (Ortiz & Cummings, 2011)

Culture and Gender

While men and women in large numbers in many nations have benefited from various forms of social and technological developments, women continue to suffer from persistent inequalities in both poor and rich societies. Women in general carry most of the burden of caring for their children and domestic work. Women often have to work in jobs with low pay and long hours to supplement family income. Empirical studies show that women also suffer the brunt of poverty and abuses due to persistent inequalities and relative powerlessness (Boserup, 1970/2007; Sen, 1990; Tinker, 1990a). Women, in both rich and poor nations, suffer various forms of institutionalized injustice and abuse, ranging from unfair employment policies and sexual harassment to physical mutilations and death. Examples of inequality in richer countries include income disparity between men and women who are performing the same work; insufficient understanding of women's needs associated with childbirth and care versus their employment; and women being often forced (due to lack of choice) to work in part-time and low-paid positions with long hours without health and retirement benefits. Enduring cultural practices and attitudes toward women have significant effects on women's status, their own health, and the well-being of their families. Consequently, this chapter first raises important theoretical and practical issues inherent in and affecting women's status and empowerment. Subsequently, it reviews lessons learned from 80 exemplary case studies of women's empowerment movements that enhanced their HRQOL. Welfare systems are conceptualized both as causal agents and as targets for reform. QOL and well-being include health as an important component; we use "HRQOL" to refer to the combination of both.

The world has witnessed an unprecedented growth of wealth and technological revolution, especially during the second half of the twentieth century. Concurrently, the overall health status in most nations has also improved (WHO, 2008). Planners, researchers, and activists are interested in understanding the relationship between wealth and health and how to maximize the synergy between the two. The steady increase in life expectancy that began in Europe in the 1900s continued virtually uninterrupted throughout the twentieth century. Most economic historians and demographers conclude that the increases in life expectancy and other health improvements are at least partially related to economic improvements resulting from agricultural and industrial revolutions (WHO, 1999, p. 1). In spite of these and other technological achievements, the majority of the world's population, the women and the poor, continue to suffer from persistent inequalities,[2] which cause preventable harm to their HRQOL. A direct relationship between human development and health status is well established by numerous reports and data sets by the WHO (*World Health Report 2013*), UNDP Human Development Report (UNDP, 2013), and individual scholars (Boserup, 1970/2007; Sen, 1990, 1999; Tinker, 1990a).

Human development is significantly and positively related to life expectancy at birth, female and adult literacy, school enrollment, family planning, and public expenditures on education and health; it is negatively related to infant mortality, and maternal mortality. These and other data at the aggregate or national level clearly show that wealth, equitable welfare systems (poverty removal and health-care access), and health development are highly correlated. Other analyses show that the health status of the population, reflected for example in the health of workers, significantly affects economic productivity (WHO, 1996, ch. 6).

The better health of population affects economic productivity through several processes:

1. reduction of production losses due to workers' illness,
2. increases in human capital by increasing the proportion of the educated public (through increased enrollment of children in schools),
3. freeing up of resources otherwise spent on the treatment of diseases for use in other developmental projects, and
4. increases in national wealth by making available natural resources and cultivable land previously not accessible due to persistent epidemics and endemic risks (International Labour Organization [ILO], 1999; WHO, 1996).

---

[2] We adopt the expression "persistent inequalities" from the title of a book edited by Tinker (1990a).

Missing Women

Women in poor nations often pay a stiff price for persistent inequality: with their lives and bodies. Maternal mortality and "missing women" are tragic indicators of preventable deaths among poor women. The range of maternal mortality across the world is simply shocking. Maternal mortality in 2013 in Sierra Leone and Chad was 1,100 and 940, respectively (per 100,000 live births) compared to only 2 and 4 in Israel and Austria, respectively (World Bank, 2014). Most of these deaths are preventable; several poor countries with lower-level human development (HDI rank) have lower levels of maternal mortality than countries that rank higher on the HDI. For instance, Malawi ranks 159 among a total of 174 countries, and Nepal ranks 144 on the HDI ranking by the UNDP (1999). Yet the maternal mortality rate in Malawi is about one-third of that in Nepal (569 and 1,500, respectively; UNDP, 1999).

One powerful indicator of the systematic neglect and abuse of women in various cultures is the estimate of "missing women," or the number of women who would be alive if they had received the same levels of food and basic health care as the men in their societies. Biologically, women are believed to be "hardier" than men, and under normal circumstances, the number of female births is slightly higher than the number of male births. More than a decade ago, the estimate of missing women globally was more than 100 million (Sen, 1999). More recently, Sen wrote:

> How have things moved more recently? At one level they have not changed much. Other data show that in spite of their significantly lower GNP [gross national product] per capita, the state of Kerala (India), China, and Sri Lanka have significantly higher life expectancies at birth than Brazil, South Africa, Gabon, and Namibia. Kerala and Gabon are the two extremes. Kerala's GNP is less than $500, but its life expectancy is over 72 years. Conversely, Gabon has a per capita income eight times higher than Kerala of nearly $4,000, but life expectancy in Gabon is only 52 years. Thus economic development, in itself, is not the primary cause of these differences in longevity. Rather, a better distribution of welfare services, with regard specifically to female literacy and access to health care, would provide better mechanisms for improving health status. (Sen, 1999)

Consequently, in a society with equal chances for survival for girls and boys, there should be more adult women than men. But this is not always the case.

Sen, who introduced the concept of "missing women" originally in 1992, stated in 2003:

The concept of "missing women," which was presented in an editorial I wrote in this journal 11 years ago, refers to the terrible deficit of women in substantial parts of Asia and north Africa, which arises from sex bias in relative care. The numbers are very large indeed. For example, using as the standard for comparison the female:male ratio of 1.022 observed in sub-Saharan Africa (since women in that region receive less biased treatment), I found the number of missing women in China to be 44m, in India 37m, and so on, with a total that easily exceeded 100m worldwide, a decade or so ago. (Sen, 2003)

In 2003, Sen notes: "and a little better in India, Bangladesh, Pakistan, and west Asia), has not altered radically in any of these countries" (Sen, 2003, p. 1297). Not only has this trend not changed substantially, but a new threat against women's survival has become more prevalent. The modern ability to detect the sex of a fetus makes it possible for many parents to have selective abortions of female fetuses. "Compared with the normal ratio of about 95 girls being born per 100 boys (which is what we observe in Europe and North America), Singapore and Taiwan have 92, South Korea 88, and China a mere 86 girls born per 100 boys" (Sen, 2003). It is noteworthy that the prevailing culture of boy-preference compels women to abort their female fetus.

Personal Empowerment: Education and Health and Quality of Life

Development studies provide overwhelming evidence about the positive effects of women's education and workforce participation on health and other aspects of QOL (Boserup, 1970/2007; Moser, 1993; Sen, 1990, 1999; Tinker, 1990a). One in-depth study in India that examined the impacts of female literacy on infant mortality, female labor-force participation, poverty (income), urbanization, and access to healthcare (Murthi, Guio, & Drèze, 1995; Sen, 1999) revealed the predominant role of women's education on health outcome. This study showed that "the powerful effect of female literacy contrasts with the comparatively ineffective roles of, say, male literacy or general poverty reduction as instruments of child mortality reduction" (Sen, 1999, p. 198). That study also examined the relative impacts of female and male education. Interestingly, the study concluded that "female literacy is found to have an unambiguous and statistically significant reducing effect on under-five mortality, even after controlling for male literacy" (Sen, 1999, p. 197). The WHO also concluded that compared to income, improving women's educational level, particularly the aspects of generation and utilization of new knowledge, has produced significantly greater impacts on several health-related outcomes, including mortality rates for children under five years of age, adult female and male mortality, adult female and male life expectancy at birth, and total fertility rates (WHO, 1999, Table 1.2). The obvious conclusion from these studies is that a welfare-reform strategy that invests in women's education, better access to health-care, and generation and utilization of relevant new knowledge (research and utilization of research) would have greater positive effects on HRQOL of the entire community—women, men, and children—compared to a strategy that focuses on wealth, technology, and modernization as goals of development.

RECIPROCITY BETWEEN INCOME, EDUCATION, AND HEALTH

Socioeconomic and political systems define welfare systems, thereby affecting our health status and QOL. At the same time, the health status of populations, epidemics, natural and man-made disasters, and QOL in turn affect economic productivity and development. Specifically, education, standard of living, access to health care, and distributive justice all have significant effects on our health status and QOL (Boserup, 1970/2007; Moser, 1993; Sen, 1990, 1999; Tinker, 1990a). WHO has long recognized that health development cannot be achieved by the health sector alone; there is a need for "beyond health" interventions (i.e., multisector collaborations) to promote health. This reciprocal relationship between health and welfare systems requires that we carefully examine how these two systems affect each other in specific populations and formulate policies and actions to promote the synergy between these processes.

Women's Perspective

Women's empowerment must be based upon the perspectives of women about what is important to them. Consequently, effective development strategies should also include leadership development, empowerment of women, and mobilization of resources from various agencies, including welfare systems. Recent sophisticated analyses focused on the relationships among income, health, education, and productivity. One reliable study looked at the relationship between income and mortality over the period from 1952 to 1992 (WHO, 1999). The study concludes:

> However important income growth may be, the changing relationship between mortality and other factors (e.g., access to health technology) is likely to be more important. ... Typically, half the gains in health between 1952 and 1992 resulted from access to better technology. The remaining half [result] from income improvements and, more importantly, better education. (WHO, 1999, p. 6)

In addition to the quality of our personal and family life, our health, job satisfaction, and occupational hazards are some of the most important domains affecting our QOL. Women are engaged in activities that are essential for bearing and rearing children and family well-being, but these activities do not produce marketable goods and services with what economists call "exchange values." Women's activities or services are not sold in the marketplace, and our societies do not value homemakers as productive members of society. Consequently, even though women often work harder than men, they do not have autonomy and control over their own lives. Ester Boserup in her original work entitled *Women's Role in Economic Development* (1970/2007), lucidly described how division of labor between men and women changed over time as economic development gradually shifted from family-based production of goods and services to specialized production of goods and services in industrialized sectors. She pointed out that rapid modernization and application of technology in economic development benefited men while it often increased women's work burden both as "family and casual labour." In the preface to her book, Boserup wrote that "in the vast and ever-growing literature on economic development, reflections on the particular problems of women are few and far between." She showed that women often did more than half the agricultural work, in one case as much as 80%, and that they also played an important role in trade. At the same time, women's contribution to overall economic development is highly undervalued. Scholarly work on gender and economic development, by pioneering researchers, has amply documented these problems (Martin, 1991).

A recent report from the ILO sums up the harsh reality of the job market for women. Worldwide unemployment and underemployment rates have increased. At the same time, "Where women are catching up with men, they are doing so because low-paid and low-skilled 'women's jobs' are growing faster than men's and because men will not do 'women's work'" (ILO, 1999). Furthermore, compared to men, "most women remain disadvantaged in terms of unequal opportunities and treatment in the labor market, unequal access to training, vulnerability to retrenchment and unemployment" (ILO, 1999). Sexual harassment on the job is common, and women are often excluded from management and decision-making positions. When women work, more often than not they are still expected to carry out their full domestic workload as housewives and mothers. Victims of domestic violence and rape are almost always women. In many poorer social strata, including in some developed countries, women head the majority of families below the poverty line and single-parent families. These women must almost always maintain full responsibility for their children without any help from a male partner; the reverse is extremely rare.

In one microeconomic analysis of power and family dynamics, Sen (1999) suggests a model of "cooperative-conflicts" that explains women's lack of "bargaining power" in family decisions (or relative powerlessness) that is rooted in our cultures. His basic assertion is that equality in women's bargaining position will only result from the removal of various forms of "unfreedoms," and enhanced empowerment of women's "agency" (their power and capacities) through education and social reforms.

Microanalyses also suggest that quality of work significantly affects the HRQOL of individuals. Occupational experience may affect QOL and the health of women workers through several processes, including: psychological dissatisfaction with monotonous work, poor pay, long and strenuous work hours, exposure to occupational hazards and accidents, sexual harassment and abuse, assault and rape (especially against street/slum dwellers, domestic helpers, and sex workers), lack of job security and advancement, inadequate daycare facilities, and absence of bargaining power and access to labor unions (ILO, 1999). The long list is familiar to most readers.

CULTURE-RELATED CRIMES AGAINST WOMEN

"Cultural crimes" are heinous offences committed against women, which are perpetuated in the name of the preservation of culture or tradition and due to the lesser value attached to women's lives. These practices are deeply rooted in culture and customs and are not due to lack of development per se; they occur in both developed and developing countries. Among the major forms of cultural crimes that threaten women's lives and health is the highly prevalent practice of female genital mutilation/cutting (FGM/C) in Africa and the Middle East, which is one example of culturally rooted extreme brutality against women (WHO, 1999). One estimate claims that FGM/C prevalence had risen by nearly 50%, from about 80 million cases in 1982 to more than 114 million in 1992. The latest estimate by the UN Children's Emergency Fund (UNICEF) is that there are 125 million women and girls who have been victims of FGM/C in 29 nations (UNICEF, 2013): "As many as 30 million girls are at risk of being cut over the next decade if current trends persist" (Geeta Rao Gupta commenting in UNICEF, 2013). In India, thousands of women become the victims of "dowry deaths" each year, when they are married for their dowry, then murdered by their new husbands. Government figures show that in 1995 there were more than 7,300 dowry deaths, while other estimates suggest a significantly higher level of prevalence (Jethmalani, 1995; WHO, 1999). Exact numbers have not been established. Dowry deaths are usually unreported, and, for each dowry death, no one knows how many more women are severely abused.

Amnesty International (AI) USA states:

Around the world at least one woman in every three has been beaten, coerced into sex, or otherwise abused in her lifetime. Every year, violence in the home and the community devastates the lives of millions of women. Violence against women is rooted in a global culture of discrimination which denies women equal rights with men and which legitimizes the appropriation of women's bodies for individual gratification or political ends. (AI, 2013)

Other forms of injustices include cultural and religious practices, which are often institutionalized as the traditional norm. Examples include laws that deprive women of their rights to vote, own and inherit property, seek employment outside the home, divorce an abusive spouse, and exercise reproductive choice. These and other forms of culturally sanctioned or encouraged practices are much too common to be considered rare examples. Changing these conditions requires culture change and the empowerment of women.

Violence Against Women

Violence against women (both physical and sexual) is highly prevalent. Box 1.1 presents selected data on violence against women (WHO, 2016). While the exact number is difficult to calculate, AI's estimate of one in three women (above) was based on a comprehensive review of 50 population-based surveys. These surveys indicate that around 10–50% of adult women have been physically assaulted by an intimate male. Because of the cultural stigma attached to the abuses and the prevailing tendency to blame the victims, between 22% and 70% of abused women interviewed responded that they did not disclose their assault and abuser to anyone prior to the survey interviews (Center for Health and Gender Equity [CHANGE]/JHU, 2000). Violence has grave long-term consequences for women's psychological, physical, and reproductive health: permanent disability, chronic pain, unwanted pregnancy leading to unsafe abortions, alcohol and substance abuse, pregnancy complications, HIV/AIDS, and sexually transmitted diseases, among others.

Sexual Exploitation and Trafficking of Women and Children

Sexual exploitation and trafficking of women and children for prostitution knows no national boundaries. It is a complex social problem, in which poverty and gender inequality play major roles. Reliable statistics do not exist; an advocacy organization estimates that more than four million women and young children are trafficked worldwide (Global Survival Network, 1999). The UNDP estimates that "The traffic of women and girls for sexual exploitation, 500,000 a year to Western Europe alone, is one of the most heinous violations of human rights, estimated to be a seven billion dollar business" (UNDP, 1999, p. 5). Cultural tolerance of the sex industry

BOX 1.1

Vulnerabilities and Violence Against Women

- Globally, as many as 38% of murders of women are committed by an intimate partner.

- Violence can result in physical, mental, sexual, reproductive, and other health problems and may increase vulnerability to HIV.

- Risk factors for being a perpetrator include low education, exposure to child maltreatment or witnessing violence in the family, harmful use of alcohol, attitudes accepting of violence and gender inequality.

- Risk factors for being a victim of intimate partner and sexual violence include low education, witnessing violence between parents, exposure to abuse during childhood, and attitudes accepting violence and gender inequality.

- In high-income settings, school-based programmes to prevent relationship violence (or dating violence) among young people are supported by some evidence of effectiveness.

- In low-income settings, other primary prevention strategies, such as microfinance combined with gender equality training and community-based initiatives that address gender inequality and communication and relationship skills, hold promise.

- Situations of conflict, post conflict, and displacement may exacerbate existing violence and present new forms of violence against women.

- Intimate partner violence in pregnancy also increases the likelihood of miscarriage, stillbirth, preterm delivery, and low birth weight babies.

- These forms of violence can lead to depression, post-traumatic stress disorder, sleep difficulties, eating disorders, emotional distress, and suicide attempts. The same study found that women who have experienced intimate partner violence were almost twice as likely to experience depression and problem drinking. The rate was even higher for women who had experienced non-partner sexual violence.

- Health effects can also include headaches, back pain, abdominal pain, fibromyalgia, gastrointestinal disorders, limited mobility, and poor overall health.

- Sexual violence, particularly during childhood, can lead to increased smoking, drug and alcohol misuse, and risky sexual behaviors in later life. It is also associated with perpetration of violence (for males) and being a victim of violence (for females).

Source: WHO (2013). Available at http://www.who.int/mediacentre/factsheets/fs239/en/. Fact Sheet No. 239 N°239. Updated November 2014. Accessed December 20, 2015.

and the selective and punitive prosecution of prostitutes (who are mostly women), while men clients go free, clearly demonstrate a double standard that punishes powerless victims. The UNDP report also concludes that illicit trade in drugs, women, weapons, and laundered money is contributing to increased crime and violence across the world. "At the root of all these is the growing influence of organized crime, estimated to gross $1.5 trillion a year, rivaling multinational corporations as an economic power" (UNDP, 1999, p. 5).

The Role of the Media, or the Role of Women in the Media

The role of the media, or the role of women in the media (or lack thereof), is an area of global concern. There is a global consensus that news and entertainment perpetuates gender inequality by (a) portraying women in subordinate positions and as sex objects, (b) depicting violence against women as a way of life, and (c) excluding women's perspectives in programs and by refusing to appoint women to policy-making positions in media establishments. In addition, with the increasing globalization of commercial and entertainment industries, people in poor countries are being increasingly exposed to media productions exported by richer countries and outside cultures. A UN Educational, Scientific, and Cultural Organization (UNESCO) study shows that the trade of media materials with "cultural content" (printed matter, music, visual arts, movies, photography, radio, and television) almost tripled between 1980 and 1991, from $67 billion to $200 billion (UNDP, 1999, p. 33). Modern communication technology via satellite has expanded very rapidly; the number of TV sets per 1,000 people worldwide almost doubled between 1980 and 1995: from 121 to 235. Multimedia industries have experienced a boom in trade in the 1990s; sales for the largest 50 multimedia companies reached $110 billion in 1993 (UNDP, 1999, p. 33). That is more than the GDP (1997 figures) of many countries, including Malaysia, Israel, Colombia, the Philippines, and Venezuela (UNDP, 1999, p. 323). Media production and sales are also becoming the monopoly of a few rich nations. For instance the biggest export sector of the world's largest economic superpower, the United States, is entertainment industry (e.g., films, music, TV programs, videos); which exceeds all other export sectors including automobiles, aircrafts, computers (UNDP, 1999, p. 33). The impact of such a rapid expansion of modern media (e.g., movies, videos, TV) propagating sex, violence, and hazardous lifestyles in Third World cultures, and in generation and gender-role conflicts everywhere, is unknown (Kar, 1999). Commercial media clearly are not welfare systems, and democratic societies uphold the value of freedom of media. Consequently, we cannot demand that media must educate and reform our societies, nor can we control the media through draconian measures. At the same time, all freedom of action and expression has its limits, which must be balanced against collective interests and utility.

Intimate Partner Violence

Intimate partner violence and sexual violence can lead to unintended pregnancies, induced abortions, gynecological problems, and sexually transmitted infections, including HIV. A 2013 analysis found that women who had been physically or sexually abused were 1.5 times more likely to have a sexually transmitted infection and, in some regions, HIV, compared to women who have not experienced partner violence. They are also twice as likely to have an abortion.

Strategies for Reform

The above discussion leads to the recognition of two universal realities:

1. *The reciprocal relationships* among health, education, and wealth; that is, each is both the means and end of the other, and therefore improvement in one improves the other (UNDP, 1999; WHO, 1996).
2. *The vast inequality* in the distribution of wealth, education, opportunities, and health between rich and poor countries, and the vast inequality within each country by differences in gender and social categories (e.g., class, race, religion, and minority status).

The imperative of the first reality is that health development and welfare reform are closely interrelated. The imperative of the second reality is that inequalities adversely affect the health and well-being of billions of people, most of whom are women and the poor. The first imperative requires multisectorial collaboration for targeted development and welfare reform for all. The second imperative requires actions to promote distributive justice, to remove barriers to healthcare and welfare services augmented by empowerment of people.

We can approach this challenge in two different ways. First, from the perspectives of those[3] who have the power to reform existing welfare systems; and second, from the perspective of those who are the victims of gender inequality. The next section of this chapter briefly reviews key issues in, and methods of, reform as they relate to women's welfare and health enhancement, particularly relating to (a) development theories and models in welfare reform and empowerment, and (b) women's empowerment case studies. The first section is based on a brief review of the seminal literature on empowerment theories and gender studies, and the second section is based on the lessons we have learned from our meta-analysis of 80 case studies of women's empowerment movements from developing and developed nations across the world (Kar, 2000b; Kar et al., 1999).

EMERGENCE OF THE HUMAN DEVELOPMENT APPROACH

Our review identified several models for development/welfare reform: welfare, anti-poverty, equity, efficiency, and empowerment (for detailed discussions of these models, see Boserup, 1970/2007; Buvinic, 1983; Moser, 1993; Sen, 1999; Thin, 1995). Boserup's contributions in this area are especially significant. Boserup, a Danish agricultural economist, is distinguished by

---

[3] Both women and men can be effective advocates of women's perspectives; the critical requirement is not the gender of the advocate, but rather the extent to which she/he is knowledgeable, dedicated, and trusted. Indeed, all successful movements require active involvement of victims and support from others who care for the victims.

her pioneering work on the role of women in human development. She demonstrated that those societies that neglect to develop women's productive capacities and exclude them from gainful employment do so at their own peril; the societies fail to develop (for more details, see Boserup, 1970/2007). The efficiency approach focuses on increased participation of women in the labor force and argues that it enhances women's status and well-being. In reality, most semiskilled or unskilled women are employed in underpaid jobs. Critics insist that these approaches do not address the basic cause of women's problems: that is, inequality and powerlessness; therefore they advocate women's empowerment as the primary model for dealing with gender inequality. It is important to note that the aim of these and other models of welfare reform is both to bring about desired structural change and address cultural diversity.

Structural change focuses on reforming specific domains of welfare systems (primarily employment, education, and health) that affect our overall QOL. The efficiency approach is currently popular with most multinational donors and national governmental agencies. It emphasizes that increased women's participation and involvement in existing programs or "mainstreaming" women in various welfare programs (sectors) is the best way to reduce gender inequality. Consequently, the efficiency approach concentrates on the enrollment of more women in existing education, employment, and healthcare programs. Critics of structural change point out that "mainstreaming" has failed to achieve equity in women's education, employment, and income. Increased employment of women in these situations reduces labor costs and thus increases production "efficiency" (e.g., the textile and garment industries and the agricultural sectors). Such mainstreaming does not offer underemployed women a decent standard of living or security. The strategy of "separate but equal programs" for women also is not very effective, because these programs cannot compete with existing welfare systems that historically favor men. Finally, categorical programs may serve specific needs, but they do not remedy the fundamental problem of inequality and often make the recipients more dependent on these agencies and welfare services (ILO, 1999; Moser, 1993; Sen, 1999; Thin, 1995; Tinker, 1990a; WHO, 1999; World Bank, 1999).

Development scholars and activists point to historical evidence and claim that prevalent welfare systems that perpetuate persistent inequality cannot be expected to reform themselves. A case in point is the failure of development programs in many nations to reduce inequity or control increasing gaps between the haves and have-nots. In order to reduce government spending, structural adjustments were introduced by many nations (in compliance with requirements of foreign and multinational donors). Structural adjustments required that national governments reduce the burden of welfare services and encourage the private sector to pick up these services and costs. This structural adjustment policy had devastating effects on the poor and the women who needed welfare services the most. It is not surprising that the scholars cited above and others, along with many feminists, insist that patriarchal systems and subordination of women are deeply rooted in culture, and that true reforms must extend beyond specific welfare reform. True reform should focus on the empowerment of women and engage in culture change to improve men's perception, attitudes, and practices toward women's rights and contributions.

THE WHO RESPONSE TO EMPOWERMENT FOR HEALTH FOR ALL

In 1978, the WHO and UNICEF jointly sponsored and led the historic Alma-Ata Conference that adopted the famous "Alma-Ata Declaration of Health for All" (WHO/UNICEF, 1978). This declaration consolidated the global consensus that health is a basic human right and that nations around the world must provide universal health care to their peoples. It identified primary health care (PHC) as the basic model that included eight basic health services, including basic sanitation, immunization, reproductive health care, health education, and various disease prevention and control services. One of the most significant conditions of the Alma-Ata declaration is that PHC must be planned and implemented with the active participation of the people. This was a historic breakthrough from the past and mandated that *public participation*, not compliance, be the key requirement in healthcare planning and implementation. Until then most health planners and professionals demanded public compliance with medical regimens as the appropriate role of the public. For instance, social scientists mostly studied why patient compliance is a problem, not why the public is not included in the planning and implementation of prevention programs. The concept of active public participation in the Alma-Ata Declaration is the seed from which the tree of empowerment for health promotion grew. The declaration emphasized that primary prevention is the central mission of PHC and insisted that PHC can only be actualized through multisectorial collaboration among health and human service agencies in both public and private sectors. More than 160 nations participated, and the notion of "health for all" (HFA) was launched.

This writer was curious why the Alma-Ata Declaration did not use the phrase "public empowerment" instead. I was fortunate to know three delegates who attended the conference. Off the record, all three delegates felt that the political climate of 1978 was not ready for that language; more than one-third of the delegates were from countries ruled by dictators and military juntas who were not fond of the concept of "public empowerment." The important point is that the Alma-Ata Declaration for the first time legitimized the public's right to participate in the programs that affect them. Since then, various WHO and UN agencies have continued to champion the public's right in the health-planning process.

Three notable declarations by WHO agencies have further expanded the right and role of the public in planning HFA policies. A brief description of this growth of the empowerment movement within the UN system is worth noting. In 1988, the WHO's regional offices for Europe and the Americas (European Regional office [EURO] and Pan American Health Organization [PAHO]) convened a conference in Ottawa, Canada, to review how the basic premises of the Alma-Ata declaration could be adapted to European and American needs and realities. This was the first international conference on "health promotion": a strategy rooted in the philosophy of the Alma-Ata Declaration but modified to suit the need of both economically advanced and less advanced societies. It adopted "health promotion" as its core strategy to meet the paradigm-shift in leading causes of deaths and disabilities from infectious diseases to health threats rooted in lifestyle and health behavior. The consensus document, the Ottawa Charter, emphasized two important concepts. First, in economically advanced and urbanized societies of Europe and the Americas, health problems are different than in poorer countries. In rich nations, the major causes of death and suffering are chronic diseases caused by unhealthy behavior and personal lifestyles. So the health programs in these societies cannot deal only with prevention and control of infectious diseases, but must also deal with chronic diseases and promote the positive dimensions of health. Second, successful health promotion requires confronting many powerful interest groups and industries that promote unhealthy products. Combating them requires more active and sustained efforts by the people (e.g., regular exercise, diet, avoiding risky behaviors). Therefore, the Ottawa Charter affirmed that "At the heart of the Health Promotion is Empowerment of the communities" (WHO, 1986; see Ottawa Charter therein). Subsequently, in 1992, the Canberra Declaration broadened the mandate to emphasize special attention on women and indigenous populations. In 1999, the WHO's South-East Asia Regional Office (WHO/SEARO, 2000) convened a conference in Kolkata, India, to review public health needs and priorities for the region in the twenty-first century. The Kolkata Declaration adopted by the delegates further broadened the PH mandate and asserted that hunger, poverty, and injustice have serious adverse effects on people's HRQOL, and consequently, PH policy and programs must empower communities to become effective partners in our struggle against the health (WHO/SEARO, 1999).

With increasing acceptance of HFA among governments and non-governmental organizations (NGOs), substantial progress has been made in improving global health since Alma-Ata. PHC, as defined by the Alma-Ata Declaration, has been adopted by most countries. Access to elements of PHC in developing countries, such as sewage disposal; safe water supply; and infant immunization against poliomyelitis, measles, and diphtheria has contributed to a decline in infant and child mortality and morbidity and to an increase in life expectancy at birth. In the past 50 years, advances in science, technology, PH, and medicine, as well as improved infrastructure, increased literacy, rising incomes, and expanded educational opportunities, particularly for women, have led to significant gains in health. The average life expectancy at birth increased from 46 years in the 1950s to 65 years in 1995 (WHO, 2000). In rich countries, the average life expectancy is 82.9 years. The gap in life expectancy between rich and poor nations narrowed from 25 years in 1955 to 13.3 years in 1995 (WHO, 2000). The mortality and morbidity due to infectious diseases have significantly decreased in many parts of the world; smallpox has been eradicated (WHO, 2000).

However, these gains have not occurred uniformly across all countries or among population segments within these countries. Based on evaluations conducted by WHO, progress toward HFA and improvement of global health overall has been hampered by a number of factors. These factors include: insufficient political commitment to the implementation of HFA, low status of women, slow socioeconomic development, weak health information systems, and lack of baseline data. Nor have the reorientation toward PH care and reduced emphasis on tertiary curative or clinical medicine occurred. Lack of expertise in health policy and management, and the dominance of clinical medicine professionals in health policy-making, continue to hamper this transition. In poor countries, insufficient funding for sanitation, health, and social services, and the governments' inability to raise funds from domestic and international sources exacerbate the problem (WHO, 2002). As a continuation of the HFA process begun in 1978, the WHO has formulated ten global health targets as part of its campaign "Health for All (HFA) in the Twenty-first Century." Set for the first two decades of the twenty-first century, these targets and priorities strive to "create the conditions for people worldwide to reach and maintain the highest attainable level of health throughout their lives." The targets are built on past accomplishments and informed by the dramatic global changes of the past 20 years, as well as the input from and consultation within and among nations. Yet the overall goals of HFA remain the same: "to achieve an increase in life expectancy and in the QOL for all; to improve equity in health between and within countries; and to ensure access for all to sustainable health systems and services."

After decades of deliberation, the UN had set the following eight MDGs (UNDP, 1999).

The eight MDGs are to:

1. Eradicate extreme poverty and hunger
2. Achieve universal primary education
3. Promote gender equality and empower women

4. Reduce child mortality
5. Improve maternal health
6. Combat HIV/AIDS, malaria, and other diseases
7. Ensure environmental sustainability
8. Develop a global partnership for development

In this volume we have reviewed key issues and factors that affect QOL (education, income, healthcare, and cultural practices), and justifications for women's self-organized movements that empower them. The review reveals that traditional human development programs bypass those who need reform the most: they do not address the basic problem, that is, excessive distress and deaths caused by gender inequality. An effective reform requires a dual approach: (a) specific health and welfare services to meet urgent needs, and (b) women's empowerment to reduce life-threatening gender inequalities. A successful movement is always a case of effective partnership involving diverse groups with distinct roles defined by their own values, assets, and constraints. The central challenge before us is to build true partnerships for health and welfare reforms, with clearly defined roles and responsibilities for those who are the participants in that partnership.

Powerlessness and poverty are major threats to our QOL. The standard economic growth model failed to reduce economic disparity between the rich and the poor. Massive foreign aid, in excess of hundreds of billion dollars per year, over several decades, has failed to help those who need it most—the poorest. The latest evidence shows that economic growth initiatives helped the rich and the middle class; but the difference between the rich and poor nations, and between the rich and the poor people within those nations, has become wider. Therefore, we need an alternative approach to reach the poorest and especially the poor women (70% of the world's poorest are women). Our review suggests that empowerment of women would be a major strategy for promoting the HRQOL of the poor and powerless families and communities. There is credible evidence that microcredit programs for poor women work (e.g., Self-Employed Women's Association [SEWA], Grameen Bank). A legitimate criticism could be that microcredit initiatives are smaller in scale and help few people. But since nothing else is working for the poorest, we should actually increase the numbers of this proven successful alternative method—the provision of microcredit to poor women–in response to the criticism; not reject a proven effective method. In health-promotion initiatives, investment in women shows a decisive advantage and return on investment. A visit to any immunization clinic would show that it is always the mothers who get their babies immunized, regardless of their social class or ethnicity.

This brief review of the global consensus declarations reveals that in a rather short period—the two decades between 1978 and 1999—the WHO and the UN have moved a long distance from advocating public participation in PHC to empowerment of the public in general, and of women in particular, to confront problems that extend beyond specific health threats. These declarations confirmed that to deal with health issues effectively, we have to go "beyond health services" and deal with deeply rooted sociocultural determinants of health, injustice, and powerlessness (Kabeer, 2010b). This conclusion is a mirror image of address both practical gender needs and long-term strategies for gender development and equity concurrently that Moser (1993) proposed decades ago. We must address the practical gender needs or problems (the symptoms) confronted by powerless women, and the strategic gender needs (or the root causes) affecting inequalities and powerlessness: Moser's *Gender Planning and Development* (1993) examines how powerless women can empower themselves, and how those who care may help.

In his foreword of the final report of the Millennium Goals by the end of 2014, the UN Secretary-General Ban Ki-moon writes:

> At the turn of the century, world leaders came together at the United Nations and agreed on a bold vision for the future through the Millennium Declaration. The Millennium Development Goals (MDGs) were a pledge to uphold the principles of human dignity, equality and equity, and free the world from extreme poverty. The MDGs, with eight goals and a set of measurable time-bound targets, established a blueprint for tackling the most pressing development challenges of our time. This report examines the latest progress towards achieving the MDGs. It reaffirms that the MDGs have made a profound difference in people's lives. Global poverty has been halved five years ahead of the 2015 timeframe. Ninety per cent of children in developing regions now enjoy primary education, and disparities between boys and girls in enrolment have narrowed. Remarkable gains have also been made in the fight against malaria and tuberculosis, along with improvements in all health indicators. The likelihood of a child dying before age five has been nearly cut in half over the last two decades. That means that about 17,000 children are saved every day. We also met the target of halving the proportion of people who lack access to improved sources of water.
>
> The concerted efforts of national governments, the international community, civil society and the private sector have helped expand hope and opportunity for people around the world. But more needs to be done to accelerate progress. We need bolder and focused action where significant gaps and disparities exist. Member States are now fully engaged in discussions to define Sustainable Development Goals (SDGs), which will serve as the core of a universal post-2015

development agenda. Our efforts to achieve the MDGs are a critical building block towards establishing a stable foundation for our development efforts beyond 2015. (Ban Ki-moon Secretary-General, United Nations)

The UN Secretary-General concludes that we need "bolder and focused action where significant gaps and disparities exist." Clearly, women's empowerment and gender equality (the third path as we call it) is an area that deserves our most attention.

2

Evolution of Global Public Health

PARADIGM SHIFTS FROM GERMS TO GENDER EMPOWERMENT
AND EQUALITY

> *Disease, grief, affliction,*
> *Captivity and calamity;*
> *Are the fruits of trees of crimes*
> *Committed by human beings.*
>
> —Sri Narayana Pandit, in *Hitopadesha*, 1675/2005

The aim of this chapter is a review of the evolution of global public health as it is defined by the world today (the UN/WHO member nations). It began with the emergence of "modern" public health (PH) and is dedicated to population-based disease prevention and health promotion (DPHP) and health-related quality of life (HRQOL) globally. While it is neither possible nor necessary to pinpoint an exact date of inception of a complex and multidisciplinary field of study such as public health, few, if any, with the basic knowledge of the health sciences would dispute that "modern" public health is a Western European innovation that began with two major scientific innovations: the discovery of "germ theory" and the invention of the microscope in Western Europe in the mid–nineteenth century. At the same time, it is important to emphasize that all notable ancient civilizations (including the Buddhist, Babylonian, Chinese, Egyptian, Greco-Roman, Indian, Islamic, Judaic, and other ancient societies) were concerned with the causes of deaths and disabilities and how best to respond to these threats to the lives and well-being of their peoples. Consequently, many ancient civilizations developed causal paradigms and healthcare systems consistent with their cosmologies and dominant health-related belief systems. Some of these health paradigms (which include theories, beliefs, and healthcare practices) are still followed and practiced as uninterrupted systems over thousands of years since their inception, and are still practiced by nearly 3 billion people across the world today. For instance, the ancient Indian Ayur-Veda (*Ayu* meaning life; *Veda* meaning science) *Charaka Samhita* (on medicine) was transcribed by Charaka in the second century BCE after it had been practiced for an undocumented for many centuries since it was conceptualized (https://www.britannica.com/topic/Charaka-samhita). Likewise, the second Ayurvedic classic, *Susruta Samhita* (on surgery), is also believed to have been transcribed in the second century BCE; it defined the science of ancient Ayurvedic surgery (http://medical-dictionary.thefreedictionary.com/Sushruta+Samhita).

These two classics from antiquity continue to inform and guide the healthcare practices of the Ayurvedic system in India and abroad, and are practiced by the majority of Indians today. *Charaka Samhita* defines in detail eight subfields of health care that continue to serve as the gold standards of Ayurveda. The government of India adopted a universal health care plan that integrated the modern allopathic (i.e., Western scientific method) and the AYUSH systems of health care for all Indians (the acronym "AYUSH" includes Ayurveda, Yoga, Unani, Siddha and naturopathy, and homeopathy). Similarly, the system of Chinese medicine that originated more than 4,000 years ago integrated other indigenous systems, including herbal therapies, acupuncture, and Tibetan medicine. They constitute Chinese medicine as it is practiced today. *The Inner Canon of Huangdi; or, The Yellow Emperor's Inner Canon* is an ancient Chinese medical text that has been treated as the fundamental doctrinal source for Chinese medicine for more than two millennia (http://www.ncbi.nlm.nih.gov/pmc/articles/PMC195056/). The work is composed of two texts, each containing 81 chapters or treatises in a question-and-answer format between the mythical "Huangdi" (the Yellow Emperor or the First Emperor of the unified China, who ruled from 246–210 BCE: http://asianhistory.about.com/od/profilesofasianleaders/p/qinshihungbio.htm/) and six of his equally legendary ministers. These two ancient Asian health disciplines from India and China have been practiced without any interruption since their inception; they have also shaped the health systems of other Asian and Western nations through the diffusion of the Hindu and Buddhist cultures and religions.

There have been other ancient healing systems, including the Egyptian medicine, the Hippocratic corpus, Mayan and Aztec healing systems, and many magico-religious shamanisms globally (e.g., Tantra, Voodoo). Modern medicine has assimilated some of these practices and replaced others with Western medical practices. Ayurveda and Chinese medicines, along with other indigenous systems such as yoga, breathing control (*pranayama*), meditation, and naturopathy (including herbal therapies) conceptualized and dealt with health and illness from a holistic perspective for several millennia before the rise of the Western Renaissance and the dawn of the Age of Reason and the empirical sciences. Modern health sciences under the influence of rational positivism and Cartesian dualism separated the physical and mental domains of health; they further subdivided "physical health" by the structures and functions of the human organs, biological subsystems of the human body (e.g., heart, lung, brain, and endocrine glands), infectious diseases, cardiovascular diseases (CVD), and cancer. Modern public health is a product of Western natural and human sciences.

Over the last five decades, China has fully integrated its traditional medicine with modern medicines delivered by traditional "barefoot doctors" in its universal healthcare system. With the combined Indian and Chinese populations of more than 2.5 billion people, plus the hundreds of millions of people in other Asian and Western nations (which is increasing), the Ayurveda and Chinese medicine are our "original and dominant" health care systems. To refer to these as "complementary and alternative medicine (CAM)" as they are called by the WHO and Western culture is a contradiction of evident truth. It is not difficult to understand why Dr. Margaret Chan, the current Director-General of the World Health Organization (Chan, 2008), recently pleaded with public health leaders across the globe to integrate CAMs into their national universal health care systems. She declared:

> Traditional medicine is generally available, affordable, and commonly used in large parts of Africa, Asia, and Latin America. For many millions of people, often living in rural areas of developing countries, herbal medicines, traditional treatments, and traditional practitioners are the main—sometimes the only—source of health care. (Chan, 2008)

Referring to traditional medicine, Chan further added in her speech:

> This is care that is close to homes, accessible, and affordable. In some systems of traditional medicine, such as traditional Chinese medicine and the Ayurveda system historically rooted in India, traditional practices are supported by wisdom and experience acquired over centuries. In these contexts where traditional medicine has strong historical and cultural roots, practitioners are usually well-known members of the community who command respect and are supported by public confidence in their abilities and remedies. (Chan, 2008)

From her analysis of traditional Chinese medicine and Indian Ayurveda, and the Global Health needs, Chan concludes:

> Other ancient medical systems in other countries, such as Ayurveda in India, offer similar approaches to health. These are historical assets that have become all the more relevant given the three main ills of life in the 21st century: the globalization of unhealthy lifestyles, rapid unplanned urbanization, and demographic ageing. These are global trends with global consequences for health, most notably seen in the universal rise of chronic noncommunicable diseases, such as heart disease, cancer, diabetes, and mental disorders. For these diseases and many other conditions, traditional medicine has much to offer in terms of prevention, comfort, compassion, and care. (Chan, 2008)

While Western medicine has integrated and assimilated the many contributions of ancient medical practices when supported by empirical evidence (especially those from the Abrahamic cultures) the Eastern medicines, especially the Indian Ayurveda and Chinese systems, have meticulously retained their original paradigms. These East–West differences are mainly due to the intrinsic natures of the two paradigms. Western positivism or rationalism chose empirical observation, experiment and refutation, and external validation of evidence as the primary methods for their sciences; the randomized double-blind assignment of subjects in clinical trials is adopted as the gold standard for Western medical research. The emphasis is to test hypotheses or establish truth from data mediated through sensory observations; this is foreign to the Eastern way of establishing knowledge or truth. The Eastern paradigms believed that valid knowledge or truths may be revealed by methods beyond empirical observations and experimentations. Consequently, knowledge gained through subjective, creative, and extrasensory methods were considered "unscientific" by Western purists.

Our objective here is not to compare the Eastern and Western scientific paradigms and methods; it is to observe how, in spite of their basic differences, these two paradigms have contributed toward the development of global public health as a field of study and action. This chapter reviews the major paradigm shifts through which public health has evolved as an independent field of study and practice; and finally reviews the transformation of public health into global public health (GPH). These paradigms do not follow on a strict linear timeline as in a relay race; one paradigm does not abruptly end before the next begins. Often two or more paradigms continue to serve people concurrently; for instance, the same population may use Ayurveda, Chinese medicine, and Western medicine concurrently. Recently, Western medical practice has begun to include some of the Eastern medicines as complementary and alternative medicines (NCCAM, 2015).

The Paradigm Shifts: From Germs to Gender Equality and Gender Empowerment

Historically, there have been five paradigms of causal beliefs and corresponding preventive and therapeutic practices. These paradigms do not follow in linear succession: some of the paradigms that originated in antiquity are still prevalent.

1. *The Age of Faith*: Before modern Western medicine and germ theory were developed in the mid–nineteenth century, Western societies believed in "miasma" (bad air) and supernatural causes of epidemics. Several ancient civilizations had sophisticated paradigms of holistic health, including Ayurveda, yoga, and meditation (India); and

Chinese, Egyptian, Greco-Roman, and Sumerian healing practices. In some traditional and isolated ethnic/tribal communities, the Age of Faith still persists: the people in these communities still believe in pre-scientific causalities and remedial and therapeutic measures consistent with their traditional ancestral beliefs. For instance, early social studies of infectious diseases in India, and in many countries in Latin America and Africa, showed that germ theory was not prevalent, and people did not believe that invisible germs caused smallpox or malaria (Dhillon & Kar, 1965; Kar & Srivastava, 1968).

2. *The Western Bio-Medical Paradigm*: The discovery of germ theory and the invention of the microscope ushered in the biomedical paradigm of health research and care. The discoveries of microorganisms as causes of major epidemics that killed hundreds of millions annually, combined with the development of vaccinations and improved sanitation as preventive measures, established microbiology and epidemiology as two core components of public health. The highlights of this paradigm include:

   a. Edward Jenner's (1796) discovery of the smallpox virus and vaccination;
   b. John Snow's rejection of "miasma" (1854) theory and his claim that waterborne microbes cause cholera;
   c. Louis Pasteur's discovery of microbes and development of the pasteurization of milk;
   d. Alexander Fleming's discovery of penicillin and antibiotics (1928);
   e. Ronald Ross's discovery of malaria parasites spread by *Anopheles* mosquitoes; and
   f. Robert Koch's formulation of "Koch's postulates" as the gold standard for confirming disease causality, and his discovery of a cholera vaccine (confirmation of Snow's theory five decades after his death). Koch, Ross, Pasteur, and Fleming were awarded the Nobel Prize (Jenner and Snow lived before the Nobel Prize was founded).

3. *The Primary Health Care (PHC) Paradigm: The Alma-Ata Declaration:* The biomedical paradigm enabled scientists and physicians to develop causal theories and preventive measures against major diseases. These developments strengthened population-based public health as the paradigm for protecting citizens, soldiers, and tradesmen as global commerce and colonization expanded. Major European and North American nations established research institutions, public health systems, and degree and diploma programs in PH in their universities. Most of these developments, however, were led by physicians/clinical scholars and based in medical colleges. There was a growing recognition that primary prevention is more

cost-effective than treatment of patients after they become sick, and that effective prevention requires proactive societal and individual actions. In 1978, led jointly by the WHO and UNICEF, the community of UN member nations adopted the Alma-Ata Declaration, which held that a community-based *Primary Health Care (PHC)* system designed and implemented through active *community participation*, and with multisectorial collaboration, is the most desirable modus operandi.

4. *The Disease Prevention and Health Promotion (DPHP) Paradigm:* Subsequent global developments revealed that as societies become richer, the leading causes of deaths and disabilities change; infectious diseases decline rapidly, and people increasingly suffer and die from diseases that cannot be prevented or cured by clinical interventions alone. The leading causes of deaths and disabilities in the world today are heart disease, cancer, stroke, and unintended injuries. Three of these top killers are attributed to tobacco use and behavior of individuals that are rooted in our cultures and lifestyles. This *epidemiological transition* implies that we must go beyond individual risk-behavior and develop effective disease prevention and health promotion (DPHP) strategies that involve appropriate cultural and lifestyle changes. The United States led in the establishment of public health schools independent of medical schools so that public health education could expand beyond the biomedical paradigm.

5. *The UN Human Development Approach (HDA) and Global Public Health (GPH) Paradigm.* The thesis of this paradigm is that good health is a basic right inseparable from human development, equitable justice, and the overall well-being of all people; poverty, injustice, and powerlessness have direct and negative effects on health. Therefore, we must go "beyond health" to address the root causes of poor health. Gender equality and empowerment are at the heart of the HDA and GPH. The HDA and GPH require multinational collaborations for: (a) removing inequalities, poverty, and powerlessness; (b) providing effective and affordable universal health care for all; and (c) increasing global commitment for sustainable growth. The global health paradigm follows this premise.

THE PROXIMAL AND DISTAL CAUSES OF HEALTH AND HEALTH-RELATED QUALITY OF LIFE (HRQOL)

The HDA and GPH paradigms extend far beyond the proximal causes of specific diseases. They both include specific germs as the biomedical causes of specific infectious diseases but expand beyond the biomedical paradigm to include behavioral, normative cultural, and environmental determinants of health and health-related quality of life (HRQOL), including lack of freedom and lack of gender equalities and empowerment (GEE). They examine the respective roles of germs, poverty, gender inequality, and powerlessness. Birth, death, health, and illness are vital functions of our lives. Depending upon the era and culture, human societies have used different paradigms or systems to explain causality of diseases and health threats and prescribe how best to respond to these threats. The earliest civilizations had systems of beliefs about disease etiologies and corresponding clinical and preventive practices as appropriate actions to take against major diseases. The aim of this chapter is not to present a confirmed historical chronology of innovations in health sciences and healing practices since antiquity, but rather to review how global public health (GPH) has evolved through several paradigm shifts and cross-pollinations.

Health historians generally recognize Robert Koch as one of the founders of modern public health paradigm. Robert Koch offered four postulates for confirming the causal agent of a particular infectious disease (http://www.life.umd.edu/classroom/bsci424/BSCI223WebSiteFiles/KochsPostulates.htm). These are:

1. The microorganism or other pathogen must be present in all cases of the disease.
2. The pathogen can be isolated from the diseased host and grown in pure culture.
3. The pathogen from the pure culture must cause the disease when inoculated into a healthy, susceptible laboratory animal.
4. The pathogen must be re-isolated from the new host and shown to be the same as the originally inoculated pathogen.

During the mid-1880s, physicians believed that cholera was caused by "miasmas"—poisonous gases that were thought to arise from sewers, swamps, garbage pits, open graves, and other foul-smelling sites of organic decay. John Snow, considered the founder of modern epidemiology, believed that miasmas could not explain the spread of certain diseases, including cholera. During the cholera outbreak of 1831 in Newcastle-on-Tyne, Snow had noticed that many miners were struck with the disease while working deep underground where there were no sewers or swamps. It seemed most likely to Snow that the cholera had been spread by invisible germs on the hands of the miners who had no water for hand-washing when they were underground. The organism that caused cholera, *Vibrio cholerae,* was not yet known and would not be until 1883, 25 years after the death of John Snow. Robert Koch, a German physician, confirmed the etiological microorganism of cholera (for more details, see Frerichs, 2015). Snow plotted the locations of the 1854 cholera outbreak on a map of London and discovered most of the patients were clustered around the Broad Street water pump in South London, and that they all used water from that source. He concluded that the water source was contaminated, and that was the beginning of the germ theory. But he had no definitive evidence of the culprit as the microscope was not yet commonly used in such investigations (although microorganisms had first been observed in 1676 by Antonie van Leeuwenhoek). After five decades, Robert Koch, armed with the microscope and his four causal postulates, conducted a series of studies that identified the causal germ of cholera. His methodology became the standard practice in public health research and established epidemiology as one of the core disciplines of public health. Koch was awarded the Nobel Prize in 1905. Since then, the success of this biomedical model for establishing the causality of diseases has been widely adopted.

THE EPIDEMIOLOGICAL TRANSITION

The biomedical paradigm of health care, along with the overall modernization that included better housing, water supply, sanitation, waste disposal, and access to immunizations and antibiotics, had significant impacts on overall health and HRQOL. Major infectious diseases that had killed hundreds of millions of people and caused misery to many more annually have been eradicated (e.g., smallpox) and/or controlled to the extent that by the end of the twentieth century, infectious diseases were no longer the major causes of deaths globally. (Figure 2.1 shows the major epidemiological transitions in the leading causes of deaths in the United States between the year 1900 and 1887.) Similar changes have occurred globally; in the year 2000, about 60% of annual deaths globally were due to chronic diseases.

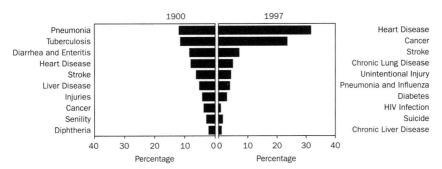

FIGURE 2.1 Epidemiological Transition.

Source: CDC (1999), Achievements of Public Health 1900–1999, MMWR Weekly, July 30, 1999, 48(29); 621–629.

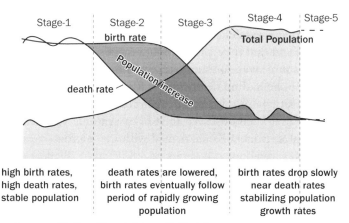

FIGURE 2.2 Demographic Transition: A Schematic Model.
Centers for Disease Control and Prevention (CDC).

DEMOGRAPHIC TRANSITION

When societies begin to modernize, death rates fall rapidly (due to a rapid reduction of infectious diseases), while birth rates do not fall as rapidly (see Figure 2.2). This demographic transition has major implications for public health and resources are needed to support the demographic changes. In addition to a rapid growth in the overall population size, since more infants survive, the proportion of children or the ratio of the dependent population increases significantly. These demographic changes create increased demands for healthcare, child health services, education, and jobs, which most poor nations cannot afford. Figure 2.2 shows the rapid decline in death rates, beginning in the first stage of the transition, followed by a decline in the birth rate many years later in stage four of a demographic transition. The solid dark area represents the size of the population increase due to the differences between the death rate and the birth rate during a demographic transition.

The WHO and Primary Health Care (PHC) Paradigm:
The Alma-Ata Declaration

Since the mid–twentieth century, visionary leaders, public health scholars, and practitioners have begun to be actively concerned with three universal observations. First, the leading causes of deaths and disabilities vary significantly between the people in rich and poor nations and between rich and poor communities within each nation. Second, the determinants of the leading causes of deaths and disabilities are consequently different between the rich and the poor nations and between economically less and more developed communities within nations. The poor more often die and suffer from diseases rooted in poverty (e.g., infectious diseases, poor sanitation), and the rich die and suffer more often from the diseases of affluence (e.g., chronic diseases, bad eating habits). Consequently, preventive strategies that are effective in the poor nations or communities may not be so in richer nations or communities. And third, contrary to the popular wisdom that prevention is better than cure, in both poor and rich nations, more resources are spent on treating diseases *after* they occur than on preventing them. A major part of this problem is that deaths and illnesses are visible as we experience these with associated pains; but diseases prevented and lives saved remain invisible. Also, the positive outcomes of a preventive behavior are often uncertain and are always delayed (e.g., the effect of not smoking tobacco on cancer rates). In response to these global concerns, in 1978, the WHO and UNICEF jointly sponsored a world conference in Alma-Ata (now Almaty, in Kazakhstan). The conference adopted the Alma-Ata Declaration, which defined and developed primary health care (PHC) as the most appropriate means for responding to these concerns. It identified eight core components of PHC; it stipulated that PHC should be planned and implemented with active community participation, and it required multisectorial collaborations between the health and non-health sectors of human development (WHO/UNICEF, 1978a).

THE EIGHT CORE COMPONENTS OF PRIMARY HEALTH CARE

The Alma-Ata Declaration defined eight essential components of PHC, which constituted the operational framework for achieving the PHC goals globally (WHO/UNICEF, 1978a). These are:

1. *Public Health Education:* Public education is the first, and one of the most essential, components of primary health care. By educating the public on the prevention and control of health problems and encouraging participation, the World Health Organization works to keep disease from spreading on a personal level.
2. *Proper Nutrition:* Nutrition is another essential component of health care. WHO works to prevent malnutrition and starvation.
3. *Clean Water and Sanitation:* A supply of clean, safe drinking water and basic sanitation measures regarding trash, sewage, and water cleanliness can significantly improve the health of a population, reducing and even eliminating many preventable diseases.
4. *Maternal and Child Health Care:* Ensuring comprehensive and adequate health care to children and to mothers, both expecting and otherwise, is another essential element of primary health care. By caring for those who are at the greatest risk of health problems, WHO helps future generations have a chance to thrive and

contribute globally. Sometimes, care for these individuals involves adequate counseling on family planning and safe sex.

5. *Immunizations:* By administering global immunizations, WHO works to wipe out major infectious diseases, greatly improving overall health globally.

6. *Local Disease Control:* Prevention and control of local diseases is critical to promoting primary health care in a population. Many diseases vary based on location. Taking these diseases into account and initiating measures to prevent them are key factors in efforts to reduce infection rates.

7. *Accessible Treatment:* Another important component of primary health care is access to appropriate medical care for the treatment of diseases and injuries. By treating disease and injury right away, caregivers can help avoid complications and the expense of later, more extensive, medical treatment.

8. *Essential Drug Provision:* By providing essential drugs to those who need them, such as antibiotics to those with infections, caregivers can help prevent disease from escalating. This makes the community safer, as there is less chance for diseases to be passed along (WHO/ UNICEF, 1978a, pp. 34–35).

REGIONAL INTERPRETATIONS OF THE ALMA-ATA DECLARATION: THE OTTAWA CHARTER FOR HEALTH PROMOTION

As expected, the Alma-Ata Declaration of 1978 generated great excitement as well as criticism. Many praised its visionary approach, its emphasis on global initiatives for dealing with problems that required global collaboration, and the importance it placed on active community participation for primary health care. The critics found it too ambitious, impractical, and indifferent to cultural, political, and economic forces that are beyond the reach of public health professionals. Most of the skepticism was from the economically advanced nations, as their health needs and priorities varied significantly from those in poorer nations. In the following year, in 1979, a follow-up conference was held in Bellagio, Italy, to define the PHC goals more precisely and in measurable ways, as well as to define and adjust strategies consistently with the levels of economic and human development in affluent and poorer nations. Subsequently, in 1986, the WHO's European Regional Office (WHO/ EURO) convened the Ottawa Conference in Canada to critically review the mandates of the Alma-Ata's PHC and to develop priorities and strategies that are most appropriate for disease prevention and health promotion (DPHP) for economically advanced nations. The Ottawa Conference adopted the Ottawa Charter for Health Promotion (November 17–21, 1986), which defined the philosophy, priorities, objectives, and operational strategies for health promotion in societies facing the emerging dominance of chronic diseases; strategies that were consistent with the spirit of the Alma-Ata Declaration. The Ottawa Charter used the term *health promotion* to describe and differentiate its strategy from the PHC strategy of the Alma-Ata Declaration. The Ottawa Charter emphasized three key requirements:

1. "Health Promotion goes beyond health care"; it includes appropriate legislation, fiscal measures, taxation, and organizational change rather than a limited focus on healthcare services alone;
2. Health promotion requires "community empowerment" instead of "community participation" as prescribed by the Alma-Ata Declaration. The Charter declared: "At the heart of this process is the empowerment of communities, their ownership and control of their own endeavours and destinies."
3. It requires "community development," which draws on existing human and material resources in communities to enhance self-help and social support (WHO/PAHO, 1996).

The Ottawa Charter is arguably the first international consensus document that stipulated that health is an inseparable part of human development and explicitly declared that "empowerment" of community is at the heart of health development. Today "empowerment" is a ubiquitous term, and it is fashionable to use this term copiously; but nearly three decades ago when the Ottawa Charter chose empowerment as a health promotion strategy, the term was rarely found in health-related literature. Those in positions of power, including the leaders of healthcare organizations, were reluctant to empower the poor and needy, and the social scientists with sincere desire to help were preoccupied with studying the reasons for lack of patient compliance with medical regimens. This change in emphasis from patient compliance to community empowerment is a notable change in the mind-sets of healthcare leaders and scholars.

In 1996, the WHO's Regional Office for the Americas (WHO/PAHO) published a volume titled *Health Promotion Anthology,* which describes the key events that transpired between the Alma-Ata Declaration of 1978 and the adoption of the Ottawa Charter for Health Promotion in 1986. In the preface of the WHO/PAHO *Anthology,* Dr. George A. O. Alleyne, the director of the PAHO, aptly summed up the prevailing spirit in these words:

> I have long believed that if we, as an international health organization, concern ourselves exclusively with a narrow vision of health, and recognize only the determinants of disease, we will do the people we serve a grave injustice. Our first task is to make it clear that we reject completely

the mechanistic view of health that harks back to the reductionism of Descartes and Newton. We must underscore again that the quest for health is an integral aspect of the eternal struggle for human development. (Alleyne, WHO/PAHO, 1996, p. vii)

This quotation represents the convergence of the views of WHO and the UN; both emphasize that health development is much more than treating the sick; it is an integral part of human development. The Ottawa Charter (1986) is an important document, and readers interested in health development would benefit from reading the full text.

The dominant theme of the Ottawa Charter is the growing imperative for changing four individual health-risk behaviors rooted in the lifestyles in affluent societies. These are: (1) tobacco use, (2) sedentary lifestyle, (3) poor nutrition, and (4) excessive alcohol consumption. With the eradication or serious reduction of epidemics of infectious diseases, several chronic diseases replaced them as leading killers. These—heart disease, stroke, cancer, and diabetes are among the most common, costly, and preventable of all health problems. The four health behaviors listed are causally linked with the leading chronic diseases; it is estimated that more than 70% of all deaths are due to chronic diseases. Heart disease, cancer, and stroke alone were responsible for more than half of all deaths in affluent nations like the United States and European nations (http://www.cdc.gov/chronicdisease/overview/index. htm). The poorer nations suffered from a "dual epidemic"; they suffered from the emerging leading killers (chronic diseases) in urban and affluent populations, while their rural and poor populations suffered from high rates of infectious diseases. For the world as a whole, chronic diseases became the new leading killers of the globe.

The WHO in 1977 organized an Internationl conference in Jakarta (Indonesia) to review the mandates and implications of previous WHO conferences (described above) for Health Promotion in South-East Asian. It is almost 20 years since the World Health Organization's Member States made an ambitious commitment to a global strategy for Health for All and the principles of primary health care through the Declaration of Alma-Ata. It is 11 years since the First International Conference on Health Promotion was held in Ottawa, Canada. That Conference resulted in proclamation of the Ottawa Charter for Health Promotion, which has been a source of guidance and inspiration for health promotion since that time. Subsequent international conferences and meetings have further clarified the relevance and meaning of key strategies in health promotion, including healthy public policy (Adelaide, Australia, 1988), and supportive environments for health (Sundsvall, Sweden, 1991). The Fourth International Conference on Health Promotion is the first to be held in a developing country, and the first to involve the private sector in supporting health promotion. (WHO, 1997a)

THE CALCUTTA DECLARATION OF 1999

In 1999, the WHO/SEARO (South-East Asia Regional Office) sponsored a conference in Kolkata (then Calcutta) on the "Future of Public Health in the 21st Century in South-East Asia." This regional conference led to the Calcutta Declaration of 1999 mentioned earlier. The Calcutta Declaration further expanded the scope of WHO's mission for poorer countries by emphasizing the effects of distal causal variables on health (including poverty, deprivation of basic freedom, injustice, and lack of adequate access to healthcare) and the need for planning strategies that are responsive to the underlying causes of poor health, especially in economically less advanced countries.

The Disease Prevention and Health Promotion (DPHP) Paradigm

While the biomedical paradigm, along with improvements in overall living conditions (including better sanitation and waste disposal systems), proved effective in eliminating or significantly reducing major epidemics and hundreds of millions of annual deaths globally, cumulative experience during the early decades of the twentieth century revealed several alarming concerns. These included three global recognitions.

First, *social gradients significantly affect the degree of health outcomes.* In spite of numerous innovations in health and medical sciences and improvements in living conditions in general, the health status disparities between the poor and rich nations, and between the poor and rich people within each nation, increased significantly. There are strong direct and inverse relationships between social status (e.g., education and income) and health status (e.g., deaths and disabilities), which cannot be narrowed by innovations in medical and clinical health sciences. These differences in health status are primarily due to social and cultural determinants that are beyond the control of individuals who are affected by them. There are excellent sources and books on the social determinants of health; the scope of this book does not permit detailed and in-depth analysis of how social and cultural determinants affect health outcomes nationally and globally.

Box 2.1 would be an excellent source on this topic.

Second, *people will always die and there will always be "ten leading causes" of deaths and disabilities.* But with the epidemiological transition, mentioned

BOX 2.1
Social Determinants of Health (WHO)

A new WHO publication entitled *Social Determinants Approaches to Public Health: From Concept to Practice* takes the discussion on avoidable and unfair inequities in health to a practical level. The book follows the publication in early 2010 of *Equity, Social Determinants and Public Health Programmes*, which analyzed social determinants from the perspective of a range of priority public health conditions, exploring possible entry points for addressing health inequities at the levels of socioeconomic context, exposure, vulnerability, health-care outcome, and social consequences.

The case studies presented in the new volume cover public health programme implementation in widely varied settings, ranging from prevention of malnutrition among girls in Pakistan and suicide prevention in Canada to malaria control in Tanzania and prevention of chronic noncommunicable diseases in Vanuatu. The book does not provide a one-size-fits-all blueprint for success; rather, it analyzes programmatic approaches that led to success or to failure. The final chapter synthesizes these experiences and draws the combined lessons learned.

These lessons include the need for understanding equity as a key value in public health programming and for working not only across sectors but also across health conditions. This requires a combination of visionary technical and political leadership, an appreciation that long-term sustainability depends on integration and institutionalization, and that there are no quick fixes to public health challenges. A common lesson learned from all the analyzed cases is to not wait to identify what went right or wrong until after the programme has elapsed or failed. Research is a necessary component of any implementation to routinely explore, gauge, and adjust strategies and approaches in a timely manner.

The book is the joint initiative of the WHO Department of Ethics, Equity, Trade, and Human Rights (ETH), Special Programme for Research and Training in Tropical Diseases (TDR), Special Programme of Research, Development, and Research Training in Human Reproduction (HRP), and Alliance for Health Policy and Systems Research (AHPSR). The 13 case studies were commissioned by the research node of the Knowledge Network on Priority Public Health Conditions (PPHC-KN), a WHO-based interdepartmental working group associated with the WHO Commission on Social Determinants of Health.

Source: World Health Organization (WHO) (2015). Available at http://www.who.int/social_determinants/thecommission/finalreport/en/ and http://www.who.int/social_determinants/en/. Accessed December 28, 2015.

---

earlier, as infectious diseases are replaced or are significantly reduced as the leading causes of deaths and disabilities, human behavior takes their place as the leading cause of these deaths and disabilities.

Third, *human behavior has emerged as the major underlying and preventable causes of deaths and disabilities.* This recognition requires an examination of "actual causes of deaths" that are often concealed behind the immediate causes of deaths as recorded in death certificates. While our conventional way of looking at this shows cardiovascular diseases, cancer, and strokes as the three leading causes of deaths, they are all significantly linked to one behavior—that is, tobacco smoking—as the underlying health risk factor. Lack of physical exercise and obesity are responsible for the next group of leading causes of deaths and disabilities. The food and tobacco industries have spent enormous sums of money disputing the research findings related to food habits and the harmful effects of tobacco use.

At the peak of this controversy, in 1964, the US Surgeon General Luther Terry released the landmark report that unequivocally implicated tobacco smoking with lung cancer (Terry, 1964). In 2014, a second surgeon general's (SG, 2014) report reconfirmed the findings of Terry's report and recommended stronger anti-tobacco policies and interventions.

Bollyky summed up subsequent developments in the United States in these words:

> Warning labels were added to cigarette packages (1965), cigarette advertising was banned on television and radio (1971), smoking on commercial airline flights was forbidden (1987), and tobacco products were put under Food and Drug Administration oversight (2009). U.S. cities and states—New York City and California in particular—led the way with bans on smoking in public spaces. U.S. criminal and civil lawsuits exposed and punished tobacco companies for decades of obfuscation and malfeasance. (Bollyky, 2014)

These initiatives, along with increased taxes on tobacco products, bans on sales to minors, movements to prevent secondhand smoke, and antismoking public education had significant effects.

> The results speak for themselves. The percent of Americans who smoke has dropped by more than half since 1964, to 18%. (Bollyky, 2014)

THE ECOLOGICAL PERSPECTIVE

A widespread recognition that effective prevention strategies should go beyond the proximal determinants of a disease and deal with the distal or underlying cultural, social, and environmental causes led to the adoption of an *ecological perspective* in disease prevention and health promotion. During the early twentieth century, social and behavioral sciences' research related to health, and applications of research knowledge in community-based disease prevention and health promotion (DPHP) perspectives, increased exponentially. Several academic and professional fields began to apply their theories and methods in health-related issues and develop fields of studies that included their respective specialties. Examples include the emergence of academic and professional degree programs in medical sociology, medical anthropology, health psychology, health economics, development economics, gender studies, social work/welfare, and public health nursing. Public health also emerged as an independent field of study. For instance, the London School of Hygiene and Public Health (LSHPH) was

BOX 2.2
Actual Causes of Death in the United States

A pioneering extensive study conducted on how "To identify and quantify the major external (nongenetic) factors that contribute to death in the United States" discovered that *human behavior* is the leading cause of mortality in the United States. The most prominent contributors to mortality in the United States in 1990 were tobacco (an estimated 400,000 deaths), diet and activity patterns (300,000), alcohol (100,000), microbial agents (90,000), toxic agents (60,000), firearms (35,000), sexual behavior (30,000), motor vehicles (25,000), and illicit use of drugs (20,000). Socioeconomic status and access to medical care are also important contributors, but difficult to quantify independent of the other factors cited. Because the studies reviewed used different approaches to derive estimates, the stated numbers should be viewed as first approximations.

Approximately half of all deaths that occurred in 1990 could be attributed to the factors identified. Although no attempt was made to further quantify the impact of these factors on morbidity and quality of life, the public health burden they impose is considerable and offers guidance for shaping health policy priorities.

Source: McGinnis and Foege (1993).

established in 1899; four of the oldest American schools of public health (Harvard, Johns Hopkins, Tulane, Yale) were established before 1920; by the middle of that century more than two dozen leading universities were offering master's and doctoral degrees in public health in the United States. Currently, there are more than 70 accredited public health schools and academic programs that are members of the Association of Schools and Programs of Public Health (ASPPH) that offer master's in public health (MPH) degrees, not counting the recent explosion of online programs. In the English language literature, Charles Edward Winslow's definition of public health (1920) became widely accepted more than 25 years before WHO offered its now-famous definition of health as a "state of complete physical, social and mental well-being; not merely the absence of diseases and disabilities" (WHO, 1948). Winslow defined public health as a "science and art of preventing diseases, prolonging life, and promoting health through organized social efforts" (1920). George Rosen's book, *A History of Public Health,* first published in 1958, and Dorothy Parker's volume, *Health, Civilization, and the State* (1993), became the most widely cited sources on the history and evolution of public health. While considered authoritative sources, in hindsight the conceptualization of the field and the history of public health in these volumes have some limitations.

1. While they acknowledged the importance of studying the growth of public health globally, their focus was exclusively on Europe and North America.
2. They neglected social determinants and cultural conditions especially (economic, ethnic, and gender effects) as major determinants of health.

3. They did not recognize contributions of ancient civilizations and healing systems to Western medicine and world populations.
4. They inadequately emphasized ecological perspectives and distal causes of health and human development.

Increased interest in public health from an ecological perspective during this phase produced a wide range of research, theories, and models, and these were developed and applied to health in general and to health-related behavior in particular. The literature became so diverse and voluminous that several health-related research organizations, including the National Institutes of Health (NIH), Centers for Disease Control and Prevention (CDC), Institutes of Medicine (IOM), and National Cancer Institutes (NCI), to name a few, constituted expert panels to review the research literature and suggest how future researchers may best navigate through disparate literatures, theories, models, and methods and apply the lessons learned in policy research and interventions. One important outcome of these efforts was the development of an "ecological model" of health behavior that is currently widely used for health and human development research. Bronfenbrenner (1977) introduced the ecological model in these words:

A broader approach to research in human development is proposed that focuses on the progressive accommodation, throughout the life span between the growing human organism and the changing environments in which it actually lives and grows. The latter include not only the immediate settings containing the developing person but also the larger social contexts, both formal and informal, in which these settings are embedded. In terms of method, the approach emphasizes the use of rigorously designed experiments, both naturalistic and contrived, beginning in the early stages of the research process. The changing relation between person and environment is conceived in systems terms. These systems properties are set forth in a series of propositions, each illustrated by concrete research examples. (Bronfenbrenner, 1977, p. 513; http://maft.dept.uncg.edu/hdf/facultys-taff/Tudge/Bronfenbrenner%201977.pdf)

The central thesis of the ecological model is that human behavior is affected by multiple determinants; and these determinants are rooted in different levels of the ecological context in which the behavior occurs. Therefore, a specific disease prevention and health promotion (DPHP) behavior cannot be understood or explained by dealing with it in a simplistic monocausal perspective (e.g., knowledge leads to desired behavior). An ecological model (e.g., of the CDC, discussed in greater detail in Chapter 5) requires that we search for behavioral determinants at several levels ranging from individual behavior to macro-level (social and cultural) determinants. More than two decades ago, McLeroy,

Bibeau, Steckler, and Glanz (1988) proposed an ecological model for health education and promotion research in these words:

> During the past 20 years there has been a dramatic increase in societal interest in preventing disability and death in the United States by changing individual behaviors linked to the risk of contracting chronic diseases. This renewed interest in health promotion and disease prevention has not been without its critics. Some critics have accused proponents of life-style interventions of promoting a victim-blaming ideology by neglecting the importance of social influences on health and disease. This article proposes an ecological model for health promotion which focuses attention on both individual and social environmental factors as targets for health promotion interventions. It addresses the importance of interventions directed at changing interpersonal, organizational, community, and public policy, factors which support and maintain unhealthy behaviors. The model assumes that appropriate changes in the social environment will produce changes in individuals, and that the support of individuals in the population is essential for implementing environmental changes. (McLeroy, Bibeau, Steckler, & Glanz, 1988)

THE DEFINITION AND SCOPE OF PUBLIC HEALTH

Public health is often misunderstood as a profession that is primarily concerned with sanitation, immunization, and the inspection of food and restaurants. The following excerpts from authoritative sources will give a better idea about the aims and scope of public health.

WHO defines the term "public health" in the following words:

> "Public health" refers to all organized measures (whether public or private) to prevent disease, promote health, and prolong life among the population as a whole. Its activities aim to provide conditions in which people can be healthy and focus on entire populations, not on individual patients or diseases. Thus, public health is concerned with the total system and not only the eradication of a particular disease. The three main public health functions are:
>
> ¤ The assessment and monitoring of the health of communities and populations at risk to identify health problems and priorities.
> ¤ The formulation of public policies designed to solve identified local and national health problems and priorities.
> ¤ To assure that all populations have access to appropriate and cost-effective care, including health promotion and disease prevention services.
>
> (Source: http://www.who.int/trade/glossary/story076/en/)

Likewise, the Institute of Medicine (IOM) of the United States defines and differentiates the field of public health from clinical medicine in terms of three primary missions of public health. These are to:

1. Prevent diseases and disabilities among the public rather than treat individual patients after they become sick
2. Conduct population-based disease prevention and health promotion (DPHP) rather than serving individual clients, and
3. Design and implement DPHP interventions with active community participation rather than the passive compliance of the public at risk.

The Five Core Areas of Public Health

Public health research and interventions are based on five "core" disciplines. These are (1) behavioral sciences and health education; (2) biostatistics; (3) epidemiology; (4) health policy and services; and (5) environmental health sciences. The key functions of public health are:

Assessment: diagnosis, surveillance, and needs-assessment, including resources available,
Policy development: evaluation of policy options, setting priorities, defining goals, and means for achieving the goals, and
Assurance of necessary health care for achieving the desired goals.

Some healthcare advocates include "policy advocacy" as a legitimate part of public health policy development (IOM, 1988). The Association of Schools and Programs of Public Health (ASPPH) defines public health thus: "Public Health is the science and art of protecting and improving the health of communities through education, promotion of healthy lifestyles, and research for disease and injury prevention."

Examples of Behavioral Risk Factors

Health risk behaviors are unhealthy behaviors people can change. "Four of these health risk behaviors—lack of exercise or physical activity, poor nutrition, tobacco use, and drinking too much alcohol—cause much of the illness, suffering, and early death related to chronic diseases and conditions" (http://www.cdc.gov/chronicdisease/overview/).

The United Nations Human Development Approach

At the conclusion of the Second World War, the world community was shaken by the massive destruction of nations, human lives, and livelihood across the world and the urgent needs for addressing the severe consequences of the war. The world powers recognized the imperative to work together for reconstruction, reconciliation, humanitarian aid, and developing mechanisms and institutions for preventing conflicts that inflict horrific devastations to the likes of World War II. Mrs. Eleanor Roosevelt presided over the process that generated the Universal Declaration of Human Rights as the moral consensus document on which the United Nations (UN) was founded in 1948 to guide world collaborations for peace and progress. It also established several UN agencies and charged these to lead UN initiatives in the key domains of human development and quality of life (http://www.un.org/en/). The World Health Organization (WHO) is one of these UN agencies. The UN includes four key organizations to lead its missions and priorities as they relate to global public health and human development:

1. The *World Health Organization* (WHO) was established as the "directing and coordinating authority for public health" within the United Nations system. The WHO is responsible for providing leadership on global health matters, shaping the health research agenda, setting norms and standards, articulating evidence-based policy options, providing technical support to countries, and monitoring and assessing health trends. In the twenty-first century, health is a shared responsibility, for equitable access to essential care and collective defense against transnational threats (http://www.who.int/en/).

2. The *United Nations International Children's Emergency Fund* (UNICEF) has the "authority to lead and coordinate" all UN efforts to protect and promote the well-being of children, including gender equality in basic education (http://www.unicef.org/about/who/index_ introduction.html).

3. The *United Nations Development Programme* (UNDP) has the mandate to develop partnerships with people at all levels of society to help build nations that can withstand crisis, and drive and sustain the kind of growth that improves the quality of life for everyone. On the ground in more than 170 countries and territories, the UNDP offers global perspectives and local insight to help empower lives and build resilient nations (www.undp.org).

4. The *UN Women* is an organization dedicated to gender equality and the empowerment of women. A global champion for women and girls, UN Women was established to accelerate progress on meeting their needs worldwide (http://www.unwomen.org/en/about-us). In addition, WHO and UNICEF have led several health-related global initiatives before and since the Alma-Ata Declaration in 1978. The evolution of the PHC paradigm owes its existence to WHO, UNICEF, and numerous governmental and non-governmental organizations (NGOs). The UNDP and the UN Women organizations

were established later and joined the notable UN efforts including those led by the United Nations Educational, Scientific, and Cultural Organization (UNESCO) in the area of preservation and promotion of cultural heritage, adult literacy, and UN-sponsored peace missions to protect and promote the survival needs of millions of innocent victims of hostilities between nations, and sectarian violence within nations. Led by WHO, these and other organizations dedicated to health-related issues are expected to work together for better health for all, in addition to supporting various "vertical programs" (e.g., stand-alone programs for the eradication of smallpox, malaria, tuberculosis, and polio).

It is not a coincidence that the three development economists who led the human development approach (HDA) movement globally are all from the Indian subcontinent (Sen, Haq, and Yunus). Two welfare economists, Amartya Sen and Mahbub ul Haq, from India and Pakistan respectively, fundamentally transformed the method of measuring HDA. An Indian Nobel laureate, Amartya Sen's theory and research established that the true measure of HDA is improved freedom; consequently, the indicators of development include better capabilities and choices to do what people value most (for details, see his book *Development as Freedom*, 1999). Sen defined the basic premise of HDA in these words: "Human development, as an approach, is concerned with what I take to be the basic development idea: namely, advancing the richness of human life, rather than the richness of the economy in which human beings live, which is only a part of it." Muhammad Yunus of Bangladesh pioneered the global microcredit programs that reduced/eliminated poverty among millions across the globe; he was awarded the Nobel Prize in 2006 for his Grameen Bank movement (discussed later in other chapters).

Based upon Sen's original research, Dr. Haq, then director of the UNDP, took the lead for developing a sophisticated and valid human development index (HDI) and a system for reporting HDA across the globe (see the *Human Development Report [HDR]*, UNDP, 2013). According to the United Nations Development Programme (UNDP, 2014):

Human development or the human development approach—is about expanding the richness of human life, rather than simply the richness of the economy in which human beings live. It is an approach that is focused on people and their opportunities and choices.... Human development focuses on improving the lives people lead rather than assuming that economic growth will lead, automatically, to greater wellbeing for all. Income growth is seen as a means to development, rather than an end in itself. (UNDP, 2014; http://hdr.undp.org/en/humandev)

The premise that has guided all subsequent HDRs is that *People are the real wealth of a nation* (emphasis mine). By backing up this assertion with an abundance of empirical data, a new way of thinking about the Human Development Report has had a profound impact on policies around the world. In his preamble of the HDR on UNDP's website, Haq continues that often what people consider valuable achievements do not show up at all in aggregate measures of economic growth, or not immediately in income or economic growth indicators: these include better education/knowledge, improved nutrition and health services, protection from crime and violence, satisfying leisure hours, political and cultural freedoms, and a sense of participation in community activities.

The 2013 HDR includes three indexes, each with three dimensions. These are (a) the Human Development Index (health, education, living standards); (b) the Gender Inequality Index (reproductive health, empowerment, and labor market participation); and (c) the Multidimensional Poverty Index (health, education, and living standards) (UNDP, 2013).

The UNDP states that:

> The work of Amartya Sen and others provided the conceptual foundation for an alternative and broader human development approach defined as a process of enlarging people's choices and enhancing human capabilities (the range of things people can be and do) and freedoms, enabling them to: live a long and healthy life, have access to knowledge and a decent standard of living, and participate in the life of their community and decisions affecting their lives. (http://hdr.undp.org/en/humandev/origins/)

Sen spoke for many when he advocated an empowerment approach in these words:

> Focusing on human freedoms contrasts with narrower views of development, such as identifying development with the growth of gross national products, or with the rise in personal incomes, or with industrialization, or with technological advance, or with social modernization. (Sen, 1999, p. 3)

Sen sums up his thesis on human development by the title of his book *Development as Freedom*. According to him, "Expansion of freedom is viewed, in this approach, both as the primary end and as the principal means for development" (Sen, 1999, p. xii).

Initially, the United Nation's HDRs used a composite HDI to rank nations on levels of human development. It combined average life expectancy at birth (as a proxy measure of health), educational attainment (adult literacy and combined school enrollment ratio as a measure of human capacities), and standard of living (adjusted per capita income as a measure of economic progress). It soon became clear that these three aggregate measures do not capture the level of pain and suffering that a large segment of people endure in both rich and poor nations alike. Even when nations as a whole show remarkable progress on these three aggregate measures, gender-based discrimination and poverty can seriously disempower people and diminish their quality of life. In recognition of this problem, the current HDI includes two additional indicators: gender equality or gender empowerment measures, and human poverty levels. These five indicators are currently used construct one composite HDI of overall quality of life (QOL) or well-being of nations. The central focus of the UN's HDA is on enhancing freedom, choice, equity, and capabilities necessary for living a healthy and meaningful life by empowered peoples.

Democracy

Freedom and democracy may be looked at as two sides of the same coin. Development is incomplete if individual freedom is diminished or does not exist. Indeed, increased freedom, political participation, economic advancement, and social progress, including equity and better health, are all integral parts of development and empowerment; they all interact. Democracy is justified on both moral (deontological) and practical (utilitarian) grounds. This book does not permit a detailed discourse on the moral bases of justification of democracy and various levels or styles of democracy. However, we present two empirical studies as utilitarian justification of why democracy is good for health and quality of life in the previous chapter, we discussed how a functioning democracy that has a free press promotes democratic processes to step in and redistribute essential food and relief services and thus prevent death and misery among the poor and enhance their life expectancy, even during the World Wars (England and Wales: Sen, 1999, pp. 13–53). We also discussed studies that demonstrate that inclusive social systems as compared to extracting systems that exploit national resources and deprive people of their basic rights and needs, promote better societies and nations (Acemoglu & Robinson, 2012). Instead of repeating these studies, we simply must remind ourselves of the importance of an inclusive and participatory democracy for enhancing freedom, which in turn enhances quality of life among the powerless poor.

Equity and Empowerment

The poor and the powerless need more investment and support than the rich and the powerful. Unfortunately, our collective experience of human development initiatives in the past decades shows that we are moving in the wrong direction; the poor become poorer and the rich become richer. This persistent inequality is a major cause of social distress and poor HRQOL. For these reasons, women's empowerment for health promotion has emerged as a policy priority. A major obligation of scholars and policy makers in the health and human service fields is to learn how we may best help empower women and better prepare our future professionals to meet this challenge. The Human Development Report released in September 2013 (UNDP, 2013) presents mixed results. While progress has been made in many aspects, the report points out that "A key message contained in this and previous Human Development Reports, however, is that economic growth alone does not automatically translate into human development progress" (Clark, 2013; in the foreword of the UNDP, 2013, p. ii). The HDR 2013 identifies four specific areas of focus for sustaining the development momentum: (a) enhancing *equity*, including on the gender dimension; (b) enabling greater voice and *participation*; (c) confronting *environmental pressures*; and (d) managing *demographic change*. The report concluded that "The rise of the South [Southern Hemisphere] is unprecedented in its speed and scale." For the first time in 150 years, the combined output of four of the world's leading economies—Brazil, Russia, India, and China (the BRIC nations)— is about to equal the combined gross domestic product (GDP) of the long-standing industrial powers of the West—Canada, France, Germany, Italy, the United Kingdom, and the United States (Summary: UNDP, 2013). It is important to remember that the UN's human development approach uses nations as the unit of analysis and ranking. The aggregate HDI does not reflect the internal diversity and disparity within a nation. Local institutions and individuals do not have direct control over their national institutions to effect change.

In 1999, the year before the UN launched its eight Millennium Development Goals (MDGs), the UN HDR emphasized several ominous global trends; these are causes of serious concern.

1. For nearly two centuries, world inequalities have been steadily increasing. For instance, in 1820 the income of the richest nations was three times greater than that of the poorest nations; in 1913 that difference increased to 11 to 1; by 1950 it was 35 to 1; in 1973 it was 44 to 1; and in 1992 it rose to 72 to 1. The richest 20% of the countries had 86% of the GDP compared to only 1% by the poorest 20% of the countries. The UNDP warns that the trend is getting worse not better.

2. On other indicators of the Human Development Index (e.g., adult literacy, school enrollment, real GDP per capita income), Gender Development Index, and Gender Power Measures, the disparities between poor and rich nations are unacceptably large (UNDP, 2013). Aggregate measures of economic developments often hide serious

threats to health and human development experienced especially by the poor, women, and other disadvantaged populations.

3. While the world as a whole needs more disease prevention using the primary health care (PHC) paradigm, both rich and poor nations tend to spend more money on sophisticated clinical interventions for treating patients and postponing deaths rather than keeping the communities healthy through community-based primary prevention interventions.

GLOBAL COLLABORATIONS FOR EPIDEMIC CONTROL

Global public health has made major progress through international collaborations for epidemic control. Discoveries between the late eighteenth and early nineteenth centuries in Europe laid the scientific foundations of pathogeneses and prevention methods of major epidemics of infectious diseases. Space does not allow a discussion of all notable applications of scientific innovations. We present three major public health threats and the role of the global collaborations of scientists, research establishments, and local governments in combatting these. These include the independent discovery of pathogenesis of cholera by John Snow in London in 1854 and Filipo Pacini in Italy in 1849; the discovery of smallpox pathogenesis by Edward Jenner in 1840; and the discovery of malaria pathogenesis by Robert Ross in India in 1888.

In 1849, John Snow in London and Filipo Pacini in Italy independently claimed that cholera is a waterborne disease. Until then, bad air or "miasma" was believed to cause cholera. In an article, David Vachon writes of John Snow's life and achievement: "For his persistent efforts to determine how cholera was spread and for the statistical mapping methods he initiated, John Snow is widely considered to be the father of [modern] epidemiology" (Frerichs, 2015). Subsequent to Snow's grand experiment in cholera control after the Broad Street Pump outbreak of cholera in London in 1854, nearly 30 years later, Robert Koch continued his clinical research testing his causal postulates of diseases (http://jmm.sgmjournals.org/content/60/4/555.full).

Cholera, which ravaged Europe in six major pandemics, swept out of India. Koch was working in Bengal Medical College in Calcutta and was able to isolate and culture the bacillus that was the causal agent of cholera in 1882. Nearly 80 years later, it was a young Indian researcher, Sambhu Nath De, who made critical discoveries on the pathogenesis of cholera that radically changed our understanding of the disease. De confirmed Koch's postulate (which says the cultured microorganism of a disease "should cause" the disease when reintroduced in a healthy body). Nair and Narain sum up De's and Chatterjee's pioneering work in greater detail in a WHO Bulletin (Nair & Narain, 2010) in these words:

Between 1951 and 1959, Sambhu Nath De made crucial discoveries on the pathogenesis of cholera that changed the course of our understanding of the disease. The discovery that cholera is caused by a potent exotoxin (*cholera enterotoxin*) affecting intestinal permeability, the demonstration that bacteria-free culture filtrates of *Vibrio cholerae* were enterotoxic, and the development of a reproducible animal model for the disease are considered milestones in the history of the fight against cholera. In this commentary, a classic article by De and Chatterje published in 1953 and its public health and research impact are highlighted by Nair and Narain (Nair & Narain, 2010, pp. 237–240)

Nair and Narain (2010) document the story:

Koch had fulfilled two of his famous postulates for proving causality, but he had yet to fulfil the third, i.e. to show that pure cultures of the comma bacillus obtained from cholera victims could cause the disease in an animal model. This third postulate remained undemonstrated for the next 75 years, until the toxin that caused cholera was discovered by Sambhu Nath De in Kolkata in 1959. De, in effect, also proved Koch's third postulate by reproducing the disease in an animal model. The full significance of De's discovery is highlighted by the fact that it took Koch just under 8 months to discover the more elusive and fastidious etiologic agent of tuberculosis, which he did in March 1882, including replicating the disease in a guinea pig model. It was the availability of an animal model for tuberculosis that enabled Koch to discover the pathogen. However, in the case of cholera success eluded him because there was no animal model to provide proof that the comma bacillus could cause the disease. (Nair & Narain, 2010, p. 238)

The pioneering 1953 article of De and Chatterjee reproduced in the original with this commentary is a classic. It was the first in a series of papers that examined the action of V. cholerae on the intestinal mucous membrane and that culminated in the discovery of the cholera toxin (http://www.who.int/bulletin/volumes/88/3/09-072504/en/). The work of De also paved the way for the discovery of entire families of labile toxins from *enterotoxigenic E. coli*, and Shiga and Shiga-like toxins from *Shigella spp.* and *diarrheagenic E. coli*. To the immunologists, De's work opened new vistas, particularly from the perspective of exploring the immune responses to the toxin and developing a vaccine containing antitoxin.

Another researcher who made unmatched contributions to malaria control was Ronald Ross:

Sir Ronald Ross, an Indian born British officer in the Indian Medical Service working out of the Bengal Medical College in Kolkata, was the first to demonstrate that malaria parasites could be transmitted from infected patients to mosquitoes. In further work with bird malaria, Ross showed that mosquitoes could transmit malaria parasites from bird to bird. This necessitated a sporogonic cycle (the time interval during which the parasite developed in the mosquito). Thus, the problem of malaria transmission was solved. (Ross, 2015)

A young Indian researcher, Kishori Mohan Bandopadhay, ably assisted Ross in this research. Ross received the Nobel Prize in 1902, and Bandopadhay received a Gold Medal from the King of England for his significant contributions to malaria research (http://www.poemhunter.com/sir-ronald-ross/biography/). Although malaria has not been fully eradicated, through national malaria control programs, India and several countries have significantly reduced deaths and disabilities and helped in global malaria control.

Smallpox existed for several millennia before Dr. Jenner's discovery of cowpox vaccine in 1796. Ridel reports that "It [smallpox] is believed to have appeared around 10,000 BC, at the time of the first agricultural settlements in northeastern Africa. The mummified head of the Egyptian pharaoh Ramses V (died 1156 BCE) bears evidence of the disease." Smallpox had been reported as early as 1122 BC in China, and it was mentioned in the ancient Sanskrit texts of India as early as the first millennium BCE. Smallpox variolation (the introduction of pus taken from fully developed pustules of a smallpox patient and inoculated into the bloodstream of healthy persons) was practiced in several nations, including North Africa, India, China, and Ottoman Turkey. India not only was a major contributor to global smallpox epidemics, but also practiced variolation as the preventive measure against smallpox long before the discovery of the modern smallpox vaccination. John Z. Holwell, a British doctor, came to Calcutta in 1732 and practiced medicine in Bengal for many years. In his book, Holwell (1767) described the variolation process performed in Bengal by special persons whom he described thus: "one would presume that they were Ayurvedic Vaidyas or their assistants" (*Vaidyas* are medical practitioners). He further reported that he was told by an Indian *Vaidya* (traditional Indian healer) that smallpox spreads through "imperceptible animalcule" (from this account one could conclude that the concept of something like germs as causal agents of smallpox was present in the Ayurvedic system long before Louis Pasteur postulated and Edward Koch confirmed the germ theory).

The variolation practice was introduced in Europe by Lady Mary Worthy Montague, the wife of the British Ambassador stationed in Istanbul, Turkey. It is believed that this process traveled to Turkey from ancient India or China. She wrote to a friend in 1717 that she had observed variolation in the Ottoman Court and had her own daughter variolized. Lady Montague later introduced it to the royal and aristocratic families in London. Soon thereafter, the practice became widespread in Europe and in North America. During the decades following the 1721 epidemic in Boston, variolation became more widespread in the colonies of New England. A prominent British physician, Dr. William Woodville, was appointed to Smallpox Hospital in London; he wrote about the significance of variolation: "At length a light was seen in the East in the shape of discovery that offered part relief and gave promise of something more" (http://www.ncbi.nlm.nih.gov/pubmed/11616267).

Several decades after variolation became widespread in Europe and America, in 1797, British physician Edward Jenner experimented on and developed the cowpox vaccine for smallpox, which was believed to cause less severe negative effects on some people than variolation. Several leading British and European physicians supported the new vaccine by Jenner, and it replaced variolation. In 1980, WHO officially declared that "Smallpox is dead." The eradication of smallpox is a historic public health success story in the world. These and similar innovative international examples confirm that effective collaborations to combat major public health threats existed long before the rise of modern public health as an independent field of study and professional practice. They also confirm that while European innovators are justly recognized with the highest level of rewards (including the Nobel Prize) for their contributions, their able collaborators from non-European nations are often ignored or forgotten.

NORTH–SOUTH COLLABORATIONS: SCHOOLS OF PUBLIC HEALTH

Credit goes to the British Empire for establishing the earliest Western medical schools in Asia. This began with the establishment of the Bengal Medical College in Calcutta in January of 1835, followed by the Madras (now Chennai) Medical College in February of 1835. The first private Western medical college, the Vellore Medical College, was established in 1902 in Tamil Nadu by Dr. Ida S. Scudder, a third-generation Christian missionary in India (the four oldest schools of public health in the United States—in Tulane, Harvard, Yale, and Johns Hopkins were founded in 1912, 1913, 1915, and 1916 respectively; the London School of Hygiene and Tropical Medicine/LSHTM was established in 1899). These and other medical colleges and institutes did make significant contributions to medical research and public health services and introduced preventive and social medicine (PSM) in medical schools by the mid-twentieth century. As discussed earlier, the Bengal Medical College made pioneering contributions to public health research in malaria, cholera, smallpox, and other infectious epidemics. During the last three decades of the British Raj, it introduced several important initiatives that have strengthened the public health research tradition. (For more information on the history and the role of the British Raj in public health in India and Asia, see http://www.ncbi.nlm.nih.gov/pmc/articles/PMC2763662/.)

Pioneering Research on Social Determinants

The Bengal Famine Inquiry Committee (BFIC) is amongst the earliest studies on the social determinants of famine and mass starvations that killed millions in 1942–1943. It was established by the British Government to determine the causes and consequences of the most infamous 1943 famine in Bengal, which killed 3–4 million people (for more on the Bengal famine of 1943, see Sen [1983]).

> This committee and other studies concluded that, contrary to popular belief, famine was not caused by food shortage per se; but by the lack of affordable food for the poor and inadequate relief services to the victims. It was primarily due to the government's refusal to admit that there was a famine and its grossly inadequate relief efforts. This was arguably one of the earliest studies of social determinants of massive human suffering and millions of deaths. This episode stirred Sen to systematically research the causes and consequences of the Bengal famine of 1943 and subsequent famines in Ethiopia and Bangladesh. From his research he concluded that these famines could have been prevented if the governments in power had taken appropriate preventive measures (price control and distribution of food) and relief measures (rationing and relief services). His pioneering research also demonstrated that during the first and second World Wars, contrary to the popular beliefs, in Great Britain and Wales, the life expectancy of the poor actually increased. He used data from England and Wales because reliable data on vital statistics and rationing during the first and second World Wars were only available from these areas. This happened because, during the two wars, the democratic government of Great Britain introduced strict food rationing, price controls, food distribution, and medical relief programs that made food and medical care more available to the poor than when there were no wars and rationing. He concluded that, in modern recorded history, no major famine occurred in a nation with a functioning democracy and a free press (Sen, 1998). These findings empowered the distinguished Indian statistician Prashata Mahalanobis (who was appointed the first Chair of independent India's Planning Commission) to persuade the first Prime Minister, Jawaharlal Nehru, and the Indian Cabinet to include anti-poverty and national family planning programs in 1950 and in subsequent Five-Year Plans. India was the first major nation in the world to launch its national family planning program based upon social science research by development economists, demographers, psychologists,

sociologists, and communication and public health specialists. (Virasia, Jejeebhoy, & Merrick, 1999).

During the early twentieth century, the social sciences flourished in North America and in Western Europe for three primary reasons:

1. Scientific innovations within individual disciplines and strong trans-Atlantic competition,
2. Research and development investments by governments in industrialized countries in several domains including military warfare, and
3. The massive exodus of creative scientists from Germany to the United States and Europe during and after World War II.

After World War II, the United States emerged as the major superpower; immigrant scientists were much sought after by research universities, and they made pioneering contributions in applications of social and behavioral science research and education programs in American universities, foundations, and industrial sectors. It is not a mere coincidence that 16 of the top 20 universities in the world are in the U.S. (*Times* University Ranking, February 13, 2014; http://www.timeshighereducation.co.uk/world-university-rankings/2013-14/world-ranking).

The Ascent of Global Public Health

Major historical developments do not start abruptly at a precise point in time; but the years of 1945 to 1948 may be considered the beginning of GPH for two important reasons. First, the members of the United Nations formally recognized public health as a major global priority and established the World Health Organization (WHO) in April 1948 to provide leadership for global collaboration for achieving "Health for All." Since then, the operational definition of "health" has expanded to encompass social issues such as freedom, justice, poverty, inequality, environment, and health threats caused by human actions. Several other multinational organizations concerned with human development also included the health status of nations both as a means and as a goal of human development. These global organizations include the UN, UNDP, UNICEF, UNESCO, International Labour Organization (ILO), the World Bank, the International Monetary Fund (IMF), and several philanthropic foundations that became increasingly involved in health and human development related initiatives (e.g., the Rockefeller, Ford, Kellogg, and Gates foundations, and the Wellcome Trust of the U.K.). The second historical development was the formal adoption of the Universal Declaration of Human Rights (1948), which serves as the foundation of all human development aspirations and initiatives. It emphasized that good health is a basic human right.

TWO MODELS OF PUBLIC HEALTH SCHOOLS

Deaths and epidemics are painfully visible, but lives saved and diseases prevented by public health efforts remain invisible to most people. In addition, from their inception, public health education programs usually remained subjugated to programs in medical schools dominated by clinical specialists. Consequently, the importance and impact of public health has remained underappreciated in our societies at large. In a tragic way, during an epidemic of deadly infectious disease or a disaster is followed by cholera or similar threats, public support for public health measures tends to increase. In the late twentieth century, the emergence of HIV/AIDS globally significantly enhanced the public understanding of the importance of population-based public health interventions.

Even when public health is considered important, the majority of the professionals in public health leadership positions do not have a professional education in public health (an MPH degree is not often required). For instance, in the United States, an estimated 70% of professionals in public health positions do not have a formal public health degree. In India, the world's largest democracy, with a population of more than 1.2 billion, until very recently there was no school or college that offered an MPH or doctoral degree in public health. The United States chose the model to have independent schools of public health (SPH) with their own deans, faculty, students, curriculums, budgets, and infrastructures. The quality of public health degrees is regulated by an independent national accreditation organization, the Council for Education in Public Health (CEPH), which is recognized by the Association of Schools of Public Health (ASPH) and the U.S. Department of Health and Human Services (US DHHS). Reflecting a true intellectual commitment to a multidisciplinary paradigm, the overwhelming proportion of the faculty in US SPHs are not physicians, and a deanship does not require a medical degree. These independent SPHs and programs represent a major development in public health education, research, and community service.

The medical school–based public health education model has been common in Europe and elsewhere (until recently). For instance, the London School of Hygiene and Tropical Medicine, the oldest school of public health in the English-speaking world, was a department of a school of tropical medicine until recently. Similarly, the oldest Asian PH institute, the All India Institute of Hygiene and Public Health (AIIH & PH), was established in 1885 and is not an independent SPH, it is an institution under the Central Ministry of Health, led by medical specialists and senior members of the Indian Civil Service. As late as 2008, there was no internationally accredited school or MPH degree in India; by the end of 2013, there were more than 30 schools and programs that offered graduate and postgraduate degrees or diplomas in public health that India considers equivalent to the MPH offered by Western universities (Sharma & Zodpey, 2011).

All MPH students in SPHs must demonstrate required level competency in all five core areas (Biostatistics, Behavioral Sciences and Health Education, Epidemiology, Health Policy and Management, and Environmental Health Sciences) described earlier. In addition, they are required to take advanced courses in their choice of specialty area (chosen from a list of the five core areas plus other specialty areas in which a degree is offered). The accreditation criteria and process are available from the Council for Education in Public Health (CEPH of USA), which is the world's largest public health accreditation organization. Although CEPH celebrated its fortieth anniversary in 2014, the previous ten years had included the most rapid growth and change in the organization's history. Between 2004 and 2013, the number of accredited schools and programs increased more than 70%, from 88 to 152 (CEPH, 2015) (http://ceph.org/assets/Newsletter_Jul2013.pdf).

In addition, there are now hundreds of universities and institutions that are offering online MPH programs; they include ranking universities (like the University of California–Berkeley and Harvard University) and lesser known entities that are not accredited by the CEPH. Another significant development is the establishment of joint graduate degree programs between schools of public health and other related academic and professional disciplines, and area or ethnic and gender studies. For instance, the school of public health at the University of California–Los Angeles (UCLA) has joint MPH programs with other degree programs in medicine, nursing, psychology, social welfare/work, sociology, anthropology, gender studies, Asian American studies, African studies, Latin American studies, Chicano studies, and urban planning. Similarly, at the turn of this century, there were fewer than half a dozen public health schools in ranking universities in Europe; the Association of European Schools of Public Health listed more than 30 member schools in 2013–2014 (http://aspher.org/). In addition, there have been significant developments in public health professional organizations in Europe.

> The Association of Schools of Public Health in the European Region (ASPHER) represents 42 European countries with more than 5000 academics and public health experts employed by its member institutions. (ASPHER, 2011; http://2011.aspher.org/pg/pages/view/17/about-aspher)

GLOBAL PUBLIC HEALTH: THE "BEYOND HEALTH" APPROACH

A new age of public health has arrived with the emergence of the GPH movement as a unifying force in research and policy development concerned with human health and well-being. By the mid-twentieth century, a convergence of eminent social philosophers and the cumulative knowledge from empirical research and policy interventions in several domains of human development led to the consensus that effective disease prevention and health promotion requires much more than well-designed stand-alone healthcare programs. The link between poverty and quality of life (QOL), including health, is not a new concept. As early as 1798, Thomas Malthus argued that the rate of population growth would exceed societies' capacity to produce means necessary for supporting population growth; if population growth is not checked, he warned, it will cause catastrophic effects. While his theory was not supported by all social thinkers and his predictions were not always proven true, his concern for the size and rate of population growth and its effect on the quality of life (QOL) is widely shared by the global community. In 1820, Scottish professor William P. Alison "described the close association between poverty and disease" (Terris, 1996, p. 34, PAHO). In 1826, Louis Rene Villerme of France demonstrated a link between poverty and deaths in various poor sections of Paris (Terris, 1996, p. 35). In Germany, Rudolf Virchow in 1847 affirmed that in industrial districts in Silesia, "the causes of epidemic were as much social and economic as they were physical" (Terris, 1996, p. 35).

In recognition of the strong negative effects of poverty and inequality on health and HRQOL in South-Asia, the WHO SEARO in 1999 convened a regional conference in Kolkata, India. The primary objective was to review the South-Asian realities, the priorities, and implications for PHC as defined by the Alma-Ata Declaration. The conference adopted what is now known as the Kolkata Declaration on Public Health. It reaffirmed the importance of a "Beyond Health" paradigm of human development advocated by the UN/UNDP as the appropriate context for health and human development in the twenty-first century. One of the main contributors of this paradigm shift that favors the human development perspective is the shifting patterns of deaths and diseases from infectious diseases to chronic diseases against which we do not have effective clinical prevention methods or vaccines: we confront new leading killers—"human behavior" or "lifestyle."

This is a global trend, and we need a much stronger global public health approach to confront these threats. The scope of the global health, as defined by several consortia of academic universities and international donor organizations, is to effectively address major health threats, including the consequences of globalization, that affect multiple nations and require global collaborations (e.g., climate change, human trafficking, HIV/AIDS).

This chapter has reviewed the evolution of global public health in five stages: from the ancient Age of Faith to the current phase of HDA and GPH. Public health concerns and prevention methods have existed since antiquity. Some of these complementary and alternative medicines (CAMs) are effective, have been continuously used for several millennia before the evolution of modern Western medicine, and are being used increasingly in the Western world as well. The Age of Faith was followed by the evolution of modern public health based on the scientific method and the germ theory, which led to the biomedical paradigm that still dominates the practice of medicine. The third paradigm focused on comprehensive community-based primary health care (PHC) espoused by WHO and UNICEF; it focused on multiple infectious diseases and often used vertical programs for specific epidemic control. The fourth paradigm focused on disease prevention and health promotion (DPHP) for controlling chronic disease caused by individual behavior and lifestyles. Finally, the fifth or current phase, global public health, goes beyond proximal determinants diseases and embraces the UN's Human Development Approach. The human development approach focuses on the distal and underlying causes of poor health and quality of life (QOL) ranging from infectious diseases, risky lifestyles, illiteracy, poverty, lack of basic health care, harmful cultural practices, gender inequality, and powerlessness.

Finally, the proponents of the UN's HDA have rightly emphasized the importance of freedom, equality, and empowerment of people as both means and ends of progress, but they are silent about the importance of social harmony and positive inter-group relationships in ethnically diverse communities as determinants of human development. In a rapidly globalizing world, where communities are also becoming more ethnically diverse as people live longer and work among others with diverse cultural origins, social cohesiveness and inter-group harmony would be necessary conditions for human development and the overall well-being of our societies. To be effective in this increasingly multicultural reality, the global public health movement has much to learn from the experiences of nonviolent freedom and empowerment movements in poorer and diverse communities (Kar, 2000; Kar et al., 2001; Penn, Kar, Kramer, et al., 1995). The emphasis placed by Tagore, Gandhi, King, Mandela, and others on the importance of intercultural and inter-gender harmony as a goal, and nonviolence and cooperation as the means for human progress, is more relevant today than ever before. Nearly a century ago, Tagore cautioned Indian educators and national leaders: "When races come together, as in the present age, it should not be merely the gathering of a crowd: there must be a bond of relation, or they will collide with one another." Events across the globe show that ethnic conflicts and violence have caused many societies to regress rather than progress and have inflicted despicable human sufferings and deaths. The success of global public health initiatives would depend to a large extent on how effective we are in creating and sustaining bonds of human relations in diverse communities.

3

Social Determinants of Health

There is nothing so practical as a good theory.

—Kurt Lewin

This chapter reviews major social and behavioral sciences research paradigms used for studying determinants of health and health-related quality of life (HRQOL). According to the National Institutes of Health (NIH) of the United States:

> Behavioral and social sciences research is a large, multifaceted field, encompassing a wide array of disciplines. Yet, behavioral and social sciences research is not restricted to a set of disciplines or methodological approaches. Instead, the field is defined by substantive areas of research that transcend disciplinary and methodological boundaries. In addition, several key cross-cutting themes characterize social and behavioral sciences research. These include: an emphasis on theory-driven research; the search for general principles of behavioral and social functioning; the importance ascribed to a developmental, lifespan perspective; an emphasis on individual variation, and variation across socio-demographic categories such as gender, age, and sociocultural status; and a focus on both the social and biological contexts of behavior. (NIH/OBSSR, 2015). When the United States Congress created the Office of Behavioral and Social Sciences Research (OBSSR) at the NIH, it mandated that the Office develop a standard definition of the field to assess and monitor funding in this area. This definition of health-related behavioral and social sciences research was developed in 1996 in consultation with behavioral and social scientists and science organizations, and benefited from the leadership of OBSSR's founding director, Dr. Norman B. Anderson (Anderson, 2015). This definition divides behavioral and social sciences research into two sections: Core Areas of Research, and Adjunct Areas of Research. The core areas of research are further divided into basic or fundamental research and applied research. Adjunct areas of behavioral and social sciences research include many types of neurological research and some research on pharmacological interventions—areas that have implications for, and are often influenced by, behavioral research (NIH/

OBSSR, 2015; http://obssr.od.nih.gov/about_obssr/BSSR_CC/BSSR_definition/definition.aspx).

Figure 3.1 presents the NIH/OBSSR model that includes the widest range of determinants, from the genomic (macro-biological) to the global and geopolitical (macro-social) levels; it further includes the time dimension over our lifespan.

In practice, however, health-related social and behavioral research and practice rarely cover such a comprehensive range of determinants and levels as those proposed by the NIH/OBSSR model. Societies conceptualize a range of causal paradigms of health and illness and develop corresponding preventive and curative responses. There are three major perspectives of studying social determinants of health; they are not mutually exclusive.

(1) *Endogenous theories and models* originated from studies of specific health issues and problems. Health and illness are studied as autonomous systems; these studies do not include cultural and social variations and influences as major determinants of health. Social organization, cultures, and contexts are exogenous to this paradigm (e.g., the biomedical paradigm, Health Belief Model, family-planning knowledge, attitude, and practice (KAP) studies, and the two dominant paradigms of alternative medicine—Ayurveda and Chinese medicine).

(2) *Adapted theories and models* originated from studies of human behavior in other domains (non-health) and are adopted or adapted to study health behaviors and outcomes. They retain the basic elements and structures of the original theory or model and adopt these to examine specific aspects of health (e.g., social-cognitive theories, social marketing or diffusion of innovation theories to explain or promote specific health-related behavior). An adapted theory could include

Macro-Social level

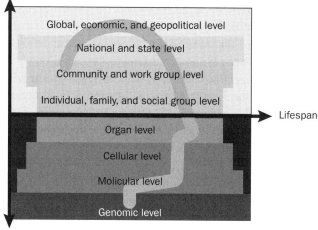

Macro-Biological level

FIGURE 3.1 NIH/OBSSR Ecological Model.

theories of natural and acquired powers (e.g., de Tocqueville's analysis of American "associations," Hobbs's types of "power," Raven and French's "Six Bases of Social Power," Sen's theory of development as "freedom" and "expansion of human capabilities," Bandura's "social learning," Kluckhohn's "value orientations," Hofstede's "six universal values," and Ingelhart's "modernization dimensions and values").

(3) *Ecological/multilevel theories and models*: These include multiple levels of systems and triangulation of methods, including temporal, historical, social, cultural, political, and geographical factors that affect health and human progress. Ecological models often integrate and apply multilevel determinants. Examples include meta-analyses of why and how civilizations rise or fall (e.g., analyses by Barbara Tuchman; Jarrod Diamonds; Amartya Sen, Daron Acemoglu, and James Robinson).

Chapters 1 and 2 presented examples of several perspectives. This chapter presents major theoretical paradigms and pioneering studies on social determinants of health. It begins with ancient endogenous paradigms by examining how two ancient civilizations had conceptualized etiologies of health and their respective responses to health threats (Ayurveda and Chinese medicines); continues with a discussion of modern Western medicine; and subsequently examines major paradigms and perspectives for studying social determinants of health.

Cultural Etiology

Two ancient and still practiced complementary and alternative medicines (CAMs)—the Indian Ayurveda and Chinese medicine—are based on a holistic cosmology (the origin and nature of the universe) and see individual life as an infinitesimal part of the eternal cosmic reality and forces. The life forces within our body are regarded as extensions of the cosmic forces of the infinite universe. When our human bodies are in harmony with the cosmic forces, we are in good health; when our bodies are not in perfect harmony with the eternal cosmic force field of energy, we become ill. It is imperative that we restore the balance or harmony between the energy within us and the "cosmic force," which is a universal and eternal phenomenon. This notion of cosmic balance is much more than the mechanistic notion of "homeostasis" that is sometimes used in modern physics and physiology to explain bodily functions or dysfunctions. The *Prana* (or Life) and the *Tao* in the Indian and Chinese systems, respectively, both mean the "life force"; it is maintained in a perfect harmony or balance between two sets of complementary forces: *Shiva* and *Shakti* in Indian and similarly the *Yin* and *Yang* in Chinese medicine cosmologies. Any imbalance between the two sets of forces is manifested as illness and changes in the five basic physical "elements" of which our human body is made. Readers interested in learning more about the basic knowledge of CAM and Yoga may find the following sources informative: Monte et al. (1993) and Broad (2012).

Table 3.1 presents a Health-Behavior Matrix showing how culturally rooted beliefs and practices that affect health related decisions and actions in three systems of medicines.

TABLE 3.1
Cultural Etiology and Health-Behavior Matrix

System	Indian Ayurveda	Chinese Medicine	Western Medicine
Oldest texts, date	*Charaka Samhita*, 1st century BCE	The Yellow Emperor's Book,	Hippocratic corpus
	Susruta Samhita, 1st century BCE, but practiced for centuries before	500–200 BCE: 1st Chinese dynasty; practiced for centuries before	2nd century BCE
Basic beliefs	Life or *prana* is an extension of the Creator. A holistic model, belief in karma and reincarnation	*Tao* or life force is a part of cosmic/holistic reality	Cartesian dualism: Mind/matter duality
Cosmic and holistic	Shiva and Shakti (male/female) balance and harmony	Complementary *yin* and *yang*, balance and harmony	Absence of cosmic/ supernatural causality
Physical attributes	Five basic elements: Earth, water, fire, air, and ether	Five-element theory: Fire, wood, water, metal, and earth	Multiple elements and causes, many unknown
Disease etiology	Imbalance of cosmic elements and *Prana* or life cause three conditions or *doshas* (these are *Tridoshas: Vata* [air and ether], *Pitta* [water and fire], and *Kapha* [water and earth]): an imbalance among these causes illness	Energies flow in body in the same way they do in nature Imbalance of energy forces causes illness	Numerous causes include germs, genes, toxin, trauma, and behavior
Health behavior	Keep/restore balance: Ayurveda, yoga, CAM	Keep/restore balance: CAM	Science- and specialty-driven
Treatment methods	Restore imbalance using ayurvedic/ holistic methods, yoga, meditation, naturopathy, etc.	Restore balance with holistic medicine, tai chi, acupuncture, naturopathy, etc.	Therapies confirmed by double-blind randomized clinical trials
Cultural adoption	Adoption of Western medicine	Adoption of Western medicine	Adoption of CAM systems
Locus of decision	Collateral: Patriarchal/ family/healers	Collateral/family/ healers	Self/MDs
Dominant Communication systems	Interpersonal/local/ some modern	Interpersonal/local/ some modern	Electronic/mass and social media

References: (NIH links).

Complementary and Integrative Medicine (National Center for Complementary and Alternative Medicine, NCCIM), http://nccim.nih.gov/news/camtats.htm;

National Center for Ayurveda medicine, http://nccam.nih.gov/health/ayurveda;

National Center of Chinese medicine, http://nccam.nih.gov/health/whatiscam/chinesemed.htm?nav=gsa.

The life force, soul, and spirit in CAM (*Prana* or *Tao*) are extensions of the "cosmic force." All preventive and therapeutic methods aim to maintain or restore the optimal balance between these. One does not see or need much of social and cultural determinants in these paradigms; the same is true for the biomedical model of Western medicine. The similarities between the Indian and Chinese cosmologies and medical foundations are remarkable, considering that there was very little overlap between their dominant cultures, languages, and religions, although historical evidence does confirm cross-pollination of these two ancient cultures. For instance, Chinese scholars spent substantive amounts of time at the ancient centers of Buddhist learning in India; these included the world's oldest university, the Nalanda University (fourth to third centuries BCE) in the state of Bihar and in Taxila, the major center for learning during the Harappa civilization (500–400 BCE). In addition, with the spread of Buddhism from India to Tibet and elsewhere in Asia, there was significant diffusion of knowledge from ancient India to China and other Asian cultures (these included mathematics, geometry, astronomy, medicine, and health sciences such as Yoga). Finally, the famous Emperor Asoka of the Mayura Dynasty (fourth to third centuries BCE) was a strong advocate of the state's responsibility in developing universal medical care; Asoka sent emissaries to promote Buddhism and Indian wisdom and knowledge to Asian nations. "The British historian H. G. Wells summed up Emperor Asoka's great contributions to the health care of the public:

> His reign for eight-and-twenty years was one of the brightest interludes in the troubled history of mankind. He organized a great digging of wells in India and the planting of trees for shade. He founded hospitals and public gardens and gardens for the growing of medicinal herbs. He created a ministry for the care of the aborigines and subject races of India. He made provision for the education of women. He made vast benefactions to the Buddhist teaching orders, and tried to stimulate them to a better and more energetic criticism of their own accumulated literature. For corruptions and superstitious accretions had accumulated very speedily upon the pure and simple teaching of the great Indian master. Missionaries went from Asoka's empire to Kashmir, to Persia, to Ceylon and Alexandria. For long centuries Buddhism and Brahmanism flourished side by side, and then slowly Buddhism declined in India and Hindu Brahmanism in a multitude of forms replaced it. But beyond the confines of India and the realms of caste, Buddhism spread—until it had won China and Siam and Burma and Japan, countries in which it is predominant to this day. (Wells, 1922)

Given this history, the similarities between Indian and Chinese medicines are not entirely surprising. India and China are two ancient civilizations making many parallel inventions and discoveries and exchanging wisdom with each other. Two additional precepts of the ancient Hindu cosmology that still affect the lives and behavior of hundreds of millions of Indians and their descendents worldwide are the beliefs in "karma" and "reincarnation" (the cycle of deaths and rebirths). What we experience in this life, happiness or misery, are the effects of our own actions (hence "karma" means both action and its effects or cosmic causality). One may find liberation (or *Mokksha*) from the endless cycles of sufferings, deaths, and births by performing the "right Karma," not by taking medicines or consulting a physician. Buddhism has a similar concept in *Dukkha* (or sorrow); it teaches that life is full of sufferings or sorrow (Buddha's First Noble Truth); and the cause of all sufferings is greed (the Second Noble Truth). The sufferings may be overcome by eliminating greed and gaining enlightenment (the Third Noble Truth); and the Fourth Noble Truth defines the various ways or paths through which one might acquire enlightenment. It is natural that those who strongly believe in the "cosmic causation" of an illness (or karma or *Dukkha*) would not choose Western preventive medicines or immunizations as their first choice of prevention of illness and disabilities (for more on Vedanta, karma, and reincarnation, see Ramakrishna, 2015). Cultural beliefs about cosmic causations affect the health-related behaviors and healing systems and paradigms.

The two previous chapters discussed the biomedical paradigm of health, which focuses on biological determinants of health and illness; primary health care (PHC); social determinants (WHO and DPHP); and the UN's Human Development Approach (HDA). This chapter presents several social science–based research perspectives that have made important contributions to the study of sociocultural determinants of health and HRQOL, as a broader background for reviewing empowerment theories and models in subsequent chapters. These are not presented in any special order, and they often overlap in their scopes; however, they may be grouped in two categories. First: those that deal with the proximal determinants of health (e.g., Health Belief Model; family-planning KAP studies); and second: those that deal with distal or more basic and universal determinants that affect our health and lives (e.g., cultural values, freedom, empowerment).

MODERN AND WESTERN PARADIGMS: BIOSOCIAL DETERMINANTS OF HEALTH

Improvement in global access to Internet (IT) technologies during the past three decades has made it convenient for interested readers to directly access the major archival sources on social and behavioral sciences theories, models, and empirical findings on health-related research and policy analysis. There are excellent summaries of this field of knowledge in highly credible sources, at no cost to interested readers, in their proprietary websites. Summarizing the contents of all social and behavioral sciences research related to health would take several volumes, and they already exist. The aim of this volume is to focus on innovative applications of empowerment theories and models related to promoting health and HRQOL and the lessons learned from them. Consequently, this chapter presents a list of the credible sources where behavioral and social sciences theories and research may be found, and important and innovative applications of social and behavioral research that have been applied widely but have not been adequately incorporated in the available archival sources on social determinants of health (WHO, 2008).

SOURCES ON SOCIAL DETERMINANTS

1. Social Indicators: Andrews (1989); Abelin, Brezinski, and Carstairs (1987); Rossi et al. (1980).
2. WHO Commission of Social Determinants of Health (the Marmot Report) 2008.
3. The NIH: OBSSR (Figure 3.1, p. 76).
4. The UNDP: *The Human Development Reports: Human Development Index* (HDI), 1990 and 2013.
5. The UNDP: *The Millennium Development Goals (MDGs)*: 1999 and 2012.
6. The CDC: *The Second Surgeon General's Report on Progress in 50 Years on Tobacco, and Health*, 2014.
7. The UNDP Sustainable Development Goals (SDGs) for 2030: UNDP 2016.

In addition, for those interested in specific theories and models for program planning and evaluation from the health promotion perspective, the two sources cited below give excellent overviews of health behavior theories and models most frequently used in health-related research and program planning. These are:

1. Glanz K, Rimer B, & Viswanath K (2008). *Health Behavior and Health Education: Theory, Research, and Practice* (4th ed.). San Francisco: Jossey Bass.
2. Green LW & Krueter MW (2004). *Health Program Planning: An Educational and Ecological Approach*. New York: McGraw-Hill.

Glanz et al. (2008) is among the two most widely read books by health education and promotion specialists in their teaching and research. It is excellent for what the authors intend to accomplish. It is therefore appropriate to briefly comment on what these two volumes cover, as the justification for not duplicating the contents of these two volumes in this book.

Glanz et al. volume presents excellent summaries of major theories and models of health behavior, which is the exclusive focus of this volume. A strength of Glanz's book is that the chapters dealing with various theories and models are written by recognized leaders in the health education and promotion fields; they share their own experience in applying the models and theories they write about. The Green and Kreuter book is also successful by several criteria. It is not a book on social and behavioral science theories and models; it focuses on a systematic approach for health education and promotion program planning, implementation, and evaluation. Most public health practitioners are not researchers; but they are involved with population-based health promotion program planning, implementation, and evaluation. Standard social science research method books do not address the key issues involved in applying theories and models for planning and evaluating health promotion interventions. Green and Kreuter have systematically gathered, analyzed, and summarized the collective experience in planning and evaluation of health promotion programs by numerous public health leaders and specialists, including their own experience over several decades. The result is a handbook on "how to plan and evaluate" population-based health promotion programs.

The two volumes mentioned above, driven by their respective objectives, do not deal with cultural diversities, dynamics of multicultural communities, ethnic and gender inequalities, or global public health such as the UN-led HDA. The readers interested in such topics would have to look elsewhere. They may begin with these three websites:

(1) WHO (2008). *Social Determinants of Health*. Retrieved February 17, 2015, from http://www.who.int/social_determinants/en
(2) WHO/Marmot Commission (2008). *Report on Social Determinants of Health*.
(3) UNDP (2013). *The Human Development Approach*. Retrieved from http://www.undp.org/content/undp/en/home/librarypage/hdr/human-development-report-2013/.

Innovative Studies of Sociocultural Determinants of Health

We mention briefly several innovative research traditions that have significant implications for health-related research, policy, and interventions.

CULTURE MATTERS

Cultural anthropology has made important contributions to our understanding of how cultures differ in terms of their deeply rooted values and beliefs and the respective healing modalities they have developed for dealing with the existential problems we all face in our lives. Susan Scrimshaw has presented an excellent summary of how anthropologists study culture and its effects on health (Scrimshaw, 2006). In addition, she has led the development of an innovative rapid assessment procedure (RAP) for improving primary healthcare intervention effectiveness through applications of anthropological theories and methods (Scrimshaw & Hurtado, 1987), which is discussed at the end of this chapter. Several leading anthropologists assume that the existential problems we face are universal, and the options available to deal with these problems are not limitless. Our values guide us to choose the option[s] available as we face our existential problems; and the options we choose make cultures different from one another. Another medical anthropologist, Marjorie Kagawa-Singer, and her colleagues have convincingly demonstrated the powerful influence of culture on cancer-related behavior and cancer care (Kagawa-Singer et al., 2010). Finally, although our values are more stable than our knowledge or attitudes about specific ends and means, our values do change over time. The rate of change and the patterns of our preferred choices for actions vary, and that also makes cultures different from one another. Cultural studies in this category focus on what people value most and how they share values or vary on these measures across social groups. Such studies also focus on how cultures and values change over time.

Cultural anthropology and social psychology theorize that people's attitudes and volitional actions are based on relatively few stable values and beliefs that they acquire from their cultures. For example, a person in a pacifist culture (e.g., a devout Hindu or a Buddhist monk) would not choose war as a means for achieving a legitimate cause; whereas members of a warrior culture or tribe (e.g., a Gurkha or a militant community) would choose to fight and die for the same cause (e.g., freedom or justice). The former Indian Army Chief of Staff, Field Marshal Sam Manekshaw (2014), best described the Nepalese Gurkhas' (the warrior tribe) valor and values in these words: "If a man says he is not afraid of dying, he is either lying or is a Gurkha" (Saighal, 2008). While a Buddhist monk may choose self-immolation in a struggle for freedom but not kill someone for his struggle for freedom, a terrorist would not hesitate to kill hundreds of innocent and helpless victims for her/his cause. Sociobiologists believe that our cultures have conditioned men to fight as the first option when they face a confrontation, while women are predisposed to seek consensus when they face confrontations. This belief led the former UN Secretary-General Kofi Annan to pronounce that women would be better for UN peace missions during international conflicts.

Anthropologist Florence Kluckhohn and psychologist Steve Strodtbeck (1961) were two pioneers in the study of cross-cultural values. They theorized that all societies must deal with a set of universal problems, and value-based solutions of these problems are not limitless. But different cultures would choose different solutions based upon their value preferences. Kluckhohn and Strodtbeck (1961) suggested five universal "value orientations" that affect our preferences and actions (http://scholarworks.gvsu.edu/cgi/viewcontent.cgi?article=1040&context=orpc); these are:

1. *Time Orientation*: On what aspect of time do we primarily focus: past, present, or future?
2. *Human and Nature Relationship*: What is the relationship between humanity and nature: mastery, submission, or harmony?
3. *Relationship with Other Humans*: How do individuals relate with others: hierarchically (which they called "lineal"), or as equals ("collateral"), or according to their individual merit?
4. *Basic Motivation*: What is the prime motivation for behavior: to express one's self ("being") to grow ("being-in-becoming"), or to achieve?
5. *Basic Human Nature*: What is basic human nature: good, bad ("evil"), or a mixture of both?

Kluckhohn and Strodtbeck's Values Orientation Theory was well received when introduced and has since been tested in several cultures. Since then, Hofstede (2010) has introduced six cultural dimensions as a framework for cross-cultural communication behaviors, and Inglehart et al. (2005) have conducted world values surveys (WVS) to study modernization processes as they affect attitudes toward gender equality across the world. These pioneering works examined how culturally acquired values vary, change over time, and promote culturally preferred patterns of responses across the world.

During the early twentieth century, social psychologists considered attitude to be the most important predictor of human behavior. The eminent psychologist Gordon Allport once described attitudes as the most distinctive and indispensable concept in contemporary social psychology. Attitude can be formed from a person's past and present actions and outcomes. Attitude is also measurable and changeable, as well as influencing the person's emotion and behavior (see Allport, 1935). In the then-emerging field of population studies and family planning, there were more than 6,000 published KAP studies by the late 1970s. One review of research on attitude-behavior consistency reported that "the consistency (or lack of it) between attitude and behavior has been a controversial issue in social psychology for the past several decades and more recently has become a focus of considerable controversy in the field of population studies" (Kar, 1978). This literature review suggested that the observed inconsistency between attitude and behavior will not be resolved by theoretical discussions, and evidence is needed from many countries at several time points to resolve this issue. Studies found, for example, several reasons why people's stated attitudes toward family planning did not always predict their contraceptive behavior. The two most important reasons were:

1. Methodological problems in defining and measuring attitudes; for instance, generalized measures of attitude toward family planning do not predict use of a specific contraceptive at a specific time; and
2. The subjects' personal attitude alone did not determine their actions; there are multiple psychosocial determinants along with one's attitude which determine whether or not one will perform a specific action (e.g., access to effective contraceptive method, monetary and psychological costs, approval/support of sexual partner, social approval/disapproval, possible negative aftereffects).

In addition, as the value orientation studies expanded in time, other scholars became involved in measuring universal values and attitudes related to fertility and health behavior.

SOCIOLOGICAL PERSPECTIVES

Sociologists Talcott Parsons, Edward Shils, and Edward Tolman (Parsons et al., 1951, p. 77) suggested that all human action is determined by five "pattern variables" or choices between pairs of alternatives. The strength of preference for a choice may vary over time and across cultures. These are:

1. *Affectivity*: need gratification versus affective neutrality (restraint of impulses);
2. *Self-orientation* versus collectivity-orientation;
3. *Universalism* (applying general standards) versus particularism (taking particular relationships into account);
4. *Ascription* (judging others by who they are) versus achievement (judging them by what they do);
5. *Specificity* (limiting relations to others to specific spheres) versus diffuseness (no prior limitations to nature of relations).

Other sociologists, including Hobbs (1909) and Parsons, Tolman, and Shils (1935), have introduced the concepts of "social class," "social role," and "social power" that are embedded in our cultures and social systems, as key determinants of our behavior. Parsons' seminal work, *Health, Illness, and Sick Role Behavior*, has stimulated considerable research on the "role" of providers and "patients" as they may affect clients' health. Raven and French led pioneering research on bases of social power and relationships and identified six bases of social power (French & Raven, 1959; Raven, 2012).

More recently, "gender role segregation" and "gender inequality" have emerged as powerful issues in health and human service–related literature. In the field of global health, the UNDP's leadership and the influence of the women's advocacy groups have led to the inclusion of "Gender Development Index" and "Human Poverty Index" as measures of overall HDI used by the UNDP to rank nations (UNDP: HDI Report, 2013). It is important to point out that the UN's HDI measures rank the country or nation as the unit of measurement; these measures do not represent the unacceptable and increasing disparities or social gradients that exist within each country. The global public health (GPH) and related human service fields (e.g., social work, community nursing, urban planning) are very committed to the issues of equality and empowerment; the mission statements of these fields clearly include gender equality and ethnic diversity and the moral imperative of dealing with these issues.

UNIVERSAL CULTURES AND VALUES

Greet Hofstede approached his research on cultural values from a different perspective. He was interested in how the various "cultural dimensions" affect workers' performance in organizations that have the same goals but are located in different cultures (e.g., International Business Machines [IBM], and one airline operating in different cultures and nations). His pioneering research served as a foundation for much later research. He was able to work with datasets on value scores of "IBM employees" in more than 50 cultures/nations between 1967 and 1973. His subsequent studies expanded to include commercial pilots and students from an additional 23 countries, civil service managers in 14 countries, consumers in 15 countries, and "élites" in 19 countries. His 2010 edition of the book *Cultures and Organizations: Software of the Mind* included in-depth analysis of results from 76 countries. This is clearly the largest longitudinal study of cross-cultural values up to that point. His "dimensions of national culture" are the values that distinguish countries from one another. The original study included four dimensions of national cultures; a fifth dimension was added in 1991. Six dimensions are included in the later Hofstede Model (Hofstede, 2010). These are:

1. *Power Distance Index (PDI)*: The extent to which the less-powerful members of society accept that power is distributed unequally.
2. *Individualism versus Collectivism (IDC)*. *Collectivism*: People belong to in-groups (families, clans, or organizations) who look after them in exchange for loyalty. *Individualism*: people look after themselves only.
3. *Masculinity versus Femininity (MAS)*. *Femininity:* The dominant values in society are caring for others and quality of life. *Masculinity:* the dominant values are achievement and success.

4. *Uncertainty Avoidance Index (UAI):* The extent to which people feel threatened by uncertainty and ambiguity and try to avoid such situations.
5. *Long-Term Orientation (LTO):* The extent to which a society shows a pragmatic future-oriented perspective.
6. *Indulgence versus Restraint (IVR):* Related to gratification versus control of basic human desires related to enjoying life.

The country scores on the dimensions are relative—societies compared to other societies. A country score is meaningless unless compared to another country.

The World Values Survey (WVS)

The mission of the WVS is: "To help social scientists and policy makers better understand worldviews and changes that are taking place in the beliefs, values and motivations of people throughout the world" (Inglehart & Norris, 2003). This global research explores people's values and beliefs, how they change over time, and what social and political impacts they have. Since 1981, the WVS has conducted six waves of studies of representative national surveys in almost 100 countries. The study has interviewed more than 200,000 subjects representing more than 90% of populations across the globe. The key cultural dimensions measured are beliefs and attitudes toward:

1. support for democracy,
2. tolerance of cultural diversity including foreigners and ethnic minorities,
3. gender equality,
4. religiosity and its role in societies,
5. effects of globalization,
6. environmental threats,
7. work,
8. family,
9. security, and
10. subjective well-being.

The WVS has over the years demonstrated that people's beliefs and values play a key role in economic development, the emergence and flourishing of democratic institutions, the rise of gender equality, and the extent to which societies have effective governments. This study identified two major dimensions of cross-cultural variation in the world: (1) traditional values versus secular-rational values, and (2) survival values versus self-expression values.

The Global Values Surveys (GVS) by Inglehart et al. (2005) show how societies are distributed on these two dimensions. Locations of the intersections of these two sets of values reflect the shift from traditional values to secular-rational values, and moving rightward reflects the shift from survival values to self-expression values. Finally, there is a predictable trajectory of change in cultural values from traditional values and survival values to self-expressive and secular values as nations and groups change over time from agrarian to modernized, and then to post-modernized societies.

Traditional values emphasize the importance of religion, parent–child ties, deference to authority, and traditional family values. People who embrace these values also reject divorce, abortion, euthanasia, and suicide. These societies have high levels of national pride and a nationalistic outlook.

Secular-rational values have the opposite preferences to the traditional values. These societies place less emphasis on religion, traditional family values, and authority. Divorce, abortion, euthanasia, and suicide are seen as relatively acceptable.

Industrialization tends to bring a shift from traditional values to secular-rational ones. With the rise of the "knowledge society" (heavy production and use of information and social media), cultural change moves in a new direction. The transition from industrial society to knowledge society is linked to a shift from survival values to self-expression values. In knowledge societies, an increasing share of the population has grown up taking survival for granted.

Survival values emphasize economic and physical security. They are linked with a relatively ethnocentric outlook and low levels of trust and tolerance.

Self-expression values give high priority to environmental protection, growing tolerance of foreigners, gays and lesbians and gender equality, and rising demands for participation in decision-making in economic and political life.

- Societies that have high scores in traditional and survival values: Zimbabwe, Morocco, Jordan, Bangladesh.
- Societies with high scores in traditional and self-expression values: the United States, most of Latin America, Ireland.
- Societies with high scores in secular-rational and survival values: Russia, Bulgaria, Ukraine, Estonia.
- Societies with high scores in secular-rational and self-expression values: Sweden, Norway, Japan, the Netherlands.

ASPIRATIONS FOR DEMOCRACY

The desire for freedom and autonomy is a universal human aspiration, but it is not a top priority when people grow up feeling that survival is uncertain.

As long as physical survival remains uncertain, the desire for physical and economic security tends to take higher priority than democracy. When basic physiological and safety needs are fulfilled, there is a growing emphasis on self-expression values. Findings from the WVS demonstrate that mass self-expression values are extremely important in the emergence and flourishing of democratic institutions in a society. With rapid industrialization and the rise of global information technology, widespread use of social media, human relations (HR) methods, and use self-expressive values become more wide-spread. Countries with authoritarian regimes come under growing internal pressure for political liberalization. This process contributed to the dramatic rise of the "third wave of democracy" in the late 1980s and early 1990s and is one of the major factors contributing to more rapid processes of globalization and democratization.

EMANCIPATION AND EMPOWERMENT

A unique aspect of the WVS is that it measures "emancipating values" and examines how they relate to "freedom," which is a central concept in works by Sen and colleagues, and the UNDP's HDA. The values of emancipation measured by the WVS are:

1. *Choices*: tolerance of abortion, divorce, homosexuality;
2. *Equality*: women's equality in politics, education, and jobs;
3. *Voice*: priority on freedom of speech and local and national issues;
4. *Autonomy*: independence vs. obedience;
5. *Individualism:* correlates strongly with emancipative values. These include citizens' rights, social movement, and innovation.

The WVS especially focuses on the cycles of empowerment and disempowerment in the evolutionary perspective. In this sense, the WVS findings and implications provide independent and empirical support for the emphasis on empowerment and emancipation of the powerless that occupies a central place in the UNDP's human development paradigm.

Human Motivation as a Major Determinant of Behavior

Psychologists have been deeply concerned with the question of what motivates people. Three psychologists whose works have been widely applied across the world are Abraham Maslow for his theory of the hierarchy of needs, Hadley Cantril for his pioneering work on patterns of aspirations, and David McClelland for his work on human motivation, which has made major contributions to our understanding of human motivation and the role it plays in social progress. Abraham Maslow theorized that, from a developmental perspective, human beings could be at one of five levels of a hierarchy of needs: survival, safety, affiliation, achievement, and self-actualization. Different people at different levels would be preoccupied with meeting the pressing needs of that level before rising to the next level of need in the hierarchy. The need hierarchy levels can be applied at the community level as well; groups of people who are struggling for survival will be unlikely to strive for long-range and higher levels of needs until their immediate survival needs are met. Similarly, a sick person's first priority would be to get well before she can seek a higher level of needs. Maslow included a five-stage hierarchy of needs in his original model; later versions by others added stages that were inferred from Maslow's work. Specifically, Maslow referred to the "cognitive," "aesthetic," and "transcendence" needs (subsequently shown as distinct needs levels in some interpretations of his theory) as additional aspects of motivation, but not as distinct levels in the hierarchy of needs. Maslow's hierarchy is as follows:

Stage 5. Self-actualization—personal growth and fulfillment
Stage 4. Esteem needs—achievement and recognition
Stage 3. Belongingness—love, affection, satisfying relationships
Stage 2. Safety needs—security, protection from harm
Stage 1. Survival—basic needs, biological and physical

Critics may argue that people do not always move higher on a linear trajectory, but that often there are upward climbs and downward falls as life goes on. In addition, as people are now living longer and there is a higher prevalence of chronic and incapacitating diseases (which are not liberating for many older people), it is questionable whether all people continue to climb higher on the ladder. Nonetheless, Maslow's needs hierarchy is an important theoretical contribution as it allows social planners, leaders, and caregivers to understand the stage at which their clients are, and deal with them accordingly.

David McClelland has identified three universal motivations that drive people's behavior. His theory of "achievement motivation" holds that individuals have three different types of needs: need for achievement, need for power, and need for affiliation; and there is a difference between people in terms of the mix of these three motivations and how that mix may influence their behavior. It is important to note that although people may possess all these needs to varying degrees, each individual is most strongly motivated by one. Consequently, leaders and managers are responsible for identifying the nature of the need for each individual member of their staff and motivating them accordingly. The same principles may be applied at the group level as well (McClelland, 1961). In 1961, McClelland published *The Achieving Society*, which articulated his model of human motivation. Arguing that commonly used hiring tests using intelligence quotient (IQ) and personality assessments were poor predictors of competency, he proposed that companies should base hiring decisions on demonstrated competency in relevant fields, rather than on standardized test scores. McClelland's ideas have become standard practice in many corporations (McClelland, 1988).

Another eminent psychologist, Hadley Cantril, completed a major international study in 16 nations on human aspirations, or "hopes and fears," to explore what people want most in their lives. The study interviewed more than 24,000 respondents between 1957 and 1963, using representative national samples. This study used a different way of measuring what people value and desire most, fear most, and how people are similar or dissimilar across the nations studied. Cantril developed a subjective "Self-Anchoring Striving Scale" that is widely used by many, including the United Nations and the World Bank as a part of their measures of human development. The scale used a two-step process: (1) First, subjects were asked to specify what do they want most or what would make them happiest, and then what would make them most unhappy in their lives; and (2) they were presented a picture of a ten-point ladder. They were asked to imagine that if everything they hoped for in life came true, they would be on Step 10 of the ladder; conversely, if everything they feared in life happened, then they would be on Step 1. Finally, the respondents were asked to decide, considering the ten-point "self-anchoring scale" (ranging between the best and the worst) where on the ladder they think they were at present; were five years ago, and expected to be five years in the future. The study asked respondents at two levels: one on aspirations for the self; and the second for their nations. The results allowed explorations of what people value for themselves and for their nations; how they stood on their scale of life-satisfaction at that time; and whether they believed that their life was getting better, remaining stable, or getting worse. Detailed explanations of the theory, methods, and results from all nations studied were presented in his book *The Pattern of Human Concerns* (Cantril, 1965). His scale and method were replicated in health-related studies in several nations and are currently used by several multinational surveys, including the UNDP and World Bank.

The Field Theory and Action Research

Many social psychologists consider Kurt Lewin the founder of modern social psychology. Lewin became involved with the Gestalt group in Germany led by Wolfgang Köhler; he also became involved with the early Frankfurt School at the Institute for Social Research in Germany. When Hitler came to power in Germany in 1933, the Institute members had to move to England and America. In England, Lewin became influential in the founding of sensitivity training through the Tavistock Clinic in London. He achieved international fame and spent several years as a visiting professor at Stanford and Cornell. He later immigrated permanently to the United States. From 1935 to 1944, Lewin worked at the University of Iowa, where he made innovative studies of childhood socialization. In 1944, he went to the Massachusetts Institute of Technology (MIT) to lead a research center devoted to group dynamics, which continued after his death. Several of his former students established the now-famous Center for Group Dynamics at the University of Michigan, which continues to lead this field of psychology.

Lewin's "field theory" is based on application of the Gestalt theory of personality and social behavior. Lewin's views influenced many leading psychologists because of the complex behaviors that can be considered in the context of Lewin's "life-space." Prominent psychologists mentored by Kurt Lewin included Leon Festinger, who became known for his cognitive dissonance theory (1956); and environmental psychologist Roger Barker. Lewin was a pioneer and founded the study of "group dynamics," organizational development, and "T–Groups" (or training groups) for professional development. His initial research program focused on the study of prejudice and behavior related to it. Studies included gang behavior and the effect of black sales personnel on sales. Lewin believed that prejudice caused discrimination, not resulted from it, and that altering that behavior could change attitudes. "He wanted to reach beyond the mere description of group life and to investigate the conditions and forces which bring about change or resist it" (Lewin, 1997; Marrow, 1969, p. 178).

Lewin's notion of "action research" transformed the goals of social science from generating knowledge about social practices by academic experts to active moment-to-moment theorizing, data-collecting, and inquiring, occurring in the midst of ongoing lives. Lewin's action research was not only a research that was meant to describe how humans and organizations behaved in the real world, but also a change strategy that was designed to help humans and organizations reflect on and change their own systems. His work significantly influenced several human sciences professions, including community psychology, public health, social work, and nursing. Theories that were developed using Lewin's action research approach include:

¤ Chris Argyris's "Action Science" (Argyris, 1970)
¤ John Heron (1996) and Peter Reason's (1995) "Cooperative Inquiry"
¤ Paulo Freire's (1970) "Participatory Action Research" or PAR

Action research is as much about creating a better life within more effective and just social contexts as it was about discovering facts and theories. It should not be surprising that action research has flourished in Latin America, Northern Europe, India, and Australia as much as, or more than, within university scholarship in the United States.

Community-Based Ecological Multilevel Interventions

A unique genre of exemplary studies of social determinants of health is that of community-based ecological research and multilevel interventions (MLI) for risk reduction in several health-related domains. The health issues of interest in these MLIs range from cardiovascular disease (CVD) and cancer research, to family planning across the world. In this section, we present six pioneering and exemplary community-based ecological/MLI longitudinal research studies to identify social determinants of health:

1. The Framingham Heart Study (USA)
2. The North Karelia (Finland) Project
3. The Stanford Five Community Project
4. The Minnesota Heart Health Project
5. Family-planning KAP studies globally
6. The Alameda County Longitudinal Study.

The first four studies focused on chronic diseases in economically developed countries, and the KAP studies focused on culturally sensitive family-planning decisions and contraceptive-promotion interventions, mostly in traditional and poorer societies.

THE FRAMINGHAM HEART STUDY: MASSACHUSETTS (1948–TODAY)

Considered to be the first major MLI, the Framingham study was embarked upon in 1948 in Framingham, Massachusetts, to explore the general causes of cardiovascular diseases (CVD) and stroke (NHLBI/NIH: http://www.nhlbi. nih.gov/resources/obesity/pop-studies/framingham.htm). At that time, very little was known about the causes of CVD and stroke, while deaths due to these diseases were rising in economically advanced nations including the United States. The aim of this community-based longitudinal study was to understand the common factors associated with CVD risks by following up participants who had no history or symptoms of CVD or stroke for a long period. The study included a sample of 5,209 men and women between the ages of 30 and 60 years old from the town of Framingham. For more than two decades, the researchers collected extensive baseline measurements through physical examinations and interviews on lifestyle behavior to identify factors associated with CVD and stroke by comparing those who developed these health problems and those who did not. The subjects were studied at two-year intervals for detailed medical history, stressful life events, and lifestyle behavior. After two decades, the study in 1971 enrolled a second generation of additional 5,124 subjects who were adult children and spouses of the original subjects. In 2002, the study entered a new phase and enrolled a third generation of respondents, including the grandchildren of the original study cohort, and members of diverse ethnic populations of Framingham (Omni Group 1 and Omni Group 2). Approximately 200 members of the original cohort are currently alive and under follow-up.

Through this extensive longitudinal and multigenerational study, researchers identified major CVD risk factors: high blood pressure, high cholesterol, tobacco smoking, obesity, diabetes, and sedentary lifestyle or physical inactivity. Although the study population of Framingham was primarily white, later studies showed that the risk factors identified by this pioneering study apply to other ethnic populations in the United States and across the world. This study has produced more than 1,200 research articles in leading peer-reviewed journals and inspired other MLIs across the world. The empirical knowledge generated is now required reading in medicine, epidemiology, public health, and allied health sciences curricula. It has also inspired numerous studies that include the role of genetic factors and cultural diversities. Its contributions have been acclaimed as some of the most important discoveries in medicine and related health sciences.

THE ALAMEDA COUNTY LONGITUDINAL STUDY

Similar findings were reported from the Alameda County Population Laboratory studies directed by Lester Breslow, a pioneer in public health and health promotion. As the then-director of the California State Health Department, he undertook a longitudinal study that followed the health habits of 6,928 residents of Alameda County for more than 20 years. Based upon these studies, Breslow (2012) reported that their earlier studies in Alameda County:

> established seven health practices as risk factors for higher mortality: excessive alcohol consumption, smoking cigarettes, being obese, sleeping fewer or more than 7–8 hours, having very little physical activity, eating between meals, and not eating breakfast. Observation now reveals that, taking into account age, gender, physical health status, and social network index in 1965, the occurrence of disability was only about one-half as great among the cohort survivors in 1974 who reported good health practices in 1965 as among those with poor health practices; those with an intermediate level of health practices experienced about two-thirds the relative disability risk of those with poor health practices. (Breslow, 2012)

Essentially similar relationships prevailed for the 1982–1983 survivors of the original (1965) cohort who, upon re-questioning, had been found to be without disability in 1974 (from the study abstract). In Lester Breslow's obituary, the *New York Times* wrote:

As an official of the California department in the 1940s and '50s, he did some of the early definitive studies on the harmful effects of smoking. Three of these studies were cited in the United States Surgeon General's landmark report in 1964 linking cigarettes to lung diseases, particularly cancer. But it was the Alameda County study that rocked the public health world, because it proved with numbers that behavior indisputably affected longevity. It's recommendations: Do not smoke; drink in moderation; sleep seven to eight hours; exercise at least moderately; eat regular meals; maintain a moderate weight; eat breakfast. (*New York Times*, April 15, 2012; http://www.nytimes.com/2012/04/15/health/lester-breslow-who-tied-good-habits-to-longevity-dies-at-97.html?_r=0)

THE NORTH KARELIA PROJECT: FINLAND

The North Karelia project, a pioneering community-wide intervention study, was designed to evaluate the effects of a systematic health promotion campaign to reduce CVD risk factors and to measure its effects. The primary objective was to evaluate the effectiveness of community-based health education and promotion interventions to reduce CVD-related risks. Reductions in cigarette smoking, serum cholesterol concentrations, and blood pressure were among the immediate objectives of this community-based campaign. An additional objective was to promote the early detection, treatment, and rehabilitation of patients with CVD. The study was carried out in the eastern Finnish province of North Karelia, a rural area of 180,000 inhabitants, with the control area of Kuopio Province, Finland. A random sample of one-sixteenth of the population between the ages of 30 and 59 years was studied, comprising 1,834 men and 1,973 women from North Karelia, and 2,665 men and 2,769 women from the control area. Kuopio was selected as the control area.

The community-based CVD demonstration program and the study cohort were followed through 1997. Five years later, a cross-sectional survey was carried out in both study areas using methods similar to those employed in the baseline survey. The sample for this second survey consisted of those between the ages of 30 and 64 years. Additional cross-sectional population surveys were carried out every five years: in 1982, 1987, 1992, and 1997. Over the more recent periods, risk-factor surveys were conducted as part of the WHO-sponsored MONICA (MONItoring of trends and determinants in CArdiovascular disease) study program. As in earlier surveys, an independent random sample was drawn from existing population registers. A comprehensive questionnaire was sent to the homes of the surveyed sample asking questions about their socioeconomic status, medical history, smoking, diet, alcohol consumption, physical activity (and attempts to change these lifestyle behaviors), and psychosocial factors. At the clinic visit examination, height, weight, skinfold thicknesses, blood pressure, and serum cholesterol were measured.

An important focus of the overall program was to reduce population serum cholesterol levels through dietary change because of their presumed role in the high CVD rates of Finland. This was accomplished through widespread reductions in saturated fat intake and concomitant increases in the consumption of vegetables and polyunsaturated fats. The intervention was originally designed to be implemented throughout the community for five years (1972–1977), but the program was gradually expanded to include the prevention of other non-communicable diseases.

This study demonstrated statistically significant changes in risk factors in study populations, which supports the value of community-based health education and promotion. Critics, however, raised important caveats concerning the cost-effectiveness and replicability of the results in larger societies with culturally diverse populations. First, Finland is a small nation with a highly homogenous population; and second, the magnitude of changes in cigarette smoking were modest and not much different from the degree of changes in the reference population.

THE STANFORD FIVE-CITY PROJECT, CALIFORNIA, 1972–1992

The Stanford Five-City Project (Farquhar, Fortmann, Maccoby, et al., 1985) was a large experimental field study of community health education for the prevention of cardiovascular disease. It was designed to answer fundamental questions in cardiovascular disease epidemiology, communication, health education, behavior change, and community organization, and to test the ability of a potentially cost-effective program to prevent cardiovascular disease at the community level. It was hypothesized that a 20% decrease in cardiovascular disease risk would lead to a significant decline in cardiovascular disease rates in two treatment communities compared with three reference communities. It included a six-year intervention program of community-wide health education and organization. Risk-factor changes were assessed through four surveys of independent samples and in a repeatedly surveyed cohort. Cardiovascular disease event rates were assessed through continuous community surveillance of fatal and nonfatal myocardial infarction and stroke (Fortmann & Varady, 1999).

Stanford, California, and the surrounding area was chosen as one of three sites to conduct community surveys on CVD. Two studies took place as part of the Stanford Community Trials: the Stanford Three-Community Study and the Stanford Five-City Project. The Three-Community Study measured the effectiveness of media campaigns and community-wide health education plus a specific high-risk intervention on cardiovascular risk-factor levels. The Five-City Project aimed a broader community-action campaign at risk-factor reduction, decline in heart disease endpoints, and cost-effectiveness measures. The Stanford Three-Community Study started in 1972 in the communities of Tracy, Gilroy, and Watsonville, California. A random sample of adults aged 35–59 was examined annually in each community with estimations of daily intake of nutrients, rate of smoking, knowledge of heart disease risk factors, and laboratory and physical measurements of cholesterol, plasma renin, urinary sodium, blood pressure, and weight. A risk score was calculated for each participant using multiple logistic function of risk. Mass media campaigns using television, radio, newspapers, and posted advertisements were launched in Gilroy and Watsonville, while Tracy functioned as a control community. The Stanford Five-City Project began in 1978 as a 13-year study. The five northern California cities involved in the project were chosen for their diversity of media outlets, populations of more than 30,000 people, and socioeconomic and ethnic similarity. In the Three-Community Study,

> a statistically significant reduction was achieved in the composite risk score for cardiovascular disease as a result of significant declines in blood pressure, smoking and cholesterol levels. This risk score decreased approximately 25% for the media-only community and 30% for the community in which media were supplemented by face-to-face instruction. (Fortmann & Varady, 1999, pp. 322–323)

In Tracy, there was a minimal decrease in risk score (less than 5% for both the total and high-risk participants). In the Five-City Project, smoking rates decreased by 14% in control communities. The intervention cities also experienced a 15% decrease in risk score based on improvements in blood pressure, physical activity, and cholesterol. Numerous sub-campaigns, including a curriculum for fourth-, seventh-, and tenth-grade students, were found effective in increasing awareness of nutrition, physical activity, and smoking cessation as essential to heart health. Strengths of the studies included random sampling from an open population and the ability to assess community for intervention. While the curriculum, counseling, and media campaigns were successful in the Stanford Community Trials, the authors were skeptical about the possibility of implementing such efforts on a national scale. Concerns articulated included lack of trained staff, overstretch of county health departments, and the decentralization of public schools.

THE MINNESOTA HEART HEALTH PROGRAM (MHHP)

The Minnesota Heart Health Program was a 13-year research and demonstration project to reduce morbidity and mortality from coronary heart disease in whole communities (1980–1993; Luepker et al., 1994). Three pairs of communities were matched on size and type; each pair had one education site and one comparison site. After baseline surveys, a five- to six-year program of mass media, community organization, and direct education for risk reduction was used for health education of communities. After two years of participation, Mankato, Minnesota, was significantly more exposed to activities promoting cardiovascular disease prevention. In this town of 38,000 inhabitants, 190 community leaders were directly involved as program volunteers, 14,103 residents (more than 60% of adults) attended a screening education center, 2,094 attended MHHP health-education classes, 42 of 65 physicians and 728 other health professionals participated in continuing education programs offered by MHHP, and distribution of printed media averaged 12.2 pieces per household. These combined educational strategies resulted in widespread awareness of MHHP and participation by the majority of the Mankato adult population in its education activities. Many intervention components proved effective in targeted groups.

However, against a background of strong secular trends of increasing health promotion and declining risk factors, the overall program effects were modest in size and duration and generally within chance levels. These findings suggest that even such an intense program may not be able to generate enough additional exposure to risk reduction messages and activities in a large enough fraction of the population to accelerate the remarkably favorable secular trends in health promotion activities and in most coronary heart disease risk factors present in the study communities. One review of several of community-based MLIs concluded:

> The core of a successful program is the community organization process. This involves identification and activation of key community leaders, stimulation of citizens and organizations to volunteer time and offer resources to CVD prevention, and the promotion of prevention as a community theme. A wide range of intervention settings [is] available for health promotion. As is true for the workplace, places of worship are receptive to health promotion programs and have access to large numbers of people. Mass media are effective when used in conjunction with complementary messages delivered through other channels, such as school programs, adult education programs, and self-help programs. Community health professionals play a vital role in providing program endorsement and stimulating the participation of other community leaders. School-based programs promote long-term behavior change and reach beyond the school to actively involve parents. Innovative health promotion contests have widespread appeal and promote participation in other community interventions. In the area of evaluation, health program participation rates are appropriate primary outcome measures in most community-oriented prevention programs. Other program

evaluation priorities include community analysis and formative evaluation, providing data to fine-tune interventions and define the needs and preferences of the community. (Mittelmark et al., 2001)

Family-Planning Knowledge, Attitude, and Practice (KAP) Studies

In the 1950s and 1960s there was a major and increasing global concern about unregulated population growth, and many national and international scholars, policy analysts, health-related organizations, and national leaders advocated robust population and family-planning policies and programs to limit the then-prevalent population growth rates; some advocated a "zero population growth" (ZPG) target, which was defined as limiting the number of children born in a year equal to the number of deaths in a defined population unit. As a result, the "rate of population growth" would be reduced to "zero" although the total population size would still increase (this is because the total population size equals the number of people alive plus the number of babies born and alive in a year). Some scholars estimated that with effective proactive programs and incentives to people for using family-planning contraceptives, it would take 20 to 30 years to accomplish ZPG. This was at the beginning of the "demographic transition" when death rates began to fall rapidly due to effective reduction of infectious diseases and epidemics, while birth rates remained high, especially in poorer countries (Berelson et al., 1966; Mauldin et al., 1971; Reynolds, 1972). The pressures to check the world's population growth became pronounced, and several international and national organizations emerged to address the challenge (e.g., the United Nations Population Fund, the Population Council, and several foundations, including Ford and Rockefeller). Outstanding scholars in reproductive science, demographers, social scientists, health management, communication specialists, and national and international leaders joined forces to address the challenge. Independently, the success of women's suffrage movements emboldened leaders of women's movements to demand that women have access to reproductive knowledge and services; they established the network of International Planned Parenthood Federations (IPPF) in several countries (the IPPF was inaugurated at a conference in Bombay, now called Mumbai, India, in 1952 by Margaret Singer of the U.S., Lady Rao of India, and leaders of the Planned Parenthood Federation from several nations). Sixty years later, the charity is a Federation of 152 member associations working in 172 countries. It runs 65,000 service points worldwide. In 2011, those facilities delivered more than 89 million sexual and reproductive health services (IPPF, 2015c).

As the international population planning movement grew, leading universities and research centers across the world joined the movement and established advanced-degree programs and undertook innovative studies related to fertility and family planning. Internationally recognized scholars took leadership in population and family-planning studies (e.g., psychologist Bernard Berelson, demographers Kingsley Davis and Ronald Freedman, sociologists Parker Mauldin and Charles Westoff, and communication scholars Donald Bogue and Everett Rogers).

A new genre of social and behavioral research focused on social determinants of fertility and family planning emerged, and became known as "family-planning KAP" studies. One estimate notes that at least 400 KAP studies were completed in 72 nations by the end of 1970; by the mid-1980s, that number had increased to more than 2,000. A KAP survey provides basic factual data on existing levels of knowledge, attitudes, and practices for the population surveyed at a particular point in time; it also measures past practices of family planning and fertility (Berelson, 1966; Mauldin et al., 1971).

In reviewing the first cohort of KAP studies from 20 countries, Berelson in 1966 wrote:

> The author believes that the answers are reliable as intragroup trends. Some generalizations were universal, such as the desire for fewer children and an ideal family size of about 25%–30% of their completed families in most Asian and African countries. Japan was the only exception, wanting larger completed families. The average family size in a country was in proportion to the desired size. From one-half to three-fourths of the people interviewed wanted no more children. Worldwide, most countries found 66%–68% of people were interested in learning about contraception; people knew very little about reproduction, and many in less developed countries did not know about contraception. The more common the practice of contraception, the earlier in life a population begins using it. The number of children desired depended on the number already born. The number of parents wanting more children decreased with literacy, income, education and urbanization. Even in developed countries, such as the U.S. where 80% use contraception, 10%–12% of the population were uninformed about contraception. The results of costly KAP surveys have been useful to correct the impression of the elite that the poor are uninterested in contraception, but the results have not generally been put to political or programmatic use. (Berelson et al., 1966)

While the volume and the enormous cost of the KAP studies increased, these studies also raised several criticisms; the most important concern was the lack of observed consistency between people's responses to questions on the measures of family-planning attitudes and their actual use of contraceptives and fertility planning in the future.

The valuable lessons learned from these worldwide KAP studies have two major implications for community-based multilevel studies. These are:

(1) *Theoretical*: A generalized attitude measure does not predict a very specific behavior in an actual behavioral context. For instance, one might think that the idea of having "good health" is desirable as a generalized goal; but that does not allow a researcher to predict whether the respondent will regularly jog or swim (specific action). The independent variable is too general, and the dependent variables are too specific and context-dependent. Similarly, a respondent may have a positive attitude toward "family planning"; but that knowledge does not allow the researcher to make an accurate prediction of a specific contraceptive use by a respondent. She might like an oral pill but not an intrauterine device (IUD). If a researcher wishes to predict jogging or using an IUD as the dependent variable, then the independent variable or attitude question should refer to (a) an intention to perform that specific behavior (e.g., "Do you intend to jog regularly?" or "Do you intend to use an oral contraceptive pill?"); (b) using a single-causal assumption when the behavior is caused by multiple determinants (e.g., approval/disapproval of sexual partner); and (c) contextual determinants (e.g., cost of, or barriers to use of, pill).

(2) *Methodological:* Weaknesses and limitations of the surveys include the measurements, sampling, and statistical procedures used. Fawcett (1973), Freedman and Berelson (1996), and Kar (1978) were among the earliest critics of the limitations of KAP studies.

In response, Fishbein proposed his "Behavioral Intention" theory—which requires measures of "intention to perform a specific act," the "perceived reference group norm," the reference group's "support for the action," and the "motivation to comply with the reference group norms" (Fishbein & Ajzen, 1975). Subsequently, this model was further developed and applied in other health problems such as smoking and HIV/AIDS; the results include Fishbein's "theory of planned behavior" and "theory of planned action" (Fishbein & Ajzen, 1975).

Fawcett, in his pioneering volume titled *Psychological Perspectives on Population* (1973) analyzed the values and limitations of KAP and psychological studies in considerable detail. Berelson (1969, 1974), Freedman and Berelson (1976), and Corsa and Oakley (1979) reviewed in-depth international programs from a macro perspective. Freedman and Berelson (1976) conducted a meticulous of evaluation of family-planning programs in 29 countries and additional case studies in 15 of these countries to examine the interactions and added effects of *program strengths* (strong to weak) and the *setting advantage* (strong to weak) to examine the program outcomes measured by contraceptive-acceptance rates and the level of fertility averted that were attributable to program inputs.

These analyses revealed complex relationships among several determinants at several levels. They concluded that program effectiveness depended on complex mixtures of these dimensions; measuring a single dimension or determinant (e.g., program strength, contraceptive attitude) would not be able to detect and explain whether or why a program was effective or ineffective. Once again, we see the importance of measuring several levels of determinants (a multilevel or ecological model) before intervention effects may be measured or detected.

Everett Rogers and his colleagues applied the diffusion of innovation and communications theories and models extensively in numerous countries. Through these they were able to develop deeper knowledge of factors that accelerate or impede adoption of modern contraceptives in pre-industrial societies (Rogers et al., 1973). Cross-national field studies in family-planning communication and education programs by this author and colleagues in India, the Philippines, Egypt, the United States, and Venezuela revealed that early, late, and non-use of contraceptive methods in these countries was mainly due to the combined and added effects of four sets of determinants. In summing up these findings, Puska, Nissinen, Tuomilehto, et al. (1996) stated: "the recent work of Kar ... has shown that in different cultures the main factors predicting health behavior (e.g., contraceptive use) are intentions, social support from significant others, and accessibility of knowledge and services" (WHO, 1966, p. 97). These and similar findings from numerous family-planning KAP studies across the world support the importance of adopting a social-ecological or multilevel model for studying the determinants of health behavior and for planning effective policy and prevention interventions.

Ecological and Multilevel Interventions

In this book, the terms *ecological research, multilevel research*, and *systems research* are used interchangeably. These terms dictate studying health behavior from a holistic perspective; the central premise is that a health behavior is caused by a combination of determinants at several levels, and therefore the most appropriate methodology is to study health behavior using a theory-based multicausal paradigm. A pioneer in using the systems approach in health-related behavior in social science was psychologist Kurt Lewin. The fundamental premise of Lewin's field theory is that a behavior is a function of the totality of determinants within the "person" (intrapersonal) and in the specific "environment" (life-space) in which that behavior occurs {$B = f \sum P \times E$}; and that a sustained behavior is maintained by "quasi-stationary equilibria" or a "force-field" within the person (where "P" is the person and "E" is the environment); or behavior is a function of the force-field consisting of forces within the person and in the environment in which the person acts. At a time when psychologists were preoccupied with studying behavior using discrete psychological constructs (e.g., attitudes, intelligence, traits, instincts, personality, motivation), Lewin cautioned that unless we understand the "force-field" in its totality that determines a behavior, piecemeal studies looking at personal characteristics will not succeed. Finally, he conceptualized the force-field as a "quasi-stationary" equilibrium analogous to the concept of "homeostasis" (in natural sciences and physiology; sounds like *Yin* and *Yang* balance). After a discussion of the concept of the reality of social phenomena, and a brief survey of topological concepts, Lewin introduced his main topic: quasi-stationary equilibria in group life, and the problem of social change.

> Various phenomena such as aggression, factory production, ability, social bond[ing], and group decisions are considered [to be] the result of interacting force fields. None of the above activities can be explained in terms of itself but only in terms of the operation of various processes which fluctuate as a function of basic forces and tensions.

Lewin's pioneering research on the effects of group discussions and decisions on various behavior, such as nutritional behavior among mothers (e.g., the use of fruit juices and organ meat), laid the foundation of *group dynamics* as a field of study and practice. The business-management field embraced his group dynamics research findings and T-Groups (Training Groups) for management and leadership development (many universities, including the University of Michigan and Columbia University, established T-Group programs and centers for group dynamics research and training). Lewin held that: "groups come into being in a psychological sense not because their members necessarily are similar to one another (although they may be); rather, a group exists when people in it realize their fate depends on the fate of the group as a whole."

Action research gained a significant foothold both within the realm of community-based and participatory action research, and as a form of practice oriented to the improvement of educative encounters (Carr & Kemmis, 1986). The use of action research to deepen and develop classroom practice has grown into a strong tradition of practice, one of the first examples being the work of Stephen Corey, who used action research and group work in educational curriculum development in 1949 (Corey, 1949b). More recently, Uri Triesman developed his MIST (Merit Immersion for Students and Teachers) model to promote math and science learning for under-performing minority students at the University of California, Berkeley (http://psycnet.apa.org/psycinfo/1948-00256-001); this was an excellent example of action research where principles of group dynamics and leadership processes were the keys through which students as learners solved academic problems with collective efforts.

Between the 1950s and 1960s, several American foundations encouraged U.S. universities and faculty members to undertake research-*cum*-action (RCA) projects in rural areas in poor countries to confront a wide range of problems in areas such as agriculture, rural sanitation, and child survival (e.g., the Gandhigram, Harvard-Ludhiana, Nazafgarh, and Singur RCA projects in India alone; similar projects were undertaken elsewhere in Africa, Asia, and Latin America). The benefits from these RCA projects were that they initiated the earliest studies on social determinants of health and trained social scientists in the area of disease prevention in poor nations.

Since then, the action research model has been widely adopted in education, health, and rural development by both poor and rich nations. For instance, reducing child mortality by two-thirds before 2015 was one of the United Nations' Millennium Development Goals (MDGs). Most of these deaths are preventable. In India, as in many developing countries, providing even basic health care in rural areas is a major challenge for the government. Analyses of India's health system have suggested that rural health care has been neglected by the government and that increasing privatization may further reduce health care in remote areas. Community-based PHC provided by trained community residents has been shown to improve child survival in areas with high child mortality. The Warmi project in Bolivia and the Society for Education, Action and Research in Community Health (SEARCH) in Maharashtra, India, have demonstrated significant reductions in perinatal and neonatal mortality. Trials in Nepal and in Uttar Pradesh, India, reported reductions in neonatal mortality of 30% and 52%, respectively (Mann, Eble, Frost, et al., 2010).

An excellent summary of Lewin's pioneering contributions and his profound influence on action research, titled: "Kurt Lewin, groups, experiential learning and action research" is available in the *Encyclopedia of Informal Education* (Smith, 2010).

In reality, however, most studies focused on determinants of individual behavior; not on multilevel determinants. In a review of 157 health promotion studies published in *Health Education and Behavior* during the last 20 years, Golden and Earp (2012) observed that:

> Overall, articles were more likely to describe interventions focused on individual and interpersonal characteristics, rather than institutional, community, or policy factors. Interventions that focused on certain topics (nutrition and physical activity) or occurred in particular settings (schools) more successfully adopted a social ecological approach. Health education theory, research, and training may need to be enhanced to better foster successful efforts to modify social and political environments to improve health. (Golden and Earp, 2012, p. 369)

The authors analyzed two dimensions of the studies: the *level* of intervention activities, and the *target* of change. Their results showed that 95% of the studies focused on the individual level of intervention activities, 67% on the interpersonal level, and 39% on institutional activities. Only about 20% of the interventions were at the community level, and a meager 6% were on the policy level. In addition, 63% of these studies included only one or two of the five levels of the ecological model. It is conceivable that if the authors had included all major journals that publish social science–based research (there are at least two dozen journals that focus on health behavior), the percentage distributions would be different.

In 2012, the NCI convened a national meeting of researchers to review the status of MLI studies in cancer control. Subsequently, a review paper on lessons learned from this meeting summarized the major findings of that review. The authors of that review paper observed that:

> MLI research is underrepresented as an explicit focus in the cancer literature but may improve implementation of studies of cancer care delivery if they assess contextual, organizational, and environmental factors important to understand behavioral and/or system-level interventions. The field lacks a single unifying theory; although several psychological or biological theories are useful, an ecological model helps conceptualize and communicate interventions. (Clauser et al., 2012)

A similar trend is prevalent in intervention studies in multicultural communities. A comprehensive literature review of "multicultural evaluation" sponsored by the California Endowment discovered that, while there is an overwhelming consensus among the authors and researchers that we need multicultural theories and models for community-based health interventions and evaluation, in reality, multicultural models of interventions and evaluations are seldom used. Most research and interventions use theories and models developed from monocultural studies and assume that these theories and models are equally valid in multicultural communities. These studies simply compare their study populations with other ethnic groups using aggregate measures; such studies do not explain the social and cultural dynamics of multicultural communities as they affect the health and well-being of entire populations (Nguyen, Kagawa-Singer, & Kar, 2003). Chapter 6 of this book is dedicated to multicultural issues and dynamics as they affect the health and quality of life of people in these communities.

In 1995, the NIH established the OBSSR to facilitate behavioral science research across the (then 24) institutes and centers at the NIH. Among the office's numerous activities and accomplishments were its efforts to foster a "levels of analysis" framework for the NIH, showing the interdependence and importance of all levels of research for accelerating advances in health science and health care. This multilevel model is most comprehensive and inclusive of all MLI models used in health-related research and interventions; not surprisingly, this MLI includes the NIH's long-standing commitment to basic biomedical research, such as its initiatives research at the genomic or macro-biological level. From the social and behavioral sciences and the global public health perspectives, the model's first four levels are more salient. These are: individual, family/close relations, community, and social organizations. It is important to note that the NIH/OBSSR model explicitly emphasizes the global levels of determinants of human health and well-being. In our current world of rapid globalization and expansion of global health initiatives, where our world is truly a "global village," exclusive focus within nations and excessive focus on individuals are inadequate both for theoretical and for practical purposes.

Through the Eyes of the Beholder

Sociocultural anthropology has made unique theoretical and methodological contributions in health-related research and our understanding of how culture affects our lives, including health behavior and outcomes. According to the American Anthropological Association (AAA):

> Research in sociocultural anthropology is distinguished by its emphasis on participant observation, which involves placing oneself in the research context for extended periods of time to gain a first-hand sense of how local knowledge is put to work in grappling with practical problems of everyday life and with basic philosophical problems of knowledge, truth, power, and justice. Topics of concern to sociocultural anthropologists include such areas as health, work, ecology and environment, education, agriculture and development, and social change. (p. 1)

The anthropological approach allows us to better understand complex social and behavioral processes affecting our health from the perspectives of the subjects (eyes of the beholder) that cannot be captured by quantitative studies from the perspective of external observers. It adopts the insider's subjective or "emic" perspective in understanding why people behave in a way rather than the outside observer's or "etic" perspective. A deeper understanding of complex health-related behavior requires a creative integration of both emic and etic perspectives and the development of innovative methodologies appropriate for such an approach.

There is an emerging consensus that health-related behavior and community-based prevention intervention requires: (a) a multidisciplinary and ecological approach, (b) triangulation of data extracted through a multi-method research design (NIH's systems science approach), and (c) combining both objective (etic) and subjective (emic) perspectives.

4

Dynamics of Multicultural Community

When races come together, as in the present age, it should
not be merely the gathering of a crowd; there must be a
bond of relation, or they will collide with one another.

—Rabindranath Tagore

The aim of this chapter is to identify social realities and dynamics of multicultural communities (MCC) as they affect the health and quality of life of the members of that community. Previous chapters emphasized the importance of social determinants of health, which include cultural and ethnic differences as they affect the health and well-being of populations. The objective of this chapter is not to summarize the results of studies on social and cultural determinants of health; the report of the World Health Organization (WHO) Commission on Social Determinants cited earlier (WHO/Marmot, 2008) and the brief review by Braveman, Egerter, and Williams, in the *Annual Review of Public Health* (2011, vol. 132, pp. 381–398) are excellent sources for that purpose. In this chapter, we focus on the unique social dynamics and forces in multicultural communities where human interactions and inter-group relations occur and affect health and quality of life (HQOL). Historically, race is defined on a biological basis when the members of a group are believed to have common biological attributes that make them distinct and different from other "races." Usually physical features, language spoken, religion, and national origin are used to place people in different groups. The concept of race was promoted by European scholars who claimed that people's inherited biological endowments of a race make them physically and behaviorally distinct from other races. There are several conceptual and methodological problems with this premise: physical features change over several generations, cultures change, behaviors also change over time, and there is a lack of decisive evidence of genomic and DNA differences among different "races" within the human species. In contrast, the concept of "ethnicity" is based on self-identified cultural groups and similarities, including language and place of origin. Ethnicity is the uniqueness of the "way of life" of groups of people who self-identify as a designated ethnic group and share common ancestries.

The concept of race lives in the minds of two types of people: those who believe in racial "superiority" (often for themselves), and agencies that must count people for public policy purposes. For instance, the white supremacists are convinced that racial hierarchy exists and that they are inherently better than others. The U.S. government uses five racial categories in census and healthcare data: (1) Black or African American, (2) White, (3) Asian, (4) American Indian or Alaska Native, and (5) Native Hawaiian or Other Pacific Islander. Research shows that these five categories do not include many who do not identify with any of these five categories; so the Office of Management and Budget (OMB), which defines rules for census, introduced a sixth residual category—"some other race," including multiple races for those who do not identify with the first five categories. In addition, the OMB recommends collecting data on "granular ethnicity"—which is defined as a person's ethnic origin or descent, "roots," or heritage or the place of birth. So while there is no decisive victory for the scientists, the concept of race is still alive. For instance, in his Foreword of the report of the IOM titled *Race, Ethnicity, and Language Data Standardization for Health Care Quality Improvement* (2009), the then-president of the IOM, Harvey Fineberg, stated:

> *The Institute of Medicine Report Unequal Treatment: Confronting Racial and Ethnic Disparities in Healthcare* (2002) called attention to poorer access to health care and worse health outcomes among certain racial and ethnic groups. According to reports from the Agency for Healthcare Research and Quality and others, disparities in the quality of care and in health outcomes persist. Accelerating progress toward eliminating these disparities depends in part on our ability to identify and track experiences in health care among individuals from a variety of racial and ethnic backgrounds and who speak a variety of languages other than English. (http://www.ahrq.gov/research/findings/final-reports/iomracereport/iomracereport.pdf)

This chapter identifies and reviews the top issues in multicultural communities (MCC) that affect health and health-related quality of life (HRQOL) of the people. In addition to those issues, this chapter discusses the importance of "trust" between ethnic groups and human service agencies as it affects health care policy and programs. The cultural anthropologists have historically studied the cultural attributes of different and often exotic populations and tribes. These studies focused on the uniqueness of the cultures they studied and often compared results with other cultures, including the dominant culture within which these ethnic groups existed as minority groups. Often these groups were isolated voluntarily or involuntarily from the dominant cultures of the nations. Anthropological studies offer us new insights, theories, and methods for examining how the implicit cultures (e.g., cosmology, beliefs, values) and explicit cultures (actions and artifacts) affect human health and well-being.

In recent decades, social scientists, including anthropologists, began to investigate cultural similarities and differences among nations and cultures across the globe. These studies focused on values, attitudes, and practices across nations and large population groups; the results are available to those interested, in several websites cited in the previous chapter. The top issues or dynamics of the MCCs that affect HRQOL are discussed below.

Ethnic Diversity

With rapid urbanization, globalization, migration, and higher fertility rates among recent immigrants (who tend to be younger persons in reproductive age), the numbers and sizes of ethnic populations living in multicultural communities are rapidly increasing. For instance, more than 90% of the U.S. population in the first census in 1790 were whites; in 1900, 88% were whites; and in the 2010 census the whites were down to about 72%. The U.S. Census Bureau projects that by the year 2050, the white population will be 52%; and soon after that whites will be one of the several minorities who constitute the total U.S. population. A recent American Community Survey in 2013 reported that in 19 out of 20 major U.S. cities, whites are a minority (ACS: US Census Bureau, 2013).

Ethnic diversity is often measured by the proportion of foreign-born citizens and residents in a country. Figure 4.1 presents the size of foreign-born populations of selected nations as a measure of cultural diversity. It ranges from 0.2% in China to 61.2% in Kuwait. But the size of the foreign-born population in a country does not represent an accurate measure of cultural diversity in our communities for several reasons. First, the foreign-born nationals are only the first generation of naturalized citizens or permanent residents; their children and descendants are born in their adopted countries and therefore are not counted as immigrants even though they are not fully assimilated, and may speak the language of their foreign-born parents and retain their personal identity as a hyphenated ethnic minority (e.g., Mexican-American, Japanese-American). Others in the community may also see them as ethnic minorities or as foreigners. Second, one may be a Native American by birth for generations and still retain one's original ethnic identity and be treated as an ethnic minority by others (e.g., Native

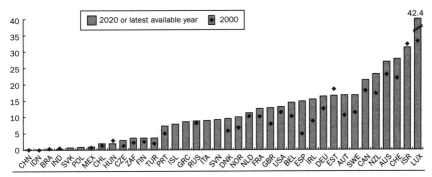

FIGURE 4.1 Foreign-Born Population. Organization for Economic Cooperation and Development (OECD).

Americans, fifth-generation Japanese Americans). Third, the ancestors of the current Chicanos, for example, were native Californians and citizens of Mexico before California became one of the United States. Fourth, the 2010 U.S. Census shows that more than 28% of Americans identify as ethnic minorities, regardless of where they were born or how many generations have lived in America.

Ethnic diversity is a major issue in a multicultural community. In our personal space, daily life, and social interactions, we must interact with people who are different from us in terms of language, religion, culture, food, music, customs, and habits.

Our perceptions of ourselves and other cultures have significant effects on the quality of life of people in a multicultural community. Available data on ethnic diversity is often misleading because people are grouped by different criteria. Some are grouped by language, some by skin color (e.g., black, white), or by geography of origin (e.g., Asians, African American). But such a classification system does not guarantee that all people in a designated ethnic group share the same cultural characteristics. For instance, Indians, Chinese, Japanese, and other groups of Asian origin in the United States are grouped as "Asian Americans", but these groups have very little in common in terms of language, religion, customs, and cultures. India is the most diverse nation in the world—it has 17 official languages (not dialects); four primary Hindu castes and several subcastes, including the former "untouchables" now called *Dalits* (means "oppressed"); and numerous tribes called *Adibashi* (or "original people"). Indians practice all major religions in numbers larger than the populations of many nations; four major world religions originated in India (Hinduism, Buddhism, Sikhism, and Jainism), and it has the third-largest Muslim population in the world. To combine Indians and other immigrants of disparate Asian origin in one pan-Asian category and call it "Asian American"

BOX 4.1

Top Ten Cities with Foreign-Born Populations

City	Country	Foreign Born (%)
Dubai	UAE	82
Luxembourg	Luxembourg	66
Toronto	Canada	52
Miami	USA	51
Queens, NY	USA	48
Amsterdam	The Netherlands	47
Muscat	Oman	45
Singapore	Singapore	43
Vancouver	Canada	40
Geneva	Switzerland	39
Auckland	New Zealand	39

Source: The 2015 World Migration Report (2015).

does not identify them or describe them; it only obscures their origin and ethnicity.

Foreign-born populations do not distribute evenly across all cities and localities in their adopted nations, and most studies do not measure the magnitude of ethnic diversity of communities. Box 4.1 shows the top ten cities with the highest percentage of foreign-born populations.

In several large metropolitan cities, the percent of foreign-born residents alone does not measure the magnitude of ethnic diversity. For instance, while the foreign-born population in Los Angeles is about 35.3%, no ethnic group has the majority. Hispanics or Latinos alone are 48.2%; an additional 14.5% are Asian, African Americans are 9.3%, and whites are 27.3% (2012 data: http://quickfacts.census.gov/qfd/states/06/06037.html).

One reliable analysis concludes that:

Cities across the development spectrum have growing mobile and diverse populations to manage. In the developed countries, one of the main sources of population diversity is international migration, while in the developing world it is most likely internal migration and, to a lesser extent, growing international South–South migration. (WMP 2015, p. 2)

Health Disparities

Global data on social determinants of health and vital statistics show significant disparities between and within countries in health status, preventive behavior, and access to modern healthcare (WHO, 2008). These disparities are universal (in rich and developing nations) and cause grave challenges to those concerned with global public health. However, because nations vary significantly on so many macro-level cultural, political, economic, and geographic conditions, and lifestyles, reliable local data from *multicultural communities* allow us to better examine the ethnic disparities in defined communities where people live and share the same healthcare systems. For this reason, this chapter uses Los Angeles County as an example of the disparities in a multicultural community.

Tables 4.1 and 4.2 present selected health indicators by ethnic groups from Los Angeles, California, to illustrate the diversities in a multicultural city where no ethnic group (irrespective of their birthplace) has the majority; this city is like many major metropolitan cities across the world where the foreign-born and ethnic minorities collectively are in the majority. The Los Angeles County Department of Health Services (LADHS) serves such a truly multicultural county. With a population of 10.3 million (2012), the city is larger than many countries. It is a true MCC on all counts. A report titled

TABLE 4.1
Los Angeles County: Ethnic Diversity

Statistics	Los Angeles County	White	African American	Hispanic	Asian American
Population in 2008	10.3 million	32%	10%	46%	13%
Life expectancy at birth/years:					
Women	82.9	82.3	77.2	84.4	86.9
Men	77.6	77.6	69.4	79.0	82.4
Infant mortality (2006)	4.8	3.9	11.6	4.5	3.7
Preterm births (2009) (from 17 to 36 weeks)	10.7%	9.5%	15.1%	10.7	9.3%
#1 cause of premature deaths (2006)	CVD	CVD	Homicide	Homicide	CVD
#2 cause of premature deaths (2006)	Cancer	Lung cancer	CVD	Car crash	Car crash
#3 cause of premature deaths (2006)	Car crash & injuries	Car crash	Lung cancer	CVD	Stroke
#4 cause of premature deaths (2006)	Homicide	Drug overdose	Liver disease	Stroke	Suicide
#5 cause of premature deaths (2006)	Suicide	Suicide	Car crash	Diabetes	Lung cancer
Mortality from all causes per 100,000 population	555.9	601.5	802.1	465.8	375.9

That is because different % with fractions more than .5 are rounded to the next higher whole numbers; less than .5 are rounded to next lower whole number. This may give a total between 99–101%; this is allowed in research documents.

Source: Data from: Fielding J et al. (2009). Leading Causes of Death and Premature Death. Los Angeles County Department of Health. Available at http://publichealth.lacounty.gov/wwwfiles/ph/hae/dca/MortalityReport2009.pdf.

TABLE 4.2

Ten Leading Causes of Deaths by Race in Los Angeles

Causes of Death: Ranks	Los Angeles County	White	Black	Hispanic	Asian
#1	CVD	CVD	CVD	CVD	CVD
#2	Stroke	Emphysema/COPD	Stroke	Stroke	Stroke
#3	Lung cancer	Lung cancer	Diabetes	Lung cancer	Lung cancer
#4	Emphysema/COPD	Stroke	Lung cancer	Diabetes	Pneumonia/influenza
#5	Alzheimer's disease	Alzheimer's disease	Liver disease	Emphysema/COPD	Emphysema/COPD
#6	Pneumonia/influenza	Pneumonia/influenza	Lung cancer	Homicide	Diabetes
#7	Diabetes	Colorectal cancer	Homicide	Pneumonia/influenza	Colorectal cancer
#8	Colorectal cancer	Diabetes	Emphysema/COPD	Colorectal cancer	Liver disease
#9	Liver disease	Breast cancer	Alzheimer's disease	Breast cancer	Nephritis
#10	Breast cancer	Hypertension	Motor vehicle crash	Alzheimer's disease	Breast cancer
Homicides per 100,000	7	2	23	7	2
Suicides per 100,000	7	11	5	4	6
HIV deaths per 100,000	3	2	11	3	...
No health insurance* (%)	28	16	21	54	50

COPD: chronic obstructive pulmonary disease
* Health insurance data (2000): *Los Angeles.*
Source: Table constructed from data in LA County Health Department: Fielding J et al. (2009). Mortality in LA County: http://publichealth.lacounty.gov/dca/dcareportspubs.htm.

"Life Expectation in Los Angeles County" (Los Angeles Department of Health [LACDH], 2010; Fielding et al., 2009) is highly revealing on the issue of health disparity. Jonathan Fielding, the director of the LACDH, noted that between 1991 and 2010, the average life expectancy at birth had risen steadily, from 75.8 to 80.3 years (Fielding et al., 2009). At the same time, he added: "While life expectancy gains have been seen across genders and each of the four largest racial/ethnic groups in the county, substantial disparities continue to exist. At the extremes, there is a nearly 18 year difference in life expectancy between black males and Asian/Pacific Islander females, 69.4 vs. 86.9 years respectively" (Fielding et al., 2009, http://publichealth.lacounty. gov/epi/docs/Life%20Expectancy%20Final_web.pdf). The data show demographic, socioeconomic, and health status differences across the major ethnic groups, which aggregate indicators fail to capture.

Life expectancy is one of the most fundamental measures of health status and quality of life, and for that reason it is universally used for health status evaluations: the United Nations Development Program (UNDP) uses it in its Human Development Index (HDI). Fielding notes: "The dramatic variation [in life expectancy] seen across the county begs the question: Why do such significant disparities exist?" Women consistently outlived men across all ethnic groups. Life expectancy varied significantly by localities; it ranged between 72.4 years in the Westmont area, to a high of 87.8 years in the La Canada Flintridge area. The study also suggested a relationship to community-level economic hardship indices; the higher the hardship, the lower the life expectancy (http://publichealth.lacounty.gov/epi/docs/Life%20Expectancy%20Final_web.pdf).

Readers interested in behavioral risk factors at various levels are advised to study the Centers for Disease Control and Prevention (CDC) Behavioral Risk Factor Surveillance System reports.

The Behavioral Risk Factor Surveillance System (BRFSS) is the largest, continuously conducted, telephone health survey in the world. It enables the Centers for Disease Control and Prevention (CDC), state health departments, and other health agencies to monitor modifiable risk factors for chronic diseases and other leading causes of death. In this survey, BRFSS collected data on the six individual-level behavioral health risk factors associated with the leading causes of premature mortality and morbidity among adults: (1) cigarette smoking, (2) alcohol use, (3) physical activity, (4) diet, (5) hypertension, and (6) safety belt use. By 1993, BRFSS had become a nationwide system and the total sample size exceeded 100,000 participants. (CDC: http://www.cdc.gov/brfss/about/index.htm)

Sources of Health Information

Ethnic groups also vary in terms of their media use and health communication sources. Sources of health information–seeking behavior across ethnic groups in multicultural Los Angeles communities illustrate ethnic diversity in health information sources. Table 4.3 presents key findings of a survey conducted by the LACDH; in 1998, they discovered that the use of prevailing communication media as sources of health information varies significantly across ethnic groups (for details on health communication in multicultural communities, see Kar et al., 2001). The LACDH survey results show that:

If only [the] overall total is looked at, it appears that people use television, doctors, newspapers, and printed materials equally as the source of

TABLE 4.3

Health Information Sources by Ethnicity: Los Angeles (%)

	Total (n = 2,054)	Non-Hispanic White (n = 924)	Hispanic (n = 679)	African American (n = 200)	Asian American (n = 251)
Television	33.7	27.5	44.3	28.5	32.1
Doctors	31.5	37.3	24.9	42.5	19.1
Newspapers	31.4	33.5	28.3	20.5	40.6
Printed materials (books, magazines, pamphlets, etc.)	31.0	31.5	29.8	37.8	26.7
Family	12.3	12.6	14.1	6.0	11.6
Friends	12.2	10.2	16.1	7.5	12.7
Radio	5.6	4.4	7.7	5.0	7.1
Hotlines	1.7	2.1	1.3	1.0	1.6
Other	7.3	7.5	9.0	3.5	5.2

Because of multiple respondent answers concerning media use, the percentages in the table exceed 100%.

Source: Los Angeles County Department of Health Services (1994). Originally published as Table 2.1: Sources of Health Related Information in Los Angeles, in Kar SB, Alcalay R, & Alex S (2001). The Emergence of a New Public Health Paradigm in the United States. In: Kar SB, Alcalay R, & Alex S (Eds), *Health Communication: A Multicultural Perspective* (pp. 21–43). Thousand Oaks, CA: Sage.

health information. However, a very different picture emerges when we examine the responses by ethnicity. Non-Hispanic white[s] rely mainly on (in order) doctors, newspapers, and printed materials for their health information (37.3%, 33.5%, and 31.5%, respectively). In contrast, television is the most frequent source of health information among Hispanics (44.3%), with printed materials and newspapers following as the next most used sources (29.3% and 28.3% respectively). African Americans, however, rely just as frequently on information from doctors (42.5%) and printed materials closely following (37.8%) and television coming in third (28.5%). For Asian Americans, information comes mainly [from] newspapers (40.6%), television (32.1%), and printed [materials] (28.5%). Family members and friends are also important sources of information. Hotlines are least frequently used by all groups, perhaps because one uses hotlines only in [an] emergency, which happens infrequently. Surprisingly, the combined use of newspapers and printed materials for health information exceeds [that of] television. (Kar et al., 2001, pp. 35–36).

Since that survey, the use of digital and electronic media (Internet, cell phones, and social media) has become more common. In spite of the ubiquitous presence of electronic media, digital divides exist between ethnic groups, urban and rural areas, and rich and poor communities.

The most recent PEW survey (PEW Research Center, 2013) of national trends in media use shows that fewer than half of adults in the following groups in the United States search online for health information: African Americans, Latinos, adults living with a disability, adults age 65 and older, adults with a high school education or less, and adults living in low-income households ($30,000 or less annual income). However, as young people, Latinos, and African Americans are increasingly using mobile devices to gather information, this could shift the patterns of electronic media use across ethnic groups (PEW Research Center, 2013, http://www.pewInternet. org/2011/02/01/health-topics-2/).

THE DIGITAL DIVIDE

There is a popular perception that everyone in the world uses the Internet; very few are aware of the digital divide that exists in this electronic information age. In Western and affluent nations, the overwhelming majority of people do use the Internet; and many believe that is true for the rest of the world. That is far from the truth. Tables 4.4 and 4.5 present selective data to illustrate the market penetration of computer and Internet communications. The number of cell phones owned by people exceeded the total global population in 2013 (many own more than one). According to the International Telecommunications Union (ITU):

> Household Internet penetration—*often considered the most important measure of Internet access* [italics ours]—continues to rise. By end of 2013, ITU estimates that 41% of the world's households will be connected to the Internet. Over the past four years, household access has grown fastest in Africa, with an annual growth rate of 27%. But despite a positive general trend, 90% of the 1.1 billion households around the world that are still unconnected are in the developing world. (ITU: http://www.itu.int/net/pressoffice/press_releases/2013/05.aspx#. U-aScfnIaUY)

Once again we find that the world's poorest are excluded from the digital world. Table 4.4 presents examples of extreme variations in Internet use. According the World Bank, in 2013, the percentages of Internet users per 100 population ranged from 1.4% in Niger and 1.7% in Sierra Leone, to 94.8% in Sweden and 96.5% in Iceland. In the world's two largest nations, with relatively higher economic growth, more than one-half of the people do not use the Internet (China = 45.8% and India = 15.1%: http://data.worldbank.org/indicator/IT.NET.USER.P2).

Internet penetration also varies significantly within in a nation by education and income levels of people. According to a Pew survey in January 2014, 87% of U.S. adults used the Internet. In 2012, 72% of those who had Internet access searched for health information online (85% of whites, 83% of Hispanics, and 81% of blacks have Internet access). Education and

TABLE 4.4

Internet Users per 100 People: Range and Selected Countries (in 2013)

Country	Internet Users (%)	Broadband Internet Subscribers (%)
Niger	1.4	0.40
Sierra Leone	1.7	NA
Tanzania	4.4	0.11
Afghanistan	5.9	NA
Papua New Guinea	6.5	0.15
Bangladesh	6.5	0.63
India	15.1	1.16
Nigeria	38.0	0.01
China	45.8	13.63
Russian Federation	61.4	16.62
Kuwait	75.5	1.40
France	81.9	38.79
Germany	84.5	34.58
Japan	86.3	28.84
United Kingdom	89.8	35.73
United States	84.2	28.54
Finland	91.5	30.90
Andora	94	34.55
Sweden	94.8	32.55
Iceland	96.5	35.15

Source: Internet Users—World Bank: http://data.worldbank.org/indicator/IT.NET.USER. P2; Broadband—World Bank: http://data.worldbank.org/indicator/IT.NET.BBND.P2

income significantly affect information technology (IT) ownership (with college education = 97%; high school or below = 77%; those with more than $75,000 income = 99%; those with less than $ 30,000 income = 77%). The Pew surveys do not give breakdowns of Internet and printed media use by

TABLE 4.5

Percent U.S. Households with Computers and Broadband, by Race (2010)

Household Type	Percent Computer Urban	Percent Computer Rural	Percent Broadband Urban	Percent Broadband Rural
All households	78	72	75	57
White: Non-Hispanic	82	72	75	60
Black: Non-Hispanic	66	53	57	41
Hispanic	67	57	58	46
Asian Americans	86	85	81	83
American Indian and Native Alaskan	74	52	66	31

Source: US Dept. of Commerce (2011). *Exploring Digital Nation.* U.S. Census Bureau Current Population Survey (CPS), November 2010 (Table 2), available athttp://www.ntia.doc.gov/files/ntia/publications/exploring_the_digital_nation_computer_and_Internet_use_at_home_11092011.pdf.

major ethnic groups; but higher proportions of recent immigrants, especially Hispanics and those from far-east Asia, tend to be from lower educational and economic strata. In some ethnic groups, the majority do not speak English at home. Consequently, in a multicultural community, a large proportion of people, if not the majority, are not likely to have a common language for communication and social interaction. In such situations, it is difficult to find a common language and media to reach all members of the community (Pew, 2014).

A report titled *Exploring the Digital Nation: Computer and Internet Use at Home* used U.S. 2010 Census data and estimated adoption of computers and broadband access at home by ethnicity, education, and income (U.S. Census, 2011). This report showed major differences in Internet penetration, ranging from 86% in Asian American households in urban areas, to a low of 31% among American Indian and Alaskan households in rural areas (USDC, 2011). For all ethnic and economic groups combined, 78% of households in urban areas and 72% of rural households had computers; 75% of households in urban areas and 57% of households in rural areas had broadband. Among all ethnic groups, blacks had the lowest level of Internet adoption; Asian Americans had the highest level of adoption of computers (86%). Adoption also varied significantly by income and education levels. Indeed, there are large digital divides, and these disparities affect multicultural communities more than monocultural communities (USDC, 2011). The results showed that even in large urban metropolitan areas, there are significant ethnic differences in the adoption and use of electronic media.

Self-Identity and Designated Identity

From the multicultural perspective, two sets of "identities" are like two sides of the same coin: they both affect our quality of life. These are our *self-identity*—how we see or identify ourselves; and our *designated identity*—how other ethnic groups, especially the majority, label or identify minority groups, often with fatal consequences. For instance, after the September 11, 2001, attack on the World Trade Center towers in New York, the Pentagon in Washington DC, and the plane crash in Shanksville PA, killed a total of 2,977; of these there were 411 emergency workers in New York City. The first person killed by a violent vigilante was a Sikh immigrant from India who was misidentified as an Arab Muslim by his killer (the Sikh religion requires that men keep long beards and wear turbans). A local newspaper reported: "On September 15, 2001, Balbir Singh Sodhi was shot and killed outside of his Mesa, Arizona, gas station by Frank Roque. Roque wanted to 'kill a Muslim' in retaliation for the attacks on September 11. Roque was convicted of first degree murder and sentenced to life

in prison for the hate crime" (http://www.saldef.org/issues/balbir-singh-sodhi/).
The victim, Sodhi, was also a naturalized U.S. citizen. But his identity as a Sikh
and his U.S. citizenship did not save him. His killer saw him only as a Muslim,
and that mis-identity cost Sodhi's life. The hate crime did not end with this
tragic event. Ten years later, the U.S. Department of Justice (DOJ) reported:

> The Civil Rights Division, the Federal Bureau of Investigation, and United
> States Attorneys' offices have investigated over 800 incidents since 9/11
> involving violence, threats, vandalism and arson against Arab-Americans,
> Muslims, Sikhs, South-Asian Americans and other individuals perceived
> to be of Middle Eastern origin. The incidents have consisted of telephone,
> Internet, mail, and face-to-face threats; minor assaults as well as assaults
> with dangerous weapons and assaults resulting in serious injury and death;
> and vandalism, shootings, arson and bombings directed at homes, busi-
> nesses, and places of worship. Federal charges have been brought against
> 54 defendants, with 48 convictions to date. Additionally, Civil Rights
> Division attorneys have coordinated with state and local prosecutors in
> 150 non-federal criminal prosecutions, often providing substantial assis-
> tance. (http://www.justice.gov/crt/legalinfo/discrimupdate.php)

This, of course, is one example and is not exclusive to one country or society; hate crimes and racial prejudices have always existed and affected our lives.
Multicultural population composition in itself cannot be held responsible for
hate crimes. The problem is rooted in deeply held beliefs and prejudices about
others who are different from us as we see them. The images in our heads about
others are the primary problem. Psychologists and social philosophers have
long pondered about the origin of social prejudice. In a pioneering study of
children's preference of black versus white dolls to play with, Kenneth and
Mamie Clark (1940) discovered that the choice of color (white vs. black) is
learned at an early age:

> Clark's results were published in a 1950 paper, "Effects of Prejudice
> and Discrimination on Personality Development," in which he con-
> cluded that institutional discrimination, including racial segregation
> in public schools, was harmful to the personality and psychologi-
> cal development of black children. His paper on the "doll tests"
> was cited by the U.S. Supreme Court in its landmark 1954 ruling,
> *Brown v. Board of Education*, which formally ended racial segrega-
> tion in American public schools. (http://www.nndb.com/people/883/
> 000115538/) (Clark, 1965)

Pride and prejudice are two sides of the same coin. The idea that we
internalize our preferences and prejudices through the socialization process in our communities as we grow up is generally accepted and serves

as the foundational principle for the desegregation of schools. When some parents explicitly and implicitly through their actions instill ethnic pride in their children, the message children learn is that their group is by definition better than others. When that belief is reinforced over time, it becomes a conviction. This conviction has serious consequences for our race relations and quality of life. In one extensive review, Janet Ward Schofield in the Education Resources Information Center (ERIC) concludes:

> The widespread concern about the impact of school desegregation and the controversy over what its effect might be have resulted in a substantial body of research. This review focuses on the impact on students themselves, presenting some conclusions that have emerged and discussing some methodological problems inherent in the assessment of the impact on students. These problems include deciding on the relevant studies, recognizing the implications of diversity, and facing the reality that much of the research is flawed. Research does suggest that desegregation has had some positive impacts on the reading skills of African American youngsters. Mathematics skills seem generally unaffected by desegregation. There is also some evidence that desegregation can help to break what can be thought of as the generational cycle of segregation and racial isolation. Evidence is beginning to accumulate that school desegregation may favorably influence such adult outcomes as college graduation, income, and employment patterns. Evidence about the impact of desegregation on intergroup relations is generally held to be inconclusive, but some positive effects are indicated. In addition, it is clear that the way in which desegregation is brought about can have effects on student outcomes. (Schofield, 1995)

School desegregation is one measure that is widely adopted by many societies; but it alone is not likely to solve the problem of race relations and ethnic prejudice. Desegregation and inclusion of ethnic groups in all domains of our communities is a second option. Disenfranchised groups are increasingly demanding equal opportunities, employment, and equal justice and protection by the law for all. The third and macro-level option is the Human Development Approach (HDA) advocated by the UN; that is, at least in principle, adopted by the majority of the UN. In reality, all three methods would have to be combined to address widespread inequalities nationally and globally.

Psychologist Gordon Allport is a pioneer who studied why (purpose served) and how (communication process) rumors spread in a community. In his classic experiment, Allport demonstrated how our prejudice affects our perception of others without our being aware of our own bias. In one famous Allport experiment, a subway scene is projected on a screen: the scene includes several people sitting on a bench, waiting for a train. In front of them, two adult men are standing facing each other, involved in a conversation. One man is a white adult with an object in his hand that could be a screwdriver, a hammer, or a shaving razor; the second man is a black adult. The first subject is called into the room and is asked to look at the projected scene. After that, the projected image is switched off, and a second subject, who has not seen the projected scene before, is called into the room. The first subject is now asked to describe the projected scene to the second subject. This process of serial reproduction continues several times. The important finding is that the story changes with successive retelling (that is what happens to a real-life rumor). Different subjects give different versions; but the versions of the story show some interesting common features. First, the story gets shorter in length (it takes less time due to a process called *leveling*); second, some details stand out and are retained (called *sharpening*); and finally, the story is put together in a coherent theme (called *assimilation*). Some versions emerge in which the two men standing are described as confronting, rather than conversing with each other, and the black man is seen to have a knife or shaving razor in his hand, threatening the white man. The storytellers distorted what they saw consistent with their racial stereotypes and prejudices; the black man is perceived to be the aggressor with a weapon in hand threatening the white man (http://www. csepeli.hu/elearning/cikkek/allport_postman.pdf). In their volume titled *Psychology of Rumor*, Allport and Postman discussed in detail their theory of rumor, their experiments, and the implications for social policy (Allport & Postman, 1947).

We all have multiple identities: in different contexts, we prefer to choose one or another identity when we present ourselves to others. How we are treated often depends upon how others see us. For instance, Amartya Sen begins his book *Identity and Violence* with a tragic episode when a group of Hindu extremists killed a poor Muslim carpenter in Dacca, which is now in Bangladesh. The victim had multiple identities: as a man, a poor laborer, a caring father who must feed his family, a Muslim, a carpenter, a resident of a community, and many more. But the gangsters chose to see the victim only as a Muslim (and ignored his other identities). Like the killer of Sodhi after 9/11, the killers of the poor Bengali laborer saw their victim through the lens of their own ethnic prejudice and racial hatred. It is our self-identity, our family and group allegiance, and the extent to which we retain the value and practices of our ethnic origin, that make us a member of a specific ethnic group, irrespective of where we were born. However, in a multiethnic community, how others identify and recognize a person of a minority group can make the difference in how that person is treated by the community. A multicultural community, therefore, has the obligation to better educate its members in cultural identity, tolerance, and mutual respect.

There are two schools of thought on how immigrants and minorities should adapt and are to be treated in their adopted countries and culture. The assimilationists claim that for the sake of social cohesion and national unity, the immigrants have the responsibility to become assimilated in the dominant culture and pledge allegiance to their adopted society. This is the melting pot metaphor. Different nations have different laws and social norms that encourage and even coerce the assimilation process. On the other hand, the multiculturalists argue that in free societies, all persons have the right to basic freedom and human dignity; they should be free to choose their personal lifestyle and religion, and allowed pursuit of happiness without overt or covert discrimination and restrictions. This is the rainbow metaphor. From global developments of the past several decades, it seems that the multiculturalists have won; our world and communities are becoming more diverse than before. One glaring proof of this trend is the proclamation by one of the best-known assimilationists—sociologist Nathan Glazer—who wrote a book titled, *We Are All Multiculturalists Now* (1998). Glazer argues cogently that multiculturalism arose from the failure of mainstream society to assimilate African Americans; anger and frustration at their continuing separation gave black Americans the impetus for rejecting traditions that excluded them. But, willingly or not, "we are all multiculturalists now," Glazer asserts, and his book gives us a clear picture of the multicultural reality and the impetus to examine our own multiple identities (http://www.hup.harvard.edu/catalog. php?isbn=9780674948365).

Dangerous Beliefs

An important meta-analysis confirms Kelman's (1987, 1997) emphasis on the influence of collective needs and fears regarding identity, security, and justice in driving intergroup conflicts. The Eidelsons begin with the premise that "much of the time, people use stable cognitive templates that produce regularities in expectations and interpretations of events. Based on their meta-analysis, the authors identify five core beliefs that individuals hold, which influence their perception and interpretation of events that affect their beliefs and behavior. These are beliefs about: (1) *superiority* (or exceptionalism); (2) *past injustice* (legitimate grievance); (3) *vulnerability* (imminent threat); (4) *distrust* (of other group/s); and (5) *helplessness*. These five beliefs, along with "cultural distance" (similarities and dissimilarities discussed earlier) among various groups in a community, could serve as a barometer of intergroup conflicts and strife.

Ethnic Diversity and Strife

Another major issue in a discourse on multicultural community is whether the more disparate (more ethnic groups) a community has, the more likely it is to have ethnic strife. Also included in this issue is the question whether one large majority group may dominate (oppress) small minorities, which fuels ethnic conflicts. Paul Collier, former director of development research at the World Bank, discusses these issues in great depth in his book *The Bottom Billion* (2007). Collier's volume is considered a tour de force by leading scholars in the field: his grasp and analysis of the problems of the poorest 1 billion people and how they may affect our world as a whole is simply profound and is supported by impeccable evidence. Collier argues that the real problem of world development is that "there is a group of countries at the bottom that are falling behind, and are falling apart" (p. 3). While rich countries are becoming richer, since 1990, "incomes in these groups declined by 5%." He identifies "four traps" that pull these countries down.

The first of the four traps is the "Conflict Trap," which includes civil war, prolonged ethnic violence, and genocide. Seventy-three percent of the bottom billion of the world's population have recently been in countries that have been through a civil war, or are still in one (he identifies 58 such countries). Naturally, a major question is what causes civil war or ethnic conflicts. The first hypothesis Collier examines is whether political oppression by a dominant majority causes civil war. He cites a major study by Stanford political scientists Jim Fearon and David Laitin, who have studied more than 200 minorities across the world: "They found no relationship between whether a group was politically repressed and the risk of civil war" (p. 23). Collier further adds: "Anke Hoeffler and I investigated the effect of income inequality, and to our surprise found no relationship" (p. 23). The contention here is not that people do not suffer from ethnic prejudices or inequalities. All too often, the really disadvantaged and powerless people are not in a position to revolt or fight back; they just suffer quietly. Collier's contention is, "Rather, some economic conditions lend themselves to being taken advantage of by gutter politicians who build their success on hatred" (p. 24). This writer has a direct personal experience that supports Collier's contention. It is true that one incident or one case study does not confirm a trend, but my experience is shared by millions of victims and many eminent scholars, national leaders, and historians. The British Raj (regime) in India had an unwritten principle of governance—that is "divide and rule." India existed for thousands of years, and even during the first 175 years of British rule, no national leader ever proposed dividing the country on religious grounds important between the Hindus and Muslims (after Indonesia and Pakistan; and has already had three Muslim presidents). But after the British Labour government decided to relinquish India, the British did everything they could to carve out regions with Muslim majorities in two states (Bengal and Punjab) to create Pakistan in 1947. I still remember with terrifying horror but never did understand why we, the Hindu children and Muslim children who played cricket and football together and studied in the same schools peacefully for years, suddenly became enemies? It was my last year in high school when India was divided and became independent. The brutal Hindu–Muslim riots that were fueled by sectarian political leaders, encouraged and supported by the British, to justify the partition of the nation. Neither the majority of Hindus nor the Muslims demanded partitioning of the country for past millennia, but it happened under the last phase of the British rule. At the least they are guilty of not stopping the atrocities when they started. In his widely popular book *The Midnight's Children*, author Salman Rushdie vividly describes the horrors of communal riots, forced migration of more than 100 million refugees, and the creation of two hostile neighboring nations (Rushdie, 1981).

Finally, to the question of whether the number of ethnic groups (degree of disparity) in a community is related to ethnic violence and strife, there is one good answer. From his extensive research on this issue, Collier (2007) concludes:

> Most of the societies that are at peace have more than one ethnic group. And one of the few low-income countries that is completely ethnically pure, Somalia, had a bloody civil war followed by complete governmental meltdown. Statistically, there is not much evidence of a relationship between ethnic diversity and proneness to civil war. (p. 25)

It is very tempting to continue quoting Collier, but I do not wish to deprive the readers the joy of reading and learning directly from this important book.

Cultural Distance and Acculturation Stress

Acculturation, by definition, means a process through which an immigrant group or persons embrace the culture of the dominant majority of their adopted nation. But the process is more complex than just moving to a different place. It often amounts to compromising one's native customs and acquaintances and often changing inherited beliefs, values, and social practices. Naturally, this process of acculturation causes considerable psychological and social stress. The more different the two cultures (the inherited culture and the culture of the adopted land, or "cultural distance") are, the greater the level of acculturation stress (e.g., religious conversion, interracial dating and marriages, belief in gender equality). Also, the level or depth of desired social relations (ranging from casual to intimate relationships) affects the acculturation stress. For instance, adopting new attire, food and drinks is easier than learning a new language and work ethic; religious conversion and developing close interpersonal relationships, including dating and marriage, would require deeper levels of change. In order to understand the social realities of MCCs, we may look at two processes that are highly prevalent in these communities.

CULTURAL DISTANCE

In order to understand multicultural dynamics, we may conceptualize a "cultural distance" scale to represent the magnitude of similarity and dissimilarity between the immigrants' culture of origin and that of their adopted countries. For instance, English-speaking Canadian Caucasian immigrants to the United States would find very little difference between their culture of origin and their adopted country; they speak the same language, are used to similar food habits, if religious follow Christianity, and are used to similar levels of affluence, modernity, and geography. They will have more similarities than differences between their core cultural practices and those in their adopted culture. They are more likely to be "accepted" by their adopted communities, and they in turn would find it easier to "identify" with their host culture. Compared to the English-speaking Canadians, Cambodian or Hmong immigrants would find major differences between their original cultures and host country in almost all major dimensions of cultural practices, including language, food, religion, gender roles, social relations, and participation in governance. The Cambodians would encounter significantly more "acculturation stress" (psychological distress and interpersonal interactions) than the Canadians would. Consequently, multicultural communities consisting of a large number of people from disparate cultures would have very different social realities, as in interpersonal interactions, community leadership and participation, social networks, social acceptance and exclusion, treatment of women and children, health-related behavior and healthcare access and utilization. It is reasonable to imagine that the magnitude of complexity of social dynamics between communities with homogenous populations compared to communities with diverse populations would be proportionate to the: (1) *size of the diverse population* or percent of population from disparate cultures and the number of diverse cultures of origin, and (2) *the sum of cultural distances* between the members' original and adopted community.

ACCULTURATION STRESS

Nearly a century ago, in 1920, American psychologist Bogardus (1933) introduced his "Social Distance Scale," which was designed to measure the level of acceptance that Americans feel toward members of the most common ethnic groups in the United States. Bogardus measured social distance by asking the subjects how much they approve or disapprove of relating with members of other ethnic groups; response categories ranged from strong disapproval of a group, to intimate personal relationships (e.g., exclude them from entering the U.S., deny residence in the same neighborhood, allow them as co-workers, approve of personal friendship with them, and welcome them in intimate personal relationships including marriage). The results showed different levels of acceptance of different ethnic groups; an interesting finding was that some subjects strongly disapproved of encounters with specific ethnic groups they had never met or known. Surveys were conducted (by different investigators, reported by Parrillo & Donoghue, 2005) five times between 1920 and 1977, with very few changes in research design. More recently, Parrillo and Donoghue (2005), consistent with prior replications, studied a random sample of 2,916 college students using the Bogardus Social Distance Scale:

> The findings indicate that the mean level of social distance towards all ethnic groups, as well as the spread between the groups with the highest and lowest levels of social distance, decreased since 1977. Mean comparisons and ANOVA [Analyses of Variance] test also showed that gender, nation of origin, and race are all significant indicators of the level of social distance towards [*sic*] all groups. (Parrillo & Donoghue, 2005)

Other replications of this scale measured several ethnic groups, including African Americans, whites, Hispanics, Jews, and Asians.

> A common finding among these studies was that individuals typically are more comfortable with others of perceived similarity and so maintain a closer social distance in interactions with them. Conversely, by evaluating their in-group more favorably, they also tend to express a self-serving bias toward dissimilar outgroups. (Hipp, 2010)

In sum, the good news is that attitudes often change favorably over time; but at the same time some ethnic groups are liked or disliked more than other ethnic groups by the dominant culture.

INTERGENERATIONAL CONFLICT

The studies above reflect people's attitudes toward other groups, not how people relate to or live with persons with different cultural values and preferences on a day-to-day basis. Family members within the same ethnicity but from different generations and genders can have major culture clashes. This is an important issue in MCCs. Usually we use the term "culture clash" to refer to two ethnic groups who are in conflict with each other, or to a clash between cultures. But in a multicultural community, the culture clash is often a clash within the families. It is an "invisible culture clash" within the family and is between the foreign-born immigrant parents and their children born and socialized in their adopted countries. This intra-family culture clash is highly pronounced between the first and second generations of immigrants and is not a new problem. Historically, all immigrants have faced this intergenerational conflict. With successive generations and acculturation, this type of intra-family culture clash tends to diminish. We see this clearly among the Chinese and Japanese groups in the United States; the same is true for early European immigrant groups. Their ancestors migrated several generations ago, but the current youths in these ethnic groups and their parents were both born and socialized in America. As a result, most of the original cultural differences diminished with prolonged acculturation. But the situation is very different for the first- and second-generation immigrants from disparate and distant cultures. The cultural distance between the foreign-born immigrant parents, who were socialized and acquired their core values several decades ago in distant cultures, and the values, behavior, and lifestyle of their children who are often living in a much more modernized MCC, is huge and immeasurably different.

Sponsored by the University of California's Pacific Rim Research Program and the Kellogg International Fellowship in Health, we conducted several exploratory studies (directed by this writer and his colleagues) on acculturation and health among Asian Americans. We surveyed more than 1,400 U.S.-born Indian (Asian), Japanese, and Korean American college students and their parents (U.S. citizens and residents of the United States) and compared them with samples of their counterparts from their countries of origin (Kar, 2000; Kar et al., 1995, 1996, 1998a, 2002; Penn et al., 1995).

We discovered highly prevalent and serious intergenerational conflicts that often remain invisible (because parents and children do not fight in public) but nonetheless cause heavy psychological and health consequences. Health behavior researchers have not explored these issues sufficiently. These studies revealed two types of intergenerational conflicts: (1) *intergenerational conflicts* between foreign-born parents and their children, and (2) *gender-role conflicts*—especially affecting the female students. The first notable inter-generational difference is the self-identities of parents and their children (students).

No Indian-born parent identified as monocultural American only; nine out of ten retained Indian identities (national or provincial). Almost a third retained their provincial identity (which is common in India; people tend to identify their state of origin as their group identity). Seventy-two percent of their American-born children used hyphenated bicultural identity; only 11% identified as Indian only. Clearly, there is a major identity shift within one family in one generation. In the study cited in Box 4.2 below, we asked Indian and Japanese respondents to name major causes of conflicts within their families (if any); about a third of the Indian and Japanese respondents mentioned "career choice" as the reason for parent–child conflict (good news is that two-thirds did not mention a career choice problem). Among the Indian students, mostly the women (seven out of ten) had their biggest conflicts with parents about marital decisions; many parents insist on choosing an Indian groom, preferably Indian-born and foreign-educated. The real issue is that the parents intend to choose the future groom or bride for their children. The acculturated young generation prefer to make that decision themselves. Fifty-seven percent of Indians would like their spouses from the same ethnicity, compared to only 21% of the Japanese. Similarly, more Indian respondents consistently prefer a spouse with the same religion. Four out of ten Indians mention their children's behavior as the major source of intergenerational conflict with their parents.

The out-marriage (marrying someone from another ethnic group) rate is a significant indicator of acculturation. Among the Japanese and Chinese Americans who have lived in the United States for several generations, the out-marriage rate (between 70% and 80%) is significantly higher than the

BOX 4.2
Indo-American Self-Identity

Self-Identity	Parents: Foreign Born (%)	Children: US Born (%)
Indian (only)	61	11
Provincial (e.g., Gujrati/Punjabi)	31	2
Hyphenated (Indian-American)	6	72
Pan-Asian (Asian American)	2	13
American (only)	0	2

Source: Data from Kar SB, Jimenez A, Campbell K, & Sze F (1998). Acculturation and quality of life: A comparative study of Japanese Americans and Indo-Americans. *Amerasia J.*, (24)1, 129–142.

BOX 4.3
Marital Preferences

Marital Preferences	Japanese (%)	Indian (%)
Same ethnicity	21	57
Same religion	32	51
Same language	18	32
Same caste	NA	26

Source: Data from Kar SB, Jimenez A,
Campbell K, & Sze F (1998). Acculturation and
quality of life: A comparative study of Japanese
Americans and Indo-Americans. *Amerasia J.*,
(24)1, 129–142.

rates among recent immigrants from Korea and India (less than 10%). We asked our respondents (students) to indicate the important criteria desired for a future spouse (see Box 4.3).

Note: the concept of "caste" in the Indian sense is not applicable in Japanese culture, but it is perhaps the most important criterion for spouse-selection among traditional Indian communities. It is interesting to note that within one generation of acculturation, caste is not important in marital choices among American-born Indian students.

Gender-Role Conflicts

Literature indicates that social values and practices common in agrarian societies undergo major changes with industrialization and moderniza-tion (Rostow, 1960); traditional cultural values such as material security, traditional authority, and communal decision-making give way to quality-of-life issues, self-expression, individualism, and post-materialism (Bell, 1973). Furthermore, levels of modernization and industrialization change gender-role segregation; in preindustrial and agrarian societies, the roles of men and women tended to be more clearly divided. Women stayed home and performed unpaid domestic and traditional roles as mothers and wives, while men worked away from home in paid jobs. This gender-role segrega-tion begins to blur with increased modernization and industrialization. As women become more educated, they begin to work outside their homes for pay and take on many jobs that men used to do, usually jobs that paid less. Women's aspirations change, and with expanded opportunities for educa-tion and employment, they begin to pursue better-paying jobs and careers. Extended families give way to nuclear families, and marriages get delayed. In agrarian societies, girls were married off at an early and younger age, before they could make their own career decisions. When they were children, they remained financially dependent on their fathers; as wives, on their husbands; and when old, on their sons.

But industrialization changes that. Inglehart and colleagues proposed and tested their revised theory of modernization empirically through their "World Values Survey (WVS)" in more than 70 countries. The results of the first five waves provide strong support of their theory, which holds that modernization brings "predictable" changes in gender roles, in two key phases:

1. Industrialization brings women into the paid workforce and dramatically reduces fertility rates. Women attain higher literacy and greater educational and career opportunities. Women are enfranchised and begin to participate in representative government, but still have far less power than men.
2. Postindustrial phase brings a shift toward greater gender equality as women rise in management and the professions and gain political influence within elected and appointed bodies. More than half of the world has not yet entered this phase; only the more advanced industrial societies are currently moving on this trajectory.

They further add that these two phases correspond to two major dimensions of cross-cultural variations. These are transitions from traditional to secular values, and survival to self-expression values (Ingelhart & Norris, 2003, pp. 10–11; http://www.doublemakemoney.com/wvs/articles/folder_published/publication_593/files/inglehart-welzel-modernization-and-democracy.pdf).

Although our study samples of Asian immigrant students and their parents were caught in a clash of values between two generations in a society that is highly industrialized, our findings are consistent with the theory that guides the WVS. Compared to the Japanese Americans, who have been in the United States for several generations, the Indian Americans are recent immigrants; more than 80% of Indian parents were foreign-born. Consequently, the Indians have had a much shorter duration of cultural contact and acculturation in the United States.

The Indian parents we have studied were mostly foreign-born and were socialized as children several decades ago, when their country was not as fully industrialized and urbanized as the United States was in the 1990s. Their family values—including the importance of obedience to parents versus individualism, marital aspirations, especially for their daughters, and gender-role expectations—were "frozen in time"; they are much more traditional than other Americans, including Japanese and Chinese Americans who have been acculturated in the U.S. for generations. The children of Asian Americans, however, were born and raised in industrialized American communities in the 1980s and 1990s, where children were encouraged to be independent and make most choices on their own. This is especially relevant in mate selection (dating and marriage) behavior. For traditional Indian parents, the biggest shock would be to see their daughter/s dating or marrying someone from a different ethnic group. About 40% report that their behavior (disobedience of parents) causes conflicts with their parents. The percentages of conflicts are much higher for the female than for the male students.

Acculturation Stress and Trauma

Multicultural communities not only consist of people of different ethnicities but also people with widely different durations and histories of residence. They range from native populations who were colonized, enslaved, displaced, or dominated, to those who came voluntarily and found freedom and security. The most recent groups are those who are responding to immigration "push" (e.g., refugees driven away from their home countries under threat) and "pull" (e.g., better opportunities). The speed and the extent of the acculturation process depends on several factors: (1) the degree of similarity between the native and adopted cultures (cultural distance); (2) the years and generation/s of residence in the adopted society (length of acculturation); (3) the migration motivation and history (push vs. pull); and (4) the level of receptivity of the host society. Consequently, in a highly diverse community, the needs and priorities of various groups vary significantly.

Let us examine these issues using the Asian Americans as an example. It is the fastest growing ethnic group in the United States and is the most diverse cultural group by any criteria. Some of them (Chinese and Japanese) have been in the U.S. for more than 150 years; their experience would be vastly different from the professionals and IT specialists who landed on American shores recently. The acculturation traumas are also very different for different groups. The loyalties of Japanese citizens were questioned and they were interned in camps during World War II. Determined to earn respect and demonstrate their loyalty, their sons joined the U.S. Army and fought valiantly.

The Punjabi farmers from India who settled in California's Central Valley in the early 1900s had different but not less acculturation trauma. Although their numbers were initially small, estimated in the few thousands, the Punjabis, who were mostly Sikh, quickly adapted to life in the farming communities of the United States, particularly in California's Central and Imperial valleys. Drawing on their extensive agricultural knowledge, the Punjabis planted peach and prune orchards, which today produce 95% of the peaches and 60% of the prunes that grow in Yuba-Sutter County, a fertile agricultural hub of California's Central Valley. Despite their contributions to California's farming industry, early Punjabi immigrants were heavily discriminated against both economically and socially. The California Alien Land Act of 1913 declared all aliens as ineligible for citizenship in the state and to own agricultural land. And although the Act primarily targeted wealthy Japanese landowners in California, the Punjabis were not considered citizens and were victimized. Strict immigrant laws also prevented Punjabis living in the United States from bringing wives from India, creating a distinct problem for the community. They would have gone to India to find brides and brought them back. But when the Asian Exclusion laws were passed, it became impossible for them to leave (http://www.faithstreet.com/onfaith/2012/08/13/punjabi-sikh-mexican-american-community-fading-into-history/20313).

The history of slavery in the Americas bears witness to centuries of discrimination and ethnic violence endured by the African Americans. For these Americans the United States has not been a land of the free. It is ironic that after centuries of discrimination and abuse, reputable modern sociologists conclude that the United States could not achieve its "melting pot" ideal, because the African Americans had not been fully assimilated in the American mainstream; this may be true but the question is who is responsible? (Glazer, 1998; Huntington, 1993; Inglehart & Welzel, 2005). The Native Americans did not do much better. Their ancestral land was taken away, they were restrained in reservations, and they are the only ethnic group in the United States that has actually shrunk while others multiplied. And since the September 11 attacks, if you have a Muslim name, you can be a target of mistrust, disrespect, and hate crime. Acculturation could be highly traumatic and stressful and it can adversely affect the HRQOL of minority groups. Given this history, it is not surprising that minority groups are suspicious of the dominant majority of other ethnicity and mutual mistrust often erects barriers between different groups.

Cultural Capitals and Paradoxes

Cultural diversity has its advantages both on aesthetic and utilitarian grounds. As the saying goes, "Variety is the spice of life." Varieties of festivals, cuisines, costumes, music, literature, various forms of art, and accumulated knowledge from other cultures immensely enrich our lives. In the health field, increasing recognition of the value of complementary and alternative medicines (CAMs) for preventing diseases and managing chronic conditions and pain is another example how knowledge and contributions from other cultures may enrich our collective well-being. Cultural paradoxes are another source of learning from other cultures. "Cultural paradoxes" may be defined as observed unique phenomena in a culture that cannot be explained by our collective wisdom and cumulative scientific knowledge.

The paradoxes are contradictions to what we know to be true. Three cultural paradoxes are presented to illustrate how we may benefit from learning from paradoxes from alien cultures: the French Paradox, Hispanic Paradox, and Asian Paradox. "Cultural capital" is defined as the beneficial cluster of beliefs, attitudes, values, and practices that differentiate a cultural group from others.

THE FRENCH PARADOX

The French paradox began with the discovery by French epidemiologists in the 1980s that French adult men had lower rates of coronary heart disease (CHD) than many European and American white men of the same age group, even though the Frenchmen smoked as much or more and had a higher dietary intake of cholesterol and saturated fat than their comparison groups in Europe and the United States. This was highlighted when in the 1990s, French epidemiologists Serge Renaud and Michel De Lorgeril published a paper in the prestigious British medical journal *Lancet* titled "Wine, alcohol, platelets, and the French paradox for coronary heart disease" (1992). In addition, the popular American TV program *60 Minutes* dedicated a segment on the "French Paradox," public interest was heightened, and CBS rebroadcast that segment. Wine sales in the U.S. increased significantly, and a flurry of research followed. These and other news media widely publicized this unique discovery— some were thrilled that you could drink yourself to better health. With epidemiological data, the authors observed that French people had a high consumption of saturated fat, and yet their mortality for CHD was lower than others in Europe and the United States. The paper noted that U.S. and United Kingdom dietary intake of saturated fat was substantially equivalent to the rate in France, but CHD rates were much higher than in Frenchmen. The authors also noted another difference: Frenchmen drank more red wine.

> Since red wine contains some protective polyphenols, such as resveratrols that come straight from red grapes, they hypothesized that higher red wine consumption could explain the apparent paradox. To further support this hypothesis, there were some striking data from three different cities within France itself. CHD mortality per 100,000 men was much lower in Toulouse compared to Strasbourg and Lille (78 vs. 102 and 105, respectively), in spite of cheese consumption being higher (51 g/day vs. 34 and 42 g/day, respectively). However, wine consumption in Toulouse was also significantly higher compared to the other two cities (383 g/day vs. 286 and 267 g/day, respectively).

These and similar observations reinforced the claim that wine consumption can "counteract the untoward effects of saturated fats," to use the words of the authors.

One nutrition expert wrote:

> In the 1990s, wine sales in Europe were inexorably declining, with many young people in traditionally wine-drinking countries steadily switching to beer, considering wine drinking an old-fashioned habit. The wine industry jumped on the "French paradox" story, promoting an epic marketing campaign which instilled in a lot of people the idea that drinking red wine is good for your heart. It was so effective that I know people who didn't drink alcohol at all, and started drinking a glass of red with their meals for fear that not doing so would increase their risk of dropping dead from a heart attack. (Stefano Vendrame, http://www.nutrition.org/asn-blog/2013/01/the-french- paradox-was-it-really-the-wine /)

Much research has followed since, and the debate is still on whether the causal link between red wine and CHD is established beyond doubt, and the implications of the French Paradox for health and nutrition education of the public. Nutrition expert Vendrame makes a very good point:

> Granted, in Toulouse they drank more red wine than in Strasbourg and Lille, while eating slightly more cheese, but they also ate a lot more vegetables (306 g/day vs. 217 and 212 g/day, respectively), a lot more fruit (238 g/day vs. 149 and 160 g/day), half the butter (13 g/day vs. 22 and 20 g/day), more vegetable fat (20 g/day vs. 16 and 15 g/day) and more bread (225 g/day vs. 164 and 152 g/day). In other words, they were eating more fruits and vegetables and they ingested more dietary fiber, less saturated fat, more polyunsaturated fat and more grains. Still surprised that their deaths were less often attributed to cardiovascular disease? If anything, the whole story proves once more the concept that the balance of diet in general is more important than any single component in preventing disease and ensuring good health. You can eat a little bit more cheese, but if you eat a lot more fruits and vegetables, you are still doing fine. (http://www.nutrition.org/asn-blog/2013/01/the-french-paradox-was-it-really-the-wine /)

The conclusion we can draw from the French Paradox is this: we may not have a 100% proof that red wine alone prevents CHD, but the observed differences in CHD rates between the French and their comparison groups are real, and the difference in their red wine intake and the better nutritional habits of the French are also real. We may learn valuable lessons on good nutrition and healthy lifestyles. These lessons from the French cultural capital can reduce CHD and deaths.

THE HISPANIC PARADOX

The Hispanic Paradox is the surprising finding that, despite having a worse risk factor profile on key health indicators, the Hispanics tend to have a better health status than non-Hispanic whites and blacks. An editorial in the *Los Angeles Times* (November 10, 2010) states:

> A recent study by the U.S. Centers for Disease Control and Prevention suggests that federal interest has been piqued. The report, released in October, found that Latinos in this country outlive both whites and blacks, with a life expectancy of 80.6 years, compared with 77.7 for the nation as a whole. (People of Asian ancestry have even longer life spans, but because of their relatively high education and income levels, those findings are not considered surprising.) Latinos tend to be less educated than African Americans and their poverty rates are similar, and [they] have a lower level of health insurance (a proxy measure of access to health care), yet Latinos outlive black people by nearly eight years. How can this be? The CDC makes a couple of guesses but offers nothing in the way of research-based explanations. Its study does not distinguish between immigrants and non-immigrants, poor Latinos and affluent, people of Bolivian heritage and those of Mexican or Puerto Rican heritage. Yet teasing out the reasons for Latino health and life expectancy might be one of the most important public-health endeavors the nation could undertake. (Hayes-Bautista, 2010; http://articles.latimes.com/2010/nov/14/opinion/la-ed-longevity-20101114)

Several meta-analyses support the overall findings about the comparative vital statistics by ethnicity. One meta-analysis found that "Hispanic ethnicity was associated with a 17.5% mortality advantage over non-Hispanics with clear differences among people who were healthy, who had heart disease, or who had a variety of other health conditions when they entered their respective studies" (Markides, 2011). Research showed that the health of Hispanics in the Southwest resembled that of whites, although Hispanics were poorer, were more likely to be unemployed, and their socioeconomic status was no better than the African Americans'. But their health status resembles the health status of non-Hispanic whites. Although early research showed that Hispanics had a similar life expectancy to whites, it was soon discovered that Hispanics actually outlived them by an average of two to three years. Hispanics also seem to survive and recover from disease quicker than non-Hispanic whites (said Dr. John Ruiz, a psychologist at the University of North Texas, http://www.dallasnews.com/opinion/sunday-commentary/20140117-decoding-the-hispanic-paradox.ece).

Several explanations are offered for the differential in health status.

The CDC suggests, for instance, that the data might simply be wrong, that perhaps people's ages at death were misstated. But Hayes-Bautista (2011), the Director of UCLA's Chicano Studies Center says that the data are always questioned at first because the results are so surprising, yet studies keep reaching the same conclusion. Another theory put forward by the CDC is that the difficulty of immigrating might lead only the hardiest people to come to the United States. In response, Hayes-Bautista points out that most Latinos are born here, and there are no huge differences in health—at least so far—between them and immigrants. The CDC also brings up what's known as the "salmon bias"—the possibility that older, ailing Latino immigrants might return home for their last months of life.

Empirical studies do not confirm the "salmon bias" hypothesis or the selective return of less-healthy Hispanics to their country of birth—on mortality at ages 65 and above. "Neither the salmon nor the healthy migrant hypothesis explains the pattern of findings. Other factors must be operating to produce the lower mortality" (Abraído-Lanza et al., 1999). One study was based on data drawn from the Master Beneficiary Record and NUMIDENT (Numerical Identification System) data files of the Social Security Administration. It concludes:

These data provide the first direct evidence regarding the effect of salmon bias on the Hispanic mortality advantage. Although we confirm the existence of salmon bias, it is of too small a magnitude to be a primary explanation for the lower mortality of Hispanic than Non-Hispanic (NH)-White primary Social Security beneficiaries. Longitudinal surveys that follow individuals in and out of the United States are needed to further explore the role of migration in the health and mortality of foreign-born U.S. residents and factors that contribute to the Hispanic mortality paradox. (http://link.springer.com/article/10.1007%2Fs11113-008-9087-4)

Hayes-Bautista responds that most elderly Latino immigrants have lived in the United States for decades and have deep family and community ties here; there is little to draw them back to their native countries. Simple genetic differences are seen as unlikely factors because, even within individual Latin American nations, people come from a variety of ethnic backgrounds.

Epidemiological data show that access to prenatal care correlates with positive birth outcomes. In other words, an increase in prenatal care should lower rates of negative birth outcomes, including infant mortality and low birth-weight babies. Use of prenatal care, in turn, depends on access to preventive healthcare, usually measured by rates of health insurance coverage. However, the insurance coverage data by ethnicity in California brings that logic into question. Fully 40% of Hispanics do not have insurance coverage, compared with 20% of African Americans in the state; the Hispanics also have the highest rate of poverty. And yet, the infant mortality rate for African Americans is four times higher than the Hispanics' (Kar et al., 2001, pp. 16–17).

The most likely and least studied causes of the Hispanic Paradox are elements of *cultural capital*—such as health-related beliefs, attitudes, and behavior, and social networks affecting health outcomes. For example, Hispanic women are less likely to smoke, drink alcohol, use drugs, or have sexually transmitted diseases than African American women as a whole. That probably helps explain the lower infant mortality rates. Finally, compared to the African Americans and the whites, a significantly lower percentage of Hispanic children are raised by single parents. The inexperienced young African American mothers, often children themselves, are prone to higher levels of health risks (e.g., smoking, drinking, drugs), and are more likely to expose their infants to greater health risks than Hispanic mothers, who are more likely to be in extended families and who get child-rearing advice and help from more experienced women in their families.

We need well-funded, cross-cultural, and longitudinal studies to answer the questions raised by the Hispanic Paradox. In the meantime, we should be guided by the lesson learned from the Hispanic Paradox—that is, a poorer and more disadvantaged group can achieve better health outcomes when their culture promotes positive health beliefs, attitudes, and behavior.

THE ASIAN PARADOX: THE "MODEL MINORITY" MYTH

Asian Americans are the fastest growing and arguably the most diverse of all ethnic groups in the United States. Figure 4.2 presents the timelines of arrival and length of acculturation of major Asian American groups in the United States. Their immigration histories are also very different; among the major Asian groups, the Japanese were the first to arrive: 1843; soon to be followed by the Chinese. Most of them were manual laborers in the agricultural, railroad, and construction sectors. The most recent immigrants are from India, the Philippines, and Vietnam. The U.S. Census Bureau reports that Indians have the highest educational, occupational, and economic achievements of all ethnic groups, including the whites. The "Asian Americans" include two extreme categories: first, some subgroups indeed have higher levels of education and income; these include the Chinese and Japanese Americans who have lived in the U.S. for several generations, and also the Indians, most of whom arrived after the Immigration and Nationality Act Amendments of 1965.

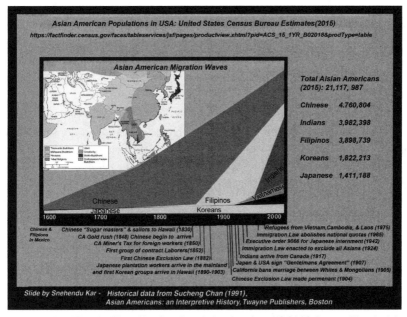

FIGURE 4.2 Asian Migration Waves Timeline. Population data from US 2010 Census: Historical data from Sucheng Chan (1991). *Asian Americans: An Interpretive History*. Boston, MA: Twayne. Figure by Snehendu Kar.

These changes allowed highly educated and accomplished Indians (doctors, scientists, engineers, IT specialists, etc.) to immigrate in large numbers. The category of Asian American immigrants at the other extreme includes poorer and less-educated groups, such as the Indochinese refugees commonly known as the "Boat People." These refugees, especially the Indochinese immigrants, came from Laos, Vietnam, and Cambodia after the fall of Vietnam in 1978. Aggregate measures combining these two extreme groups into one group of Asian Americans hide the great differences in education, income, and health status of various subgroups. This leads to what is called the "Model Minority myth," or a false perception that all Asians are successful and highly educated. It gives the false appearance that the Asian Americans as a whole do not have any problems; the reality is just the opposite. For instance, according to the Asian American Studies Center at the University of California–Los Angeles (UCLA), Asian Americans speak at least 29 distinctly different languages (not dialects, but languages) and practice all major religions of the world.

India alone prints its currency notes in 17 different languages (Indians speak more than 300 distinctly different dialects as well). "Asian Americans" also include such disparate groups as the Hmong, Mongolians, tribes from

Indonesia, and the Afghans. Putting such extremely diverse groups into one ethnic category does not describe their own identity, nor do most of them identify with the synthetic category of the pan–Asian American ethnicity imposed on them (most identify as a hyphenated bicultural group that includes the name of their country of origin (e.g., Japanese-American, Chinese-American, Indo-American).

The Asian Paradox is that, based upon limited knowledge of a few subgroups (almost entirely about their educational and economic achievements), Americans have an image of all Asian Americans as a highly successful, problem-free, and happy minority group. The Asian American are often called as the "Model Minority" who are successful, hard-working, loyal, law- abiding, and free of problems; implying that theirs is a model that other groups should follow. This stereotype hides two serious realities: first, not all Asian Americans are successful and affluent; and second, a large number of subgroups, if not all Asian Americans, suffer from serious existential problems, including poverty, racial discrimination, and crimes including hate crimes (historically, Japanese internments, Asian exclusion laws, exclusion from local and national-level political participation; and currently, real poverty among several subgroups). And yet they are not recognized as a disadvantaged "minority group" with serious problems needing help. This is the Asian dilemma. Table 4.6 presents some data to dispel this "Model Minority" myth.

The poverty data from a U.S. household survey (2008) show 23.1% of Asian Americans (compared to whites, 9.4%) have suffered a poverty spell lasting two months or more. In 2009, about 26.1% of Asian Americans were

TABLE 4.6
Educational Achievements by Ethnicity (age 25+)

Ethnic Groups	Percent with Less than High School Education	Percent with Bachelor's or Higher Degree
U.S. population:	19.6	25.9
African Americans	28.7	14.2
Hispanics	48.3	10.3
Whites	16.6	25.9
All Asian Americans	19.4	42.7
Chinese Americans	12.5	43.3
Japanese Americans	8.6	40.8
Indian Americans	12.6	64.4
Cambodian Americans	52.0	9.1
Hmong Americans	59.0	7.4
Lao Americans	49.0	7.6
Vietnamese Americans	38.0	19.5

Table constructed from U.S. Census 2000 data.

without health insurance for at least one month in the previous year. These studies also ignore that some subgroups are indeed doing inexplicably well in spite of their serious socioeconomic handicaps and hardships that cannot be explained by conventional research and theories. We may learn something new by studying them that could help other struggling groups. Researchers who have seriously studied such subgroups have interesting stories to tell about how *cultural capital* helped children of Indochinese refugees achieve scholastic success. News coverage of the extraordinary academic achievements of the children of refugees aroused the curiosity of researchers at the University of Michigan. Caplan, Choy, and Whitmore (1991) conducted a pioneering multisite study of the academic performance of Indochinese students and reported their findings in *Children of the Boat People: A Study of Educational Success*. Their study began in 1981 in Boston, Chicago, Houston, Seattle, and Orange County in California. They studied the academic performance and conventional socioeconomic measures of the children of the Boat People from Indochina: Vietnam, Laos, and Cambodia.

The Boat People were extremely disadvantaged, uneducated, poor farmers and laborers who were forced to flee from their native countries after the fall of Vietnam to the Communist army and when the Khmer Rouge of Cambodia began its reign of terror in that country. These refugees were denied entry into their neighboring countries, and they had no safe means to escape by land or air. Consequently, they had no option but to sail for overseas refuge on highly risky, makeshift boats. Thousands perished by drowning, lack of food or water, and medicines for the sick. When they arrived on foreign shores, including the United States, they were starving, sick, poor, penniless, jobless, unable to speak local languages, and had no place to go. Things could not be worse even for the homeless people on U.S. streets. When these refugees found shelters, they had to accept the worst living conditions in slums with crimes, drugs, gangs, and underperforming schools. Their children had been out of school for multiple years before they enrolled in neighborhood schools, and everyone expected them to do poorly in school. But within two to three years, the children were performing at the top of their classes. The Michigan researchers discovered astonishingly high levels of educational success measured by grade point average (GPA), standardized test scores in math and science (California Achievement Test [CAT], Scholastic Aptitude Test [SAT]), and other measures including the rate of high school completion, admission to colleges, spelling bee awards, and the number of valedictorians among them. Box 4.4 shows the academic performance scores of boat children.

Schools in Orange County reported that fewer than 20% of their students were children of Boat People; and yet 12 out of a total of 14 valedictorians were from this group. They were also "doubly over-represented" at the upper end of the CAT scores. Another surprising finding was a positive

BOX 4.4

Academic Performance of Boat Children

Grade	GPA Overall (%)	GPA Math (%)	GPA Science (%)
A	27	47	26
B	52	32	40
C	17	15	29
Below C	4	6	4

Source: Data from Caplan, Choy, and Whitmore (1991).

correlation between family size (number of siblings) and GPA. At the general population level (all ethnic groups combined), there is an inverse relationship between GPA and family size; the GPA drops in families with three or more children. This was not the case with the children of Boat People. Also, research on substance abuse and related problems of adolescents showed that parental supervision and participation has significant protective effects with regard to substance abuse and the legal problems of teens (Kar et al., 1999, *Substance Abuse Prevention: A Multicultural Perspective*). The Boat People, due to their own lack of education and English-language proficiency, could not directly supervise their children's homework or participate in any community- or school-based drug-prevention programs. The absence of parental supervision did not affect the teens' academic performance or other problem behavior common among other teenagers. The Michigan researchers statistically tested the academic performance of these students while controlling for the effects of standard socioeconomic variables (e.g., parental education, income, occupation, area of residence, English-language competency); none of the standard measures of socioeconomic variables explained the high levels of academic achievements. The researchers concluded that "family and cultural heritage" must be in play here; they collected some qualitative data on family structure and dynamics and cultural heritage, such as respect for one's elders and compliance with parental expectations, recognition of parental sacrifice for children's education, the belief that a good education is the only opportunity they have to lift their families out of poverty and misery. The Confucian values of duty and family obligations may also have influenced the outcomes.

One point must be made clear; while the children of the Boat People are doing well in school, this does not mean that they or their families and communities are happy, healthy, or well. They are suffering from levels of poverty, hardship, poor health, crimes, indignities, and racial and gender discriminations that are unacceptable in civil societies. However, the imperative of this study is that we should understand the cultural capital and culture-specific processes that prevent health risks and promote quality of life, and learn from them. They can teach us lessons that benefit the entire community; this is a gift of multicultural communities.

Relative Priorities

There are several other issues in a multicultural community that we should be aware of. One of these is that because the community consists of diverse cultures, different ethnic groups may have different priorities. In addition, depending upon the immigration history, within the same ethnic group recent immigrants will have different priorities than the previous generations. For instance, in the 1990s, the Kellogg Foundation via this writer's Kellogg Foundation fellowship encouraged us to develop a community-based participatory community-development program in South Central Los Angeles. From our past involvements in the community, we chose the Holmes Avenue Elementary School and the neighboring communities that send their children to that school. The African American principal of the school was highly respected by the community, he was very committed to his community, and we had established a trusting and productive working relationship with him and his staff. He was instrumental in our ability to form a partnership with his school, the Parent–Teacher Association (PTA), other community-based organizations (CBOs), and local leadership. In order to understand the community dynamics, it is relevant to describe them briefly.

The school was in close proximity to King Hospital, which was established in 1972 after the Watts riots of 1965 as an answer to the long-ignored complaint that the county's white-run health system neglected the black community. By the mid-1980s, "South Central L.A.," was synonymous with black Los Angeles. But by the early 1990s, middle-class African Americans began to move out to communities that once were all white. Asian Americans, who had congregated in enclaves near downtown, began to move into suburban communities.

Widespread unemployment, poverty, and street crime contributed to the rise of street gangs in South Central, such as the Crips and the Bloods.

The "Mapping L.A." project of the *Los Angeles Times* reported that the ethnic breakdown in 2000 was: Latino, 56.7%; black, 38%; white, 2.2%; Asian, 1.6%; and Other, 1.5%. In the area of our UCLA project, about 70% were Hispanics, about 22% blacks, 5% were Asians, and 3% whites. The large Hispanic population was further divided in two segments; U.S.-born Hispanics whose families had lived in California for generations and who had working knowledge of the English language; and recent Hispanic immigrants, including undocumented aliens, who had limited or no English-language proficiency. In communities like these, we had to become used to several realities that are not typically found in a stable community with a dominant majority. First, the once-dominant blacks with a substantive local majority and political experience with the civil rights movement and subsequent grassroots movements had developed a social network that they could summon for their common causes. Even after the black populations moved out and were replaced by a Hispanic majority, the black leaders retained their social and political capital. The Hispanics, although they constituted the largest group, were diverse within; they came from different countries, some were recent immigrants, others were native born, often non-citizens, and included undocumented persons as well. The Hispanics were not only handicapped by their limited or nonexistent English competency, but were also lacking social capital or organized political leadership that could protect and promote their needs. One credible reporter quoted Ron Wakabayashi, executive director of the Los Angeles County Commission on Human Relations.

> That is b.s. Diversity simply is. The core question is how do we extract its assets while minimizing its liabilities? To be sure, the new immigrants have renewed old neighborhoods, created new businesses and enriched the culture of Los Angeles. But the exploding diversity also has changed the nature of racial conflict and drawn new groups into battles that once were waged almost exclusively between blacks and whites. Here, black and Latino civil servants square off over public jobs. Black activists and Asian store owners fight over control of local businesses. And Latino and Asian gangs battle for control of their turf. (Fletcher, 1998; http://www.washingtonpost.com/wp-srv/national/longterm/meltingpot/melt2.htm)

Through our initial needs-assessments, we discovered that the majority in the community did not identify with the established black leadership, and that the existential priorities of different groups were very different. We conducted focus groups separately with different groups (at their request) and held four "town hall" open meetings with the entire community (at the Holmes Avenue School auditorium). The differences in priorities articulated by the community members were substantive.

Box 4.5 shows that recent immigrants are more concerned with language, immigration status, and jobs; while the established immigrants are more concerned with children's education and safety issues. Health is not the top priority for either. The lower priority assigned by new immigrants to children's issues is not because they were less concerned with children, but because recent immigrants were relatively younger in age, and fewer of them had school-aged children. The second major finding is that the recent immigrants

BOX 4.5
Relative Priorities of Recent and Established Immigrants

Recent Immigrants (Mostly Hispanics)	Established Immigrants (Mostly Second Plus Generation in the US)
Immigration assistance (46%)	Children's education (62%)
Language education (42%)	Protect children from "Harms" (52%)
Employment (36%)	Safe neighborhood (40% children and family)
Better schools (35%)	Better health care (38%)
Medical and health (32%)	Equal pay for equal job (32%)
Family relationship (25%)	Career, education, advancement (28%)
Race relations (24%)	Elderly care (16%)

Source: Kar SB & Jain S (1999). *SAHARA Needs Assessment Study.* UCLA: The Public Health Practice Office.

were more concerned with not having their own voice and leadership (they were reluctant to discuss this openly), and consequently we chose not to do a quantitative assessment of this item because publishing the findings may have created internal discord.

What Unites Us?

We have discussed in some detail the issues that can divide a multicultural community. We should also be asking "What unites us?" We need ongoing discourse on this issue. A better understanding of what divides us; how some multicultural societies maintain and promote ethnic harmony; and how to develop better opportunities for meaningful contacts, including planned desegregations, in various domains of our lives are some of the means. Professor Collier's brilliant analysis (2007) discussed earlier dispels several myths about what causes ethnic strife. Sen's book *Identity and Violence* also looks at violence from a human development and macro-level perspective. Enhancing personal "freedoms" and "capabilities" through human development measures would reduce inter-ethnic strife and promote community capacities to deal with conflicts. The UN/WHO and the Committee on the Elimination of Discrimination Against Women (CEDAW's) initiatives to promote gender empowerment and equality and to reduce the "culture of violence" against women are notable initiatives.

From a micro-level (individual) perspective, psychological approaches used to understand prejudice deserve serious review. More than 50 years ago, psychologist Gordon Allport published his landmark volume *On the Nature of Prejudice* (1954), in which he laid the foundations for subsequent research on the nature of prejudice, its cause and consequences. His famous "contact hypothesis" suggests that intergroup strife and violence may be reduced and intergroup cooperation may be enhanced by carefully designed "contact" experiences in serving a common cause. On the fiftieth anniversary of that publication, the Fetzer Institute sponsored a conference to review the field of research on Allport's legacy. Forty-four scientists gathered to review the research on prejudice and suggest a future course of action. That conference summarized the state of the science (and art), which led to a volume titled *On the Nature of Prejudice: Fifty Years after Allport* (Dovidio et al., 2005). This is an excellent source to review the psychological theories and research addressing some of the key issues raised by Allport in his original book. Among these issues, two have especial significance to health-related discourse. The first is Allport's contact hypothesis, or sociocultural approach to reducing interracial stereotypes and hostility; Allport described his "contact hypothesis" in these words:

> Prejudice may be reduced by equal status contacts between majority and minority groups in the pursuit of common goals. The effect is generally enhanced if the contact is sanctioned by institutional support (i.e., law, custom, or local atmosphere) and provided it is of the sort that leads to the perception of common humanity between members of two groups. (Allport, 1954, p. 281)

Second, Allport's social-cognitive approach suggests that a stereotype serves a function: it is an irrational process that is learned and can be unlearned. It seems that these two propositions are supported by fifty years of research and deserve serious attention by researchers and health professionals involved in multicultural communities. Our experience from the Kellogg project in the Holmes Avenue community supports Allport's contact hypothesis.

In the previous section we discussed the relative priorities of disparate groups in that community. For the sake of brevity, we will skip the prolonged group processes we used through which we could come to agree on a common goal. What we discovered should have been obvious to all, but it took some time before everyone was willing to restructure their thoughts and agree that the project should be to protect children from "harms" ("harms" is their choice of term—they were not accustomed to speaking in medical, epidemiological, or legal terms to define project goals). When the community realized that if they could not agree upon a single goal, the project would not be funded at all, they did find an option they could agree with. So many members were willing to forego their top priority and settle for the next priority rather than not get anything. The overwhelming majority of the community had children, and as parents, they were convinced that preventing harms to their children would be an important gain. Also, anyone who has worked in communities knows that it is the women and mothers who are more willing to volunteer for a cause to promote children's interests, and when mothers volunteer, the rest of the community will not stand in their way. In summary, their strong motivation to prevent harms to their children unified the community. Finally, the active participation of a group of women and mothers (WAM) as eager volunteers is a much more agreeable way to get something done that helps the community rather than fighting for separate priorities by different segments of the community.

We found the same to be true in another project when we recruited Latina WAM as *promotoras* ("promoters") from the community to increase childhood immunizations in underserved communities in Los Angeles (our "Rescatando Salud" or Rescue Health project), which more than tripled the timely and complete childhood immunizations coverage and received a national award for reducing ethnic disparities in health in 2001. In sum, a program designed to protect all children in the community with the help of WAM from that community is an effective way to unite the community for a common cause. In such a case, WAM of disparate ethnicity come in direct contact and work together for a common cause that is valued by all. Protecting children from danger is a strongly unifying force, and the involvement of "nonpolitical" mothers makes such an initiative highly credible.

MUTUAL TRUST AND THE "BOND OF RELATIONS"

Mutual trust and a "bond of relations" are the two essential elements of a peaceful and unified community. Trust-building and maintenance is the first requirement for all community-based work. No population-based initiative will succeed unless the groups affected trust one another and the agency professionals who are involved in their community. For the professionals, it is tempting to become task-oriented and see Trust Building and Maintenance (TBM) steps as optional activities or even as a waste of time. This is far from the truth. TBAM is an essential component of any work in a multicultural community that consists of several ethnic groups who may not fully understand one another. If one ethnic group perceives an outreach professional to be more supportive of another group, that may cause mistrust for the professional. Unfortunately, there is no simple manual or guide that tells us how to build trust and maintain it. Examples from three projects in disparate cultures and problems are used for brief illustrations of key issues; some of these issues will be discussed in greater depth later (e.g., cultural competency, transformative leadership, and evaluation of participatory research and action) in the last chapter of this volume.

At this point, let us focus on the trust issue. The first example is from a smallpox eradication campaign in early 1960 in India. The second example is from population and family planning issues in the early 1970s at a major American university. And the third example is from childhood immunization promotion in the 1990s in Los Angeles.

The Smallpox Eradication in India

WHO declared in 1980 that "smallpox is eradicated." Until then, smallpox was a deadly annual epidemic in India (and in several poor nations). This author's first assignment with the Indian Health Ministry was to join a small-pox-prevention team and visit the rural areas in the state of Bihar. Bihar was one of the least developed states. My responsibility was to study the social and behavioral determinants of the epidemic; more specifically, to answer this question: since primary vaccination was required by law and it was a free door-to-door service, why were many villagers not having their children vaccinated? Adults were also not getting re-vaccinations as recommended. The smallpox team soon discovered that the lack of knowledge or access to free vaccination services were not the problems. The problem was that, at that same time, the Indian Government was also vigorously promoting family planning, and there was a rumor going around that the Indian Government, under the pretext of giving smallpox vaccinations, was injecting antifertility drugs. Naturally, villagers were concerned and wanted to determine whether the vaccination team members had had smallpox vaccinations, too. It was an issue of trust; can the team be trusted? After consulting with the team doctor and finding out that another booster shot would not harm us, we decided to organize a "vaccination fair" and have the team members vaccinated in front of the villagers. We did just that, and most villagers concluded that vaccination was harmless, otherwise we would not have taken it. The lesson learned here is that the people had a legitimate concern; and our obligation was to demonstrate to them that we were not deceiving them. Trust-building required that we practice what we preach. (The story is much more complex, and the entire problem was not solved by one demonstration. There were other objections to vaccination. We are limiting ourselves here to the issue of trust.) While smallpox is gone, the issue of trust is still alive in other programs and situations.

Population Planning

In the late 1960s, I joined the University of Michigan at Ann Arbor as a young assistant professor with a joint appointment between the Center for Population Planning and the Department of Health Behavior and Education. At that time, a population-planning initiative was widespread across many universities and nations of the world. A major goal of population planning was to achieve "zero population" growth (that means the number of babies born is equal to the number of deaths per year) as soon as possible. With zero population growth (ZPG), the cumulative absolute population size will still grow, but the "rate of growth" will be "zero." Demographers calculated that to achieve ZPG, each couple should have an average of 2.2 children. One of the very first questions the smart graduate students in population planning would ask was: How many children do the population-planning faculty members have? Here again, the students were verifying whether the faculty practiced what they taught. Well, the program director and the two most senior faculty members had four or five children. These faculty members justified their support of ZPG the following way: they had their children before the population-planning movement began, and also had learned the consequences of having a large family. So, they argued, the students should learn from their experience and not emulate them. Although the number of children the faculty had did not directly affect the students, they wanted to confirm whether the faculty believed in what they taught.

The Rescatando Salud (Save Health) Immunization Program

Los Angeles has pockets of very poor and disadvantaged populations. Many are in heavily Hispanic areas and do not speak English well. They also include unknown numbers of undocumented immigrants. For these and other reasons, they are suspicious of non-Spanish-speaking professionals probing into and roaming around their neighborhoods. They were afraid of Immigration and Nationalization Service (INS) agents and plainclothes policemen searching for illegal immigrants, gangs, and drug dealers. In short, they were afraid of anyone who did not look and speak like them. They also had a very low coverage of timely childhood immunizations. By the time the children enter public schools, by law they are all supposed to be immunized; but prior to that, many children did not have timely immunizations. Not having timely vaccinations means children are exposed to periods of "needless risk"; by adding up all the periods of needless risk, one gets a measure of the total duration of exposure to risks. Ralph Frerichs, a professor of epidemiology at UCLA, estimated that more than seven out of ten children were exposed to long periods of "needless risk." The biggest challenge the County Health Department faced was how to reach the parents of these children and immunize them at the recommended times.

In 1999, the Public Health Practice Office at UCLA (UCLA-PHPO) started a four-way Rescatando Salud (Save Health) collaborative project for promoting the timely immunization of Hispanic children; the four collaborating agencies were UCLA-PHPO, the LA County Health Department Immunization program (LACDHIP), La Esperanza Community Housing project (LECHP), and the South Central Community Health Center

(SCCHC). The project had access to all birth records by project years, but when we attempted to contact the mothers on the phone numbers on the records, we could reach just a very, very small number (fewer than 9%) of the women. We used Spanish-speaking graduate students and outreach workers, but still most of the women could not be contacted. A majority of those we could reach on the phone hung up the phone when they did not recognize the voice of a friend or neighbor they trusted. Door-to-door visits by Spanish-speaking outreach staff of LACDHIP and UCLA graduate students did not produce better results. Most of the mothers would not open the door, would hide their children, or would claim the person we were looking for did not live there. We exhausted all the methods in the community survey textbooks but failed to reach more than 10% of mothers with a child born in the past three years. We faced a huge trust barrier.

Finally, we launched a project called "Empowerment of Women for Health Promotion" that recruited local Hispanic WAM from these communities as *promotoras* ("promoters"); we helped them plan and conduct the door-to-door visits and arrange immunization street fairs and camps; and we sent them to the community clinics for immunizations. By integrating the women's empowerment and children's immunization initiatives, in two years the "complete timely immunization rate" more than quadrupled.

Unlike numerous *promotora* programs, we did not use the women as low-paid aides or outreach workers for our project. Instead we had a quid pro quo agreement. They agreed to work as *promotoras* to promote childhood immunization in their community, and in exchange we paid for their training for an income-generating career. For instance, they would be trained and certified as a phlebotomist, hair stylist, secretary, dressmaker, home health care provider, etc. The idea is, when our project ended, they will have skills that will allow them to earn for many years. The community trusted them because they were known to the community and part of it; and the *promotoras* trusted us because they could see we were there to promote their well-being and the health of their children. Several of the first cohort of our *promotoras* later found full-time paid positions and advanced in their careers through further job training, and four of them now own homes in low-income housing development projects (a 14-minute video that describes the project is available on YouTube: http://www.youtube.com/watch?v=OXRp7LzuKdE).

These examples show that when trust is lacking, people's protection motivation steps in and erects a barrier between us and the community we intend to work in. Each barrier is different and requires a different solution. The important point is to remember that establishing and maintaining trust is not a luxury we cannot afford; it is so essential that we cannot afford to ignore it.

5

Key Issues in Empowerment Theory

THE EMPOWER MODEL

*Despite progress made since 1994, the empowerment of women
and girls and gender equality remain unfulfilled and discrimination
against women is evident in all societies. Women's empowerment
and gender equality are pivotal to creating the enabling conditions
in which half the global population can define the direction of their
lives, expand their capabilities, and contribute fully to societies.*

—United Nations (2014) Conference on Population
and Development Report

This chapter reviews key philosophical and conceptual issues in empowerment theory and action and presents the EMPOWER model for research and
action. The EMPOWER (acronym) represents the seven *empowerment methods* used by the 80 case studies of our meta-analysis of empowerment movements. The EMPOWER model and its implications are discussed at the end
of this chapter.

The first four chapters of this volume reviewed the justifications for wom-
en's empowerment, social determinants of health, the emergence of global
public health (GPH) as a new paradigm, and the global consensus on the
human development approach (HDA) led by the UN and WHO, while the last
chapter reviewed the realities of multicultural societies that affect the health
and well-being of people.

Literature reviews conclude that culture matters (Sen, 1999; Inglehart &
Norris, 2003; WHO, 2008). Causes of powerlessness, and various forms of
abuses, including violence against women and domestic violence, are deeply
rooted in cultural practices. Consequently, the current global consensus explicitly stated in the UN's Millennium Development Goals (MDGs) is that gender
equality and women's empowerment (GEE); poverty reduction; and the elimination of culturally rooted values and practices that promote violence against
women, including domestic violence, are among the most important priorities
of the HDA (United Nations Development Programme [UNDP] 2014). Within
this context, some of the broader issues in current empowerment theory and

research requires collective critical thinking about our current discourse on empowerment. The goal of this chapter is to stimulate critical thinking on how to make contemporary empowerment theories, models, and research more consistent with our universal aspirations reflected in the UN's Declaration of Human Rights (UN, 1948) and the existential realities of our increasingly multicultural societies across the globe.

Philosophy of Empowerment

People's empowerment (or lack of it) has been a source of concern among philosophers, scholars, social reformers, and above all among the victims themselves. Our literature review identifies five determinants of powerlessness: Poverty, Patriarchy, Prejudice, Political exclusion, and Psychophysical limitations. This section briefly reviews the developments in our modern history, especially since the mid–nineteenth century (most human sciences and services professions emerged during this period) that have inspired women's empowerment as a global priority.

GLOBAL CONSENSUSES ON EMPOWERMENT

A confluence of philosophical positions has profoundly influenced the philosophy of women's empowerment theory and action. These are:

1. *Five global consensuses on Universal Human Rights* (e.g., UN's Declaration of Human Rights, Alma-Ata Declaration, Ottawa Charter, Committee on the Elimination of Discrimination Against Women [CEDAW], and the UNHDA)
2. *Nonviolent movements* (e.g., those led by Gandhi, Tagore, King Jr., Mandela, Havel, Suu Kyi, Walesa)
3. *Women's rights movements* (e.g., women's suffrage, the National Organization of Women [NOW])
4. *Human service professions' shared values* (e.g., public health, social work, community health sciences)

Our own meta-analysis of women's empowerment focuses on women's self-organized movements (see chapters 6–10 of this volume). It is important to note that these five types of consensus and forces do not work in isolation; more often than not, effective movements reinforce and support one another.

Five major UN declarations and charters spelled out the global consensus on human rights and women's rights. The first was the Universal Declaration of Human Rights (UDHR). After the horrific atrocities perpetrated by Nazi Germany during World War II came to light, many nations in the world community unified to prevent similar tragedy happening again. During the war, the Western Allies adopted the "Four Freedoms" proposed earlier by U.S. President Franklin Delano Roosevelt in his State of the Union address on January 6, 1941: freedom of *speech*, freedom of *religion,* freedom from *fear*, and freedom from *want*. The UN commissioned a committee to draft a charter of universal human rights— that commission included Australia, Belgium, Byelorussia, Chile, the Republic of China, Egypt, France, India, Iran, Lebanon, Panama, the Philippines, the United Kingdom, the United States, the Union of Soviet Socialist Republics (USSR), Uruguay, and Yugoslavia (the commission included a spectrum of nations that were capitalist, communist, socialist, militarist, and imperialist). In recognition of her commitment to human rights advocacy, Eleanor Roosevelt, First Lady of the United States, was appointed to serve as the chairperson of the UN Commission on Human Rights. More than 50 member nations participated in drafting the declaration. The final UN UDHR was adopted in 1948; it committed all member states to promote universal respect for, and observance of, human rights and fundamental freedoms for all without distinction as to race, sex, language, or religion. This was a historic global consensus which defined the four pillars of freedom for all. It recognized that vulnerable populations and groups have the rights to these freedoms and the world community of nations has the obligation to help and empower them (UNDHR, 1948).

The second global consensus is the 1978 Alma-Ata Declaration of Primary Health Care (PHC), which was discussed in greater depth in Chapter 2; for that reason the discussion is not repeated here. It is important to reemphasize that this declaration identified "community participation" and "intersectorial collaboration" as the central imperatives for developing comprehensive healthcare. This is the beginning of a healthcare paradigm that goes "beyond medicine" for better health for all.

The third global consensus, once again led by the United Nations, specifically addressed the importance of women's freedom and empowerment when the UN established the CEDAW. The CEDAW in 1979 declared that "Equality of rights for women is a basic principle of the United Nations. The Preamble to the Charter of the United Nations sets as one of the Organization's central goals the reaffirmation of 'faith in fundamental human rights, in the dignity and worth of the human person, in the equal rights of men and women' (UN, 2000–2009). CEDAW, established in 1979, is composed of 23 experts on women's issues from around the world and charged with monitoring progress and recommending appropriate actions thereon by the UN. According to the CEDAW:

The Committee's mandate is very specific: it watches over the progress for women made in those countries that are the States parties to the 1979

Convention on the Elimination of All Forms of Discrimination against Women. A country becomes a State party by ratifying or acceding to the Convention and thereby accepting a legal obligation to counteract discrimination against women. The Committee monitors the implementation of national measures to fulfill this obligation.

In January 2008, the CEDAW reported:

The Committee celebrated the twenty-fifth anniversary of its work last year (1982–2007). Since the inaugural session at the United Nations Office at Vienna in October 1982, the Committee has held 39 sessions, the most recent one in August 2007 at United Nations Headquarters in New York.

In his message on International Women's Day, the UN Secretary General, Ban Ki-moon said, "We are highlighting the importance of achieving equality for women and girls not simply because it is a matter of fairness and fundamental human rights, but because progress in so many other areas depends on it. (Moon, March 26, 2014)

The UN's Women's Rights Division concludes that

Despite great strides made by the international women's rights movement over many years, women and girls around the world are still married as children or trafficked into forced labor and sex slavery. They are refused access to education and political participation, and some are trapped in conflicts where rape is perpetrated as a weapon of war. Around the world, deaths related to pregnancy and childbirth are needlessly high, and women are prevented from making deeply personal choices in their private lives. Human Rights Watch is working toward the realization of women's empowerment and gender equality—protecting the rights and improving the lives of women and girls on the ground. (UN Human Rights Watch 2015)

The fourth world consensus is the Ottawa Charter of 1986 (WHO, 1986), which explicitly stated that "Health Promotion works through concrete and effective community action in setting priorities, making decisions, planning strategies and implementing them to achieve better health for all. At the heart of this process is the empowerment of communities, their ownership and control of their own endeavors and destinies" (WHO 1986). To the best of our knowledge, the Ottawa Charter is the major international consensus document that explicitly declares that community empowerment is at the heart of health-promotion strategies; previously, most social scientists and healthcare providers were preoccupied with the lack of compliance by the community and patients as the main barrier to effective community health intervention.

The central thrust of the Ottawa Charter is that with the elimination and/ or control of many traditional infectious diseases, people are increasingly suffering and dying from chronic diseases that are primarily caused by unhealthy behaviors (e.g., tobacco abuse, high-risk sexual behaviors, domestic violence, dietary habits). There are no vaccinations against these health threats; human behavior is at the root of these problems and these can only be reduced or controlled by sustained adoption of health promotion and disease prevention (HPDP) practices by individuals in their social contexts. The Ottawa Charter advocates community empowerment as the key to effective HPDP strategies.

The fifth international consensus and philosophical foundation for women's empowerment is the development and adoption of the UN's HDA in 1990 and the adoption of CEDAW in 1979 by the UN General Assembly. CEDAW "is often described as an international bill of rights for women"; it explicitly includes gender equality and empowerment as required indicators of Human Development Indices. In 2000, the global community, under the UN, adopted eight MDGs to achieve by 2015. Two additional WHO-sponsored internal consensuses supported the expanded mandate of the HDA to include poverty elimination and gender empowerment: these are (1) the Jakarta Declaration on Health Promotion (WHO/WPRO, 1997), and (2) the Kolkata (Calcutta) Declaration on the Future of Public Health in the Twenty-first Century (WHO/SEARO, 1999).

These five global consensus documents prompted several activities across the world. However, in the ten years since the adoption of the MDGs, as the UN Secretary-General Ban Ki-moon reported, we still have a long way to go (UN/ICPD [International Conference on Population and Development], 2014a: *Beyond 2014* report). It is important to note that these consensuses have set a global agenda to promote women's empowerment for the benefit of all people, not just for women—as a pathway for progress for all (UN/ICPD, 2014a).

The Apostles of the Nonviolent Empowerment Movements

We begin with four "apostles" of nonviolent empowerment and freedom movements and their messages before discussing other theories and models of empowerment. The philosophies of these four men had a global impact that no other empowerment theory or model can match. These are Mahatma Gandhi, Rabindranath Tagore, Martin Luther King, Jr., and Nelson Mandela. The twentieth century witnessed several innovative and successful applications of nonviolent movements. The concept of nonviolence, or in Sanskrit *Ahimsa*, goes back to antiquity in Indian philosophy; it occupies a special place in Hindu, Buddhist, and Jain theologies. Gandhi popularized the Sanskrit phrase *Ahimsa Parama Dharma* or *"Ahimsa is the supreme duty"*; it guided his philosophy and nonviolent struggles for India's freedom.

Nonviolent liberation movements provided a sound philosophical foundation and strategic lessons for empowerment movements. Gandhi and Mandela struggled to earn freedom from their oppressive foreign colonizers; King Jr. struggled for civil rights, equality, and dignity for African Americans in a free nation that denied them their basic and equal rights; and Tagore struggled to liberate the minds of hundreds of millions of people in India through educating and unleashing the *Atma-Shakti* or self-power of the poor and the powerless masses (in Sanskrit, *Atma* meaning self; *Shakti* meaning power or strength). Mandela placed special emphasis on forgiveness and reconciliation (not revenge) with their adversaries as a precondition of an empowered nation. After 27 long years of imprisonment in Robben Island, when he became the president of South Africa, Mandela was most interested in "truth and reconciliation" with his former oppressors and the leaders of the white minority of his new nation. Social harmony played an important role in community empowerment for Gandhi, Mandela, and Tagore. For instance, Gandhi's favorite prayer chant includes this line: "You are both the God and the Allah; please guide the peoples of all religions to live in harmony."

Martin Luther King, Jr. promoted racial harmony by leading his nonviolent civil rights movement. Through this movement he called for an end to racism. He insisted that people should judge others by "the content of their character rather than the color of their skin." He also preferred nonviolent civil-disobedience movements to achieve the dreams that he spoke of in his famous speech in Washington, D.C., in 1963.

Tagore was especially committed to a secular social system wherein peoples of different religions, cultures, and races might retain their separate identities but live in peace and harmony. In the national anthem of India, written and composed by Tagore, a stanza that sounds like a prayer says:

> *Your call has reached everyone.*
> *The Hindus, Buddhist, Jains, Sikhs,*
> *Parsees, Muslims, and the Christians,*
> *from the East and the West,*
> *have gathered around your throne,*
> *with garlands woven with love.*

(Note: Tagore also wrote a second national anthem of Bangladesh)

Tagore named all major regions of India in his "garland" of love; social harmony was very important in his philosophy of human development. He was also a strong advocate of the empowerment of women. More than

100 years ago and several decades before the women's liberation movements began in the West, Tagore promoted women's empowerment through his numerous teachings, poems, short stories, essays, and novels. As early as 1929, in an aptly named poem *"Shabala"* (*Sha* meaning own or self; *bal* meaning power; and *"a"* is added at the end to make the term feminine), Tagore had his protagonist ask:

Dear Lord, tell me why
a woman should not be allowed
to seek her own fortune
with power of her own?

Gandhi and Mandela were highly educated and successful lawyers before they began their freedom movements; they were dedicated to human rights and became full-time political and national leaders. Tagore was a full-time philosopher, poet, educator, and artist who was deeply disturbed by the powerlessness of the poor and by how badly the British Raj (regime) treated its powerless subjects. He renounced his knighthood from the British King in protest and disgust when the infamous Jallianwala Bagh massacre occurred. This massacre happened when British General Dyer ordered his soldiers to shoot and kill hundreds of unarmed and nonviolent demonstrators, including children and women, who were trapped in an enclosed compound and had no way to disperse. Tagore was never a professional politician, but he dedicated himself to liberating the masses in a more profound way; he chose empowerment, education, rural reconstruction, and microcredit as early as 1905—as means for his movements. He commanded deep respect from citizens, scholars, and national leaders alike. He was, of course, committed to earning India's independence from the British Raj, but he was more concerned about liberating the minds of the masses and instilling *Atma-Shakti* and self-reliance in them. As a social philosopher, he believed that education involves much more than learning to read newspapers and sign one's name; education must empower the people to become productive, earn a living, live with dignity, and actualize their full potentials. Tagore was not interested in creating a class of literate but unemployed citizens.

King Jr., was a Baptist minister who became a full-time champion of civil rights and justice for African Americans in the United States. He was committed to racial equality, integration, and nonviolence as the central principles of his civil rights movement and was dedicated to the Gandhian ideology of *ahimsa* (nonviolence).

In spite of their differences, they all were fully committed to nonviolence as the modus operandi for their respective liberation struggles. All four shared a philosophical position that included these principles: freedom, nonviolence, empowerment, equality, self-reliance, and *Atma-Shakti*. These principles constitute the philosophy of empowerment as they taught and practiced it. A few excerpts from these men and scholars who wrote about them are presented here to illustrate their philosophy and work. A discussion of empowerment without their ideology and inspiration would be incomplete.

MAHATMA GANDHI

The Mahatma (the "Great Soul") said at the end of an address: "*Satyagraha* is search for truth; and God is Truth. *Ahimsa* and nonviolence is the light that reveals that truth to me. *Swaraj* for me is a part of that truth" (Gandhi's speech at the Indian National Congress held at Belgaum in 1924). "You cannot bring peace through violence. The most effective answer to violence is nonviolence," Gandhi said in one of his articles in his newspaper *Harijan* (1938; Gandhi, 1916).

Philosopher Karl Jasper in *The Future of Mankind* (1958) wrote: "Today we face the question of how to escape from physical force and from war, lest we all perish by the atom bomb. Gandhi, in words and deeds, gives the true answer: only a supra-political force can bring political salvation" (see Jasper, 1958). "This is the voice of the world conscience and this is an echo of the voice of Gandhi. The voice may not reach all ears. But they have reached at least some ears. What is strange is that Germany, a country responsible for the Second World War, is the country which is now stressing the need for Gandhian nonviolence in the modern world" (Dasgupta, 2015, p. 1).

Werner Heisenberg, arguably the greatest physicist after Einstein, in an essay on Gandhi says, "Gandhi's teaching of nonviolence could prove to be stronger than the vague impersonal conception of an international court of justice. Gandhi's unique example shows that a true personal involvement together with the total rejection of force could be very successful politically" (cited by Jasper). Several Nobel laureates who successfully led nonviolent freedom movements confirm Heisenberg's prediction.

> Gandhi's spiritual and moral approach to our political problem is particularly important today after the US declaration of war on terrorism. To realize this we have to value Gandhi's idea of reflection on ourselves and see what we are. The Pentagon's fire-power will not end terrorism. It will only make violence more rampant. Let us hope that the people of America, once nursed on the idealism of Emerson, Thoreau and Whitman will soon begin to understand Gandhi and will abandon the spirit of revenge which now regulates the policy of dealing with terrorists. You cannot bring peace through violence. The most effective answer to violence is nonviolence. (Dasgupta, 2007)

Nelson Mandela best summarized the power and promise of a Gandhian approach in these words: "As we find ourselves in jobless economies, societies in which small minorities consume while the masses starve, we find ourselves forced to rethink the rationale of our current globalization and to ponder the Gandhian alternative" ("The Sacred Warrior," *TIME: Person of the Century,* December 1999).

"The essence of nonviolent technique is that it seeks to liquidate antagonism but not the antagonists," said Gandhi. While introducing Gandhi to the world, the British Broadcasting Corporation (BBC) paraphrased Gandhian philosophy thus: "Non-violence doesn't just mean not doing violence; it's also a way of taking positive action to resist oppression or bring about change" (BBC, 2014).

The concept of nonviolence goes back to antiquity in India; it was Gandhi's genius to make it an effective means for political goals in the modern age. At least eight national leaders who followed the Gandhian nonviolent method were awarded the Nobel Peace Prize: Martin Luther King Jr., Lech Walesa of Poland, Vaclav Havel of the Czech Republic, Nelson Mandela, Aung San Suu Kyi of Myanmar (Burma); Ellen Johnson Sirleaf and Leymah Gbowee (of Liberia) and Tawakkol Karman (of Yemen; the last three were joint winners in 2011). And yet, the most famous champion of nonviolence in the modern world, Gandhi, was never awarded the Nobel Peace Prize (there are many speculations on why; when the Dalai Lama was awarded the Nobel Peace Prize in 1989, the chairman of the committee said that this was "in part a tribute to the memory of Mahatma Gandhi"). The ultimate irony is that most of the popular textbooks on community organization and development by Western scholars do not include Gandhi; experts on community empowerment, organization, public health, and human development in Western cultures do not find Gandhi and Tagore worthy enough to include in their writings and teaching.

Tagore sums up his vision of freedom and liberty in this song:

Rabindranath Tagore on Unity, Truth and Freedom

Where the mind is without fear and the head is held high;
Where knowledge is free;
Where the world has not been broken up into fragments by narrow
domestic walls;
Where words come out from the depth of truth;
Where tireless striving stretches its arms towards perfection;
Where the clear stream of reason has not lost its way into the dreary
desert sand of dead habit;
Where the mind is led forward by thee into ever-widening thought and
action—
Into that heaven of freedom, my Father, let my country awake.

—Rabindranath Tagore (1913)

Tagore was deeply disturbed by the lack of literacy, extreme poverty, power-lessness, and sufferings of the uneducated populations. Tagore's idea of rural development is captured in this quotation:

> If we could free even one village from the shackles of helplessness and ignorance, an ideal for the whole of India would be established. Let a few villages be rebuilt in this way, and I shall say they are my India. That is the way to discover the true India. (Tagore, 1928, p. 8)

Tagore firmly believed that a sound education is the necessary foundation for developing self-reliance of the people. To achieve his vision of education, self-reliance, and global peace, Tagore established a world university, the Santiniketan ("The Adobe of Peace") in 1921 with this primary mission:

> To seek to realize in a common fellowship of study the meeting of the East and the West, and thus ultimately to strengthen the fundamental conditions of world peace through the establishment of free communi-cation of ideas between the two hemispheres. And, with such ideals in view, to provide at Santiniketan, a centre of culture where research into and study of the religion, literature, history, science and art of Hindu, Buddhist, Jain, Islamic, Sikh, Christian and other civilisations may be pursued along with the culture of the West, with that simplicity in externals which is necessary for true spiritual realisation, in amity, good fellowship and co-operation between the thinkers and scholars of both Eastern and Western countries.

Subsequently, in 1922, Tagore established Sriniketan ("The Adobe of Pro-sperity") for promoting rural education and reconstruction with these two goals:

> To win the friendship and affection of villagers and cultivators by taking a real interest in all that concerns their life and welfare, and by making an effort to assist them in solving their most pressing problems.
>
> To initiate a dialogue between academic study and research of rural economy/culture and on-field experience. (Visva-Bharati http://www.visvabharati.ac.in/Mission_Vision.html. Accessed December 28, 2015)

An excerpt from a Tagore scholar Basu (2009b) says:

> Tagore's concept of sustainable development of India is rooted deep in rural regeneration, since the majority of the population of India resides in villages. It has two major planks: (i) Cooperatives and (ii) Panchayats (Village Councils). In both the cases, Tagore calls for revival of the spirit of the rural masses so that they could be self-suf-ficient and free from dependence on outside assistance ("to approach

the authorities with begging bowls," so to say) for their economic and social empowerment. Tagore lays greatest stress on instilling the spirit of self-confidence and unity in the minds of the rural folk (through proper education) so that they could, on their own, fight off the maladies afflicting rural India. (Basu 2009b, p. 58)

Tagore advocates self-organized bottom-up empowerment processes and warns that: "If cooperatives and panchayats are thrust on the rural folk from without (say, by the government, political parties or vested interest groups), they would miserably fail to generate and support the process of sustainable development. Tagore holds that success can be found only by inspiring the rural masses to form cooperatives and panchayats by their own efforts." (p. 58). Evangelical community organizers and activists may ponder over Tagore's philosophy of empowerment and his last caveat. (Basu, 2009b)

NELSON MANDELA

In his address to a joint session of the U.S. Congress on October 16, 1994, Mandela proclaimed that: "each one of us as nations ... should begin to define the national interest to include the genuine happiness of others, however distant in time and space their domicile may be." That same month, in an address to the UN General Assembly, Mandela urged "The empowerment of the ordinary people of our world freely to determine their destiny, unhindered by tyrants and dictators." Mandela's democratic sentiments were echoed by his foreign minister, Alfred Nzo, who told the Eleventh Conference of the Non-Aligned Movement in Cairo in June 1994 that "human rights are the cornerstone of our government policy and we shall not hesitate to carry the message to the far corners of the world. We have suffered too much ourselves not to do so" (Nzo, 1994, quoting Mandela in his 1994 UN speech). Mandela's philosophy of empowerment education was guided by three basic principles. First, education should instill the unshakable conviction in us that nonviolence is the best way to struggle for our freedom and liberation from our oppressors; it is a strength that our oppressor does not have. Second, we must learn our responsibilities toward others, especially those who are less fortunate than us. And, third, we must cultivate a mindset of "community thinking" (King Jr. & Nelson, 2012).

MARIN LUTHER KING, JR.

Dr. Martin Luther King Jr. summarized his philosophy that guided his nonviolent civil rights movement. "I have a dream that my four little children will one day live in a nation where they will not be judged by the color of their skin but by the content of their character" (King Jr. & Nelson, 2012). He also held that the fundamental aim of education is to be able to think intensively and critically. He hopes that the basic content of our character and our ability to think critically will inform our action in a civil society.

RABINDRANATH TAGORE

Gandhi, King, and Mandela are well known to Western populations, but unfortunately, Tagore either remains unknown or he has been forgotten. No serious discussion of empowerment of the poor, and the importance of education for empowerment and freedom, would be complete without Tagore's ideas and his exemplary contributions to empowering millions of the poor and powerless. For that reason, Tagore deserves a somewhat longer introduction than does Gandhi, Mandela, or King.

Rabindranath Thakur (or Tagore) was a contemporary of Gandhi's; they respected and inspired each other. Gandhi named him *Gurudev* (*Guru* means "wise master" or a sage, and *Dev* means "God" or "godly"); ever since, millions of people in India and abroad have called him "Gurudev." Tagore called Gandhi a *Mahatma* ("Great Soul") and the world calls him Mahatma Gandhi.

Tagore was born to a progressive and affluent Bengali family in India. Most of those who know of him remember him as a great Indian poet. He was the first non-Westerner to win the Nobel Prize in Literature (in 1913) for his exquisitely lyrical and spiritual book of poems named *Geetanjali* ("Offerings of Songs"). In the foreword of *Geetanjali*, the Irish Nobel Laureate poet W. B. Yeats wrote, "… these prose translations from Rabindranath Tagore have stirred my blood as nothing has for years" (Yeats, 1913, foreword, *Geetanjali*).

Tagore is the only poet in human history who wrote the lyrics and composed national anthems for two independent nations (India and Bangladesh). He was as great a musician as well: he created a new genre of music called "*Rabindrasangeet*".

Tagore also wrote novels, short stories, and essays on critical social issues. He was a prolific author; his collected works fill more than 40 volumes. He was also a successful artist; his paintings were exhibited in prestigious galleries in Europe, including London, Paris, and Berlin, to name a few.

Above all, Tagore was a philosopher, an innovative educator, and social reformer; he was decades, if not a century, ahead of his time. It is this facet of Tagore that is germane to the topic of this book. To Tagore, education is much more than learning the three "Rs"; it is "essentially an awakening of the mind; not merely an awakening of the hunger for knowledge, but an awareness of belonging to a social setting—micro and macro at the same time" (Majumdar, 2009, p. 8). In Tagore's own words, "The highest education is that which does not merely give us information but makes our life in harmony with all existence" (cited by Majumdar, 2009, p. 8). His emphasis on education is on awakening a deep understanding of our place in the larger reality, and our interconnectedness with nature and disparate cultures that determines our quality of life.

If Gandhi was first a nationalist, Tagore was a secular universalist. He saw the world as one extended family of humans, and believed that the purpose of education is to promote self-knowledge. He wrote several songs in the Baul tradition that began with words like: "*If I do not know my own mind, how can I know others' minds?*" He used the Sanskrit term *Atma-shakti* or self-power to describe the goal of education; education is the pathway to awakening our *Atma-shakti* and reaching our ultimate potential as humans (some may see a similarity here with Abraham Maslow's concept "Self-Realization"). Tagore deeply believed in *e pluribus unum* or "out of many, one"; he argued that we empower ourselves by establishing a "bond of relations" with people of different cultures and "races" (when Tagore wrote, the term "ethnicity" was not commonly used in English; well-known scholars including William Jones, Max Muller, and Mortimer Wheeler used the term "race" to designate different groups of people who were believed to be distinctly different in their cultural heritage. Also at that time, the theory of an "Aryan invasion" into the Indian subcontinent, which historians now reject, was believed to be a proven fact and was promoted by European scholars). Tagore was a leading multiculturalist (although this term was not in the common vernacular either) educator and believed that just knowing another language or learning about other cultures is not enough. He used this phrase "bond of relations" several times; in 1925 he cautioned us: "When races come together, as in the present age, it should not be merely the gathering of a crowd; there must be a bond of relation, or they will collide with each other" (Tagore, 1925, "On Education," in *Talks in China, Visva-Bharati*, p. 216).

As a philosopher he recognized that one standard model of education would not be appropriate for all people, especially in poor and impoverished nations. He proposed and actually practiced three types of education (O'Connell, 2003; Tagore, 1929). At the top level there would be "world universities" or open universities that attract outstanding scholars from across the world. It would be a residential campus where eminent scholars, authors, leaders, scientists, artists, and others would live, think, work, and learn from their fellow scholars, especially from those with disparate cultural heritages. It would be something like the Institute for Advanced Studies in Princeton, New Jersey, where physicist Albert Einstein and other eminent scholars lived and worked. The goal is more than gaining knowledge; it would be to study the best from other philosophies and cultures, and develop bonds of relationship among people who have the potential to make a difference in the world. In 1905, Tagore established the Visva-Bharati ("World University") in his Santiniketan ("Abode of Peace") in West Bengal in India as a seat of global learning; it is still thriving, and decades ago it was elevated to the status of national university.

Tagore's second model of education would be for the younger generation or the future citizens and their leaders: like colleges and universities, he designed this model for graduate education, except that the students would not be bound by a rigid discipline-based curriculum. Its educational philosophy and method were driven by the ancient Indian model of *Guru–Sishya Parampara*. A *guru* is a wise master, the *Sishya* is the learner or novice, and *Parampara* is the system of learning used in ancient ashrams, where teacher and learner lived together in a fully committed relationship devoted to learning away from external distractions. For instance, this is how the famous Indian sitar master Ravi Shankar learned his music; he lived in the house of his guru Ustad Alauddin Khan (Shankar was a Hindu and his guru was a Muslim) for many years learning Indian classical music. The *Guru–Sishya Parampara* refers to the unique relationships and bonds between the teachers and their students, which are often more involved than those the students have with their own biological families and parents. Living together on campus, they practice a two-way educational exchange of learning and education. This may sound like a Freirean praxis (the practice of special teacher–student relationships involving joint studies and live-in arrangements), but Tagore began his own *Guru–Sishya* praxix more than a decade before Freire was born (in 1921). The focus is on learning: tests and exams are not used to measure learning. Many parents concerned with providing the best education they can offer to their children send their offspring to Tagore's Santiniketan. For example, Nobel Laureate Amartya Sen studied there. So did Indira Gandhi, the daughter of India's first prime minister, Jawaharlal Nehru; decades later, in 1971, she became India's prime minister herself.

Tagore's third type of education was for the poor and uneducated masses. The great social disparities between the poor and the rich deeply disturbed Tagore. He focused on education as the primary means for his "rural reconstruction" in India; he chose rural areas because at that time more than 80% of Indians lived in rural areas. Extreme poverty, powerlessness, and disparities alarmed him.

For a short but insightful summary of Tagore's philosophy and contributions, see Amartya Sen's review in Alam and Chakravorty (2011), *Essential Tagore.*

Tagore's philosophy of "empowerment education" included three basic principles: enlightenment, empowerment (*Atma-Shakti*), and elimination of extreme disparities. His rural reconstruction experiments focused simultaneously on three empowerment methods: mass education, developing income-generating micro-enterprises, and cooperative banks for financial self-reliance. This approach will be discussed in greater detail under the topic of the microcredit movement in the last chapter of this book (O'Connell, 2002).

Women's Empowerment Movements

Arguably, the earliest women's equal rights movement began when Gautama Buddha's foster mother led several hundred women who were keen on becoming *Bikkhunis*, or women monks. The women implored Lord Buddha to grant them permission to become monks. That was about 2,500 years ago. These women had already taken vows of celibacy and adopted the lifestyle and practices of monkhood (shaved their heads, wore saffron robes, meditated and lived like monks in Ashramas). Queen Maha Pajapati was Buddha's foster mother. After Buddha's biological mother died, soon after his birth, Pajapati nursed him and raised him like his natural mother would have. After the king (Buddha's father) died, Queen Pajapati desired to follow the teaching and the practice of Buddha seriously and requested to be ordained as a Bhikkhuni. But when she approached and asked for permission, Buddha simply said, "Please do not ask so."

> Maha Pajapati was unshaken in her decision. She, along with 500 Bhikkhunis (women novices) from the royal court, shaved their heads and donned the yellow robes. They followed him on foot until they arrived at Vesali where Buddha resided. Upon arriving at the *arama* (residence), they did not ask to have an audience with Buddha for fear of being rejected again. Ananda, the Buddha's cousin and personal attendant, found them at the entrance covered with dust, with torn robes and bleeding feet. Many of them were miserable and in tears of desperation. He learned from them of their request, and on their behalf approached Buddha. Again, Buddha forbade Ananda in the same manner, "Ananda, please do not ask so." (Kabilsingh, 1991)

There are several speculations about why Buddha declined their request:

> First of all Maha Pajapati was a queen who, along with 500 ladies of the court, knew only the life of comfort. To lead a reclusive life, allowing them only to sleep under the tree, or in the cave, would be too hard for them. Out of compassion the Buddha wanted them to think it over. The fact that these women followed him on foot to Vesali is a proof of their genuine commitment to lead religious lives and removed

the doubt that their request might be out of [a] momentary impulse. (Kabilsingh, 1991)

Pajapati and the hundreds of *Bhikkhunis* refused to leave the premises where Buddha resided until their request was approved (like a modern day sit-in or a vigil). Ananda became deeply concerned about the safety and well-being of the women; he pleaded to Buddha that his foster mother and hundreds of devoted women who had already embraced monkhood with unquestionable devotion deserved compassion.

This continued rejection did not diminish the women's commitment to monkhood; they requested Ananda to plead to Buddha on their behalf for a third time. Upon Ananda's third return and request for the women to be ordained, Buddha is said to have agreed after reflecting and determining that rejecting the women again would cause mental anguish for Ananda (Dhammananda Bhikkhuni; Kabilsingh, 1998).

Buddha was initially concerned that the life of monkhood in forests would be too harsh for women to bear. But his foster mother and other women who aspired to the path of monkhood prevailed. The women earned the right to become monks with the blessing from Lord Buddha. They lived a simple life, equal to that of a *Bhikkhu* or monk, and quite different from that of other women. A *bhikkhuni* wears orange robes, shaves her head, lives near the *Sangha* (a monastic community), learns and practices Buddha's teaching and listens to *Dhamma* talks every 15 days (Dhammacaro, 2013; *Dhammapitaka*, Buddhist Dictionary).

In the modern era, women's empowerment movements may be traced back to centuries. Some scholars say that one of the earliest claims made for freedom and equal rights was by an uneducated black slave woman named Mum Bett in Massachusetts. In 1781, Bett successfully sued the state and earned her freedom from slavery. She inspired many black men and women to follow her example to freedom. Toypurina (1760–1799) was a Kizh/Gabrieliño Native American medicine woman, who led the revolt of enslaved and abused native Indians in the San Gabriel mission in California, for which she was severely punished and forced to marry a Spanish soldier (Matsumoto & Allmendinger, 1999). Another pioneer was Mary Wollstonecraft (1759–1797), a British author best known for her book *A Vindication of the Rights of Woman* (published in 1792). She was a forceful advocate for women's equal rights and inspired generations of authors, feminists, and activists.

Men, too, have actively promoted women's rights. Raja Ram Mohan Roy (1772–1833), a prominent Bengali educator and social reformer, successfully led social movements for the education and emancipation of women. He was the chief force behind the movement that convinced the then–Governor General of India, Lord William Bentinck, to legally abolish the horrible practice of "*Sati* immolation" in 1829. The practice required a newly widowed woman to immolate herself on the funeral pyre of her husband. The widow had no choice. This practice dated back to Vedic times in 17,500 –500 BCE. Roy also denounced the caste system, polygamy, and child marriages, and wrote extensively about these issues in self-published newspapers. He also actively supported another eminent educator and social reformer, Ishawar Chandra Vidyasagar, in the successful movement for the right of widows to remarry. In Britain, in 1903, Emmeline Pankhurst founded and led the women's suffrage organization, the Women's Social and Political Union (WSPU). During the First World War, the WSPU mobilized thousands of volunteers and supported the British govern- ment's war efforts. In 1918, voting rights were granted in Britain to women over 30 years old; and ten years later women 21 and over were granted voting rights.

In the United States, Elizabeth Cady Stanton organized the women's movement and led the first women's conference in Seneca Falls, New York, in 1848. Two other prominent feminist leaders, Susan B. Anthony and Lucretia Mott, united with Stanton and provided the leadership for the women's suf- frage movement.

> During the 1850s the women's suffrage movement began to expand; but the Civil War intervened and diverted the momentum away from this movement. Soon after the Civil War ended, the US Constitution ratified the 14th and 15th Amendments to address the issues of constitutional protections and voting rights of citizens. In 1868 the 14th Amendment confirmed Constitutional protection to all citizens, and in 1870 the 15th Amendment guaranteed black men the right to vote. But the constitu- tion defined "citizen" as men. These two amendments energized the women's suffrage advocates to demand for a truly universal suffrage. In 1869, the women's movement formed the National Woman Suffrage Association to fight for a constitutional guaranty for women's right to vote. In 1920, almost fifty years after the 15th Amendment granted black men the right to vote, the 19th Amendment granted women the right to vote in Federal elections. While some states had granted voting rights to women in local and state election before the 19th Amendment was ratified, equal rights of women still remains as a goal yet to be reached. (Source: https://www.nwhm.org/education-resources/history/ woman-suffrage-timeline)

Existential philosopher and author Simone de Beauvoir serves as a major force in analyzing the philosophical issues and existential dilemmas of women in her seminal book *The Second Sex* (1942). She was perhaps the most important feminist philosopher since Mary Wollstonecraft. *The Stanford Encyclopedia of Philosophy* introduced de Beauvoir in these words.

> Unlike her status as a philosopher, Simone de Beauvoir's position as a feminist theorist has never been in question. Controversial from the

beginning, The Second Sex's critique of patriarchy continues to challenge social, political and religious categories used to justify women's inferior status. Though readers of the English translation of The Second Sex have never had trouble understanding the feminist significance of its analysis of patriarchy, they might be forgiven for missing its philosophical importance so long as they had to rely on an arbitrarily abridged version of The Second Sex that was questionably translated by a zoologist who was deaf to the philosophical meanings and nuances of Beauvoir's French terms. The 2010 translation of The Second Sex changed that. In addition to providing the full text, this translation's sensitivity to the philosophical valence of Beauvoir's writing makes it possible for her English readers to understand the existential-phenomenological grounds of her feminist analysis of the forces that subordinate women to men and designate her as the Other. (Source: https://plato.stanford.edu/entries/beauvoir/)

From the philosophical perspective, the most important thinker on women's issues is Germaine Greer. In 1970, Greer published *The Female Eunuch,* which made her a highly influential spokesperson for women's liberation in the United States, Australia, and Europe, and identified her with the new women's liberation movement that was then emerging in the West. For Germaine Greer, the goal of women's liberation was not to obtain equality with men. She rejected simple equality with men and complete assimilation of gender roles that require women to behave like men. Such assimilation for women would make them only the equals of enslaved men. To Germaine Greer, women's liberation should take the form of accepting gender differences in a positive light. Women should gain freedom by defining their own value system and gaining sovereignty over their own fates.

In *The Female Eunuch* she attacked the social conditioning of women in which the roles and rules taught from childhood to feminize girls also deform and subjugate them. While feminists since Mary Wollstonecraft have explored the limitations placed by society on women's knowledge, behavior, and education, Greer looked at the mystery and shame surrounding the knowledge of women's bodies and the constrictions placed on their sexuality. Women, she argued, are conditioned under pressure from the "feminizers" to abandon their autonomy and embrace a stereotyped version of femininity. The result is helplessness, resentment, a lack of sexual pleasure, an absence of joy.

There are several other prominent women thinkers whose ideas were integrated collectively by the feminists as they defined the central issues of what we know as the feminist movement today. The feminist philosophy analyzes the condition and status of women and men to develop a better understanding of how to improve women's lives.

At a more pragmatic level, Betty Friedan of the United States and Sarojini Naidu of India led movements that produced structural changes that helped millions of women. Ms. Sarojini Naidu was a Gandhian who was elected president of India's powerful Congress Party, which led the country to independence and ruled India for more than six decades after independence. One of Naidu's most visible contributions was a controversial culture change; she abolished the *purdah* system that restricted Muslim women because many could not go out in public; if they did, they were required to wear a "purdah" (veil, hijab). This meant that many Muslim women could not take part in education or work outside their homes. As she was a Hindu woman, it was not an easy task for Naidu to abolish a Muslim cultural practice, which antagonized orthodox Muslims.

Betty Friedan addressed the issues of women empirically and led an action plan to mobilize the "second wave" of the women's liberation movement after the women's suffrage movement; while the suffrage movement was primarily about women's voting rights, the second wave led by Friedan was about women's equality in several domains. In her book titled *The Feminine Mystique* (1963), Friedan spelled out empirically the existential problems women encountered and drew a plan of action to deal with these; she led the movement and founded the NOW in 1966. At the fifteenth reunion of her Smith College graduating class, Friedan discovered that most of the women of her graduating class were not happy with their lives. She did a systematic survey of her former classmates. They were all full-time housewives and mothers and had had to abandon their personal dreams. Their job was to keep their husbands and children happy; and they were expected to be happy being housewives. She described her findings in her book, and that was the beginning of the second women's liberation movement. Friedan defined "the feminine mystique" as a "highly idealized image of women" to which they must fully conform despite of their lack of personal fulfillment. Women were expected to perform "perfect housewife roles" ascribed to them by the male-dominated society. This deprived them of all other opportunities of self-fulfillment, which made them unhappy. Women were asking: "Is that all?" that is: What is the meaning of life and what makes a good life?

This is the basic existential question that Beauvoir was asking as a philosopher. The 1950s were a time of regression on several counts. It was just after the end of World War II and the Great Depression; consumerism and material prosperity were on the rise. Fewer women were attending colleges, more were getting married earlier and having babies before they had had the opportunity to explore options or think seriously about what they wanted out of life. More importantly, their roles and responsibilities were structured by men without even asking them what they really wanted.

After Friedan's book created a major impact, especially on educated women, she was appointed to the President's Commission on the Status of Women. She effectively made the best use of her position on the Commission to launch NOW. Friedan and 28 other women met and drafted a statement that became the road map for NOW. The four issues that feminists were concerned with were:

1. Gender differences
2. Gender inequality
3. Gender-based discrimination
4. Structural oppression (e.g., capitalism, patriarchy, and racism)

NOW's current top six priorities are (http://www.now.org/about.html):

1. Advancing reproductive freedom
2. Promoting diversity and ending racism
3. Stopping violence against women
4. Winning lesbian rights
5. Achieving constitutional equality
6. Ensuring economic justice

Gloria Steinem was another powerful voice in women's struggles for equality. She began her illustrious career writing for the television show *That Was the Week That Was*. Subsequently Steinem and Dorothy Pitman Hughes founded an organization called the Women's Action Alliance. In 1972, they published their own magazine on feminism, called *Ms.* In 1972, *McCall's* magazine named Steinem "Woman of the Year." Steinem argued for legal abortion (which was codified in the Supreme Court case *Roe vs. Wade* in 1973), founded *Ms.* Foundation of Women, the Coalition of Labor Union Women, and the National Women's Political Caucus, and published *Outrageous Acts and Everyday Rebellions*; *Marilyn: Norma Jean*; *Revolution from Within: A Book of Self-Esteem*; and *Moving Beyond Words* in 1983, 1986, 1992, and 1994, respectively. Steinem continues her activism internationally on diverse issues that affect powerless poor people and women, including preventing human trafficking and prostitution. As recently as January 11, 2014, Steinem wrote from India, "India taught me how to organize from the bottom up when I came here only a decade after independence and walked through villages with the land reform movement. It changed my view of the world. Now that social justice movements must be as global as the vast inequalities we are trying to change, Ruchira and I and many others are working together" (Steinem, 2012). Ruchira is a leader in the current movement for preventing violence against women in India, and Steinem could not resist the opportunity to join. Steinem is also supporting movements led by other woman leaders such as Dr. Vandana Shiva, in her struggle for the poor farmers who faced financial disaster after they were lured to buy expensive cotton seed from Monsanto. The multinational giant promised that their seeds were pest-resistant and free from weeds. The result was a disaster for the poor farmers; the new seeds produced super weeds and super pests, and the farmers went broke. It is estimated that at least 75,000 farmers committed suicide after their crops failed. This is what Steinem wrote about their struggle:

> On Vandana Shiva: *Today*, she is bringing news of another genetically modified seed scandal. Like the expensive cottonseed from Monsanto that promised immunity from pests and weeds—yet produced super pests, super weeds and such high costs that many Indian farmers suffered financial disaster and at least 75,000 farmers committed suicide—a genetically modified banana is about to be pushed by global interests. The agro industries promised that if the farmers buy this seed that will replace India's 200 varieties of homegrown bananas, they will supply more iron to pregnant women. Of course, its iron content is less than that in turmeric, a common Indian spice. (Gupta & Steinem, 2015)

Academic and Professional Disciplines

Several professional fields, including public health, global health, social work, and community nursing, had deepest involvements in women's empowerment. These programs focused on studying cultural values, power asymmetry, inequalities in opportunities, gender roles, freedom of choice, social bases of power, and empowerment theories and models.

San Diego State University was the first in the United States to establish a women's studies program, in 1970. Professor Lois Kessler was an important contributor to the founding of the first Women's Studies Department there. A nurse, Lois Kessler had degrees in nursing and health education and was a strong advocate of autonomous programs in women's studies. When San Diego State established the department, many other universities were offering some classes in women's studies. By the mid-1970s, there were at least 80 women's studies programs across the United States, and the *National Women's Studies Association* (NWSA) was established in 1977. Its primary objectives were promoting and supporting the production and dissemination of knowledge about women and gender through teaching, learning, research, and service in academic and other settings.

Shortly after San Diego State, Cornell University established a Women's Studies Department that same year (Cornell's program was renamed "Feminist, Gender, and Sexuality Studies" in 2002). As of 2013, the NWSA had listed more than 500 women's studies programs in the United States alone. According to one count, there are more than 900 women's studies programs in the world with registered websites.

Among the various professional disciplines, public health, social work, and community/public health nursing have a strong commitment to population-based empowerment strategies in their own missions and agenda statements; these three have more in common than any other human service professions. Public Health, Social Work, and Community/Public Health Nursing begin with the premise that:

1. Women are parts of families and communities; they do not make decisions alone;
2. Even those in the poorest communities, including women, have the capacity to improve their lives;
3. Empowerment is better than offering short-term charity or help;
4. People have the capacity and right to make informed choices, and
5. Education and social support are the best way to promote empowerment and lasting change.

Community-based empowerment for health-promotion intervention is a win-win collaboration. The community is empowered and gains something tangible; while women gain self-efficacy and measurable knowledge and competencies that may help others.

The words from two eminent educators and inspirational leaders from professions would sum up the essence of how we should approach the issue of community empowerment. The first is Prof. Dorothy Nyswander; she is to health education what Margaret Mead is to cultural anthropology. She is considered to be the mother of health education around the world. Nyswander began her career as a psychologist and activist. In 1946, she established the Health Education graduate program at the University of California–Berkeley School of Public Health; it is now considered to be one of the best in the world. She "retired" in 1957 but was active in inspiring students and colleagues until her death at the age of 104. Nyswander also mentored many GPH leaders, and had an illustrious career spanning more than six decades at the international, national, regional, and community levels. She was ahead of her time in advocating for equality and justice for all people, and was one of the first to introduce the concept of an "Open Society" in public health. This is what she had to say about it:

An open society is one where justice is the same for everyone; where dissent is taken seriously as an index of something wrong or something needed; where diversity is respected; where pressure groups cannot stifle and control the will of the majority or castigate the individual; where education brings upward mobility to all; where the best of health care is available to all; where poverty is a community disgrace not an individual's weakness; where greed for possessions and success is replaced by inner fires for excellence and honor; where desires for power over men (and women) become satisfactions with the use of power for men (and women). (Nyswander, 1966)

More than 65 years ago, Nyswander was advocating for equality, justice, respect for diversity, and elimination of poverty as our professional duties. It is gratifying to note that the United Nations has operationalized Nyswander's vision of the "Open Society" in the UNDP's HDA and its MDGs. As a young graduate student, this author had the good fortune to have the opportunity to know her closely, especially after she retired. Her deep insights and keen dedication to empowering neophytes were astounding. This reflects her own values as a person; her sage-like grace and humility inspired everyone. One of her mantras was "Start where the people are." Her message was not fully clear then, but as decades have passed and professional challenges across the world have taught us some sobering lessons, her message is becoming clearer.

There is a remarkable parallel between Nyswander and the eminent social work scholar Barbara Solomon, the author of *Black Empowerment: Social Work for Oppressed Communities* (1977). In her review of the history of social work in the United States, Solomon informs us that the idea of empowerment was dominant in the American social work ethos since the 1890s. In the preface of her book, she writes: "Social work's commitment to helping marginalized and impoverished people empower themselves is as old as the occupation itself." She goes on to say that, in social work, the professionals "have viewed clients as persons, families, groups, and communities with multiple capacities and possibilities, no matter how disadvantaged, incapacitated, denigrated or self-destructive they may be or have been" (1977, p. 1). Solomon presents the concept of "empowerment" as a goal of problem-solving with clients who belong to a stigmatized group. The manner in which the negative evaluation of such individuals leads to feelings of powerlessness and reduced social effectiveness is described. Criteria are suggested for measuring whether a particular professional intervention is likely to lead to empowerment. The sociohistorical context that influences problem-solving with black clients is discussed, and specific philosophical and scientific issues relating to the empowerment concept are evaluated. The effects of the negative images of blacks are traced as they operate in major social institutions such as the family, peer groups, and schools. These effects are connected to the emergence of characteristic personal and social problems encountered in black communities.

Solomon's book, the role of the social work professional is examined through practical exercises and discussions.

The historical record will show that the professions of public health, nursing—especially community or public health nursing (PHN), and social work, grew out of a deep concern for the suffering of the poor and powerless, and the sick and wounded soldiers in war. In 1853, Florence Nightingale began her professional career as the superintendent of the newly established Hospital for Invalid Gentlewomen in London. At the request of the British government, she led a team of 38 nurses to Turkey as the Superintendent of Female Nurses during the Crimean War (1854–1856). She was deeply shocked by the lack of healthcare and hygiene that the British soldiers had to endure. She returned from the war permanently sick and invalid, but continued to promote nursing care for the poor and unfortunate. Grateful to her for her services in the Crimean War, Britain raised funds and established the first School of Nursing in London. That philosophy and spirit of caring for the sick, especially among the poor and powerless, still drives the nursing profession across the world. The Civil War laid the foundation of nursing education and the profession in the United States. At that time, there were no American nursing schools or scholastically trained nurses (Egenes, n.d.; see also Kalisch & Kalisch, 1995). Neither the Union nor the Confederate armies had nurses to take care of the wounded or sick soldiers. In fact, more soldiers died of sickness than from battle wounds. It is estimated that more than 3,000 women volunteers joined the Civil War as nurses, but they had no formal training. After the Civil War ended, some of these women were instrumental in establishing the first school of nursing. Dorothea Dix and Kate Cummings served as the superintendents of nursing for the Union and Confederates armies, respectively. Other pioneers included Clara Barton, also a volunteer nurse during the Civil War: she later founded and became the first president of the American Red Cross; and the famous poet Walt Whitman, who served as a volunteer in the Union Military Hospital in Washington, D.C. (for a history of the evolution of nursing, see Egenes, *History of Nursing*, n.d.).

Currently, the field of nursing is undergoing a major transformation. The Institute of Medicine (IOM) in collaboration with the Robert Wood Johnson Foundation (RWJF) has undertaken a major initiative on the future of nursing.

The initial cornerstone of the program is a major study whose goal is to produce a transformational report on the future of nursing. The initiative began with a serious examination of four issues, with the goal of identifying vital roles for nurses in designing and implementing a more effective and efficient health care system. These are:

"1. Reconceptualizing the role of nurses within the context of the entire workforce, the shortage, societal issues, and current and future technology;

2. Expanding nursing faculty, increasing the capacity of nursing schools, and redesigning nursing education to assure that it can produce an adequate number of well-prepared nurses able to meet current and future health care demands;

3. Examining innovative solutions related to care delivery and health professional education by focusing on nursing and the delivery of nursing services; and

4. Attracting and retaining well-prepared nurses in multiple care settings, including acute, ambulatory, primary care, long term care, community and public health."

Robert Wood Johnson (August 31, 2010) http://www.nationalacademies.org/hmd/Activities/Workforce/Nursing.aspx. Accessed January 6, 2017.

(Note: Item 4 includes primary care and community and public health as components of nursing as well.)

In Figure 5.1, the intersection of the three circles in the Venn diagram contains the key words or principles that are commonly found in the mission and priority statements of these three professions: (1) public health (PH) including global health; (2) social work (SW); and (3) Public Health Nursing (PHN).

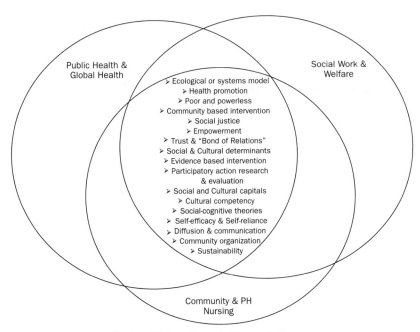

FIGURE 5.1 Shared Professional Values. Figure by Snehendu Kar.

The shared values identified from websites of three professional associations—Public Health (PH), Social Work (SW), Public Health Nursing (PHN)—are summarized in Figure 5.1. They believe:

1. in using a "systems" or "ecological" or "multilevel" approach for diagnosis and action
2. in working with communities and families outside clinical settings
3. in helping the powerless and disadvantaged groups
4. in respecting cultural diversities, freedom of choice, and dignity of people in distress
5. that even the poorest have social and cultural capitals that can be mobilized for progress
6. that even the poorest and weakest with help have the capacity to improve their destiny
7. that empowerment is an important goal and better than offering short-term charity or help
8. that we (professionals) should learn how to be more humanistic in multicultural communities
9. in evidence-based and participatory action research, implementation, and evaluation
10. in building mutual trust and "bonds of relations," especially in multicultural communities
11. in a two-way learning and development from participatory empowerment action
12. in accountability and respecting professional codes of ethics.

Self-Organized Women's Empowerment Movements (SOWEM)

A major goal of this book is to examine whether and how "women's self-organized movements" promote health and quality of life in communities, and how human service professionals may support these movements. Chapters 1 and 2 provided evidence that traditional economic development tends to bypass the poorest, and the record of human development programs shows similar neglect for the poorest who need help most. Under these circumstances, women's self-organized movements, when supported by human service professionals, can play an important role as a third force for social progress.

Generic Issues in Empowerment Research and Action

This section reviews the generic issues in empowerment before analyzing women's empowerment. Considering the importance of empowerment in GPH, several issues deserve serious deliberations (the phrase "public health" is used both as a societal goal and to designate a multidisciplinary professional field). A widely accepted definition of *empowerment* by Rappaport (1981) states that it is a process by which people gain mastery over their lives. He has also wisely added elsewhere something like: This is true; and because of this, it is useful to identify several philosophical issues related to adopting empowerment as an operational option.

In their theory of the "social bases of power," eminent theorists Raven and French (Raven 2012, French & Raven 1959) define *social power* as the ability of people to influence other people's beliefs, attitudes, and behavior; they identify six bases or domains of social power through which leaders may influence others. There is a consensus in the literature that empowerment philosophy is based upon the premise that people have the *capacity*, should have the *freedom* to make informed choices consistent with the *values* they have internalized freely, and have the *responsibility* to accept the consequences of their own choices. If we accept this position, then we need to clarify several related issues.

First, how freely have people internalized the values and cultural practices that affect them? The "missing women" often do not have the freedom to make choices that would protect them and keep them alive. Millions of young, poor, uneducated girls do not have the freedom or capacity to refuse female genital mutilation or cutting (FGM/C). Millions of girls and women are lured away from the shelter of their families with lucrative jobs offers by criminal human traffickers: should these women be held responsible for the consequences of their actions? Collier, in his global study of the "Bottom Billion" people, concludes that most of the poorest people are so helpless that they are unable to fight back or organize to empower themselves. There are numerous situations like these when external negative forces in the culture or environment are much too powerful for the victims to overcome. Such situations require more than education; they require strong societal and structural measures.

Second, our cultures often tolerate, if not encourage, heinous crimes in the name of the preservation of cultural traditions. Intimate partners perpetrate most of the heinous crimes and violence against women, and other crimes are perpetrated under the pretext of "cultural practices." A UN study cited below and women activists conclude that a pervasive "culture of rape and violence" exists in many societies; they allow, if not encourage, these heinous crimes. These cultural elements should be effectively eliminated, which calls for culture change; focusing on empowering abused women alone will not do it. Within this context, we need to ask: If all people have an equal right to practice their respective religions and traditional cultural practices (some of which disempower or abuse their people; e.g., FGM/C, child marriage), then what right do we have to stop the abusers? How do we decide which cultural practices should be removed? The answer comes from the global consensus, the UDHR, and the basic values and rights stated in the governing constitutions of numerous nations. Abusive cultural traditions that contradict the values that are protected by global consensus would be legitimate targets of removal, especially if the traditional practices are perpetrated with brutal force against powerless victims. The example below should clarify this point.

> A 2013 UN multi-country study on Men and Violence in Asia and [the] Pacific found that nearly half of the 10,000 men interviewed reported using physical force and/or sexual violence against a female partner, ranging from 26–80 per cent across sites. Nearly a quarter of men interviewed reported perpetrating rape against a woman or girl, ranging from 10 per cent to 62 per cent across the sites. (UN, *IPCD Report*, 2014)

It is important to ascertain when individual/psychological empowerment of the victims alone is not effective. There is a tendency among scholars and educators to believe that psychological empowerment is always good and effective, regardless of whether the root cause of a problem is primarily within the victims or contextual (or in the social or physical environments). Several meta-analyses suggest that more than 90% of studies focus on the individuals at risk—not on organizations and social conditions—to determine where the problem is (Multilevel Intervention/National Cancer Institutes [MLI/NCI] 2011 Golden & Earp, 2012). When local situations are dreadful and violations of human rights occur notwithstanding whether constitutional or legal guarantees from the state are in place, and when the victims are too weak to protect themselves, then focusing on empowering potential victims only is not sufficient: structural changes are needed.

In such the situations, the protection of the victims from the abusers, structural changes to restrain the abusers, and removal of the root causes of victimization should supersede empowerment education for the victims. Psychological empowerment of victims alone would be at best a symbolic act, and at worst, tantamount to victim-blaming (like telling a rape victim she invited the problem and "educating" her after the crisis).

THE GUIDING PRINCIPLES FOR EMPOWERMENT RESEARCH

Analyses of literature identified the following guiding principles that may serve as the philosophical foundations of empowerment research and intervention.

Ecological Approach

Empowerment study and interventions require a holistic—that is, by definition, a multilevel—approach. Holistic medicine requires treatment of the whole person, taking into consideration physical, social, cultural, and environmental factors, rather than treating just the physical symptoms of a disease. Similarly, empowerment research and interventions must study the individuals who are at risk within the social and environmental contexts that cause or exacerbate a problem. Gestalt psychology and Lewin's "Field Theory" are examples of looking at a "person" within the "total environment"; not just studying qualities within a person such as instinct, motivation, or cognition. Most social and behavioral sciences endorse this in principle. It is encouraging to note that the National Institutes of Health (NIH)/ National Cancer Institute (NCI) has adopted an Ecological Model for research and multilevel intervention (MLI) model; in 2011, the NIH sponsored a scientific meeting to review MLI in cancer research. Their review concluded that, while the concept of MLI is accepted widely, in practice more than 90% of the studies focused on the individual level. Similarly, a recent meta-analysis of health education and promotion research published in a leading journal in the field discovered that about 95% of studies dealt with the individual level (Golden & Earp, 2012).

One widely accepted tradition of empowerment theory defines *empowerment* at three levels: individual, organization, and community. Our review shows that a holistic approach to empowerment should include five levels: individual, relationship/family, organization, community, and the macro environment.

Interactive Process

The five levels of the ecological model (discussed under "Ecological Model," below) are not separate; rather, like a biological system or a human body (e.g., circulatory, neurological), model has several subsystems that work together to perform a common function. A *system* is defined as "a set of things working together as parts of a mechanism or an interconnecting network of a complex whole" (*Oxford American English Dictionary*). If one subsystem fails, that affects the entire system; if the heart fails to pump blood as required, the whole person dies. If a family has a setback (e.g., Father loses his job), that affects a child and the family as a whole. Consequently, even if an intervention is designed at the individual level, such as empowering one family member with a self-efficacy problem, a family-level trauma will affect that individual and the intervention process.

Reciprocity

Reciprocity is closely related to interaction; if a child is expected to attend a school-based empowerment program, the mother or father would have to drive the child to school. In return, the teacher/empowerment agent would have to educate, and the child is expected to learn and perform a certain way (e.g., babysit a younger sibling). At home, parents may have to help the child with homework. The principles of interaction and reciprocity mean that even though the aim of an empowerment intervention may be at the individual level, the intervention may have to be at several levels (e.g., family, school, community). Consequently, we need to define clearly whether this is an individual intervention or an MLI that requires different levels of inputs and outputs with considerable interactions among them. Also, the outputs at one level may be inputs for another. For instance, the National Alliance for Mental Illness (NAMI) educates and empowers the family members (caregivers) of mentally ill persons; the family members gain knowledge, skills, and self-efficacy about better care for the ill; and the ill family members get better care. It is hard to imagine any successful empowerment that can be restricted to one level of the ecological model (e.g., individual, organizational, or community level).

Simultaneous Inputs and Outcomes

Often an MLI requires simultaneous inputs at several levels with expected outcomes at more than one level. Let us say that a couple (two live-in partners) are having serious personal conflicts (e.g., marital breakdown or domestic violence). Dealing with that would involve several levels of inputs and expected outcomes (counseling, legal referral help, and financial support). The empowerment agent may choose to work on the problem only at the level s/he chooses and ignore other problems.

The IOM's ecological model is based on Breslow's premise, described by the IOM thus:

> Breslow's approach is less reactive and less directed at problem solving (i.e., treating and preventing) and more forward looking than other approaches. From this point of view, health is more than merely the absence of disease; it is a resource that allows people to live full, productive, and satisfying lives. This perspective is aligned with the World Health Organization's definition of health as a state of complete physical, mental, and social well-being and not merely the absence of disease or infirmity. (Liburd & Sniezek, 2007)

Two points are worth mentioning about the ecological model it includes five levels (Figure 5.2):

1. First, the model includes family or close relations as an important level of determinant of health; this is a separate level from the community level which focuses on people, social networks, and organizations in a defined community.
2. The second level examines close relationships that may increase the risk of experiencing violence as a victim or perpetrator. A person's closest social circle—peers, partners, and family members—influences their behavior and contributes to their range of experience.

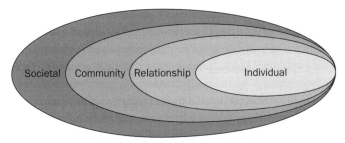

FIGURE 5.2 The Social Ecological Model: Centers for Disease Control and Prevention (CDC).

The first issue in adopting an ecological perspective is to answer this question: "What are the *critical levels* of determinants?" Empirical research on social determinants of health, global consensus statements and charters on health and human development, and social sciences research on human behavior clearly articulate that "family and culture matter." Several modern social and behavioral scientists have made groundbreaking contributions in empowerment and motivation theories: in keeping with our scientific tradition, they have proposed their causal theories and models as generalized and universal propositions and structured these theories and models as context-independent universal realities. This context-independent research paradigm (CIRP) may be appropriate for research in physical and natural sciences, but it is legitimate to ask how valuable is behavioral science research that ignores the causal influences of our family and culture on individual behavior and lifestyles.

In current health-related research, several prominent empowerment theories/models conceptualize three levels of empowerment: individual, community, and organizational levels. Most of the contemporary researchers, who have done pioneering work and deserve credit for making empowerment an important area of research, have proposed three levels: family and culture are not included. The three-level model has been helpful for defining the input levels or actions for empowerment and the outcome levels where an empowerment effect is intended and measured. But current mainstream empowerment theories, as practiced in health-related research (with the exception of the feminist theories and ethnic/cultural theories) do not include *family and culture* as separate levels of determinants. These two are treated under the *ceteris paribus* ("all other things being equal") assumption. Important causal levels of family, gender, and culture are subsumed under exogenous factors (some researchers statistically "control" for these factors, but statistical controls do not explain the processes through which causal factors work; besides, we cannot build a theory if the causal variables are excluded from the model).

Cultural Appropriateness

We need to rethink this critical issue of cultural appropriateness in empowerment theory and actions for health. From a multicultural perspective, we need to measure not only the outcome level of empowerment but also the intervention level/s required for that outcome. While using an ecological model, we must ask what other levels of determinants could affect the intervention. When we use the "ecological" perspective to study social determinants of health, which has emerged as the modus operandi for population-based health programs and is advocated by health research establishments (e.g., WHO, NIH, CDC, IOM), it requires that we use a systems approach that includes all levels of determinants. *Family* is a basic social unit that has a critical influence on human lives, from conception to death. Similarly, *culture* affects our health and quality of life; therefore, empowerment strategy should be culturally appropriate. Empowerment theories and models diminish their own relevance by excluding family and culture from their conceptual parameters.

Gender Inequality

Gender inequality is another universal reality deeply rooted in our cultural values and practices. The international human service organizations such as the UN, WHO, and UNDP have all determined that gender inequality and violence against women are almost always rooted in the cultural attitudes and values of our societies concerning women. For instance, WHO sponsored a six-nation survey of sexual violence against women (cited in Chapter 1), which has revealed shocking levels of culturally endorsed violence against women, including rape. CEDAW and UN Women, among other groups and activists, have coined a new term, "the rape culture," to describe and draw the world's attention to the cultural conditions that allow rapes to happen in the first place and then to blame the victims. A rape culture is defined as:

> an environment in which rape is prevalent and in which sexual violence against women is normalized and excused in the media and popular culture. Rape culture is perpetuated through the use of misogynistic language, the objectification of women's bodies, and the glamorization of sexual violence, thereby creating a society that disregards women's rights and safety.

A Five-Level Ecological Model for Empowerment

Based on a critical review of related literature, we propose a five-level empowerment model: (1) Individual; (2) Family; (3) Community; (4) Organization; and (5) Society/Culture (macro system).

Figure 5.2 presents the CDC ecological model with *four levels* that have been widely used in health-related human development studies and movements globally by public health, SW, community/PH nursing, and other professionals. There are several ecological models proposed by health-related research organizations with some variations in terminologies and diagrams; but they are similar in their basic premises. Human service professions do overlap in their scopes, conceptualization of problems, and philosophies of action. For instance, PH, SW, and nursing are each deeply concerned with marginalized and powerless communities; and their interests and actions overlap considerably. These fields are philosophically and professionally committed to the empowerment of the helpless. Therefore, there are more similarities than differences between these professions. Table 5.1 below

TABLE 5.1
Empowerment Theories by Ecological Levels

Empowerment Levels	Theories, Models, and Methods
I. Individual level	
1. *Hierarchy of needs* Maslow (1943)	Humans are driven to action by five levels of needs
2. *Achievement Motivation* McClelland & Winter (1969), Cantril (1965)	Humans are driven by three needs: need for achievement, need for affiliation, and need for power
3. *Six Bases of Social Power* Raven (1992), French & Raven (1959)	Social power is the potential to influence others' behavior. The six bases of social power
4. *Community Psychology* Rappaport (1987), Perkins & Zimmerman (1995), and Wallerstein (2006)	Enhancement of individual capacities: cognitive, motivational, and behavioral competencies and skills
5. *Yoga and Mindfulness* Indian and Buddhist innovation	Enhancement of higher level of consciousness, renunciation of greed, and spiritual growth liberates from sorrow and illness
6. *Behavior Modification* Skinner (1953)	Operant conditioning theory
7. *Leadership and T-Groups* Lewin, Benne, & Zander	Based on group dynamics and organizational research
II. Family and dyadic level	
8. *Theory of Cooperative Conflict* Sen (1999)	Culture influences women to define self-interest much broadly in a way that makes them vulnerable
9. *Equity Assistance Centers* U.S. Department of Education	Helps parents provide a better home for early childhood development and school performance
10. *National Alliance for Mental Illness (NAMI)*	Largest voluntary organization supports families with mentally ill members. Provides education and tangible support
11. *Family-Centered Help-Giving Practices* Dunst, Trivette, & Hamby (2007)	Meta-analysis study of effects of FCHGP (Family-Centered Help-Giving Practices)
12. *Parental Empowerment*	Parents of children with developmental disabilities; peer-to-peer matching

Nachshen (http://29303.vws.magma.ca/publications/journal/issues/vol11no1/download/nachshen.pdf)

(continued)

TABLE 5.1

Continued

Empowerment Levels	Theories, Models, and Methods
13. *Domestic Violence Prevention* UN, UNDP, CEDAW	One out of three women suffers violence perpetrated by intimate partners (IPV). Prevention is UN's priority
III. Community level	
14. *Community Organization* Freire (1968), Alensky (1971), McKnight (1978), Minkler (1992)	Several models by scholars and activists—their guiding principles and methods vary
15. *Mass Grassroots Movements* M.K. Gandhi, M.L. King Jr., N. Mandela, L. Walesa, V. Havel, Suu Ki Yi	Organized by recognized leaders CBOs, civil rights movements, NOW, race and gender equality, LGBT, organized by community leaders
16. *Self-Organized by Powerless Victims* Organized and led by ordinary and often stigmatized victims	Mothers Against Drunk Driving (MAAD), Sonagachi (sex workers) movement, Women's Dalits, NOW, IPPF, ACT UP
17. *Micro-Enterprise loans* Tagore (1966), Bhatt (2007), Yunus (2010), et al.	Economic autonomy through small microcredit loans
IV. Organizational level	
18. *Leadership and T-Groups* Lewin (1951), Benne, & Lippit	Leadership, group consensus (e.g., Delphi), scenario building, participatory planning
19. *Learning Organizations* Lewin (1951), Triesman (1992), Senge (2006)	Group as the target and medium of change, the "Learning Organization," "Hole in the Wall"
20. *Globalization of Federations*	Successful local and national organization become federation for global reach
21. *Voluntary Organizations*	Federations of national nonprofit HIV/AIDS, Heart, Red Cross, IPPF, philanthropy, Cancer
22. *Economic Development*	World Bank, IMF, OECD
V. Cultural and societal level	
23. *Human Development Approach (HDA)* UN, UNDP, WHO, etc.	UN MDG, global consensus and action plan, HDI monitoring
24. *Global Action Initiatives* Various donors and global federations	Global health, consortiums of nations and CBOs, charitable and missionary organizations
25. *Modernization and Culture Change* Global studies, research, innovations, higher education and disseminations	UNESCO, World Value Surveys (WVS), cultural exchange initiatives for inclusion of stigmatized populations, academic and religious institutions
26. *National Governance, Liberation, and Development*	Governments, CBOs, structural reforms including governance (democracy, freedom, and inclusion)

presents theories and models that are frequently used for social determinants and empowerment research and interventions.

LEVEL 1: THE INDIVIDUAL LEVEL

This level is considered as the first level of empowerment of a person. Several scales are used to measure individual empowerment. It deals with motivation as an important determinant within the individuals. The major motivation theories/models applicable at this level are as follows.

Abraham Maslow: Theory of Hierarchy of Needs

Five human needs range in a hierarchical order of "stages" in Maslow's theory. This theory helps assess the level where the people are, and helps them move to a higher level. It is widely used in counseling and organizational leadership development. Critics say that the stages are too broad and open to different interpretations, that not everyone reaches the peak, and that they may even slide downwards (Maslow did not say this).

David McClelland: Motivation Theory

Humans are driven by three motivations: the need for achievement (nAch), the need for affiliation (nAffil), and the need for power (nPow). People have these needs in different combinations, which determine their behaviors. Organizational leaders can learn about these needs and develop leadership styles for better outcomes. This theory is widely used in management and leadership development research and education.

Bertram Raven and John P. French: Theory of Six Bases of Social Power

The six bases of power are: Informational, Reward, Coercion, Legitimate, Expertise, and Referent (identification). The model explains the nature of each base of power and its potential effects; consequently, it is very helpful in designing empowerment research and interventions. This model integrates elements of social psychology and group dynamics and is widely used by social psychologists and management specialists. The original model did not include the Informational base; fortunately, Raven's insight led him to expand the model by including it. In this age of ubiquitous information technology and social media, the model with six bases is more relevant to a wider audience.

Hadley Cantril's Levels of Aspirations (Cantril's Self-Anchoring Striving Scale)

Cantril (1965) designed a ten-point subjective ladder or scale; 10 is the highest possible level of achievement or satisfaction in life, and 0 is the most unhappy or opposite of happiness. Respondents are asked to describe what constituted 10 (highest) and 0 (lowest) level for them; estimate where they think they are now; where they were five years ago, and where they think they will be on the ladder five years in the future. The scores represented their level of aspirations and achievements as judged by them.

The Cantril Self-Anchoring Striving Scale (Cantril, 1965) has been included in several Gallup research initiatives, including Gallup's World Poll in more than 150 countries, representing more than 98% of the world's population, and Gallup's in-depth daily poll of America's wellbeing (Gallup-Healthways Well-Being Index; Harter & Gurley, 2008). The World Values Surveys (WVS) and the World Bank also use this scale to measure and monitor subjective life satisfaction across nations.

The Cantril Scale, which has been used by a wide variety of researchers since its initial development by Hadley Cantril, is an example of one type of subjective well-being assessment. At the same time, scholarly research has revealed that measurement of well-being is multifaceted, including a continuum from judgments of life (life evaluation) to feelings (daily affect). Different measures of well-being provide different perspectives on the process by which respondents reflect on or experience their lives. The Cantril Scale measures well-being closer to the end of the continuum representing judgments of life or life evaluation (Diener, Kahneman, Tov, & Arora, 2009). Research conducted across countries around the world (Deaton, 2008) indicates substantial correlations between the Cantril Scale and income. This contrasts with measures of feelings or affect that appear to be more closely correlated with variables such as social time (Harter & Arora, 2008). We know that one's level of education, including professional education, has a strong relationship with one's income and quality of life; in fact, one of the UN's and the Sustainable Development Goals (SDGs) and MDGs for 2030 is to promote gender parity in education.

But the individual category is not about formal education; it focuses on seven types of non-formal education and practice to develop mental and behavioral skills:

1. *Mindfulness*-based stress reduction (MBSR) through yoga and meditation; the NIH have recently sponsored several projects on this. Eastern cultures such as India, China, and Tibet have been practicing this for millennia;
2. *Anger-management/negotiation skills* to prevent or manage interpersonal conflicts;
3. *Behavior modification* through incentives and disincentives based on B. F. Skinner's "operant conditioning";
4. *Public health education* and mass literacy targeted at the promotion of specific preventive behavior such as tobacco use prevention and contraceptive use;
5. *Leadership development or "T-Groups"* based on Kurt Lewin's group dynamics and management development models. Major PH agencies

and donors have been sponsoring PH leadership programs for leaders in the field who are highly accomplished in a specialized area (M.D., Ph.D., etc.) but have no education as chiefs of the complex organizations they must lead; and

6. *Self-help and education*—people at various types of risks, or their caregivers, organize themselves into groups where they may learn from others who have to increase self-efficacy—the NAMI, Alcoholics Anonymous, La Leche League, and poor women's microfinance movements are examples of how peer-to-peer help and education can have significant empowering effects.

LEVEL 2: FAMILY AND INTIMATE RELATIONS

Demographers often tend to group persons between 0–15 years of age as children; and dependent children and adults living together as a social unit or a family. Specific research studies, census, and population studies define demographic groups based upon the specific purposes of these studies. Social capital as a construct is often used to describe the capacities and resources a family has at its disposal for its needs and well-being. Research on human development shows that the quality of our family environment fundamentally affects our lives from conception through death. The gestation condition of a mother and her behavior may have irreversible effects on the mental, physical, and emotional health of her baby. Parental involvement and supervision of children's education have significant effects on better school performance and reduced high-risk behavior, including substance abuse and delinquency. On the positive side, we have seen how parental role-modeling can positively affect the academic performance of children of recently immigrant parents.

Domestic violence and abuse happen in families in much greater magnitude than is generally known. Most adult parents would do everything for their children, but some abuse the helpless children. In short, empowerment of parents and adults in families affects the quality of family life. And yet family is not even considered by several prominent theorists as a legitimate level of empowerment. Our review identifies five domains of family life that affect the members of that family.

1. Structure: single parent, nuclear, same-sex, joint, and joint/multigenerational;
2. Marriage and family dynamics (in the U.S., about 50% of marriages end in divorce, and conflicts leading to separation negatively affect the family);
3. Domestic violence interventions (one out of three women report they have experienced domestic violence);

4. Self-care and help from family members; and
5. Empowering caregivers of chronically ill members in the family.

With the emergence of nuclear and single-parent families, mothers in these families do not have access to social support that mothers in extended families (with grand-parents, cousins, multiple experienced elders, and others relatives) do. Consequently, the mothers in nuclear and single-parent families, more often have to depend on help from others outside their families for performing their important roles as the primary care giver. Thus, family structures and dynamics have significant effects on our social relations and HRQOL. Yet, community psychology and sociology often do not give adequate attention to family as an important level of empowerment. For instance, several important scholars of empowerment, including Rappaport (1981) and Zimmerman (1989), advocate use of social support and resources for community empowerment, but do not include "family" as a separate level of empowerment.

Dunst et al. (2007) found a strong relationship between help-giving styles and empowerment in Australian and American parents of preschool children with disabilities who were participating in early-intervention programs. Despite a significantly higher level of enabling practices and empowerment in the American sample, the relationship between enabling practices and empowerment was the same. In both samples, enabling practices accounted for the largest percentage of variance in empowerment and was the only significant predictor variable. Demographic variables (parent age, employment/education status, and child age), locus of control, and the frequency of parental contact with the child's school did not significantly predict empowerment of children. Furthermore, enabling practices accounted for significant variance of empowerment once the other variables were taken into account. The authors assert that both relational and participatory components of help-giving are crucial in the facilitation of empowerment, regardless of cultural and demographic differences. It will be important to determine whether this relationship will continue to hold true for parents whose children do not have a developmental disability.

A United Nations Children's Emergency Fund (UNICEF) study of the level of happiness in industrialized nations (Organization for Economic Cooperation and Development, OECD) found that Danish children and adults are the happiest in the world. The study discovered that parents in Denmark work the fewest hours per week, spend more time with their children, place less pressure on children's academic performance, and have very family-friendly social policies and services from the state (maternal/paternal leave, day-care assistance, and health care). Their children also perform at the top of the list on GPA and standard academic tests—with the exception of a few Asian nations including Singapore, Japan, and South Korea. They also pay a very high level of income tax to support family-friendly state policies (Nordic countries routinely top the lists of happiness rankings, and they all share similar characteristics with Denmark. The U.S. ranks 26th and the U.K. 23rd among the 29 OECD nations [CNN, 2014]). These studies show that children raised in good and happy families and adults in these families have the happiest and best subjective measures of happiness. It is high time for policy planners and scholars to take seriously the importance of parental and family empowerment for promoting the quality of life of families in communities.

The first two chapters of this book reviewed how the field of PH has greatly expanded beyond disease-based paradigms; under the leadership of the United Nations, various donor agencies, development studies, ethnic and gender studies, and GPH initiatives, we have moved beyond the health-promotion paradigm and are now involved in the HDA; according to the HDA, the quality of human relations affects our health and quality of life. This new HDA paradigm requires that we conceptualize the human family as a holistic system consisting of different subsystems or units of human sub-systems ranging from living alone, in dyads, nuclear families, extended families, and various other modalities of family systems. These units offer or deny us the basic conditions in which we expect to live, actualize our human needs, rights, freedom, equality, justice, health, and peace. The three-levels empowerment (individual, organizational, and societal) espoused while still useful in many situations, is not sufficient in responding to the imperatives of the HDA paradigm.

LEVEL 3: COMMUNITY DEVELOPMENT

The third level of empowerment is organized communities or localities. Community organization and development have been popular methods of activism in both traditional and modern societies alike. Scholars, activists, and the victims all have been forceful in advocating nonviolent and constructive community organization and development models, especially after World War II. Historically, scholars and activists have been energized by their ideological and altruistic human values of freedom, equality, and justice. Victims were motivated by their desperation. In the human service fields, public health, SW, and community/PHN have a long tradition of community-based interventions; they list four dominant modes of community-based movements:

1. Community organization and development,
2. Grassroots movements—various "liberation movements",
3. Self-organized movements by victims, and
4. Microenterprise or microcredit movements.

Our review shows that scholars of empowerment in modernized and affluent countries (with the exception of the women's movement) have been indifferent to two vulnerable populations: women and ethnic minorities. Their writings do not differentiate the existential suffering of women and minorities. They, especially male scholars, were concerned about poor and marginalized people in general as oppressed people, but they do not go deeper into empowerment of women or multicultural issues as they affect racial disparities. Our review shows that women's equality and racial-equality movements were mainly organized by the victims and women scholars themselves (e.g., Mary Wollstonecraft, Simone de Beauvoir, Dorothy Nyswander, Betty Friedan, Esther Boserup, Irene Tinker, and Martha Naussbam).

LEVEL 4: ORGANIZATION

Empowerment at the organizational level frequently focuses on the leadership and group dynamics of an organization that affect the productivity, performance, efficiency, and morale of the members of an organization. The tendency has been to recruit the "best" person/s to lead the organization and to provide her/him on-the-job training to develop the most effective leadership style. One of the key issues from the HDA and women's perspectives is that not enough women are educational, occupational, and political hierarchy to rise to top in leadership positions. The central argument is that women should have the opportunity to rise to the level of leadership in professional organizations, business corporations, public media, and political and governmental establishments. For instance, psychologists such as Kurt Lewin, Warren Benne, Ronald Lippit, Alvin Zander, and Davis McClelland have been most interested in looking at leadership and empowerment within the context of defined organizations. In the 1990s, Peter Senge introduced the concept of "learning organizations"; he argued that we should look at organizations as units of learning, just as we consider individuals as learners. The focus of this approach is on education and learning by an organization as a whole, not on training the individuals/leaders. Bandura and other social cognitive theorists focused on beliefs, perceptions, roles, personality, and social learning (vicarious learning) in organizational development. At the macro-level, the UNDP's HDA, development economists, gender studies specialists, and activists focus on the rapid advancement of women in leadership positions in professions, social institutions, academia, corporations, mass media, and politics and elected offices. These opportunities truly empower women, and these women can also serve as role models. According to this philosophy, several countries, especially the Nordic nations, use a reserved quota for women in leadership positions to remedy centuries of discriminations against women. India, for instance, adopted a quota system to reserve a percentage of positions for women and *Dalits*. One may debate the ethics of a quota system, but it empowers those who were systemically excluded and marginalized.

LEVEL 5: SOCIETAL-CULTURAL LEVEL

By definition, this level of change is beyond the scope of individuals and isolated communities. Consequently, empowerment movements at this level require national and multinational organizations and collaborations among them. Modernization is one process through which societies and cultures change over time. Anthropologists have studied how isolated cultures changed through cultural contacts and the acculturation process and the diffusion of ideas and innovations between cultures. Developmental economists, sociologists, and social psychologists have studied culture change and acculturation processes from their respective theoretical paradigms. Since the end of World War II, various authors who have made significant contributions in this area include Lipset (1959), Rostow (1960), Deutsch (1964), Bell (1973), Inkeles and Smith (1974), Hofstede (1980), Inglehart and Welzel (2005), Sen (1998), Boserup (1981), and Triandis (1993). Feminist scholars argued for gender equality from a moral and utilitarian perspective. With the establishment of the UN, the UNDP and various other UN organizations (e.g., WHO, CEDAW, UNESCO, UNICEF, World Bank, International Monetary Fund [IMF]), the world community as a whole began to develop initiatives to promote freedom, equality, health, economy, and the well-being of societies. The focus has changed from individual country efforts to collective global movements under the leadership of the UN organizations.

CULTURAL LEVEL

Culturally accepted and internalized barriers to empowerment are the norms of patriarchal social systems, including inheritance laws, traditional roles of women as caregivers, women's unpaid work at home, women working on their husbands' land or for their business, arranged and child marriages, "honor" killings, FGM/C, dowry systems, male-child preference, purdah, polygamy, and traditional role-modeling. Proponents of gender equality argue that in addition to legal and economic reforms, men's attitude toward women's contributions and worth must also change before substantial progress can be made. Women should be treated as "social capital" and assets, not as dependents, burdens, and free laborers. Research shows that cultural factors, including the devaluation of women, are the primary cause of violence against women, which is highly prevalent in many if not most cultures. There are laws against violence that are ignored, and the perpetrators go free. Studies also show that women's education and empowerment along with cultural changes can enhance quality of life for all, even for those in nations with lower levels of economic development; the Kerala State (in India) model, the UN study on sexual violence, and the happiness study by UNICEF along with several studies discussed earlier support this contention. The cultural perspective also includes the education and training of professionals to develop their "cultural competency," to develop "culturally responsive" intervention strategies, and to develop "participatory action research and evaluation" by professionals and organizations working in multicultural communities. External change-agents and organizations depend on professionals for outreach work; professionals may be well-trained in their field but may lack the cultural competency to be effective in a minority or high-risk population. Reciprocal trust is an important issue; a community may or may not trust an external organization or change-agent in spite of the intentions of those willing to help. This is especially true in marginalized and multiethnic communities where people do not even share a common language with external change-agents or organizations. Such multiethnic communities are common and increasing. The dynamics of multicultural communities discussed in Chapter 4 are particularly relevant in this context.

INDIVIDUAL EMPOWERMENT PERSPECTIVE

Their emphasis is on enhancement of personal/individual (intrapersonal) competencies and peer-support (interpersonal) systems. Literature reviews show that social and behavioral scientists grossly over-subscribe to this perspective. Our reviews in this and previous chapters should persuade us that some of the major problems are deeply rooted in our cultures, distribution of opportunities and resources, and social injustice. There is no doubt that individual empowerment enhances the quality of life of the people involved in such interventions and brings some indirect benefits to their families, but it is important to remember that deep social and cultural barriers that cause powerlessness will not go away if we only focus on individuals who are fortunate enough to have access to empowerment initiatives.

COMMUNITY EMPOWERMENT PERSPECTIVE

This perspective is widely discussed in the literature and is the second most frequently adopted perspective after the individual approach. It includes two categories:

1. *Community organization and community development*: movements developed by agents or organizations from outside the community dedicated to the cause of a community. In this case, the leadership and impetus originate from outside the community; and
2. *Self-organized (bottom-up) movements*: organized and led by the victims themselves.

It is important to make this distinction for several reasons. *First*, external agents or organizations have their own agendas and priorities. When an organization hires a person or funds a specific program (say, obesity control), that initiative may or may not be the top priority of a community. The community may be more interested in job creation or violence reduction. In this situation, a community organizer or her organization does not have the flexibility of switching their own priority; the stated goals of a funded project drive the empowerment agenda. So there is an issue of consistency and inconsistency between two sets of priorities between the community and the external funding agency/organization. Consequently, many issues that a community considers most important may be ignored. The *second* issue is that of the cultural competency of the agency and its employee. *Third*, a clear articulation of who benefits from an externally induced change process is an important issue. If there is a win-win combination, then an externally induced change would be optimal. But our reviews show that the problems of the poor and marginalized are getting worse, not better. We see this reflected in the growing health and income disparities between the rich and poor countries and between the rich and the poor within countries. The inference is clear; over time and across the globe, the rich are getting richer and the poor are getting poorer. Obviously, the problems of the poor and marginalized are being ignored by those in power. In such situations, how long should the poor wait for external agents and agencies to make their lives better? It is therefore not surprising that positive changes often originate from self-organized movements by the powerless victims themselves.

SOCIAL ACTION LITIGATION (SAL)

This perspective focuses on legal activism and the robust application of existing laws to punish ("dis-incentivize") those who violate the rights of others, conduct surveillance, conduct case-management with victims, and advocate and enact new laws and social norms. Examples are vigorous legal and social actions against families, local police, and others who are involved in dowry deaths in India and legislative activism in other nations against "honor" killings, FGM/C, and child marriages. A UN-sponsored study conducted in six South Asian nations interviewed 10,178 men to understand the social determinants of sexual violence and intimate partner violence (IPV), including rape. The findings are alarming. The prevalence of IPV perpetration ranged from 39.3% in Sri Lanka to 87.3% in Papua New Guinea.

Factors associated with IPV perpetration varied by country and type of violence. On the basis of population-attributable fractions, we show factors related to gender and relationship practices to be most important, followed by experiences of childhood trauma, alcohol misuse and depression, low education, poverty, and involvement in gangs and fights with weapons. (Fulu et al., 2013)

Laws against IPV were in place in these countries. However, in spite of laws against IPV, "factors related to gender and relationship practices" are most important determinants of IPV. Activists forcefully argue that cultural factors promote IPV, and existing laws are not implemented in most cases. Similarly, dowries were banned in India in 1961, but according to recent official crime records, dowry murders are increasing.

In 2010, 8391 dowry death cases were reported across India, meaning a bride was burned every 90 minutes, according to statistics recently released by the National Crime Records Bureau. A decade earlier this number was 6995, but climbed to 8093 dowry deaths in 2007. Dowry, although banned by law in 1961 but never seriously enforced, is an ancient tradition prevalent amongst most Indian families. (Bedi, 2012)

One can only speculate how many cases are not recorded. Activists are rightly insisting that it is essential to change men's attitudes about the "culture of rape and violence"; protection of women, and strict enforcement of the laws on the books, should be our priorities. This perspective appropriately shifts the focus onto the real social determinants of violence against women, not on blaming the victims or on passing more laws while existing laws are ignored.

MACRO-ECONOMIC PERSPECTIVE

Esther Boserup, Tinker, Nussbaum, Sen, Huq, and others have argued that the exclusion of women in economic development initiatives not only harms the women themselves, but also hinders the overall economic development of societies and nations. This recognition has led the UNDP to use a Gender Development Index (GDI) and gender empowerment measures (GEM) to monitor and rank women's status across the UN's Member Nations. Gender development scholars and activists have played key roles in the movement.

The macro-economic perspective looks at one of the distal or root causes of powerlessness at the macro-level; economic empowerment and bringing home a paycheck enhance a woman's position and self-efficacy. Reduction of gender inequality, and support for women's education, career opportunities, paid employment, income parity with men, women's leadership in governance and a free press, legal reforms, and the removal of social and cultural "unfreedoms" are central to this perspective. The UN, WHO, World Bank,

IMF, UNICEF, UNESCO, CEDAW, major donors, and nonprofit multinational organizations are most active in this domain.

MICROENTERPRISE PERSPECTIVE

Critics of the standard or conventional macro-economic development perspective forcefully point out that the last five decades of economic development efforts led by the IMF, World Bank, and other donors have failed to benefit those who need help the most. Income disparities continue to increase. This recognition has led to the development of innovative micro-economic or microfinance initiatives (MFI) directed primarily at poor women, which have shown remarkable success; recent examples include Ahmedabad's SEWA (Self-Employed Women's Association) and Bangladesh's Grameen Bank initiatives. This perspective focuses on increasing "freedom" and gender-emancipating values and practices at the local level. The central theme of this perspective is organized local action to meet a global problem. It subscribes to the overall philosophy of the human development movement. One local indicator of human development is increased personal income and freedom for poor women, which allows them to take better care of their children and families (not material gains alone). Microenterprise movements in India, Bangladesh, and other poorer countries have demonstrated that, even in poor, traditional, and Islamic cultures, which tend to have greater gender inequality, micro-enterprise projects work; contrary to the concerns of their critics, they do not create a clash between the two genders and between traditional and modern cultural values.

The MFI has become a global movement, and it is now difficult to find a nation where MFI has not been adopted (including rich nations like the U.S.). The emphasis is on the enhancement of women's employable skills, equitable employment, and sustained income-generation. One legitimate criticism of the MFI program is that it only benefits a small number of women and families. Given that the two other alternatives combined (economic development [ED] and the human development approach [HDA]), have failed to reduce disparities between the poorest and the richest, our communities would be better served if we invest more efforts and resources to promote self-organized development movements (the third path). The case studies and meta-analyses of self-organized women's empowerment movements presented in this volume clearly demonstrate that poor, powerless, and ordinary women, with little help from dedicated professionals, can and do lead empowerment movements that fundamentally transform their life and well-being. The Grameen Bank project began with a few families in one village; now it is transformed the lives of millions of families in several countries. The SEWA initiative began in one town in India; now it has the biggest MFI and cooperative organization in India. Both have received numerous international recognitions, including a Nobel Prize for the founder of the Grameen Bank, Muhammad Yunus, and the UN Medal for Ila Bhatt, the founder of SEWA. Both projects have been adopted by several nations, including economically advanced nations for their pockets of poor people.

John Rawls (1971) and Amartya Sen (1990, 1999), two preeminent contemporary social philosophers, hold somewhat similar views. Rawls' theory defines "justice as fairness." He holds that in a pluralistic society, there may never be full equality among all members in every aspect of life. Rather, a just society must find a "fair" process for distributing its goods and opportunities (which he calls "primary goods") among its members. The five primary goods are basic liberty, freedom of movement and choice of occupation, powers and prerogatives of social position, income and wealth, and social bases of respect. According to Rawls, fundamental fairness in distribution of these primary goods is more important than numerical equality. Furthermore, for the sake of such fairness, sometimes we must treat people differently in special circumstances (e.g., maternity leave, special privileges for the disabled). Rawls gives us a useful framework to look at important domains where reform is needed. Clearly, by Rawls' criteria, women are not treated fairly. According to his theory of justice, women deserve several special treatments, not as a favor to them, but as a just society's obligation to treat all with equal justice and fairness.

Sen's (1999) model of "cooperative conflict" describes the conditions and acculturation processes that deprive women of their basic power and bargaining position within the family and society. Society perpetuates conditions or "unfreedoms" that are deeply rooted in our cultures; these conditions place women in no-win situations. Consequently, empowerment of women requires a fundamental culture change resulting in men's favorable perception of women's contribution as the prerequisite for any social reform. Reforms of specific welfare systems, in the absence of women's overall empowerment and culture change will not be effective in remedying the exploitation of women.

According to Rawls, Sen, Haq, Moser, Boserup, and others, lack of freedom and unfair treatment of the disadvantaged underlie all social and welfare inequalities. Until the sources of these "unfreedoms" are removed and women are empowered, true social welfare will remain elusive. The Beijing Declaration and the UN Platform of Action echo this position when they insist that we must "intensify efforts to ensure equal enjoyment of all human rights and fundamental freedoms for all women and girls who face multiple barriers to their empowerment and advancement because of such factors as race, age, language, ethnicity, culture, religion, or disability, or because they are indigenous people" (Beijing Declaration, paragraph 32, UN 1996). According to the UN Secretary-General's report in February 2014, we have not yet met the MDG of gender equality targeted for 2015.

The EMPOWER Model

This chapter concludes with the self-organized EMPOWER (acronym) model that is based on our ongoing meta-analysis of self-organized women's empowerment movements across the world. The EMPOWER acronym stands for the seven *most frequently used methods* by self-organized empowerment movements. These are:

1. E = Empowerment training and leadership development
2. M = Media use, advocacy, and support
3. P = Public education, participation, and grass roots movements
4. O = Organizing networks including cooperatives, unions, affiliations, and associations, etc.
5. W = Work training, cooperatives, unions, and MFI (microfinance initiatives)
6. E = Enabling services, emergency aids, crisis intervention, and
7. R = Rights protection and promotion, including SAL (social action litigations).

TWO-STEP METHOD

Our Self-Organized Women's Empowerment Movements (SOWEM) research and interventions consist of two phases. The first is a meta-analysis of 40 case studies which led to the development of an EMPOWER model, first published in 1999 in our seminal paper "Empowerment of women for health promotion: A meta-analysis" (Kar et al., 1999). This first meta-analysis included only four case studies that primarily focused on health promotion; others were on human rights, equal rights, and MFI (Microfinance Initiatives). Four cases on health promotion is too small a sample size for any statistical analysis and inferences. Consequently, in the second phase, we added 40 health promotion (HPDP) cases and completed an expanded meta-analysis with 80 case studies. The second meta-analysis served as the background paper for the first World Conference on Women and Development, sponsored by WHO, at the Kobe Center in Japan in 2000 (Kar, 2000a).

Figure 5.3 presents our EMPOWER model, which consists of the following: (1) five empowerment *levels;* (2) initial condition and four *stages* of

I. FIVE EMPOWERMENT LEVELS (Units) : Individual, Family, Organization, Community, and Nation/Society

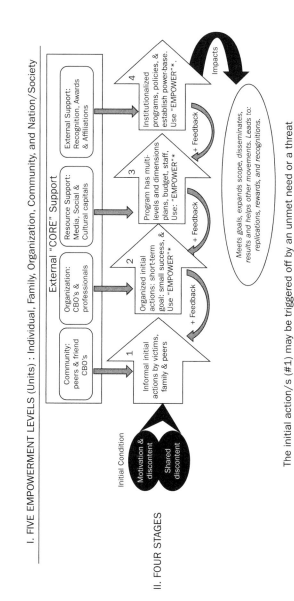

The initial action/s (#1) may be triggered off by an unmet need or a threat

* The "EMPOWER" (acronym): the seven empowerment methods (dimensions)

E = Empowerment training and leadership development
M = Media use for support and advocacy
P = Public education and participation
O = Organize partnerships: cooperatives, coalitions, and federations
W = Work and job training including Microfinance initiatives (MFI)
E = Emergency and enabling services
R = Rights protection and promotion

III. SEVEN DIMENSIONS
(Actions)

FIGURE 5.3 The EMPOWER Model.

empowerment processes; (3) seven EMPOWER *dimensions* or categories of empowerment methods; and (4) four sources of CORE *supports* required for successful empowerment movements. It is important to note that while there are five levels of empowerment theory, intervention and impact evaluation, the level of public health intervention is the community or the "public"; not an individual.

EMPOWERMENT DOMAINS

There are four empowerment *domains:* (1) human rights (HR), (2) equal rights (EQRT), (3) economic development (ED), and (4) health promotion and disease prevention (HPDP). Several case studies suggested a fifth domain— spiritual empowerment. However, the case studies analyzed do not include operational definitions and standard measures of a spiritual dimension; consequently, at this point empirical measures and analysis of the "spiritual" domain of empowerment is not included in the EMPOWER model. In our next phase we are exploring this missing domain.

EMPOWERMENT STAGES

The EMPOWER process consists of an initial discontent or motivation for change, followed by the following four processes: (1) initial individual spontaneous actions by victims; (2) organized actions by victims and peers with local support; (3) a multilevel intervention (MLI) for empowerment movements with its own objectives, methods, and budget; and (4) self-organized methods for institutionalization, expansion, and replication of an effective movement, leading to national and international recognitions and awards.

EMPOWERMENT CORE SUPPORT

The EMPOWER model identifies four CORE (acronym) supports: (1) *Community* and peer-support; (2) *Organizational* support from CBOs and local agencies; (3) *Resource* support, including seed money, social and cultural capital; and (4) *External empowerment* support, needed for carrying out specific EMPOWER movements.

EMPOWER DIMENSIONS

EMPOWER dimensions include seven categories or types of methods, which make up the acronym.

The next chapter (Chapter 6) presents a description of the meta-analysis of 80 SOWEM case studies using the EMPOWER model, the key findings, and implications. There are 86 case study summaries (in chapters 7–10)—six of these did not have complete information on all research questions, but are included in this book as they are interesting and innovative. These six are excluded from the meta-analysis, however.

6

A Meta-Analysis of Self-Organized Women's Empowerment Movements (SOWEM)

It is not for themselves, it is for the children. And that
is the key to everything because when one woman
defends her own child, she defends them all.

—Maria Elena Moyano, assassinated leader of *ollas communes* (the community kitchen movement, Peru; Intermon, 1997)

This chapter presents the meta-analysis of 80 self-organized women's empowerment movements from across the world that were initiated and led by ordinary women to address major existential threats confronted by them and their families. The significance of women's empowerment and the theoretical issues that drive this meta-analysis have been presented in the previous chapters; the implications of the important findings will be discussed in the last chapter (Chapter 11) of this book, along with the major findings and implications of the results from a review of all chapters of this book.

Our study included 86 case studies. The Meta-analysis used a two step process: the first step is a meta-analysis of 40 exemplary case studies that met our selection criteria; but there were only four health promotion (HPDP) case studies. This small number was not adequate to compare whether the EMPOWER methods used in HPDP movements varied from case studies in other three domains. Consequently, in the second step we added 40 HPDP case studies and completed our final Meta-analysis. The statistical results presented are from the Meta-analysis of 80 case studies. In addition, there were six innovative case studies from hard to reach populations (e.g. human trafficking, sex-workers, domestic violence) but these did not provide the required quantitative data to answer all six research questions. For this reason, these six were included in descriptive discussions but excluded from the statistical analyses.

The four chapters immediately following this one (Chapters 7–10) present a brief summary of each case study so that the readers will have a glimpse of each movement, with comparable information on each, and sources to consult for further information. The case studies are grouped into four empowerment domains: Human Rights, Equal Rights, Health, and Income. The aggregate statistical analyses do not convey the rich information on the dynamics and uniqueness of the cases; the case study summaries will allow the readers direct access to the basic and qualitative information on these 80 self-organized empowerment movements. Perceptive readers may draw their own conclusions from these case summaries and may choose to follow up the developments in the movement/s they are interested in. It is rare for a reader to find a source that presents a range of 80 self-organized women's empowerment movements across the world, with comparable information on each, from which they may derive implications for further study or action. This chapter describes the EMPOWER model as an acronym of the seven methods most frequently used by the women to address their problems and empower themselves.

In times of dire need and in times of relative stability, women and mothers (WAMs) offer their toil and sweat to keep their families healthy and happy, and their environments livable as best they can. Any threat to a woman and her family compels her to initiate protective and preventive action. Results confirm that even the most disenfranchised and deprived WAMs do their best to improve the quality of life of themselves and those around them. Impoverished women in all countries, rich and poor, lead and organize movements, set up small businesses (microenterprises), build infrastructure, and struggle to change or better implement existing laws that ameliorate their situation, and through these processes empower themselves. At times when those in powerful positions ignore the plights of the poor communities and victims of injustice, ordinary women and mothers, in rich and poor nations alike, mobilize themselves to initiate actions and add strength to public health movements to prevent or reduce threats to their children and families (e.g., prevention of drunk driving, gun violence, and the AIDS epidemic). In addition to movements for women's suffrage and gender equality, women across the globe, from poor and rich nations and diverse sociocultural and political systems, are confronting institutional and cultural barriers that perpetuated violence against women and children for centuries (e.g., prevention of domestic violence, dowry deaths, female genital mutilation/cutting or FGM/C, child marriage, polygamy, "honor" killing, human trafficking, and victimization of sex workers). The recent example of the 15-year-old Afghan girl Malala's courage to advocate girls' right to education, in spite of life-threatening opposition—actually being shot in the face—by the extremist Taliban in Pakistan, is an inspiring example; her life-threatening assault by the Taliban did not frighten her into quitting. Indeed, her inner convictions and the worldwide support she has received have emboldened and empowered her.

Although this is a dramatic example, it is not uncommon. We have found several examples of courageous women, including those who are young and illiterate, leading bold movements that fundamentally transform the lives of those they fight for and in that process become empowered. Examples include: 14 semi-illiterate women in Argentina leading the *Madres de Playa Mayor* movement against the brutally oppressive military junta regime, demanding news of the whereabouts, and the release of, their "disappeared" sons and relatives (some of these women were assassinated); the then youngest Nobel laureate, Rigoberta Manchu of Guatemala, leading the struggles of the indigenous Quince Indians' right to keep their ancestral farming land (she was only 29 when she received her Nobel Prize for peace; her father was killed, and her mother was raped and killed); uneducated mothers organizing against violent gangs to protect their children and families against gang- and drug-related violence; the Sonagachi sex-workers' movement in Kolkata (Calcutta), which organized against abusive police and pimps and demanded preventive care against HIV/AIDS as a legitimate sex-worker's right (they also organized the first annual international sex-workers' conference and gained protective support from local government and the municipal public health department (Swendeman et al., 2009). A similar movement that was led and organized by sex workers in Tijuana, Mexico, was documented by Dr. Sonali Chaudhuri at UCLA).

These and similar examples led us to ask the question: Are these rare exceptions, or can and do ordinary women self-organize movements that transform their lives for the better when the "powers that be" do nothing to help them? This question was the genesis of our meta-analysis project.

Six Research Questions

This chapter presents the meta-analysis framework, methodology, and key lessons we have learned from our meta-analysis of the 80 case studies of women-led "successful" movements that have significantly reduced threats to themselves or enhanced the quality of life (QOL) of their children, themselves, and their families. We asked *six research questions*:

1. Can and do ordinary women self-organize and lead successful movements that significantly improve health and quality of life (QOL) of their families and communities?
2. If yes, what are the characteristics of these women?
3. What problem/s motivate them to organize and act?
4. What methods are used by the successful movements?
5. Who and what kinds of support or opposition do they encounter?
6. What are the intended and unintended outcomes of these movements?

We also collected relevant information on the larger social context of the movements that may affect the movements and their outcomes. The contextual information includes the overall historical, socioeconomic, cultural, political, and serendipitous events (e.g., change in ruling party, war, natural disasters, and unplanned events that may affect the overall context). The chosen case studies represent women from disparate cultures and from poor and rich nations who successfully improved their overall QOL.

We studied "successful" self-organized empowerment movements to discover whether and how often various empowerment methods are used by these movements, because people normally write and publish success stories. Consequently, well-documented success stories are more readily available. Our content analysis and statistical methods required that we have sufficient information on all six research questions and the relevant contextual information for each case study (we had to exclude several successful case studies that did not meet this inclusion requirement). Ideally, we would have liked to have an equal number of case studies of movements that have failed so that we might have robust statistical comparisons between the successful and unsuccessful empowerment movements. Unfortunately, in spite of our best efforts over several years, we could not find more than three case studies of failed movements that met our criteria of inclusion (i.e., sufficient information on all six research questions). This is a limitation that is beyond our control. (We have initiated a project that identifies failed movements and uses "key informant" interviews to collect information and document these cases. It would take some time before we would have enough failed movements for statistical comparisons.) Without a sufficient number of well-documented unsuccessful case studies, it would be impossible to statistically test and draw inferences on similarities and differences between methods used in successful and unsuccessful movements. So the primary purpose of this chapter is to examine and learn the lessons from successful cases about "what works"; these successful case studies tell us what worked in similar situations, not why movements failed. Given this caveat, we believe that the benefits of knowing what works from a meta-analysis of a large number of case studies far outweighs the limitations of this approach. The alternative is to ignore available knowledge and base intervention policies on personal preferences and unexamined collective experience; that is a far worse option.

In this study, "success" is defined as accomplishing the stated goal of a movement and inspiring others to join and/or adopt a movement's goal and methods elsewhere. For example, the Mothers Against Drunk Driving (MAAD) movement began with one mother's struggle against prevention of drunk driving in California and now has more than 600 chapters in several nations; similarly, the Grameen Bank in Bangladesh began in one small poor village and has inspired similar microcredit movements in many countries worldwide.

A final note about the inclusion criteria is warranted here. Of the 80 case studies included in our meta-analysis, all except one (the Grameen Bank's microcredit movement) were initiated and led by women to enable themselves and other women like them to cope with existential threats faced by them or their families. Although the Grameen movement was started by a man, the movement itself was intended to help women. It was organized in small groups of village women, more than 97% of borrowers were women, and the loans were given to women organized in small working groups as collective loan guarantors (not as individual women seeking a loan). The women were required to perform tasks and manage their loan-related activities as a group. We believe that the primary reason for the initiative's remarkable success (more than 97% repaid their loans on or before the deadline and increased their family income) was the self-organizing workgroups of women and their motivation to succeed in order to benefit their needy children. Thus, although the project was initiated by a man, the Grameen Bank movement meets our criterion of a women's movement organized by women and for themselves.

Finally, we define the "ordinary woman" as someone who is not a person occupying a powerful position, inherited or earned (e.g., wife or daughter of a head of state or a leader of a major political party, or a president/CEO of a major organization). For instance, as of our last count, there have been more than three dozen women heads of state in the world; most of them were the wives or daughters of heads of state or ruling political parties, such as Indira Gandhi (India), Benazir Bhutto (Pakistan), Sirimavo Bhandaranaik (Sri Lanka), Begum Khalida (Bangladesh), and Isabela Peron (Argentina), to name a few. They were women, but not ordinary women; they were *extra*-ordinary women from established political dynasties. Our study is about ordinary and powerless women as they organize and lead movements that empower themselves and promote their family well-being.

METHODOLOGY

In order to identify suitable cases for the meta-analysis, a literature review was performed. Through an extensive bibliographical search (MELVYL, ORION), the authors uncovered relevant resource materials related to women's empowerment during the last three decades. Other investigative methods included telephone and personal interviews with members of national and international agencies; international, national, and local women's organizations including key informants when possible; review of graduate-level course syllabi and master's and doctoral theses dealing with community organizations and development; consultation with professionals and scholars; lists of participants in conferences related to gender, health, and human development; and website searches for information on relevant organizations and contact persons.

The case studies that met the following criteria are included in the meta-analysis.

1. *Availability*: of reliable written descriptions from authoritative published articles, papers, books, etc., from credible publishers or organizations.
2. Information on all six research questions and the overall context must be available for data extraction and comparative analysis.
3. *Representativeness:* case studies represent economically developed and less developed countries and culturally diverse societies.
4. *Domains*: case studies represent all four domains: human rights (HR), equal rights (ER), economic development (ED), and health promotion and disease prevention (HPDP).
5. *Impact:* there must be measurable information on the level of problem/s or a baseline condition before the movement began and the outcomes/impacts of the movements at later date/s.
6. *Empowerment:* there must be objective and subjective indicators of empowerment with clear description of the efforts and methods used by the movements that can be attributed to the movements (Kar, 1989).
7. *Uniqueness*: the movements should be effective and innovative. Effectiveness is defined in terms of the degree to which the intended goals were achieved; innovative movements must be original, not used by others before, and then adopted.

Content Analysis of Case Studies

For each of the case studies, we conducted a content analysis to extract basic and comparable data on seven predetermined categories or dimensions of information, using the EMPOWER model and the six research questions and contextual background.

Content analysis extracted and quantified data on the following components of movements:

1. *Identifiers*: case study name, location, year of founding, rich/poor country (using the World Bank's classification: Low income, Lower middle income, Upper middle income, and High income); website/phone/contact for follow-up; source of original description/report.

2. *Problems:* what motivated the movement? Description of the problem, and the state of affairs before and after the program.

3. *Leadership and beneficiaries:* who started, led, and sustained the movement, and who followed, their demographic characteristics, what motivated them, and costs/benefits.

4. *Empowerment methods*: how often and which of the seven empowerment methods (EMPOWER) were used. Description of the process of empowerment efforts and the movement's impacts both objective (quantitative efforts) and subjective (self-assessment or self-efficacy).

5. *Support/Barriers:* description of the nature of support received and opposition encountered. Description of the four types of the CORE support (Kar, 200b): support (capacity development, training, coalitions, and cooperatives).

6. *Macro-environment:* macro-social context and historical developments (exogenous) that affected the movement.

7. *Effects/Impacts:* intended and unintended outcomes, extent to which original goal was reached, sustainable and institutionalized impacts, and national and international recognition.

Box 6.1 presents the overall framework for quantitative and statistical comparisons for the meta-analysis of movements using the framework of the EMPOWER model.

RESULTS

Individual vignettes of each of the 80 case studies are presented in chapters 7 through 10 and categorized by domain. The cases are broken down as follows: 11 cases on HR (Chapter 7); 14 cases on ER for women in the social, economic, and political spheres (Chapter 8); 8 cases on ED (Chapter 9); and 47

BOX 6.1
The Meta-Analysis Framework

EMPOWER Dimensions: The meta-analysis compared and analyzed the extracted data from the 80 individual content analyses. Group comparisons are used to examine whether and how the EMPOWER dimensions/methods used by the 80 cases vary: first, across four empowerment domains for all cases (Tables 6.1 and 6.2); second, comparisons by levels of industrialization (Table 6.3); third, how the seven EMPOWER dimensions or methods vary between the health-promotion (HPDP) domain versus the non-HPDP domains (human rights, equal rights, and economic development). Table 6.4 presents the EMPOWER methods for only the health-promotion domain, broken down by level of industrialization.

Note: Content analysis deals with qualitative or descriptive information from each case study; Meta-analysis deals with quantitative and statistical analyses of data from all/large number of case studies.

cases on health promotion (Chapter 10). Each vignette provides a brief description of the seven dimensions of the case:

1. problem,
2. impetus,
3. leadership for change,
4. empowerment method/s used,
5. supporters and opponents,
6. macro-environment or context, and
7. outcome or current status of the initiative.

The EMPOWER Model

Our content and meta-analysis identified seven categories of empowerment methods or dimensions that were most frequently used (activities and who performed these) by these women-led movements.

Cochran's Q test (Cochran, 1950) was used to determine whether the frequency of use of the seven empowerment methods varied significantly across the case studies. This test is used in a block design with dichotomized responses. The observations in different blocks are assumed to be independent, but the responses within each block may be related. In this case, the 80 case studies represent the blocks. The use or non-use of each empowerment method by these cases represents the observations. Cochran's Q test confirmed that the frequency of the seven methods used by the cases varied significantly ($Q = 80.75$, df = 6; $p < 0.01$). [Q stands for percentage of users; in this case 80.75% of movements used this method very often or often. The methods used varied significantly, from a very high use of *enabling* services (87.5 %) to *work-related training and microenterprise* (27.5%).

In descending order, the seven EMPOWER methods were utilized as follows (Table 6.1): Enabling services and assistance (87.5%), rights protection and social action reform (73.8%), public education and participation (73.8%), organizing partnership (65%), empowerment training and leadership development (55%), media use (48.8%), and work-related training and microenterprise (27.5%).

Women used the method of "empowerment training and leadership development" to educate WAMs about their rights, privileges, and opportunities, and to develop the leadership and organizational skills necessary to navigate within their respective sociopolitical systems. This method was used by more than half of the cases (44 cases or 55%, Table 6.1). A significant difference was detected among the four different domains (Chi-square = 12.95; $p = 0.005$; see Table 6.2). Members of Mahila Milan (Case No. 33), an Indian organization of slum-dwellers, learned the correct procedure to file grievances against

TABLE 6.1
EMPOWER Dimensions/Methods (All Cases)

EMPOWER Dimensions/Methods	Count (N = 80)	Percentage
Empowerment training and leadership development	44	55
Media use and advocacy	39	48.8
Public education and participation	59	73.8
Organizing cooperatives and partnerships	52	65
Work-related training and microfinance initiative (MFI)	22	27.5
Enabling service and support	70	87.5
Rights protection and social action litigation (SAL)	59	73.8

*Chi-square analysis was performed for each method to determine statistically significant differences between levels of industrialization. Cochran's Q test confirmed that the frequency of the seven methods used by the 80 cases varied significantly (Q = 80.75, df = 6; $p < 0.01$). The methods used ranged significantly from a very high use of enabling services (87.5%) to work-related training and micro-enterprise (27.5%).

the police and other formal organizations. The group successfully sued the Bombay Municipal Corporation for destruction of their makeshift shelters, and the local police for theft of their belongings, thereby gaining the respect of the community (Gahlot, 1993). Leadership training was used by the *De Madres a Madres* (Case No. 45) to train volunteer mothers in Houston, Texas, to become community health promoters and to educate peers about prenatal care (McFarlane & Fehir, 1994).

Media use and advocacy included using television, radio, newspapers, etc., to accomplish two complementary objectives: (a) to gain media support for an existing movement; and (b) to influence public policy, mobilize

TABLE 6.2
EMPOWER Methods Used by Four Empowerment Domains

EMPOWER Methods	Human Rights n = 11	Equal Rights n = 14	Economic Development n = 8	Health Promotion n = 47	TOTAL n = 80	Chi-square* (.05 level) p>
Empowerment training and leadership	2 (18.2%)	12 (85.7%)	6 (75%)	24 (51.1%)	44 (55%)	0.005
Media use and advocacy	6 (54.5%)	7 (50%)	0 (0%)	26 (55.3%)	39 (48.8%)	0.035
Public education and participation	8 (72.7%)	11 (78.6%)	3 (37.5%)	37 (78.7%)	59 (73.8%)	NS
Organizing partnership	6 (54.5%)	12 (85.7%)	7 (87.5%)	27 (57.4%)	52 (65%)	NS
Work/job-training and microenterprise	0 (0%)	7 (50%)	6 (75%)	9 (19.1%)	22 (27.5)	<0.001
Enabling service and assistance	9 (81.8%)	13 (92.9%)	8 (100%)	40 (85.1%)	70 (87.5%)	NS
Rights protection and social action/reform	11 (100%)	13 (92.9%)	4 (50%)	31 (66%)	59 (73.8%)	0.016

*Chi-square analysis was performed for each method to determine statistically significant differences among domains.

public opinion, or generate public support for action. To achieve the first objective, the media draws attention to a specific organization or movement by publicizing a landmark action or other newsworthy event. Nearly half of all our cases used this method (39 cases, or 48.8%). In this context, it is important to note that it takes a long time, often decades, before it is possible to determine whether an empowerment movement has been successful or not. For instance, the pioneering Self-Employed Women's Association (SEWA) project in India began in 1972, and the Grameen bank project in Bangladesh began in 1976. Ela Bhatt, the founder of the SEWA, received her first major international award in 1984, from the Right Livelihood Award Foundation of Sweden (www.rightlivelihood. org/sewa.html). That was 12 years after she founded the SEWA. Since we studied "successful" case studies, many of these case studies were initiated decades before the Internet and social media became ubiquitous. Consequently, while recent social movements (e.g., the "Arab Spring") have used social media heavily, most of the case studies in our meta-analysis began before the advent of its massive use. The significant points to note here are that successful women's movements tend to use the mass media that are most prevalent and accessible to them; and consistent with the prevalent "digital divide" between rich and poor societies, the poor tend to use mass/social media less frequently than the urban, affluent, and younger generations (Table 6.3 confirms this; it shows that media use varies significantly between more and less industrialized countries 66% versus 24%, respectively). Interestingly, the case studies we included have incorporated modern media in their recent activities, and several poor communities (e.g., Bangladesh, Indonesia) are now using cell phones as their microenterprise entrepreneurships, including phone services for a fee for those who do not have cell phones.

In the United States, the National Organization for Women (NOW; Case No. 13) garnered media support through community-based protests, demonstrations, and speeches by NOW leaders. In the 1970s, NOW members captured the attention of the media by invading the regional office of the Equal Employment Opportunity Commission (EEOC) carrying bundles of classified advertisements bound with red tape to symbolize the sexual discrimination faced by women in the workplace (Davis, 1991). In the 1990s, the women's health movement *La Casa de la Mujer* (Case No. 42) alerted the press to its planned protest of a recent tragic event: a Bolivian family had died from eating food made of flour contaminated by a nearby garbage dump. Attracted by the media attention, the city mayor came to the protest to address the problem (Paulson et al., 1996). In Argentina, the *Madres de Plaza de Mayo* (Case No. 4) mothers were protesting the "disappearance" of thousands of their male family members, with no success. Knowing that members of the world press were in Buenos Aires covering the 1978 World Cup soccer tournament, the mothers staged an impromptu protest that drew the attention of the press, finally gaining international recognition for their cause (Kusterer, 1993).

Other cases directly relayed the organization's message through more controlled media campaigns, press conferences, and press releases. For example, the Women's Health Care Foundation (Case No. 39), a Filipino organization that fights for women's reproductive health rights, actively uses the media by writing to newspapers, appearing on radio and television, granting interviews to the press, and holding press conferences (Family Health International). When comparing cases by level of industrialization, a significant difference was detected between cases in more industrialized (66%) and less industrialized nations (24.2%) (Chi-square = 13.5; $p < 0.001$; Table 6.3).

The "public education and participation" method was utilized by 59 of the 80 cases, the second most frequently used method along with "rights protection" (73.8%, Table 6.1). This method entails informing and educating the general public and community leaders of organizations that serve affected communities such as churches, temples, and volunteer and human service agencies. The primary objective is to raise awareness about relevant issues, generate material support for programs, and inspire public action and participation. Specific activities include using speakers' bureaus, public service announcements, websites on the World Wide Web, distribution of printed media such as newsletters or brochures, and the development of ethnic networks such as advisory councils or boards that enlist public support for specific programs and initiatives.

TABLE 6.3
EMPOWER Methods Used by Level of Economic Development

EMPOWER Methods	More Advanced $n = 47$ Count (%)	Less Advanced $n = 33$ Count (%)	TOTAL CASES $n = 80$ Count (%)	Chi-square* (.05 level) p>
Empowerment training and leadership development	26 (55.3%)	18 (54.5%)	44 (55%)	NS
Media use and advocacy	31 (66%)	8 (24.2%)	39 (48.8%)	<0.001
Public education and participation	40 (85.1%)	19 (57.6%)	59 (73.8%)	0.006
Organizing partnership, cooperatives, and coalitions	30 (63.8%)	22 (66.7%)	52 (65%)	NS
Work/job-training	8 (17%)	14 (42.4%)	22 (27.5)	0.012
Enabling service and assistance	41 (87.2%)	29 (87.9%)	70 (87.5%)	NS
Rights protection	35 (74.5%)	24 (72.7%)	59 (73.8%)	NS

*Chi-square analysis was performed for each method to determine statistically significant differences between levels of economic development.

A significant difference was found in the use of this method between cases from more industrialized and less industrialized nations (85.1% vs. 57.6%, respectively; Chi-square = 7.6, p = 0.006; Table 6.3). Perhaps because of the relatively high cost of such activities in terms of financial and resource costs, less industrialized nations are unable to use this method as frequently as affluent nations. Furthermore, among less industrialized nations, community needs are often localized and well known to the community. Therefore, formal or structured ways of communicating these issues to the public are not necessary (see Table 6.2). Cases from the health-promotion domain conducted speakers' bureaus on such topics as family planning among rural Korean women (Mothers' Clubs, Case No. 36); breast and cervical cancer among Asian American and African American women (National Asian Women's Health Organization [NAWHO], Case No. 53, and Sisters Network, Case No. 55); and domestic violence among South Asian women (Narika, n.d., Case No. 64, and Sakhi, 2015, Case No. 63).

More than half of all cases (52 cases, or 65%) made use of the "organizing partnership" method. No significant difference was found in the frequency of use of this method across four domains. These cases created formal and informal organizations that united individuals with similar needs, demands, or problems. In many of the case studies, lack of money and other resources posed a major barrier to poor women in their struggle to improve their QOL. Formal cooperatives, unions, and associations provide protection against abuse and exploitation by employers and a power base for bargaining from a position of strength. SEWA (Case No. 26) established cooperatives of dairy workers (and other occupational groups) to pool resources and strengthen their bargaining power (Rose, 1993). Cooperatives allow members to obtain financial, legal, and technical assistance. In some cases, such cooperatives enable participants to satisfy basic survival needs. The community kitchens in Peru (Case No. 31) provided severely low-income women with at least one healthy meal per day by pooling needed ingredients (Kusterer, 1993). The Mothers' Clubs (Case No. 36) in Korea carried out many cooperative efforts such as joint cooking, shared childcare services, and collective rice plantation and harvest (Kang, 1998). These collectives reduced members' total dependency on their exploiters while supporting members' rights and privileges. A member of Mahila Milan, a slum-dwellers' organization in India (Case No. 33) that established a collective savings fund for housing and daily emergencies, describes how organizing helped her cause:

> Nobody listened to us when we're alone but now we're organized and strong. Singly, we were thin sticks, which could be easily broken. Together, we are like a thick bundle. Unbreakable. (Women's Feature Service, 1992, pp. 138–143)

Grassroots organizations often form coalitions with other like-minded community organizations in order to strengthen their base of support and further their cause. Equality Now (Case No. 10) is part of the Women's Action Network, a coalition of nearly 2,000 groups and individuals from 65 nations that gathers and shares information about HR abuses and violations around the world so that concerned parties can take necessary action (Bouvard, 1996). For example, Mothers of East Los Angeles (MELA; Case No. 9) joined citywide coalitions to protest undesired construction of various projects that threatened the safety and integrity of its community (Bouvard, 1996). The Coalition Against the Prison enabled community groups to join forces in successfully fighting the proposed construction of a state prison near the heavily populated Boyle Heights community and its 33 schools. In fact, several cases in the health-promotion domain have built community partnerships in order to achieve their specific goals. NAWHO (Case No. 53) collaborated with tobacco control agencies and community groups in a nationwide anti-smoking program for the Asian American population.

The "work/job-training and microcredit" method refers to training in work-related skills, and income-generating microcredit enterprises. Job-training gives women the opportunity to master skills necessary for paid employment. The Union of Women Domestic Employees (Case No. 14) from Brazil offers training in cooking, laundry, and food preparation (Anderfuhren, 1994). Jordan's Noor Al Hussein Foundation (Case No. 32) created training programs and projects to teach such employable skills as growing herbs, appliance repair, and computer use. This method was the least frequently used method of all (22 cases, 27.5%). A significant difference was also found by level of industrialization (Chi-square = 6.28; p = 0.012), with less industrialized nations (42.4%) using this method more frequently than more industrialized nations (17%) (see Table 6.3). A significant difference was also found among domains (Chi-square = 18.43; p < 0.001; Table 6.2); and between the health-promotion domain (19.1%) and non–health-promotion domains (39.4%) (Chi-square = 5.3; p = 0.046; Table 6.4). In most cases, lack of gainful employment or job-related problems were the primary issues being addressed, and so the necessity of this method is evident. This suggests that the cases from poorer nations are in greater need of an economic intervention. Many of the health-promotion cases held job-training or supported income-generating projects. Step Up on Second (Case No. 79), a center for recovering mentally ill adults in California, offers its clients the opportunity to learn on-site job skills at its mini-market, and assistance from vocational counselors to find permanent positions at local businesses (L. Mansouri, personal interview, November 17, 1998). Sakhi (Case No. 63), a New York–based domestic violence support group for South Asian women, created an "economic justice project" that provided skills in job-hunting, budgeting finances, and starting small businesses, as well as information about sexual harassment on the job

TABLE 6.4

Empowerment Methods Used by Health Promotion and Other Domains

EMPOWER Methods	HPDP n = 47 Count (%)	Non-HPDP n = 33 Count (%)	TOTAL N = 80 Count (%)	Chi-square* p = .05
Empowerment training	40 (85.1%)	30 (90.9%)	70 (87.5%)	NS
Media support and use	26 (55.3%)	13 (39.4%)	39 (48.8%)	NS
Public education and participation	37 (78.7%)	22 (66.7%)	59 (73.8%)	NS
Organizing partnership	27 (57.4%)	25 (75.8%)	52 (65%)	NS
Work/job-training and micro-enterprise	9 (19.1%)	13 (39.4%)	22 (27.5)	0.046
Enabling service and assistance	31 (66%)	28 (84.8%)	59 (73.8%)	NS
Rights protection and promotion	13 (27.5%)	11 (33.3%)	26 (32.5%)	NS

*Chi-square analysis was performed for each method to determine statistically significant differences between HPDP and non-HPDP domains.

and employees' rights. Income-generating projects raise money for its participants through small-scale activities such as crafts and agriculture (Sakhi, 1999). Members of the Mothers' Clubs in Korea (Case No. 36) engaged in income-generating projects such as cattle-breeding, beekeeping, and fruit-tree plantation (Kang, 1998).

Microenterprise programs, such as the SEWA program in India (Case No. 26) and the Grameen Bank in Bangladesh (Case No. 27) provide small, collateral-free loans to needy women who possess traditional skills in knitting, basket-weaving, rug-making, and other handicrafts (Bornstein, 1996; Rose, 1993). These loans enable the women to buy raw materials at bulk rate and produce handicrafts to sell in local markets. As a result, poverty-stricken women are given the opportunity to earn income (some had never actually touched money before), to improve their QOL, and to raise their self-efficacy. The Working Women's Forum (Case No. 28) of India began as an experiment of well-known political activist Jaya Arunachalam who helped 30 women get small loans for starting or expanding small businesses. By 1994, the Forum owned its own cooperative bank and had 225,000 members in nine branches (Bangasser, 1994). In Jordan, a prototype women-in-development program was so successful that the Noor Al Hussein Foundation (Case No. 32) established the Small and Micro Enterprise Development Unit, devoted entirely to providing credit to microentrepreneurs throughout the country. Microenterprise has even been adopted internationally and in affluent nations including the United States to assist their poorer communities by enhancing autonomy and internal loci of control. By tapping into the rich resources that a woman possesses, her family and community can reap the benefits.

It is important to set the record straight and give due recognition to the originator of the microfinance initiatives (MFI) programs in Asia as we know them today. While Prof. Yunus was justly awarded the Nobel Prize for successfully applying and popularizing the MFI in Bangladesh, it would be incorrect and unfair if we do not acknowledge the originator of this important movement. In 1905, 100 years before the year of Yunus's Nobel award, the concept was introduced by another Nobel laureate, Indian poet, philosopher, social reformer, and educator Rabindranath Tagore, in the village Patisar (now in Bangladesh). Tagore established the first well-documented Kaligram Krishi Bank (means "Farmers' Bank") with his own funds and introduced the ideas of "collateral-free," "group borrowing," and "cooperatives" (he called these "rural societies") as essential requirements to ensure that poor farmers could benefit from this program. The small surcharge or interest of 4.6% he collected for program cost was remarkably low compared to much higher interest rates claimed by many current MFI programs today.

Tagore recognized that the traditional banking system that is designed with a profit motive was not suitable to help poor farmers; the goal of setting up a bank for the poor must be to alleviate the financial burden of the poor and to empower them financially. In such a situation, one must harness the inner talents (they have many traditional skills) of the poor and their ability to self-organize in problem-solving groups. At a time when rich Indians sent their sons to study law or medicine in England or Germany, Tagore sent his son, Rathindranath Tagore, to the University of Illinois in Urbana, Illinois, to study agriculture (in 1906) so that he would have an in-house agricultural specialist to help the rural cooperatives and banks that Tagore had established. The Sriniketan established by Tagore is still thriving near Santiniketan in India; it is dedicated to rural and cottage industries to promote the rural economy (Mondal & Peters, 2011; O'Connell, 2003).

I am baffled by the fact that Tagore's name is not mentioned in any serious discussion of microcredit or the MFI movement. I am similarly puzzled by the lack of any mention of Gandhi in textbooks written by Western social scientists in discussions of community organization and development. Gandhi's nonviolent civil disobedience movement or *Satyagraha* ("seeker of truth") is the largest known nonviolent freedom movement in human history; it has demonstrated its power in India's independence movement and has inspired many prominent national leaders in the last century such as Martin Luther King, Jr., Nelson Mandela, Lech Walesa, Vaclav Havel, and Aung Sun Su Kyi; all five won the Nobel Prize for Peace; Gandhi never won the Nobel Peace Prize. Popular textbooks in community organization used at top U.S. universities do not mention Tagore or Gandhi.

In 1972, Ila Bhatt, a lawyer in Ahmedabad (India) was the next to use MFI, in the SEWA (Case No. 26) movement we mentioned before. She was the lawyer for the labor union of the textile industries and noticed that the workers' wives who desperately needed work as part-time workers to feed their families were abused, forced to suffer inhumane work conditions without medical or health benefits, and often were sexually harassed or abused. It became obvious to Bhatt that these women desperately needed money. Litigations against employers for abuse, while necessary, did not feed the women and their families. This realization led Bhatt to introduce a microcredit program and workers' cooperative to economically empower these women. The SEWA movement has won several international awards and laurels as an exemplary women's empowerment movement.

In the same year in 1972, the Bangladesh Rural Advancement Committee (BRAC) introduced a collateral-free microcredit program within its multi-faceted strategy designed to promote the health and well-being of the rural Bangladeshi population (Mondal & Peters, 2012). The BRAC has also won several international awards and recognitions.

The Grameen Bank was initiated in 1976, more than seven decades after Tagore's Krishi Bank was founded, and several years after SEWA and BRAC introduced microcredit programs. The Grameen Bank has helped a large number of women and families and has earned a wider recognition. The recognition is fully deserved, and we applaud Yunus for his exceptional leadership in empowering millions of women and their families. Let us hope that the microcredit program becomes an integral part of the community empowerment discourse.

The method of "enabling service and assistance" was most frequently used by all empowerment cases (70 cases or 87.5%; Table 6.1). In each domain, at least 80% of all cases used this method; all eight cases in the ED domain used this method. Enabling service and assistance directly provide essential services in crisis-intervention and create opportunities for the members and beneficiaries of the program or organization. The basic services offered—counseling; legal, financial, and medical aid; and provision of material aid such as food, housing, or clothing; and victim protection—often enable the recipients to initiate or maintain other activities. For example, the Asian Immigrant Women Advocates (Case No. 24) of California offer literacy and English-speaking classes (Andrews, 1996). Black Sash (Case No. 2), an anti-apartheid group in South Africa, established several Advice Offices across the country in order to counsel and advocate on behalf of black women accused of breaking the restrictive "pass laws," which required black women to carry passes at all times (Bishop, 1991). Black Sash was the only resource for these women at that time. Former factory workers of the Export Processing Zone (Case No. 18) set up a women's center that offers legal and medical assistance, library facilities, and seminars in women's rights (Martens, 1994). *De Madres a Madres* (Case No. 45) of Texas established a community center for the volunteer health promoters to meet and share information (McFarlane & Fehir, 1994).

Other cases formed mutual support groups that let members share experiences, lean on one another for emotional support, and interact socially; they are excellent examples of the power of self-organization in action. *Agrupación* (Case No. 3), the Chilean women's organization for the "disappeared," has a folklore group in which members collectively sing and compose songs about their lives as single women (Agosin, 1993). ATABAL/La Esperanza (Case No. 20) of Mexico formed its own folk-dancing troupe that provides entertainment for its social events (Lazarini & Martinez, 2001). The support groups held by the Supportive Older Women's Network (Case No. 49) focus on the issues that matter to older women: stereotypes of aging, widowhood and bereavement, health care, and financial management (Kaye, 1997). Still others provide services for the community as a whole, especially to youth. The women of Innabuyog (Case No. 23) of the Philippines set up day-care centers and organized early childhood education seminars to train the caregivers (International Institute for Sustainable Development, 1997). MELA (Case No. 9) runs a lead-prevention program for poor children, a water conservation program, a community clean-up project, and a scholarship for needy students.

Among the health-promotion cases, health promotion and direct health services are provided. The South Carolina AIDS Education Network (Case No. 72) develops and distributes AIDS pamphlets, mini-seminars, and AIDS educational materials designed for children (Sumpter, 1990). Nigeria's Girls' Power Initiative (Case No. 44) teaches young girls age-appropriate lessons about self-esteem and reproductive health (International Women's Health Coalition, 1993). The Over Sixty Health Center (Case No. 47) offers medical and social services to its elderly clientele (Squatriglia, 1995), while the Traditional Child Bearing Group (Case No. 37) offers maternity services to African American women (Waite, 1993). The Creative Health Foundation (Case No. 80) provides an alternative type of mental health care for individuals with severe mental illness.

"Rights protection and promotion" was the second most frequently used empowerment method (along with "public education and participation"). In 59 of the 80 cases (73.8%; Table 6.1), promotion of the rights of individuals (human, equal, or health) was the primary modus operandi. This category includes all social, political, and legal actions taken by women and their supportive organizations to improve their living conditions. Actions aimed at rights protection and social and legal reform include demonstrations, passive resistance, confrontations with authorities, disruptive pressures (strikes), political and voter registration campaigns, lobbying for legislative reforms, and SAL.

The organizations that utilized this method have had varying degrees of success. Through a nonviolent demonstration, Mahila Milan (Case No. 33) persuaded local officials to issue ration cards (which are needed to get subsidized food and to establish identity and place of residence) to families they had originally refused (Gahlot, 1993). On the other hand, Call Off Your Old Tired Ethics (COYOTE; Case No. 15), the prostitutes' rights organization, was not as effective when it picketed hotels used by police to "entrap" prostitutes. Their protest did not succeed in changing police behavior, but it did generate local media coverage (Jenness, 1991). A significant difference was found among domains (Chi-square = 10.36; p = 0.016; Table 6.2). All HR and 13 out of 14 ER cases used this empowerment method. For three cases in our meta-analysis, namely the Chipko Movement (for trees) (Case No. 67), Chipko Movement for Water (Case No. 69), and the Arrack Ban (Case No. 61), rights protection was the *only* empowerment method used to successfully achieve their objectives.

Other types of sociopolitical action use more formal avenues of advocacy, such as sponsoring legislation and lobbying politicians at the local, state, and national levels through hearings and testimonials. Many of the health-promotion cases were involved in legislative struggles to make living and working environments safer and healthier. For example, Mothers Against Drunk Driving (MADD) (Case No. 57) has been instrumental in enacting several anti–drunk driving laws in the United States, including the law standardizing the legal drinking age in all 50 states to 21. Much of MADD's success is attributable to the bereaved families and victims of drunk drivers who offered powerful and poignant testimony before Congress (Lord, 1990). The *Comite Por Rescate de Nuestra Salud* ("Committee to Rescue Our Health") (Case No. 68) successfully fought to make Puerto Rico's powerful industrialists accountable for the dangerous working conditions in an industrial park (Muñoz-Vázquez, 1996).

Social Action Litigation (SAL) refers to landmark lawsuits undertaken in local, state, and federal courts, and initiated by women's organizations. SAL serves three important functions: (a) it is a deterrent against HR violations; (b) it provides victims and their families with a means of seeking retribution and punitive damages; and (c) it generates pressure to comply with existing laws. Such lawsuits are often filed against individual violators, corporate employers, and governments that fail to protect HR. The movement against dowry deaths in India (Case No. 7) is a good example of SAL. Women's Action Research and Legal Action for Women (WARLAW), a women's organization founded by a group of female lawyers, successfully prosecuted perpetrators of dowry deaths in more than 85 cases, representing a conviction rate of more than 90% (Jethmalani, 1995).

The overall findings suggest that no matter what the empowerment method or combination of them, if used well, they have empowering effects. These and other findings confirm, as empowerment theory holds, that empowerment occurs at multiple levels and reinforce each other. Furthermore, there are strong interactions among various dimensions of an effective empowerment process. Success with one empowerment method can set the stage for, and in some cases, facilitate the use of, another method. Based upon our meta-analysis, three key themes common to the 80 exemplary cases were noted: the empowering effects of involvement; the role of individuals; and the influence of the context or macro-environment.

Empowering Effects of Involvement

Regardless of their specific goals, methods, or outcomes, involvement in social action movements yields empowering effects in two ways. First, participation enhances the women's subjective well-being, self-esteem, and self-efficacy. As a result of their involvement in even small-scale self-help initiatives and local programs, WAMs gain confidence in their ability to initiate change for the betterment of their lives. Second, as women acquire technical skills, communication networks, and organizational skills, their social status is significantly enhanced. As programs or projects continue to grow, many of the women assume positions of responsibility as supervisors, trainers, and managers; some find full-time paid employment. Members of the Centro de Infomacíon y Desarrollo de la Mujer or CIDEM (Case No. 40) share information about reproductive health with relatives, friends, and neighbors in informal settings. Emilia Gutiérrez boasts that she has become a family planning evangelist:

> We've gotten used to talking about these things, and now when I see a pregnant woman with a baby on her back and another holding her hand, I just want to go right over and talk with her. Sometimes we talk a little, just joking, or conversing like this, and sometimes it works out, and she gets interested. Even at parties, or anywhere at all, I talk about family planning. My family laughs at me, but I've managed to influence all of my sisters and sisters-in-law, too. They've all ended up with only two or three children. (Paulson et al., 1996, p. 38)

Many of these women-led programs are considered pioneers in the field of women's empowerment and development and regarded as inspiration for grassroots and community-development movements worldwide. The "impact" section of each vignette illustrates these kinds of empowerment effects at various levels. For example, the Boston Women's Health Book Collective (BWHBC, Case No. 46), best known for authoring the widely acclaimed book *Our Bodies, Ourselves (OBOS)*—a collection of valuable medical information about women's health from a woman's perspective—has inspired women across the world to pen their own culturally specific books on women's health. In addition to the more than 20 translated versions of

OBOS, several similar books (not direct translations) about women's health have been published in Denmark, India, and Egypt (BWHBC, 2000).

Role of Individuals

Individual leadership can play a crucial role in building grassroots movements. Although it is not possible to isolate an individual's impact from the total effect of the movement in quantitative terms, our meta-analysis revealed, in case after case, the catalytic role of individuals in initiating and sustaining social movements. Sections entitled "Leadership Impetus" and "Partners/Opposition" in our case summaries identify such individuals and their roles. Often these individuals are outside professionals who care about the powerless and are powerful enough to lead a movement without fear of personal harm. Yunus of Grameen Bank (Case No. 27) and Jethmalani of the anti-dowry-death movement (Case No. 7) are examples of external leaders. In the case of the Grameen movement, a major barrier faced by the village women was lack of confidence and refusal by local banks to loan them money, which they sorely needed for their income-generating projects. Yunus took out a personal bank loan to provide seed money for the villagers' projects. A local cooperative bank was subsequently established to manage the cash flow of the successful financial ventures (Bornstein, 1996). This example illustrates the role of individual leadership in overcoming a formidable obstacle. In other cases, victims within the community have provided effective leadership that is essential in planning and institutionalizing empowerment movements. For instance, Aurora Castillo, one of the founders of MELA (Case No. 9), articulates her impetus for organizing:

> You know if one of your children's safety is jeopardized, the mother turns into a lioness. ... We have to have a well-organized, strong group of mothers to protect the community and oppose things that are detrimental to us. ... Mothers are for the children's interest, not for self-interest. (Castillo, 1988)

Angela Gomes of *Banchte Sheka* ("Learn to Survive") in Bangladesh suffered stigma, insults, and social exclusion because she was a single woman doing social work in a conservative Muslim culture; she was perceived as a woman with "bad moral character" who wanted to corrupt the minds of young girls and convert them to Christianity (Gomes, 2015a; *Banchte Shekha* website: http://word.world-citizenship.org/wp-archive/1118).

Often, individual leaders, especially those from powerless communities, have suffered enormous personal loss and havoc. Members of the *Madres de Playa de Mayo* and the community kitchen movement were murdered for their beliefs and actions (Kusterer, 1993); Nobel laureate Rigoberta Menchú's parents were brutally tortured and murdered in Guatemala, forcing her to escape to Mexico to save her life and to sustain her struggle (Menchú, 1983). Despite these personal threats and costs, two trends are noted.

First, all effective movements were initiated by individuals—either victims themselves who were determined to fight for their own cause, or more powerful individuals who identified with the cause of the oppressed and were determined to join the struggle. Second, in order for a movement to continue and succeed, it must attract a critical mass of individuals; from them a core leadership can emerge. A successful movement requires its participants to perform many organizational tasks that require both technical skills and leadership qualities. As Table 6.1 revealed, more than 50% of the cases used leadership development and empowerment training to enhance individual capacities.

Influence of Context or Macro-Environment

Although the descriptive text of the case studies does not allow a quantitative evaluation of context effects, we believe that the social context or macro-environment of each case significantly affects the overall movement and outcomes. The macro-environment may either present a set of barriers to the women's empowerment movement or (less frequently) support a movement. The sections entitled "Macro-environment" in the 80 vignettes illustrate the elements of the context or macro-environment, which affect empowerment movements and outcomes. For example, women in several cases were met with skepticism from the established organizations and male community members. The women of the *ollas communes*, or community kitchens (Case No. 31) in Santa Maria, Peru, faced a major barrier. Men held a stereotype of Peruvian women as weak, indecisive, dependent on men, socially ineffective, lacking organizational ability, and unable to handle the pressures of leadership (Macera & Oyola, 1997). Yet, as a result of their actions, the women were able to dispel cultural stereotypes and win recognition from the men as equals:

> *Machismo* exists because men do not want to recognize women as *compañeras*; instead women are treated as servants. The only difference between men and women is that men cannot become pregnant, and women can. Because everything else you can both do—work, earn money and raise children [*sic*]. (Intermon website, 1997: http://www.intermon.org, translated by Macera & Oyola).

TRANSFORMATION OF MEN'S ATTITUDES

A change from male chauvinism to acceptance of women as partners was noted in several cases of our meta-analysis. *Agrupacion* (Case No. 3) illustrates the influence of context in shaping women's roles.

> [During the military regime in Chile in the 1970s] and its political, as well as economic, consequences, it is not surprising that women, as the mothers, wives, sisters, daughters and grandmothers of the victims of repression, were the first to mobilize in opposition to the dictatorship. Men were the victims of abuse more often than women. Women during the socialist regime of Salvador Allende tended to play what were considered marginal or secondary roles in the targeted organizations, principally political parties and trade unions. It was precisely women's traditional invisibility which allowed them to become politically visible during a time when it was extremely dangerous for anyone to do so. (Agosin, 1993, p. 87)

Our overall conclusions derived from this meta-analysis are that powerlessness has direct, independent, and adverse effects on our health and QOL; consequently, empowerment is both an essential goal and means for health promotion and enhancement of QOL. Empowerment is a multidimensional and multilevel (MTL) construct; there are at least five levels of empowerment that affect our health and QOL. These are: (a) individual, (b) family and intimate relations, (c) community, (d) organizational, and (e) sociocultural. These levels interact and have a combined effect on the empowerment process and outcomes. Furthermore, investment in the empowerment of women has a significantly greater return on comparable investment on men for community-based health promotion. Finally, while women are relatively more powerless than men, even the most impoverished and powerless women can and do, with a little external help (from the community and professionals), lead self-organized movements that significantly improve the health and QOL of their families and communities.

Empowerment is a dynamic process and it has moving targets or goals; after the initial success, empowered people tend to set new and higher goals for themselves. This process may further empower them which may have positive effects on other domains of their lives that they did not dare to expect initially. Traditional program evaluations tend to focus on measuring the program objective-driven outcomes and ignore the outcomes that were not originally planned but emerged from the increased self-efficacy and capacities of the empowerment process. For instance, the original objective of the Grameen Bank was to increase the income of a small group of poor village women; as the movement progressed, female literacy and better health services were demanded and added. After two decades, the goal of many original Grameen participants now is to have their children earn college degrees. Empowerment evaluation should be sensitive to these emerging goals and outcomes; often these emerged goals and outcomes may far outweigh the original modest goals. Box 6.2 presents ten axioms or propositions related to the discourse on empowerment theory and action. Based upon our results and discussions above, we offer ten propositions that may serve as a set of guidelines for planning community-based interventions that empower disenfranchised populations and enhance QOL and health. While these propositions refer to social actions that empower women and mothers, they would be relevant to empower other groups as well.

By integrating key findings from our meta-analysis, we have conceptualized a multilevel empowerment movement. We observed some parallels between the theories of chaos and complexity and self-organized empowerment movements. According to these theories, complex self-organizing systems (such as a grassroots movement) can undergo "spontaneous self-organization." Dynamic systems have an inherent capacity to self-organize

---

BOX 6.2

Ten Empowerment Axioms: Lessons Learned from the Meta-Analyses

---

1. **Maternal motivation** to prevent harm to their children and families is a driving force for social action by them. Women's and mothers' deep commitment to protect and promote the well-being of their children and families often serves as a unifying force for action that transcends ethnic, political, and social barriers. We observe this phenomenon in case after case.

2. **A just struggle for basic survival needs** is likely to engender wider public support even in societies under authoritarian rule and military dictatorships; when women lead struggles for minimum survival needs (e.g., a minimum wage, human rights violations) it is less threatening because they are not demanding a regime change.

3. **Struggles led by non-political women** for their children's well-being, safety, and prevention from harms are likely to generate wider public and social approval and support. Case studies suggest that even corrupt military and gang members respect their own mothers. Women are not seen as threats to political positions by those in power.

4. **Public participation and involvement** have empowering effects. Involvement as participants in any movement has empowering effects independent of tangible individual gains. Initially, involvement in self-help initiatives at the local level enhances self-esteem and self-efficacy. Subsequently, involvement in empowerment programs enhances social status, professional competence and leadership, leading to an improved QOL for the participants, their families, and their community. Most violations of rights are deeply rooted in cultural practices; therefore changing men's perception of women and abusive behavior are essential targets of change.

5. **CORE support** at the early phase of a local self-care initiative is essential for developing a viable enabling program. CORE is an acronym of four types of essential supports: (a) Community support, (b) Organizational support from community-based organizations (CBOs), (c) Resource support—local resources

(either cash or in-kind) for initial efforts, and (d) Empowerment support—various instrumental support and empowerment methods. CORE support may come from citizens, volunteers from neighborhood religious institutions (churches, temples, etc.), and from community-based organizations (CBOs).

6. **Enabling services and assistance** are essential in allowing victims protection against abuse and means necessary to sustain their struggles. Fear of retaliation by abusers often deters victims from seeking help and/or resisting abuse. Enabling services and assistance help victims deal with traumatic experiences and empower them with the knowledge that they have protection against future abuse. These services enhance the likelihood that the abused will join the struggle against their tormentors.

7. **Leadership training and development** have empowering effects on both individuals and organizations and significantly influence program outcomes. This method is critical in enhancing women's competency to organize programs for themselves. Non-formal leadership education includes: (a) educating and informing the public to generate community approval and support for an initiative (in turn, such approval and support from the immediate community translate into positive public opinion, cash and in-kind instrumental support, and community-based activities), (b) education and training of WAM in survival and income-generating skills, and (c) training in organizational and leadership skills.

8. **Media use, support and advocacy** complement program efforts and may significantly enhance their effectiveness. Movements involve two types of media use: (a) "Media support" as the effective use of available media including communication media (both modern and indigenous) to support and promote an existing policy or program, and (b) "Media advocacy" as effective use of modern media, especially social media, to bring public opinion to bear on policy reform and on better implementation of existing policies and laws.

9. **External recognition and support** enhances institutionalization and wider adoption of innovative local initiatives. Recognition from credible national and international organizations legitimizes a struggle and empowers those involved. It also helps to generate resources, stabilize and expand the program and enhances its diffusion through networking and collaborations.

10. **A non-violent social action movement** for a just cause is likely to gain social approval and thus enhance its effectiveness. The Gandhian *Sarvodaya* (*sarva* meaning "everyone" and *udaya* meaning "arise") movement for India's independence, the civil rights movement led by Dr. Martin Luther King, Jr. in the United States, and Argentina's Madres de Plaza de Mayo are but a few of the many remarkable examples that attest to the effectiveness of non-violent civil disobedience movements. In addition, seeking genuine truth and reconciliation may have greater positive effects on community empowerment than seeking justice and revenge through the use of force (e.g. Mandela's South Africa). Violent armed conflict, sectarian strife, and international terrorism that disempower victims are caused by forces that are often beyond the scope of local solutions (regardless of whether movements are led by men or women); however, women's movements produce positive effects on relief and restitution efforts to help victims.

---

and transform from an apparent chaos toward a new order. These "complex self-organizing systems are *adaptive*, in that they don't just passively respond to events the way a rock might roll around in an earthquake. They actively try to turn whatever happens to their advantage" (Waldrop, 1992, p. 11).

Similarly, the meta-analysis of the 80 grassroots movements has revealed a common pattern. One does not have an action plan or a project proposal or an agent to direct the emergence of a self-organized system; the case studies show that no one had a premeditated "action plan"; they all had a strong motive (initial condition) and an urgent need to change the initial condition. Actions were often triggered by a sense of desperation or outrage. There were others who were in the same situation but there was a spiral of silence; they felt weak and isolated and believed they were alone and powerless. Initial actions by a critical mass of persons sharing the same initial condition breaks the spiral of silence, and brings them together to form informal networks; chaos leads to self-organization and to movement or action for change. This pattern is made of common components, including a series of four developmental steps.

Illustrated in Figure 5.3 the proposed conceptual model describes the progress of a grassroots movement; it begins with an initial condition that the victims or unhappy folk are motivated to change, followed by actions through four stages: first, initial individual actions; second, organized collective actions (movement gains momentum); third, an articulated program with a structure and multiple planned actions; and fourth, an established and institutionalized program with its own structure, resources, and power base.

Successful movements need and receive critical support from others at different stages and use different combinations of the seven EMPOWER methods as described in several tables of this chapter. All movements do not necessarily progress easily from one step to the next. Numerous barriers stand in the way. Many movements collapse in the face of these barriers, and they are not well documented or publicized. This meta-analysis identified five types of barriers:

1. **Traditional cultural attitudes** and gender role segregation are major barriers to women's QOL, and discourage social action by women. Cultural reforms are as important as structural changes for enhancement of the personal capabilities of women.
2. **Gender inequality**, devaluation of women as people with legitimate rights and capacities, and devaluation of their contributions to social progress not only harm the women, they also diminish the overall well-being of a society. Inadequate opportunities for developing the personal capabilities of women are a major challenge in both rich and poor nations.
3. **Lack of access to structural support** and institutions to protect the vulnerable and to promote the women's legitimate cause. Often self-efficacy and objective capacities may not be consistent and motivation is not enough. The underprivileged need structural support to

remove barriers and create opportunities to enhance their capacities. This is where professionals and social policies are most helpful.

4. **Lack of public awareness** of the problems and support for removal of real/distal causes of powerlessness. Our socialization processes condition us to treat people differently who do not appear similar to us.

5. **Strong opposition from the oppressors** and abusive systems who gain by exploiting women.

In the final analysis, these 80 movements demonstrated that ordinary women can and do lead exemplary movements, with a little help from their supporters and professionals. The important lesson we need to learn from these cases is that, as professionals, we need to study these and similar movements carefully and empower ourselves to be able to support their struggles more effectively.

7

Human Rights Case Studies

The Chapters 7–10 present summaries of case studies used in our Meta-analysis. Before we present the summaries, it is important to highlight the characteristics that transcend individual movements or case studies. First, these movements were organized and led by ordinary women who have accomplished extraordinary goals and in so doing inspired others to follow their examples. Second, these women were not driven by personal achievement or self-actualization motives; they were motivated by their unconditional love and concerns for the well-being of their children, families, and other victims like them. Third, all important movements attract strong external supporters and opponents; and these women had to sustain their struggles sometimes for decades (the median age of the movements is 26 years). In some cases (e.g., Grandmothers of Playa de Mayo, Grameen) projects continued for multiple-generations. This finding implies that one should not expect immediate success nor abandon a struggle too soon. Fourth, the women had to had to pay a heavy price including death-threats, violence including death, and severe physical, psychological and financial harms. In spite of these serious threats, they were not afraid to persist. Fifth, they were all victims of serious inequality and injustice; but their self-interest was not limited to personal advancement; they believed that there must be a collective success. For this reason, the victims developed a strong bond among themselves which encouraged them to work as in cohesive groups; it promoted cooperation rather than competition. Sixth, human development involves progress in several domains concurrently; these domains affect one another. The case studies reflect this reality. We find that while initially some of movements focus on a single goal (e.g. MADD, Dowry Deaths), other movements begin with multiple goals across domains. In addition, after initial progress, some movements expand their original scope and include additional important goals (e.g. SEWA began with protecting women from work-site abuse and Grameen Bank began with poverty reduction in village women; both movements added health care, literacy, and gender development goals). This reality means that many movements have multiple goals when they begin and others expand and include multiple-goals as they progress. For this reason, some case studies may be listed in more than one domain; but in our the statistical Meta-analysis, the total number of cases studies is eighty. Six additional cases are included in discussions only because these did not have quantitative data required for statistical comparisons.

The research questions, criteria of inclusion of case studies in four domains, methodology used for the meta-analysis, and the key findings of quantitative comparisons of 80 case studies across the four categories were presented in Chapter Six.

Some readers may look at the year when a movement began and conclude whether the case study is old or outdated. We hold the position that, if a movement is still active, or has inspired new movements, then the earlier it began and the longer it continued to meet the empowerment needs of people, the stronger is that movement, compared to a more recent one about which no one knows whether it will last long or succeed. The press and public may forget when such an established movement was initiated, or they may remember more recent events. But a longer period of operation and replications of an innovation by others are valid criteria of the success and sustainability of a movement. Similarly, Margaret Sanger began the women's reproductive rights movement (and was imprisoned for that) in the first decade of 1900; she soon led the planned parenthood and sex education movement; a half- century later, in 1952, that movement led to the foundation of the International Planned Parenthood Federation (IPPF), which continued to promote and protect women's sexual and reproductive rights in more than 172 countries. In this study, we do not call these "old" and "outdated" movements because they began decades ago.

These cases are neither old nor obsolete; these are exemplary and prove successful empowerment movements.

Before we present the case study summaries, it is important to highlight several characteristics that transcend individual case studies. First, these movements were organized and led by ordinary women who have accomplished extraordinary goals and in so doing inspired others to follow their examples. Second, these women were not driven by personal achievement goals or self-advancement motives; they were motivated by their love and concerns for the well-being of their children, families, and other victims like them. Third, these women had to sustain their struggles sometimes for decades (the median age of the movements is over 20 years). In some cases projects sustained over multiple-generations (e.g., Grandmothers of Playa de Mayo, Grameen). This implies that one should not expect a quick success nor abandon a struggle too soon. Fourth, all important movements attract supporters and opponents; the women had to pay heavy personal price including suffering from death-threats, violence including death and grave physical, psychological and financial harms. In spite of these, they were not afraid to persist. Fifth, they were victims of serious inequality and injustice; they firmly believed that they must work together for their collective their success; that individually they were powerless to overcome the barriers they face. For this reason, the victims developed a common identity and strong bond among themselves which encouraged them to work in cohesive groups. This solidarity promoted cooperation rather than competition. Sixth, human development requires progress in several domains concurrently; these domains affect one another. These case studies reflect this reality. We find that while initially some of movements begin with a single goal (e.g., MADD, Dowry Deaths), after initial progress, some movements expand their original scope and include additional important goals (e.g., SEWA began with protecting women from work-site abuse and Grameen Bank began with poverty reduction in village women, both movements added health care, literacy, and gender development goals). For this reason, some case studies may be listed in more than one domain; but in our the statistical Meta-analysis, the total number of cases studies is 80 but some of these fall in more than one domain (in addition six innovative cases are included in discussion only).

Human Rights: Case Study Summaries

CASE STUDY #3: *AGRUPACIÓN DE LOS FAMILIARES DE DETENIDOS-DESAPARECIDOS* ("ASSOCIATION OF THE RELATIVES OF THE DETAINED AND DISAPPEARED"), CHILE, 1974 (HR)

Problem

The major problem being addressed is the disappearance of men during a period of political unrest following the coup of Salvador Allende in Chile.

Leadership Impetus

Agrupación de los Familiares de Detenidos-Desaparecidos (Agrupación) was formed in 1974 in response to the political repression by the military junta as a way to find out the whereabouts of detained and disappeared family members. Women of disappeared loved ones united after their individual efforts of searching prisons, hospitals, and government offices failed. Realizing that they were not alone in their struggle, these women began to trust each other for emotional support. With the assistance of the Committee for Peace, they formed Agrupación. The objectives of the group are to obtain information about their family members, raise awareness of the disappearances to the public, and demand justice for those responsible for the crimes. When the women were asked why they participated in Agrupación, they replied, "Because we are the women and mothers of this land, of the workers, of the professionals, of the students, and of future generations" (Chuchryk, 1993, p. 94).

EMPOWER Methods Used

¤ Rights protection and social action/reform
¤ Enabling service and assistance
¤ Empowerment training and leadership development

Both traditional means of protest (such as *habeas corpus* and court depositions) and more drastic measures (such as hunger strikes and chaining themselves to the gates of the government palace and Supreme Court) were performed by Agrupación members to raise public awareness. In 1983, Agrupación formed a folklore group, where women collectively sang and composed songs about their lives as single women. As a form of protest and expression of their despair, folklore members also perform the *cueca sola*, a variation on Chile's official national dance, at public demonstrations. Traditionally, most *cuecas* are about the man's struggle to win the woman's love and are performed by a couple. However, a *cueca sola* is performed by a single Agrupación member and depicts the woman's search for the missing man as well as the struggles of her country.

Other political activities include a folk group designed to engage in protest campaigns and provide mutual support for its members; the creation of *arpilleras*, or burlap tapestries, that illustrate the current Chilean political and economic circumstances; a youth group for the children, grandchildren, nieces, and nephews of the members; and workshops in political education, public relations, and leadership training.

Partners/Opposition

The Committee for Peace, an inter-church organization headed by Roman Catholic Archbishop Raul Silva Henriquez, was formed shortly after the overthrow to aid victims of repression. It was this organization that initially helped Agrupación to organize itself. After it was forced to disband by the government, the Committee for Peace was subsequently replaced by the Vicariate of Solidarity—a Roman Catholic organization directly under the authority of the Archbishop of Santiago. Agrupación is also currently a member of the Latin American Federation of Associations of Relatives of the Detained-Disappeared (FEDEFAM). Because of the nature of their work, many members of Agrupación have been arrested, and they continue to be at risk. Returned husbands of members may also oppose their wives' participation in the political group.

Macro-environment

The period surrounding the founding of Agrupación was one of intense political repression and economic troubles marked by the 1973 military overthrow of the democratically elected government of Salvador Allende. It was a violent time in which thousands were exiled, executed, imprisoned, and tortured. Men were the targets of abuse more often than women, due to women's secondary roles in the political parties and trade unions that were at risk of persecution from the military junta. Since the mid-1970s, there has been significant development of non-governmental women's organizations in Chile, such as the Women's Department of the National Trade Union Coordinator and the Women's Committee of the Chilean Human Rights Commission. Yet, as in many Latino countries, Agrupación exists within a society of machismo, which can often serve as a barrier to women insofar as participating in the political arena is concerned.

Impact and Remarks

Even after the reestablishment of democracy in Chile, Agrupación continued to be active in the political arena, in such acts as demanding trials for the military junta. There are roughly 150 members of Agrupación, only two of whom are men. They range in age from 15 to 70 years old and are primarily middle- and working-class housewives and mothers. The members of Agrupación report that they have gained "a new sense of themselves as political beings ...[and as] occupying a public political space that had not [been] occupied previously" (p. 95). In some cases, women have continued to participate in the organization even when it resulted in the dissolution of their marriages due to their returned husbands' opposition to her involvement. Many women look to Agrupación as a form of liberation and personal growth. They are also part of a more generalized political awakening where women are beginning to more actively define their own roles in the political process.

CASE STUDY #7: PREVENTION OF DOWRY-DEATH MOVEMENT, INDIA (HR)

Problem

The major problem being addressed is dowry-related violence and death, including wife-burning, abetted suicides, rape, and sexual harassment in India. In 1995, the National Crimes Records Bureau reported that an average of 17 dowry deaths occurred each day in India (i.e., more than 6,000 per year).

Dowry is a traditional practice in Indian marriages when usually the groom's family demands large sums of cash and/or expensive items during marriage negotiations. The more socially desirable the groom, the higher the dowry demanded. Often, the initial demands are beyond the financial means of the bride's family or beyond what they are willing to pay. Like many negotiations, some original demands are dropped during negotiations. Dowry, although illegal now for decades, is still a common practice; many greedy and unscrupulous grooms' families continue to put pressure on and abuse the newlywed brides to extract more dowry money or items from the brides' families even after the marriages. What begins with verbal abuse often escalates to physical abuse, and in extreme cases, ends with the victims being killed: this is called "Dowry Death." Dowry deaths are murders of brides by their husbands or in-laws who continue to abuse the brides to put pressure on the brides' families for more dowry money and/or items that were demanded earlier but were not agreed to by the brides' parents during the dowry negotiations. Common methods of killing include pouring kerosene oil (commonly used as a cooking fuel) on a victim and setting her afire or by hanging the bride by the neck. The grooms' families claim these "accidents" as suicides. After the death, the grooms are free to marry again with new demands of dowry.

The NCRB statistics show that 91,202 dowry deaths were reported in the country from January 1, 2001 to December 31, 2012.

In spite of all the stringent laws and campaigns against dowry, statistics on dowry-related deaths in the country during the past 12 years from 2001 released by the National Crime Records Bureau (NCRB) last week show that such deaths have only increased over the years.

The NCRB statistics show that 91,202 dowry deaths were reported in the country from January 1, 2001, to December 31, 2012. Out of that 84,013 were charged and sent for trial and the rest were either withdrawn by the government during the course of investigation or not investigated. Of this, 5,081 cases were reported to be false after investigations.

While 6,851 Dowry deaths were reported in the country in 2001, the figure reached 7,618 in 2006 and touched 8,233 in 2012.

State wise break-up provided in the statistics show that the highest incidence of dowry deaths was in Uttar Pradesh and Bihar. During the period, 23,824 dowry deaths were reported in Uttar Pradesh and 19,702 sent for trial. In Bihar 13,548 cases were reported during the period and 9,984 sent for trial.

These numbers exceed the national averages by about four times.

Dowry offenses continue despite the passage of the Dowry Prohibition Act of 1961, as well subsequent amendments issued in 1983 and 1986.

Leadership Impetus

Beginning in the late 1970s, women's organizations intervened in dowry-death cases brought to court. Led by a Supreme Court advocate, Rani Jethmalani, a group of organizations collectively called "Solidarity with Women" were involved in a number of landmark cases of dowry deaths. In fact, the term "dowry death" first became used around 1977–1978 by women's organizations when investigations revealed that deaths of married women were actually murders or abetted suicides associated with dowry demands.

EMPOWER Methods Used

- Rights protection and legal activism
- Emergency services using case-management
- Public education
- Media use

Social action litigation (SAL) is a common legal strategy used by family and women's organizations to aid in dowry-death cases as well as in other cases of injustice. When the aggrieved person is detained or cannot file a petition herself, any person, such as the bride's family or a women's organization, can move the court on her behalf. The court then intervenes to protect the rights of the disadvantaged and vulnerable. "Specifically, the court insists that the laws must be followed; in those cases where there is a failure to implement the law, either through acts of commission or omission, then the court... can intervene and correct the executive actions and when any law takes away or abridges any rights, [can] declare such law void and correct the legislative action" (Jethmalani, 1995, p. 24).

Partners/Opposition

Established in 1992, WARLAW (Women's Action Research and Legal Action for Women) provides free legal services to victims of dowry violence (Jethmalani, 1995). WARLAW was directly involved in several landmark cases of public-interest litigation in general and dowry-death cases, in particular. Women's organizations and women lawyers have also filed petitions and held demonstrations to further the cause. In terms of posing opposition to the anti-dowry-death movement, the lax attitudes of the police and the judicial system often trivialize the dangerous nature of dowry murders. Despite laws that prohibit dowry, the practice is not seen as immoral. Rather, dowry, along with the associated violence committed by the bride's family, is widely accepted. "Dowry-related deaths were usually dismissed as suicides or accidents. In fact, prior to 1983, every form of violence committed within the family, either in the natal or spousal home, was not considered criminal. Law did not enter the private sphere of the home" (Jethmalani, 1995).

Macro-environment

In Indian society, patriarchal values reign, and male members dominate female members. The internalization of these values by women can be seen in the crimes perpetrated by women on women, such as a mother-in-law or sister-in-law abusing or killing the bride. Dowry is a commonplace practice among all classes, communities, religious groups, and castes. Since women are considered an economic liability within their natal homes and husbands' home, a dowry (money or property) is given to the bridegroom or parents as compensation for the bride's "non-productive" status.

Impact and Remarks

Because of the assistance of women's organizations such as WARLAW and Solidarity with Women, several amendments have been made to Indian laws that were insufficiently punitive in dealing with dowry deaths. For example, as a direct result of an important case involving the dowry death of Satya

Rani Chadha, the definition of "dowry" was amended in 1983 to include a demand for money at any time after the marriage, rather than only previous to the marriage. In addition, the Supreme Court accepted WARLAW's petition that challenged India's non-compliance with the UN Committee on the Elimination of Discrimination Against Women (CEDAW). According to Hindu Personal Law, individuals who give or take dowry can now be tried in court. Despite the legislative gains pertaining to dowry death and dowry-related abuse, the problem remains deeply rooted in the cultural norms of the society. However, legislative change does set the standard of behavior and can help shape public opinion. According to the founder of WARLAW, "The acceptance of [WARLAW's] petitions regarding male-biased laws is a big step towards empowerment." In addition to amending the constitution of India, WARLAW efforts have exposed the lack of gender sensitization among ruling judges and investigating officers.

CASE STUDY #2: BLACK SASH, CAPE TOWN, SOUTH AFRICA, 1955 (HR)

Problem

The major problem being addressed is apartheid in South Africa and HR violations perpetrated against black and colored people in South Africa.

Leadership Impetus

> It started when six middle-class white women—Jean Sinclair, Ruth Foley, Elizabeth McLaren, Tertia Pybus, Jean Bosazza, and Helen Newton-Thompson—met for tea on 19 May 1955 to discuss how to oppose the specific Parliamentary Bill designed to increase the number of National Party representatives in the Senate in order to pass the Separate Representation of Voters Bill.

As a result of the initiative of six white women who were against a crucial change in the South African Constitution, the Women's Defense of the Constitution League was created in 1955. A newly introduced Senate bill would have filled the Senate with its supporters in order to guarantee the needed two-thirds majority to change the Constitution, barring "colored" people (i.e., neither white nor black, and usually of Indian descent) from voting. In response, the six women recruited other women to join them in obtaining 3,000 signatures on a petition required to call a public meeting. On the day of the meeting, thousands of women supporters marched to city hall where the mayor greeted their arrival. The group later became known as "Black Sash."

The Black Sash continued their anti-apartheid protests in a wide variety of ways, but within a decade of its establishment, in 1964, Nelson Mandela and other prominent national leaders were imprisoned. Between the 1960s and the 1980s, oppression, discrimination, and violence in the apartheid nation escalated; in 1985, the Black Sash Advice Office Trust was established to raise funds to support their mission. In 1990, Mandela was released from prison and he declared the Black Sash the conscience of South Africa. In 1995, the Black Sash was awarded the Danish Peace Foundation's Peace Prize (Black Sash, 2015, p. 1).

EMPOWER Methods Used

- Rights protection and social action/reform
- Enabling service and assistance
- Media use
- Public education and participation

During the 1960s, the Black Sash had a two-pronged focus. The first was to protest the introduction of certain legislation. A common demonstration of protest was the "silent stand," during which women stood in place while carrying placards. In 1962, the government banned all demonstrations within one mile of the city hall and within a certain radius of Parliament in Cape Town. Therefore, the Black Sash resorted to writing letters to the newspapers. However, at first the media was not receptive to such protest, and it was only after much struggle that the letters or articles were published. The second focus was to provide various types of assistance such as counseling support via the Advice Office. The first Advice Office in Cape Town originated as a bail fund to get black women out of prison who had refused to carry passes (needed to leave townships and go into white areas to work). Being released from jail would allow these women to be with their children until the trial. Gradually, other offices opened in other cities as the Black Sash gained a better understanding of the pass laws. Laws required black men and women to carry passes at all times. Punishment was usually a fine or 70 days in jail. Black Sash members essentially became experts on pass laws in the entire country. Practicing lawyers were uninformed about the specifics of the pass laws. Therefore, the Black Sash was often the only source of such information for the press, and by the 1960s, the press was more open to publishing their materials. Black Sash members monitored the Langa Pass Law Court on a regular basis in order to provide on-the-spot counseling as needed or help in obtaining an attorney. Visitors were brought to the courts in order to expose the unjust process of the pass laws. The Black Sash also searched for missing people after police raids on squatters (clusters of homeless people living in temporary and makeshift huts or cottages).

The Black Sash has focused on the issue of forced removals of black people from their homelands (black South Africans were often expelled from their homes by force by government authorities). Although the Black Sash movement tried to expose the forced removals of black people from their homes for a long time, it was only after various denominations of South African churches got involved in this movement, that the white majority and other nations of the world became aware of this major problem.

Partners/Opposition

Not only was the press reluctant to print letters written by the Black Sash, the editor of *Rand Daily Mail* once told the Black Sash president "that it was very foolish to keep this organization going and that she should rather be working [for another political organization]" (Duncan, 1991, p. 316). Black Sash workers often faced the threat of arrest and even attempts on their lives. For example, one of the leaders of Black Sash was arrested several times for being in black areas without permits. Tear gas was fired at her home. Her car was burned in front of her house. She received threatening phone calls. She was also involved in a suspicious car accident, which resulted in the death of her husband as well as a well-known female activist. To this day, some suspect that the "accident" was a deliberate act perpetrated by the government as a scare tactic.

Macro-environment

During the 1960s there was very little opposition to the South African government outside Parliament. Repression of political activity and the declaration of a state of government in 1960 succeeded in preventing black resistance for nearly ten years. Also during this time, the government practiced the policy of forced removals of black people from their home-lands to resettlement camps. Resettlement camps often had no water or sewer facilities, and sometimes no shelter was provided at all. Because the people lost their means of survival and income, the people became impoverished and were forced to join the migrant labor system. An esti-mated 3 million people were forced to move, including about 700,000 white, colored, and Indian people. Although Black Sash and others tried to expose the issue, it was not until the 1970s that the government was directly challenged. According to Black Sash, "As the force of Apartheid strengthened in 1970, so did the determination of the Black Sash to end it. The members protested vigorously against the Bantu Homelands Citizenship Act, which stripped African people of their South African citizenship" (Black Sash, 2015; http://www.blacksash.org.za/index.php/our-legacy/our-history).

Impact and Remarks

By the end of 1995, the Black Sash had evolved into its current struc-ture of a professionally staffed non-governmental organisation, led by a National Director, and accountable to a Board of Trustees. Currently the Black Sash works in three areas in the social protection arena, with an emphasis on women and children: rights-based information, education and training; community monitoring; and advocacy in partnership. (Black Sash, 2015).

The Black Sash proved to themselves and the immediate community that women have an equal contribution to make in terms of society and political work. The organization empowered its leaders to positions of authority that they might not have gained if not for this organization and the fight against apartheid. The Black Sash represented real opposition to the HR violations perpetrated by the former government through their unrelenting efforts, even in the face of physical danger to their own lives. The plight of non-white people in South Africa was exposed to white communities both in South Africa and elsewhere in the world.

CASE STUDY #5: COMADRES OF EL SALVADOR (COMMITTEE OF MOTHERS AND RELATIVES OF POLITICAL PRISONERS, DISAPPEARED, AND ASSASSINATED OF EL SALVADOR MONSEÑOR ROMERO, 1977 (HR)

Problem

The major problem being addressed was the disappearance of individuals and other HR violations in El Salvador during the revolutionary conflict and repression of the Duarte regime.

Leadership Impetus

The committee of CoMadres was founded on Christmas Eve, 1977, when Monsignor Romero invited a group of approximately nine grieving women with missing relatives to supper, and proposed forming a committee for victims of political repression. Of the founding members, some were politically aware and active, while others were not. They were united by the goal of protection of fundamental HR as well as the discovery of the facts surrounding the thousands of disappearances and political killings that had occurred since 1972.

EMPOWER Methods Used

- ¤ Enabling assistance and service
- ¤ Rights protection and social action/reform
- ¤ Media use
- ¤ Public education and participation
- ¤ Organizing partnership

A group of mothers and relatives of the disappeared persons organized and named themselves as CoMadres to address this problem:

Comrades (CoMadres) is the committee of mothers and relatives of prisoners, the disappeared and the politically assassinated of El Salvador.

> It was established in December 1977, with the help of the Catholic Archdiocese of San Salvador and the Archbishop Óscar Romero, to discover the truth behind the missing relatives of the membership. Among their activities are the distribution of flyers to get out the message, and the occupation of government offices to elicit the help of foreign nations in pressuring the Salvadoran government. By 1993, there were an estimated 500 or more members. A leader of this organisation was María Teresa Tula. (Tula, 2015)

Its activities included taking over the Salvadoran Red Cross building, organizing a hunger strike and nonviolent occupation of the UN building in San Salvador, as well as public demonstrations in parks and plazas. Since then, the organization has grown, and the CoMadres have organized their activities by assigning specific tasks to individual groups. For example, one group provides material aid, such as weekly rations of rice, beans, sugar, and milk, to prisoners and victims' families. It also conducted outreach to individuals living in shantytowns by investigating their cases and getting legal assistance for them. Another group facilitated media coverage on the CoMadres by writing news bulletins and press releases and broadcasting information about political prisoners on the Catholic Church radio station for 20 minutes each day. This group also organized monthly masses in commemoration of Monsignor Romero's assassination, bi-weekly sit-ins at the Ministry of Justice, and other demonstrations (Acosta, 1993; CoMadres, 2015; Tula, 2015). Other groups were responsible for maintaining relations with the labor unions, political organizations, government offices, and the press; organizing delegations of CoMadres to Costa Rico, Mexico, and Canada; arranging press conferences with foreign and national journalists; and investigating and keeping track of denunciations presented to the CoMadres. The CoMadres maintained communication with political prisoners so that family members, who were often forbidden to see the prisoners, could send food or other items. The group also kept track of kidnappings and deaths. In order to inform others of the atrocities taking place and the role of CoMadres, representatives of CoMadres were delegated to special conferences. In El Salvador, CoMadres were constantly informing people of the latest crimes through public talks and flyers distributed in egg crates at the public markets.

Partners/Opposition

CoMadres are affiliated with and supported by the Roman Catholic Church. Monsignor Romero, the Archbishop of San Salvador, spread the word about the CoMadres through his preaching to the community and even gave the organization money from his own savings to buy medicine and food for the political prisoners and to pay for the press releases.

In 1981, several Latin American organizations formed by relatives of the disappeared formed a collective HR federation, *Federacion de Familiares de Detenidos-Desaparecidos* (FEDEFAM). Beginning in the mid-1980s, "Friends of CoMadres" solidarity organizations were established in the United States, Australia, Switzerland, Germany, Mexico, and Canada. These groups raised funds and served as political watchdogs for HR violations in El Salvador. Yet, in El Salvador, the CoMadres faced continual danger for their open protest against the government. Their offices have been bombed at least five times. A majority of the most active members were arrested, tortured, and raped. Five were killed and three disappeared. One pregnant CoMadres member was kidnapped, raped, and stabbed by Death Squad soldiers. A few weeks later, she was placed in jail where her baby was born. In addition to governmental opposition, many husbands of the CoMadres were opposed to their participation; some of the women were beaten because of their activism.

Macro-environment

During the 1970s, Latin American women were organizing themselves around issues of labor and consumer demands, HR issues, and other gender-, age-, and ethnic-related problems. El Salvador, in particular, was embroiled in a civil war (1979–1992) that further added to the problem of HR violations. El Salvadorans were being threatened by an organized terror on society that systematically eliminated any opposition to the militarist regime.

Impact and Remarks

Currently, there are approximately 700 CoMadres members from poor, working, and middle classes. Mothers of soldiers who disappeared in action are now also invited to join. CoMadres are known internationally, with offices in Mexico, Costa Rica, and Canada. To honor their efforts, the CoMadres were given the Robert F. Kennedy Human Rights Award in the United States and the Bruno Kreisky award in Austria. Even though the CoMadres is primarily a HR organization associated with the Roman Catholic Church, it now serves an important role in the political process of El Salvador. For example, the CoMadres demanded a peace settlement between the two fighting political and military forces that were engaged in a civil war: the U.S.-supported Christian Democratic Duarte government, and the Democratic Revolutionary Front–Farabundo Martí National Liberation Front (FDR-FLMN) coalition of politico-military groups that used guerilla tactics.

Patricia grew up in a Christian base community that was persecuted during the 1980s and was forced to flee the country at a young age. She had aspirations of becoming a nun, but unable to return to her community after discovering her parents were murdered by the Salvadoran military, she joined the CO-MADRES at the tender age of 10 years old at the suggestion of Archbishop Oscar Romero, who visited Salvadoran refugees in Mexico where she was in exile.

Upon joining CO-MADRES, she immediately became involved in their orphanage, attending to children rescued from bombarded rural areas of El Salvador. CO-MADRES members often remarked that, "she took care of the children when she was just a child." As the CO-MADRES work grew and became more visible, many of their members became targets of military persecution and violence. Patricia was no exception and was captured, brutally raped and tortured twice. During the telling of her testimony, she humbly remembered how she was rescued moments before her execution through international solidarity efforts and direct intervention from then U.S. Senator Edward Kennedy in 1990.

Patricia became a nurse, working in the same profession as her adoptive mother, CO-MADRES co-founder, Alicia de Garcia, and dedicated her life to the defense of human rights. She taught first aid and literacy classes in rural areas, assisted in refugee resettlement and advocated for political prisoners during the war. She also worked, as so many CO-MADRES did, on the investigation and documentation of cases of the disappeared, assassinated and imprisoned, and organized countless marches and protests against the brutality of the Salvadoran military regime. Through her work in the church, she also carried on Archbishop Oscar Romero's legacy of consciousness-raising and self-determination of the poor through liberation theology. She leaves behind her four children, devoted sister Blanca Garcia, and over 300 members of CO-MADRES who will carry forward the work that she led with wisdom, strength and undying faith. (Friends of CoMadres, 2014)

Over the years, the needs of CoMadres have evolved from the reappearance of their loved ones to the liberation of their country and the protection of all HR, including women's rights. They have demanded that women be included in formal political decision-making bodies, and discussed issues of domestic violence, rape, women's lack of control over their own sexuality, and women's oppressive gender roles. An important and common attribute of all human rights movements is they begin with the goal of protection against immediate threats, promotion of freedom, and survival needs in powerless societies; however, it takes several decades before tangible and substantial progress is accomplished by these movements in terms of the enhancement of empowerment in any one or all five levels (individual, family, community, organization, and sociocultural).

CASE STUDY #10: EQUALITY NOW, UNITED STATES, 1992 (HR)

Problem

The major problem being addressed is the violation of women's HR around the world and the lack of attention given to this problem by international organizations, national governments, traditional HR groups, and the press. Issues of concern include rape, trafficking of women, domestic violence, female infanticide, genital mutilation, and sexual harassment.

Leadership Impetus

In 1992, Jessica Neuwirth (an American lawyer), Navanethem Pillay (a South African lawyer), and Feryal Gharahi (a Muslim lawyer) created Equality Now as an organization dedicated to securing the civil, political, economic, and social rights of women and girls around the world. The founders envisioned an organization with two main components: detailed and accurate documentation of violations, and for the HR of women. Equality Now is a volunteer-based movement that targets ordinary people, rather than "professional" activists, so that they will be motivated to express some form of protest against HR violations.

EMPOWER Methods Used

- ¤ Public education and participation
- ¤ Rights protection and social action/reform
- ¤ Media use
- ¤ Organizing partnership

Equality Now operates largely through the Women's Action Network, which is composed of more than 4,000 groups and individuals in more than 100 nations around the world. This network gathers information about abuses and violations from an international network of activists and organizations. Appropriate responses and strategies (appeals) are then formulated in conjunction with local experts and communicated to the public through the network. Often letters or petitions are written by individuals from around the world to express protest against a particular case of abuse.

Equality Now organized a worldwide protest on behalf of women's reproductive rights in Poland by contacting doctors and medical associations around the globe and expressing opposition to the Polish Medical Society's decision to prohibit abortions. Equality Now has successfully used the media in at least two cases. First, Equality Now published an editorial in the *Christian Science Monitor* on behalf of a Saudi Arabian woman who had sought asylum in Canada on the basis of gender discrimination and who was later threatened with deportation back to her home country.

She was subsequently allowed to stay in Canada; Canada also established national guidelines on gender-based political asylum. Second, Equality Now persuaded several American public television networks (e.g., Link TV) to initiate an awareness-raising campaign of the problem of female genital mutilation.

From 1994 to 1996, Equality Now had a monthly letter-writing column in *Spin* magazine, a music magazine for a young adult audience. This forum generated many letters of protest from its readership on behalf of the violations featured in the column. Equality Now has an advisory council which comprises prominent activists including Gloria Steinem and Rose Styron, widow of novelist William Styron.

Partners/Opposition

In addition to the support provided by the Women's Action Network, Equality Now has received assistance on specific issues. For example, there has been collaboration with the Polish Federation for Women and from Planned Parenthood and the IPPF in the fight for reproductive rights in Poland. Equality Now has also worked with the BATIS/AWARE Center for Women in the Philippines (*Batis* means "spring" in Tagalog) and the HELP (Housing in Emergency of Love and Peace) Asian Women's Shelter in Tokyo, Japan, in order to raise awareness about the potential dangers to Filipino women working in Japan's entertainment industry. Young women allured to big cities with the promise of a movie/modeling career but who end up as "call girls" or victims of trafficking as sex-slaves are euphemistically called entertainment industry workers. Both these organizations are dedicated to helping women in distress and human trafficking victims (BATIS/AWARE, 2015).

Macro-environment

Despite the fact that most abuses committed against women fall within the purview of the United Nations' 1948 Universal Declaration of Human Rights, these violations are often ignored by the Member governments because they often fall within the private sphere (such as domestic violence) and are therefore not considered legal offenses.

Impact and Remarks

Equality Now prides itself on striving to represent women's issues from many different nations as demonstrated by the international membership of the Women's Action Network. It also tries to structure its organization to be democratic and decentralized by relying on the collaboration between professionals and laypersons around the globe. By channeling local efforts to protest a particular HR abuse, varying cultures can unite on common issues of concern. Through such solidarity, women have been both empowered and inspired to engage broad HR efforts.

CASE STUDY #6: FORWARD INTERNATIONAL (FOUNDATION FOR WOMEN'S HEALTH RESEARCH AND DEVELOPMENT), LONDON, ENGLAND, 1980 (HR)

Problem

This case study falls within the domain of HR. The major problem being addressed is the continued practice of female genital mutilation/cutting (FGM/C) in many African countries. Described by one anti-FGM/C activist as a complex social practice that is performed to suppress and control the sexual behavior of girls and women (Dorkenoo, 1994, p. 4), FGM/C can have serious physical and mental health consequences such as chronic pain, bleeding, infection, infertility, and loss of sexual responsiveness.

Leadership Impetus

The Women's Action Group Against Excision and Infibulation (WAGFEI) was formed by African, Arab, and British men and women in the wake of international interest sparked by a 1980 FGM/C report published by the Minority Rights Group (MRG). The MRG is an international research unit registered in the United Kingdom as an educational charity organization. The report, entitled *Female Circumcision, Excision and Infibulation: The Facts and Proposals for Change*, contained contributions from a number of African women campaigners. Subsequently, FORWARD (now known as FORWARD International) developed from WAGFEI into an independent international organization in 1983. Registered under the UK Charity Act, it is dedicated to the promotion of health among African women and children, and anti-FGM/C education and actions.

EMPOWER Methods Used

- Rights protection and social action/reform
- Enabling service and assistance
- Media use, support, and advocacy
- Public education and participation

Efua Dorkenoo, a founding member and director of FORWARD International, first introduced FGM/C as a HR issue to the United Nations Commission on Human Rights in 1982. Since then, FORWARD International has lobbied the government on a number of different issues concerning FGM/C. Operating at the grassroots level, FORWARD International combines community action, emergency child protection measures, professional guidelines, and training in order to prevent FGM/C. It produces and disseminates training manuals for professional and community workers that are widely used in several countries. FORWARD International operates a consultant service for policy-makers, local and health authorities, and agencies such as WHO, the World Bank, the Royal College of Nursing, and the Swedish Board of Health and Social Welfare.

In 1989, it held the First Study Conference on Genital Mutilation of Girls in Europe. Attended by representatives of the UK Department of Health, UK local authorities, community group leaders, and professionals from Europe, the United States, and Canada, this conference pushed the issue of FGM/C outside of Africa onto the international agenda. As a result of these efforts, the Commonwealth's "London Declaration" established a framework for the eradication of FGM/C in Western countries, which has been adopted by other European countries and Canada.

FORWARD International has served as consultant to several television documentaries and radio programs seen internationally, including a 1993 ABC production called *Scarred for Life,* which dealt with FGM/C in Gambia. Other notable projects initiated by FORWARD International include an anti-FGM/C training conference for men in Africa; a counseling service for young girls in the United Kingdom; fund-raising for the anti-FGM/C campaign encouraging concerned individuals of non–FGM/C-practicing communities to support the cause; and a periodic newsletter called *Forward Links.*

Partners/Opposition

Lord Kennet, a member of the House of Lords, assisted FORWARD International in introducing the first (yet unsuccessful) FGM/C-prohibition bill into the UK Parliament. (A 1985 law would later prohibit FGM/C in the United Kingdom.) Lord Kennet also helped the organization obtain funding for education of the immigrant women from countries where FGM/C practices are prevalent. In the United States, FORWARD International works with Equality Now (Case Study #10) in order to brief senior staff at Congress and the U.S. Agency for International Development (USAID) on FGM/C policy. It also served as an advisor to Congresswoman Pat Schroeder on FGM/C related bills and deliberations in the U.S. Congress.

FORWARD International collaborates with governmental, non-governmental, and international agencies, including the UK Department of Health, WHO, and the UN Center for Human Rights. It networks with community organizations, health and social work professionals, and women's organizations around the world, as well as African campaigning groups such as the Inter-Africa Committee on Traditional Practices. It also supports grassroots projects with training and educational materials, funding, or lobbying efforts. For example, in Ghana it funded the first research conducted on FGM/C in the Upper East Region of Ghana and lobbied for the Gambian Women's Bureau to obtain research funding (Walker & Parmar, 1993).

Macro-environment

More than 125 million girls and women alive today have undergone some form of female genital mutilation in the 29 countries in Africa and the

Middle East where the harmful practice is most concentrated. It is however, a global health issue, and can have devastating physical, psychological, and social consequences for women and girls. (WHO, 2015)

A recent WHO estimate concludes that more than 125 million girls and women in Africa and Middle East have undergone FGM/C (WHO, 2015). It is a major global health threat. Twenty-eight African countries are reported to practice one or more forms of FGM/C. According to recent WHO data, the estimated prevalence rates of FGM/C among girls and women between the ages of 15 and 49 years of age in Africa is between 97.9% in Somalia (in 2006) and 0.8% in Uganda (in 2006); in seven countries, the prevalence is greater than 80% (WHO FGM/C, 2015). Outside Africa, FGM/C is practiced in Oman, both North and South Yemen, and the United Arab Emirates (UAE) as well as in other Arab countries, including Bahrain, Qatar, and some areas in Saudi Arabia. Clitoridectomy (the removal of the clitoris often called female circumcision) has been reported in South America by some indigenous groups in Peru, Colombia, Mexico, and Brazil; female circumcision is practiced by Muslim populations of Indonesia and Malaysia and by Bohra Muslims in India, Pakistan, and East Africa. In Western countries (Europe, Australia, Canada, and the United States), immigrant women from areas where FGM/C is practiced are reported to be genitally mutilated, but no prevalence studies have been conducted, nor have studies been done on the numbers of girls at risk.

Impact and Remarks

In 1989, FORWARD International was instrumental in the passage of a child-care law that includes FGM/C as a form of physical abuse. Its model for FGM/C prevention has been tested with the African immigrant communities in the United Kingdom and adopted by the UK Department of Health and local authorities.

Despite these successes, elimination of FGM/C in traditional societies requires action on different levels, networking, and multi-national collaborations.

CASE STUDY #8: *GRUPO DE APOYO MUTUO* ("MUTUAL SUPPORT GROUP") FOR THE REAPPEARANCE OF OUR SONS, FATHERS, HUSBANDS, AND BROTHERS (GAM), GUATEMALA, 1984 (HR)

Problem

This case study falls within the domain of HR. The main problem being addressed was the deaths and disappearances of hundreds of thousands of people during the 1970s and 1980s in Guatemala, the highest number of such *desaparecido* cases in Latin America as of then. Without an internal HR monitoring group, the government policies and abuses were left unchecked.

According to a critical report by The American Association for the Advancement of Science (AAA) (Ball et al., 1999):

> "During Guatemala's 36-year armed conflict, the State killed hundreds of thousands of citizens and displaced a million more. The enormity of the numbers involved creates the danger that the terror in Guatemala, as in Stalin's Russia, will be remembered as statistics and not as human lives cut short." [But inverting Stalin's quote,] "statistics can also establish the patterns of what is both a tragedy and a crime, in this case a deliberate and drawn-out policy of extra-judicial murder by the Guatemalan government." (Ball et al., 1999)

Leadership Impetus

Three women formed the Mutual Support Group in Guatemala (known as the GAM) on June 5, 1984 (GAM, 1985). Searching for their loved ones, they had frequently met one another at the morgues, cemeteries, police stations, and hospitals, or at the University of San Carlos. The women began to meet regularly at the local headquarters of Peace Brigades International. Inspired by an audiotape recorded by the CoMadres, the group of mothers of missing Salvadorans, the Guatemalan women decided to follow suit. Several of the original members were relatives of 19 university students and professors kidnapped in 1984. Two-thirds of the GAM members are poor indigenous women without previous organizing experience (GAM, 1985).

EMPOWER Methods Used

- Rights protection and social action/reform
- Enabling service and assistance

Knowing full well the dangers of challenging the government, GAM did not make overt accusations in the very beginning of their fight. In 1984, GAM requested meetings with the national police chief and foreign minister, to no avail. At the same time, the group started to keep detailed records of the disappearances revealed to them by their members. In all, 416 such cases were reported, most of whom were men aged 20–40 years old, some women (several pregnant), and children aged 6–16 years old. GAM also held public demonstrations and protests. After many entreaties, President Mejía Victores finally met with GAM on August 1, 1984. Despite promises to investigate the incidents and to establish a tripartite commission to do so, the president told them that the missing persons had joined the guerillas or left the country. Because of the continued lack of institutional support afforded to their cause, GAM increased their level of pressure exerted on the government through several forms of protest. They publicly charged divisions of the security forces with direct blame for the disappeared persons; petitioned the tri-partite commission to let them testify; protested the Public Ministry (by blocking traffic; playing flutes, whistles, and drums); demanded the results of the alleged investigations; and occupied the National Constituent Assembly so that political prisoners would be recognized in the new Guatemalan Constitution.

Partners/Opposition

In direct response to GAM's public protests, the Mejía Victores administration discredited and terrorized GAM members. In November of 1984, 72 hours after GAM's fourth meeting with the chief of state, two of those listed as missing were found tortured and dead. In March of 1985, the departmental governor of Guatemala City asked four members of GAM to sign a document stating that "provoking public disorder was a subversive act" (p. 43). The president publicly announced his suspicion that GAM was being manipulated by the communists and subversists who were making trouble in an otherwise peaceful nation. After GAM publicly refuted the charges, Héctor Gómez, one of the few men on the GAM directorate, was kidnapped and later found tortured and dead. At his funeral, a wife of a disappeared student leader openly commemorated his death. Later, she was also found dead along with her younger brother and infant son.

Macro-environment

Guatemala had a over 30-year history of government violence, an oppressive affluent minority, and of the highest number of disappearances in Latin America. Aside from a few citizen groups that formed to voice their protest against the government's action (the first one being the Committee of Relatives of Disappeared Persons in 1967), Guatemala does not have an internal HR group that can monitor rights violations. In 1976, following a major earthquake in Guatemala, indigenous-*ladino* (*mestizo*) organized through an umbrella labor organization called *Comité Nacional Department Unidad Sindical*, linking unions and peasant groups in their fight for better working and living conditions. The government responded with death squads that killed union, peasant, and political leaders, as well as others suspected of "dangerous" opinions. This "Reign of Official Terror," which also led to the massacres of more than 50,000 indigenous peasants, destruction of hamlets, and forced relocations, clearly showed the government use of violence.

Impact and Remarks

By January of 1986, then-president Cerezo agreed to establish an independent investigatory commission, even though he had previously rejected responsibility for the past governmental actions and orally agreed to an amnesty law. In May of 1986, the new Supreme Court gave list of 1,367 cases to a single criminal court for investigation. The judge in charge of the investigation reported that 105 cases had common explanations; most were declared dead without specific causes; and 19 had been issued passports from the Immigration Office. None of the cases were reported to be involved with any security forces or military officials.

In June 1986, members of the Christian Democratic Party met with a presidential assistant to talk about the Law of Social Service, which offered financial aid to the widows and orphans of the missing. Fewer than 12 GAM members accepted the money; those who did were expelled from the group. Although GAM was one of the last resistance groups to organize in Latin America, in the 1970s and 1980s, it was the first HR group to survive amidst the intense repression of Guatemalan military regimes. GAM continues to fight for the memories of their disappeared loved ones despite enormous obstacles.

CASE STUDY #4: MADRES DE PLAZA DE MAYO, ARGENTINA, 1977 (HR)

Problem

This case study falls within the domain of HR. The main problem being addressed is the disappearance of an estimated 30,000 individuals during the 1970s, a period in Argentina that was marked by political instability and extremism. In 1976, certain right-wing factions of Peronism tried to subvert guerilla activity by kidnapping, torturing, and executing suspected leftists. However, the government refused to even acknowledge most of these *desaparecidos* or disappearances. According to Madres de Plaza de Mayo, there were 15,000 murdered in the streets, 30,000 disappeared without a trace, 8,900 political prisoners, and 1,500,000 refugees in other countries. International Institute of Social History (2017), https://socialhistory.org/en/collections/madres-de-plaza-de-mayo (For more see: "Marguerite G, Revolutionizing Motherhood: the Mothers of the Plaza de Mayo," Wilmington, DE: SR Books, 1994, pp 24-27, 256. Accessed January 16, 2017).

Leadership Impetus

The mothers of the first *desaparecidos* who were reported missing between the years of 1974 and 1975 spoke individually to the government officials, the police, the Roman Catholic Church, and politicians in order to find out about their missing children. Some even visited the jails and churches to search for them. As the number of *desaparecidos* increased, the mothers found themselves bumping into one another in police stations and on the streets. In mid-1977, a group of 14 women protesting the disappearance of their sons, husbands, and brothers gathered in a square in Buenos Aires. At first, no one took much notice of their gathering. The government labeled them as terrorists, their families were despised by the community. Yet they returned each week to meet, support one another, and share their experiences. The mothers decided to divide their ranks and have small groups visit the Ministry of Interior and the police stations. The rest would go door-to-door in order to encourage other mothers to join them at the plaza. They wrote letters to keep in touch with one another when they were not meeting. When the number of mothers involved in the movement reached around 60–70, the police told them they could no longer congregate in the plaza; they were ordered to, then forced to, move. Instead of retreating home, the mothers began to march around the pyramidal monument in the center of the Plaza de Mayo. On a couple of occasions, the police demanded to see one of the mothers' identity papers. On one occasion, the women handed the police officer more than 300 identity papers for each one of the mothers present at that time. The mothers stayed in the plaza until each of the papers was returned. This action allowed them to remain in the plaza for more than two hours, whereas before they were only able to stay for a few minutes at a time. Eventually, these women became known as Las Madres de Plaza de Mayo. As more people disappeared, more women joined the march every day—grieving publicly and calling attention to the increasing number of disappearances.

EMPOWER Methods Used

- ¤ Media use
- ¤ Organizing partnership
- ¤ Enabling service and assistance
- ¤ Rights protection and social action/reform
- ¤ Public education and participation

The Madres' first gatherings did not attract media attention. However, the mothers took advantage of certain opportunities to make their cause known. For example, when the press was in the plaza covering the visit of the U.S. Ambassador to Spain, Terence Todman, the mothers gathered in the plaza, where armed soldiers tried to forcibly remove them from the area. At this moment, the mothers yelled to catch the attention of nearby journalists, who later reported the incident in the international media.

The mothers bonded with other grassroots organizations by participating in protest marches. In order to stand out from the crowd, the mothers decided to don white triangular shawls (really their children's old nappies or diapers) on their heads, which became their trademark. At one of the marches, 300 protesters were arrested, including some foreign journalists who would later report on the incident of the mothers taking action in honor of their missing children. The mothers, along with another grassroots organization called "Familias," wrote a petition that was published in the local newspaper. While in the midst of preparing another petition, three of the mothers were kidnapped. Despite these intimidation tactics, the mothers returned to the plaza to demonstrate their outrage.

In 1978, the year Argentina played host to the World Cup soccer tournament, the repression of the mothers' efforts in the Plaza de Mayo increased. They were thrown in jail, beaten, attacked by police dogs, and even tear-gassed. Because of the increased patrolling of the plaza during this time, the mothers began meeting in churches. They were afraid that if the police found them they would be thrown out of the churches as well. In part due to the World Cup event, the media provided much coverage (both positive and negative) of the mothers' protests in the Plaza.

After the World Cup, some of the mothers traveled to Europe and the United States trying to gain international support from government officials, the press, and other HR organizations. When these delegates returned to Argentina, the treatment of the mothers had worsened: mothers were being arrested every week. If one mother was arrested, all the mothers would accompany her in a show of solidarity! The "official" Association of Mothers of Plaza de Mayo was formed on May 14, 1979, in the presence of a public notary. In 1980, with the financial support of women's organizations in Holland, the mothers opened their own office to hold their meetings. During this year, they also published their first bulletin to inform the public of their activities. Their slogan became *Aparición con Vida* ("Reappearance with Life"). The mothers also wrote a book of poems expressing their despair and outrage toward the dictatorship.

Today, after more than 30 years of struggle, the mothers and grandmothers remain active by attending HR conferences, publishing a newspaper, giving speeches, and maintaining a website in four languages, in addition to their ongoing protest activities. They have also lent support to international political activities outside of Argentina. (For more details, see the three websites cited at the end of this case study; Las Madres Playa de Mayo, 2015.)

Partners/Opposition

The military government attempted to suppress the feminist movement by outlawing certain feminist groups and emphasizing the importance of traditional values. Women's participation in politics was strongly discouraged. The mothers' activities were subject to intense repression from the police. The mothers gained international recognition and support in 1978, when the international press came to Argentina to cover the World Cup. When the story broke worldwide, the women became a symbol for HR in general, and the conscience of the nation in particular. As a result of increased media coverage, women's groups in Europe lent tremendous support to the mothers' efforts.

Macro-environment

The role of women in Latin American society has largely been influenced by the cultural phenomenon of machismo, which can be loosely defined as an overemphasis on the "male" attributes of strength and sexuality. The female complement to machismo, known as *marianismo*, encourages women to assume passive roles in society and to focus on the home and family. In many Latin American countries, these stereotypes have been reinforced by the government, the Catholic Church, and the women themselves. While this type of gender stereotyping certainly limits women's choices and behavior in Latin American society, the concepts of machismo and *marianismo* ultimately provide women with a unique power of their own. For example, in Latin American culture, women are believed to be morally superior to the Latin male. Motherhood is highly respected, and mothers are revered by both sexes. Viewed from this perspective, gender stereotypes have served as a tool as well as a barrier to the feminist movement in Latin America.

Impact and Remarks

At first, the government ignored the Madres and later tried to discredit them by calling them crazy old women. But the women were able to use their image as caring, loving mothers to gain the attention of the public. Once the government realized that these women were having an impact, they tried to instill fear in the women by outlawing the groups and threatening them physically. Interestingly, the women realized that their position in society, as dictated by traditional values and the concept of *marianismo*, offered them not only respect, but protection. This knowledge gave them the courage to continue their vigils in defiance of the military mandate to stop the demonstrations. In fact, when some of the women were arrested or abducted, the public grew increasingly supportive of the women and more suspicious of the government. What began as group of grieving mothers became a revolutionary political movement. Today, the organization has 2,000 mothers all around the country and 20 supporting groups all around the world.

In 1986, 12 mothers formed *La Linea Fundadora de las Madres de la Plaza de Mayo* ("The Founding Line"). The remaining mothers are now known as the Association of the Mothers of the Plaza de Mayo and continue to locate missing children. With key differences in perspective and methodology, the Founding Line made nonviolence a key component of their philosophy. Formed in much the same way as the Madres, the *Abuelas de Plaza de Mayo* ("Grandmothers of Plaza de Mayo") protest the disappearance of children. The grandmothers are devoted to finding children separated from their biological families who were either given or sold to members of the armed forces, or abandoned or given to orphanages. These children were born during the "Dirty War," the period from 1976 to 1983 when Argentina was under a brutal military reign. By making appeals to the community and putting advertisements in the newspapers, the grandmothers continued to locate their grandchildren. They also stand vigil in the Plaza de Mayo wearing white masks or white shawls inscribed with the names of the missing children. Through their vigorous efforts, they have found 59 of the 230 children that they were searching for; seven were killed, 31 were returned to their biological families, and the remaining children keep in close touch with the grandmothers.

Several international awards received include:

> For numerous national and international awards received by this movement see: Tompkins C and Foster DW (2001), Notable Twentieth-century Latin-American women, Santa Barbara, CA: Greenwood Press.

Today's Heroes (2015). http://www.womeninworldhistory.com/contemporary-07.html. Accessed on July 3, 2015.

Las Madres Home (2015). http://www.madres.org/navegar/nav.php. Accessed July 3, 2015.

CASE STUDY #9: MOTHERS OF EAST LOS ANGELES (MELA), UNITED STATES, 1985 (HR)

Problem

This case study falls within the domain of HR. The primary problem addressed is the social and political injustices suffered by Mexican Americans in East Los Angeles, which in turn can have a direct impact on their quality of life. Specifically, proposals to build a prison, an oil pipeline, and a hazardous-waste incinerator in East Los Angeles communities threaten to displace community members from their own neighborhoods.

Leadership Impetus

The Mothers of East Los Angeles (MELA), also known as the *Madres del Este de Los Angeles*, was formed in 1985 to protest the proposed construction of a state prison near the heavily populated community of Boyle Heights and its 33 schools. Founding members consisted of mothers who were long-time residents of East Los Angeles, most of whom had previous organizing skills through activity in churches, schools, or labor support groups. In fact, Juana Guitiérrez, president of the Santa Isabel chapter (MELASI), had previously organized a neighborhood watch committee in order to eliminate drug deals and gangs from their area. It was precisely because of her successful grassroots efforts that then–State Assemblywoman Gloria Molina informed Gutiérrez of the proposed prison, knowing that Gutiérrez would initiate action. Also hearing of the proposal, Father Juan Moretta of the Resurrection Church told the women of his East L.A. congregation about the prison. Gutiérrez, along with Aurora Castillo and other concerned mothers, formed MELA to fight the environmental injustices facing East Los Angeles residents.

EMPOWER Methods Used

- Rights protection and social action/reform
- Media use
- Public education and participation
- Organizing partnership
- Enabling service and assistance

MELA informed community leaders, members, and local organizations of the proposed prison site through word of mouth and informal meetings. Even though the Department of Corrections had first considered the site more than a year before opposition was raised, the community itself was never notified. Nine hundred signatures were gathered among local church parishioners; and the Coalition Against the Prison was formed, which consisted of organizations such as Boyle Heights, Lincoln Heights, and El Sereno Chambers of Commerce; the Central City Business Association; the Boyle Heights Kiwanis Club; and the Rotary Club of Boyle Heights. In order to obtain their own information about the issue, MELA and the Coalition launched a research and information campaign. Weekly candlelight vigils and press conferences were organized to attract media attention and garner more support for the cause. MELA lobbied state legislators in Sacramento for political support, telling them that there were already too many prisons near East L.A. schools. With the assistance of fundraisers by local Chambers of Commerce and buses donated by a local bus company, MELA also lobbied the California Department of Corrections and the governor in state and local arenas.

MELA fought against other environmental "intrusions" in the East Los Angeles community, including an oil pipeline and a municipal waste incinerator. In 1987, MELA joined a citywide coalition that defeated a proposal to build a pipeline from Santa Barbara County to Long Beach. In order to avoid affluent coastal communities, the pipeline was to detour through East Los Angeles, including one stretch that would be built 3 feet under an East L.A. junior high school. In 1988, MELA threatened to sue the City of Vernon and California Thermal Treatment Systems when they proposed to build a toxic waste incinerator. MELA also staged protest marches and attended public hearings to prevent the air-polluting facility from being built. The incinerator proposal was abandoned in 1990.

MELA continues to participate in community health issues that affect their families and neighbors, such as lead poisoning in poor children, the lack of jobs for local students, and lack of scholarships to keep students in school. MELASI runs a water conservation program that is sponsored by the Department of Water and Power, Metropolitan Water District, and Central Water Basin. MELA gives away low-flush toilets and recycles old, water-guzzling ones. The money earned from recycling the toilets is used to fund other programs including MELA's scholarship fund. More than $20,000 was raised in one year for college scholarships.

Other programs run by MELASI employ community youths while offering important services to the community, including a lead-poisoning–education project that employs ten youths, and a graffiti removal program that employs 15. The Lead Poison Awareness Program hires local high school students to go door-to-door and educate the community about the dangers of lead poisoning. The students also make referrals to local county health clinics to test children for poisoning. The internationally known Graffiti Abatement Program hires students to keep the community clean. Along with the Mono Lake Committee in California, MELA sponsors annual outings to Mono Lake for community youths. These visits provide a valuable opportunity for city youths to explore areas of natural wildlife. MELASI publishes a biannual newsletter—Las Madres del Este de Los Angeles—Santa Isabel Newsletter to inform the public of its activities, programs, and events. MELA also offers assistance to other communities that are embroiled in their own environmental issues and is a member of the Mentor Task Force in the Building a Healthier Community Program at White Memorial Medical Center in Los Angeles. In August 1998, MELA built an eight-unit housing project for low-income, first-time homeowners. Named after MELA leader Aurora Castillo, the Villas de Castillo housing project provided affordable housing in overcrowded East Los Angeles. The housing project was funded by the L.A. County Community Development Commission.

Partners/Opposition

MELA often joins forces with other community groups to fight the environmental injustices occurring in their community. Ironically, one prominent Eastside group—the United Neighborhood Organization (UNO), did not join the Coalition because they thought it was a lost cause. However, when MELA and the Coalition were gaining ground, UNO joined at the last minute. During the fight against the pipeline construction, groups in the East Los Angeles community formed a coalition to stand up to the powerful and wealthy companies who were sponsoring the pipeline. In 1989, MELA united with Huntington High School students to protest the construction of a toxic plant located across the street from one of the largest high schools in the Los Angeles Unified School District.

Macro-environment

Often lower socioeconomic communities are targeted as construction sites for waste-to-energy facilities or other "undesirable" facilities such as prisons because of their assumed lack of political voice as opposed to higher socioeconomic status (SES) areas who have more political sway with the local politicians. In fact, a report by an L.A.-based consulting firm for the California Waste Management Board explicitly suggested that middle and higher SES areas should not fall within the one-mile or five-mile radii of the proposed site, and that older people with less than a high school education are the least likely to oppose a facility. Labeled by some environmental activists as "environmental racism," these practices are common among racial minority communities. Latino residents have traditionally been ignored during the period when such projects are being proposed. In the United States, three out of five African Americans and Latinos live near toxic waste sites, and three of the five largest hazardous-waste landfills are in communities with highly concentrated Latino populations.

Impact and Remarks

Largely because of the tremendous efforts of MELA, the California State Senate defeated the bill authorizing construction of the East Los Angeles prison that had been passed by the state assembly. In fact, a bill was later passed declaring that no state prisons could ever be built in Los Angeles County. Other victories for MELA and the East Los Angeles community include the defeated proposals for the hazardous-waste incinerator and the oil pipeline. As a result of the concerted efforts of concerned community groups, Assembly Bill 58 (Roybal-Allard), which provided all Californians with the minimum protection of an environmental impact report before the construction of hazardous-waste incinerators, was passed. MELA and other grassroots activists played an important role in making sure this law is enforced.

MELA has been recognized nationally for its successful efforts, including by President Clinton. Gutiérrez won the Mujer Award in 1995, a national honor given by the National Hispania Leadership Institute—an organization that trains Latinas in leadership skills. One of the original MELAs, Aurora Castillo, was the first Los Angeles resident, the first Latina, and the oldest person to receive the $75,000 Goldman Environmental Prize in 1995. MELA's mission statement sums up the vision of this influential grassroots organization: "Not economically rich—but culturally wealthy, not politically powerful—but socially conscious, not mainstream educated—but armed with the knowledge, commitment and determination that only a mother can possess" (http://web.archive.org/web/20080406123621/http://www.mothersof eastla.com/).

CASE STUDY #11: OKINAWAN WOMEN ACT AGAINST MILITARY VIOLENCE, OKINAWA, 1995 (HR)

Problem

This case study falls within the domain of HR. The major problem being addressed is the U.S. military presence in Okinawa and the burden that it lays on Okinawa citizens. Okinawans have endured hundreds of rapes, homicides and crimes, air and noise pollution, hazardous wastes, coral destruction, dangers from live-fire exercises, and forest fires as a result of the military presence. It is reported that US forces in Okinawa are responsible for an average of 23 crimes and that between 1972 and 2010 there were a total of 9,838 crimes committed, including rapes, by US forces (Reversion Affairs Division, Executive Office of the Governor Okinawa Prefectural Government 1-2-2 Izumizaki, Naha, Okinawa, Japan, 2015).

Leadership Impetus

In 1995, three U.S. servicemen raped a 12-year-old Okinawan girl. This tragic event prompted concerned women led by Suzuyo Takazato, Naha City Council to form the group known as the Okinawan Women Act Against Military Violence (OWAAMV) in September of 1995.

EMPOWER Methods Used

- Rights protection and social action/reform
- Public education and participation
- Organizing partnership

On October 21, 1995, following the founding of OWAAMV, members drew worldwide attention to the rape of the 12-year-old girl and other violence perpetrated against Okinawan people. An estimated 85,000 individuals gathered at a rally in Ginowan Seaside Park in Ginowan City. This was the largest demonstration against the U.S. military presence since the Reversion of Okinawa to Japanese rule (post–World War II) in 1972. In addition to protesting the rape, demonstrators were demanding a review of the U.S.-Japan postwar Status of Forces Agreement (SOFA). The rally was organized by 53 Okinawan municipalities, by political parties, and by 120 associations such as labor unions and women's groups.

In February 1996, Takazato led the same group of Okinawan women (also known as the "Okinawan Women's America Peace Caravan") on a visit to the United States in order to oppose the U.S. military presence in Okinawa. The Caravan traveled to San Francisco; Washington, D.C.; New York; and Honolulu to share information with American women, U.S. Congresswomen, citizens, and members of the UN Commission on the Status of Women and the Human Rights Commission, and discuss common concerns for peace. In November 1997, Takazato participated in the International Conference on Violence Against Women in War and Armed-Conflict Situations in Tokyo, which reported to the UN Special Rapporteur on Violence Against Women. Responding to this critical need, the Rape Emergency Intervention Counseling Center–Okinawa (REICO) volunteer hotline and counseling program was established (Doktor, 1996).

In October 1998, a delegation of 13 women traveled to Southern California to campaign for the dismantling of the 42 U.S. military bases located on Okinawan soil. Members spoke with city and state officials, college students, community activists, and church congregations. The delegation also traveled to Washington, D.C., to lobby congressional and State Department officials, as well as to Japan's mainland.

Partners/Opposition

According to a U.S. Defense Department spokesman, the United States is very receptive to and seriously considers the concerns of the Okinawan people, but feels that the American troops are necessary in order to preserve the security and stability of the Asian-Pacific region. In contrast, Johnson (2002), the cofounder of the Japan Policy Research Institute, a nonprofit group devoted to the study of Japan and transpacific issues, believes that the U.S. military installations are a collusion between the United States and Japanese governments. He feels that these governments are only serving their own interests while making Okinawans bear the costs of the military presence.

Macro-environment

According to the Okinawan Women, the U.S. military presence has disturbed life on the island of Okinawa for 53 years and turned their home into a *de facto*

U.S. military colony. The 50,000 U.S. troops, civilians, and military dependents exert an unwanted influence on Okinawan culture and society. Okinawans are treated as third-class citizens by mainland Japan and the United States. Although Okinawa constitutes less than 1 percent of Japan's land, Okinawa is home to 75 percent of all American military facilities in Japan. A total of 27,000 U.S. troops and 23,000 U.S. civilians and military dependents live on the island. According to Okinawan government statistics, there have been 130 aircraft accidents and 154 brushfires caused by military exercises since 1972. According to a delegate of the Naha City Women's History Project, more than 200 Okinawan women and girls have reported being raped by U.S. Servicemen since 1972. This is most likely an undercount of rapes due to the shame on the part of the rape survivors. An Okinawa government study revealed that babies born near Kadena Air Base had the lowest birth-weight in Japan. Another study of 933 preschool-age children living in five communities adjacent to military bases reported that the sample population had poorer concentration and suffered more colds, emotional problems, headaches, and stomachaches than children in areas not located near military bases.

Impact and Remarks

The formation of the OWAAMV has raised worldwide awareness of the problems associated with the military occupation of Okinawa. By pooling their resources and collaborating with other Okinawan HR groups, OWAAMV has voiced their concerns about a continued military presence in their homeland and expressed outrage about the countless crimes perpetrated against their people.

CASE STUDY #85: APNE AAP, P. 267: SEX-WORKERS' HUMAN RIGHTS AND INTERNATIONAL ANTI-TRAFFICKING MOVEMENT, INDIA (RUCHIRA GUPTA AND GLORIA STEINEM) 2015 (HR)

Apne Aap was founded by twenty-two women from Mumbai's red light district, with a vision of a world where no woman could be bought or sold.

The twenty-two women who founded were the subject of Ruchira Gupta's Emmy award winning documentary, 'The Selling of Innocents," which exposed trafficking of women and girls from Nepal to India. During the production of the film, the women formed a connection with each other that ended their isolation and gave them the strength to resist their situation. When filming completed, the group continued to meet informally in parks. The respect they received when acting as a group and the strength of their collective bargaining inspired them to create a legal structure to support their vision. Apne Aap registered as an NGO in 2002 in Mumbai, India. Through the efforts of a board member, Apne Aap was given a room in an abandoned municipal school on Falkland Street, the heart of Mumbai's red light area. This room was a safe place to converse, sleep, repair torn clothes, bathe and receive mail. It was also a place to hold meetings and classes.

In the following years, Apne Aap's vision and impact grew. Members reached out to other women trapped in prostitution and organized self-empowerment programs in Bihar, Delhi and West Bengal, where Apne Aap is currently working in local communities. (Apne Aap Website)

The feminist leader Gloria Steinem is one of the strongest supporters of Apne Aap and is personally involved in this movement. (For more details, see Shah, 2014; for a summary of Apne Ap ["On your Own"] founded by Ruchira Gupta and joined by Gloria Steinem, see Apne Ap, 2015b.)

This case study is not included in the meta-analysis because quantitative data were not available for all the six required dimensions. It is mentioned here to inform the readers about Apne Aap's innovative strategies that has attracted active involvement of internationally renowned leaders including Gloria Steinem and Vandana Shiva. It focuses on antitrafficking and sexual abuses of powerless women including involuntary sex workers. For further details, visit their website: Apne Aap (2015a, "On Your Own"): http://apneaap.org/

8

Equal Rights Case Studies

> In 1995, at the UN Fourth World Conference on Women
> in Beijing, 189 nations agreed to an ambitious "Platform
> for Action" that called for the "full and equal participation
> of women in political, civil, economic, social and cultural
> life." At this conference, Secretary Clinton memorably
> declared that "women's rights are human rights."
> —The Clinton Foundation, 2014

A 20-year follow up of the 1995 Beijing Declaration by the Clinton Foundation
and Gates Foundation concluded that:

> Nearly 20 years later, progress has been made, with greater
> participation in public life and nations enacting public policies
> to promote full equality. *Yet for all of this progress, women and
> girls still comprise the majority of the world's unhealthy, unfed,
> and unpaid, and hard-won rights and legal protections remain
> elusive on the ground. Advancing the status of women and girls
> remains the unfinished business of our time* (emphasis mine).
> —The Clinton Foundation, 2014

> *We need to push for what we want, not just what we can get.*
> —Eleanor Smeal (2003)

Several countries including Brazil, Canada, India, Mexico, the Philippines,
Sri Lanka, the United States, and a group of several Muslim countries exemplify women and mothers' (WAM's) determination to gain status equal to
men. Half of the cases center on issues of gender discrimination in the workplace (from factory workers, to domestic workers, to sex workers). For example, the Asian Immigrant Women Advocates (AIWA) of Northern California
(Case #24) are fighting for better working conditions for electronics assemblers and other low-income, limited–English-speaking women. The other half
of cases, including the groundbreaking National Organization for Women

(NOW) of the United States (Case #13) and the multinational YWCA (Young Women's Christian Association) founded in 1849 (Case #12), address issues of gender oppression in their daily lives. One group, known as the Women Living Under Muslim Laws (Case #21), advocates for Muslim women whose personal rights are severely restricted by institutional and cultural practices. As these cases show, women who fight for equal rights are fighting not only for themselves but for the rights of future generations of women.

Forty-seven cases represent 11 nations, including Bolivia, Canada, China, India, Jamaica, Korea, Nigeria, the Philippines, Puerto Rico, South Africa, the United States, and three multinational organizations. WAMs have organized themselves around issues of reproductive health/prenatal care (12 cases), drug and alcohol abuse (6 cases), environmental health (5 cases), AIDS and HIV (5 cases), violence (5 cases), and mental health (4 cases). One of the most famous efforts began in 1980 when a pair of grieving mothers founded Mothers Against Drunk Driving (MADD); 20 years later, alcohol-related fatalities had dropped 40% in the United States. This successful campaign has inspired countless WAMs to political and social action. One of the most recent examples is the "Million Mom March" in Washington, D.C., a grassroots lobbying effort for stricter gun laws. The march, which was slated to take place on Mothers' Day in 2000, was the brainchild of one New Jersey mother. She had been motivated to action after seeing television news footage of preschoolers being led away from a Los Angeles community center after a shooting spree killed one and wounded five.

CASE STUDY #24: ASIAN IMMIGRANT WOMEN ADVOCATES (AIWA), CALIFORNIA, 1993 (EQRT)

Problem

This case study falls within the domain of equal rights (EQRT). The major problem being addressed is the poor working conditions faced by Asian immigrant women. A credible investigative report concludes that:

> California sewing factories employ over 100,000 sewing machine opera-tors, most of whom are Asian and Latina immigrants. Health and safety violations are common in the mostly small factories that employ these minimum wage workers. This report is based on the clinical findings and survey results from sewing machine operators seen at the Oakland-based Asian Immigrant Women Workers Clinic (AIWWC), a free clinic for gar-ment workers sponsored by Asian Immigrant Women Advocates (AIWA) and the University of California San Francisco (UCSF). A total of 66% of the garment workers in this study reported "poor" or "fair" health. This is three to four times higher than the rate for women in California. (Lashuay et al., 2002, p. 3)

More than a third of the women have not seen a physician in the last three years. About 97 percent of them were eligible for filing for workers, compensations for their injuries but they did not claim it either because they were unaware of their rights or afraid to do so, or both (Lashuay et al., 2002, p. 4).

Similar conditions prevailed in other work situations as well.

Leadership Impetus

AIWA is a community-based organization established in 1983 by three female activists: Elaine Kim, Pat Lee, and Young Shin, a female Korean lawyer. Through education, leadership development, and organization, AIWA seeks to empower low-income, limited–English-speaking Asian immigrant women who work as seamstresses, hotel room cleaners, electronics assemblers, nursing home workers, and janitors in the greater San Francisco, Oakland, and South Bay areas.

EMPOWER Methods Used

¤ Rights protection and social action/reform
¤ Enabling service and assistance
¤ Public education and participation
¤ Empowerment training and leadership development
¤ Media use

AIWA sponsors a number of advocacy campaigns for women workers in an effort to encourage Asian women to exercise their rights and develop the skills needed to advocate for justice and dignity in their lives and workplace. The Environmental Health and Safety Project educates and organizes approximately 200 Korean immigrant women electronics assemblers in the South Bay. The project focuses on education about toxic chemicals and hazards in the industry. Sixty women and their families participate in workshops focusing on working with hazardous chemicals and identifying safe alternatives; affecting public policy in the electronics industry; and women's health.

When a sweatshop in Oakland's Chinatown area closed in May 1992, some of the displaced seamstresses sought help from AIWA. They had not been paid wages for their labor at the sewing company. In response to this injustice, AIWA founder Young Shin and the women forged the Garment Workers Justice Campaign. This campaign and the women who were fighting for their rights gained considerable support from the public, media, churches, and county and city officials. The Garment Workers Justice Campaign targeted corporations in order to improve working conditions in the garment industry through media campaigns, picketing, and a community hearing in which both local and state officials and their aides listened to the women's testimony. In March of 1996, AIWA signed a historic agreement with Jessica

McClintock, Inc., to uphold worker protection. The Garment Workers Justice Campaign directed their protest campaign at Jessica McClintock, Inc., because it had one of the sewing company's exclusive contracts.

In addition to AIWA's protest efforts, the organization offered workplace literacy classes in Oakland and San Jose. In the initial years, more than 530 classes are offered to 120 Chinese and Korean immigrant women annually. The classes included basic English skills and focused on the rights of immigrants, women; workers, as well as on occupational safety and health issues; and on political participation through citizenship and naturalization. As a part of the workplace literacy curriculum in San Jose, California, the women completed a risk-mapping exercise of their workplaces. The women located and labeled where certain hazards were. They told each other where the chemical smells were the worst, where the machine noise was the loudest, and where they would be working all day. This activity provided an opportunity for the women to share stories of workplace hazards and began brainstorming ideas on how to protect themselves from these hazards (Lashuay et al., 2002):

> Working conditions in garment factories are frequently substandard. Approximately 94% of patients reported one or more problems with their workstations including inadequate seating (90%), awkward bending and twisting (67%), breathing problems due to fabric dust (48%), less than adequate rest breaks (40%), and being yelled at by their bosses (36%). Garment workers typically work over 40 hours per week for low pay and no benefits. Patients reported earnings of $6.32 an hour, 25% less than the poverty level for a family of four. Only 22% of patients had health insurance and only 12% reported paid sick leave. (Lashuay et al., 2002)

In order to teach AIWA members leadership skills, AIWA holds leadership development and training sessions. AIWA trains more than 50 Chinese and Korean immigrant women in communication, immigration and social history, organizing skills, advocacy, economic literacy, and network-building with other women workers on issues affecting immigrant women's working conditions. With their newly gained skills, AIWA members can participate in AIWA's membership board and project committees. Approximately 35 low-income immigrant women workers collaborate to plan and implement many of the projects of AIWA. There are four project committees; namely, Outreach, Education, Events, and Fundraising. Collectively, the committees provide outreach and bilingual services; participate in developing workplace literacy class curricula and teaching immigrant women; organize educational field trips, conduct leadership development training and various social events, and assist in writing grant proposals and conducting grass roots fundraising for AIWA's projects.

AIWA keeps its members abreast of pertinent issues through a quarterly newsletter that is published in Chinese, Korean, and English. AIWA also publishes educational brochures about health and safety and workers' rights in these languages. Immigrant women and their families also receive multilingual information and referrals on a variety of issues affecting immigrant women's lives through phone consultation, workplace outreach, and peer counseling. AIWA holds an annual celebration for the women and their families, and makes an annual report at the event. That, coupled with the classes, where wives learn about workers' rights and share the information with their husbands who are immigrants also, has led to growing support for AIWA among the men.

AIWA has received media coverage on their efforts to improve the working conditions of their members. In particular, the Korean news media, such as *Korea Times* and Han-Mi Radio, covered an ergonomics training led by AIWA peer trainers in San Jose. The peer trainers used an informative and interactive teaching style that was well received by the participants, who were electronics assemblers. The information and stress-relieving exercises introduced at the training were compiled in a Korean newsletter that was distributed to more than 200 AIWA Korean members in Santa Clara County. The print and radio media coverage reached the broader Korean community in the San Francisco Bay area. In another instance, the *New York Times* ran full-page ads about the Garment Workers Justice Campaign.

Partners/Opposition

AIWA's work through the Garment Workers Justice Campaign has received support from elected officials in the San Francisco Bay area, as well as women's, immigrant rights, labor, and religious communities across the country. For example, the Public Media Center in San Francisco helped the women launch a public relations operation. Several unions in San Francisco joined AIWA and the garment workers in picketing. Workers in ten cities, including New York, Chicago, and Los Angeles, also rallied in support of the campaign. The Board of Global Ministries has given AIWA various forms of support, including a mission intern and grants from the Women's Division to assist AIWA in empowering disenfranchised Asian immigrant women who work in garment manufacturing, food service, electronics, hotel cleaning, and nursing homes (Andrews, 1996; Lashuay et al., 2002).

AIWA continue to face resistance from the industries employing Asian immigrant women. Despite AIWA's research indicating that there are safe alternatives to harmful workplace chemicals, such as lead solder used by electronic assemblers, the industry is not willing to use these alternatives due to their higher cost.

During the protests forged by the Garment Workers Justice Campaign, the San Francisco Superior Court placed restrictions on their free-speech rights in protesting garment manufacturer Jessica McClintock Restrictions included an injunction that limited the picketing efforts of the garment workers and their supporters. For example, protesters had to march at least six feet away from the entrance of McClintock's store, and only two people could march in front of McClintock's residence.

Protesters also fear that openly picketing will jeopardize their opportunities to find jobs in the industry, or that they will be blacklisted as troublemakers. Some women even wore masks to conceal their identity. The limited English skills of some immigrants also make finding a job in other sectors very difficult.

Macro-environment

Anti-immigrant legislation in California and in Washington has made AIWA's advocacy efforts even more vital to immigrant women workers. Racial discrimination and exploitation also play a role in the Asian immigrant women's lives. In order to combat these larger issues, groups that had previously been one-issue organizations need to work together on the larger issue of basic human rights. Immigrants have played a significant role in the history of labor in the United States. In the 1800s, immigrants were among those who established an eight-hour day, fought for the right to organize, and for the right to have the few labor laws which protect workers.

Contributing to the problem of poor working conditions are trade agreements such as the North American Free Trade Agreement (NAFTA) and the General Agreements of Tariffs and Trade (GATT) Treaty. Production in the garment industry is being moved out of the country. In order to keep production of their garments in the United States, manufacturers must keep costs down. Generally, it is the workers who suffer the cutting-cost measures though low wages, unsafe working conditions, and longer hours. Contractors who run sweatshops must vie for contracts in a very competitive business, often making very low bids. Cultural factors also contribute to the discriminatory atmosphere experienced by these women. For example, Asian cultures tend to encourage submissiveness among females. Husbands often object to the empowerment of these women.

Impact and Remarks

The Washington Office of the United Methodist Board of Global Ministries' Women's Division bestowed on AIWA and its executive director and co-founder Young Shin the Letelier-Moffitt Human Rights Award for a domestic human rights (HR) program. A three-year effort to seek justice for the group of seamstresses involved in the Garment Workers Justice Campaign resulted in a March 1996 agreement. The agreement held that the manufacturer would pledge to provide scholarships, a fund for former workers, bilingual publications about labor standards, toll-free numbers in Cantonese and English about wage and hour laws, as well as monitor wages and conditions.

In March 1997, AIWA announced the conclusion to meetings with the executives of three prominent garment manufacturers in the Bay Area: Allan Byer, president of Byer California; Bob Tandler, president of Fritzi California; and Jay Margolis, chief executive officer (CEO) of Esprit de Corp. These companies agreed to maintain their already existing monitoring programs and to implement toll-free, confidential hotlines to protect garment workers' rights in the workplace. These hotlines will allow workers to report problems without fear of being fired or identified as a troublemaker. Over 2,500 garment workers in the Bay Area can voice their concerns to these manufacturers (Lashuay et al., 2002).

Current Status

AIWA is still active and includes several initiatives on the youth, social justice, and community leadership development. "AIWA youth initiated a Biliteracy Campaign (2009–2011) to formally recognize all students who can demonstrate proficiency in two or more languages. This campaign encouraged the development of all global citizens while raising awareness of the contributions and talents of immigrant youth. To strengthen and deepen social justice movement building efforts, AIWA began to share our leadership model CTOS (Community Transformational Organizing Strategies) (Labor/Community Strategy Center, 2015) with other organizations, academia, supporters and allies locally, nationally and globally. AIWA began to document CTOS Grassroots Leadership program (2008–2013) and assess its socioeconomic and political impact for the past 25 years, which produced three published articles in KALFOU (2010), SIGNS (Asian Immigrant Women Advocate [AIWA], 2015) and Immigrant Women Workers in the Neoliberal Age (2013).To foster a broader dialogue about the importance of grassroots leadership development and to shift social paradigm to put priority on the full and equal development of grassroots leaders from the disadvantaged communities toward building a just and inclusive society, AIWA began a multicity tour (2014) by showing AIWA's new film *Becoming Ourselves* (2014) and sharing CTOS model (AIWA, 2015).

CASE STUDY #20: ATABAL COLLECTIVE AND LA ESPERANZA,
MEXICO CITY, 1986 (EQRT)

Problem

This case study falls within the domain of equal rights (EQRT). The main problem being addressed is lack of organization among domestic workers. The poor working conditions (discrimination, sexual abuse, maltreatment by the employer family, and little communication with employers); poor living conditions (little or no access to cultural, sporting, or recreational activities); and overall undervaluation of domestic work are also issues of concern.

Leadership Impetus

In April of 1987, the ATABAL Collective for Support and Promotion of the Organization of Domestic Service Workers was created in Mexico City by two political activists and one of the founders of the Domestic Servants' Center, a social service center with child-care facilities and mutual support. The ATABAL Collective was officially recognized as an association in September of 1992. Its feminist political purpose was to fight for the social and political rights of domestic-service workers as well as to incite domestic employees to organize in pursuit of these rights.

Within the structure of training workshops given by ATABAL, a group of female domestic servants working in private households (mostly unmarried mothers) self-organized to form their own domestic workers' group, called *La Esperanza* ("Hope") which that is to establish a trade union. The two groups are interdependent but autonomous entities, directly involved with each other's activities and projects.

About 2.1 million Mexicans are employed as domestic workers, with women accounting for about 90 percent of such employees, and the majority lack employment contracts, are not registered in the *social security* system and are subjected to discrimination, long work days, poor pay and other forms of abuse, the National Council to Prevent Discrimination, or Conapred, said.

The figures come from a survey of domestic workers that was conducted in association with U.N. Women and the International Labor Organization, or ILO, Conapred said in a report presented to the Senate.

The 2010 National Survey on Discrimination in *Mexico*, or Enadis (National Council to Prevent Discrimination), found that 38 percent of domestic workers consider excessive work and low pay the main problems facing them, while 19.3 percent complained of mistreatment and discrimination, among other abuses, as well as the lack of labor rights. (Encuesta Nacional sobre Discriminación en México (Enadis)/UNICEF, 2010)

EMPOWER Methods Used

¤ Empowerment training and leadership development
¤ Public education and participation
¤ Media use
¤ Enabling service and assistance
¤ Work/job training and micro-enterprise
¤ Rights protection and social action/reform
¤ Organizing partnership

In response to the women's concerns, ATABAL holds training workshops regarding workers' rights, the female identity, women's role in society, human relations, methods of organization, and trade unions. ATABAL also offers advice to La Esperanza in regard to training and organization; provides human, financial, and infrastructural resources; and assists the group in achieving recognition from the community's domestic employers, employment agencies, lawyers, legislators, government labor authorities, non-governmental organization (NGO) support centers, women's organizations, rural workers' organization, trade unions, Christian organizations, political parties, academics, researchers, students, and educational institutions.

La Esperanza strives to develop its own capacity (members, skills, and knowledge) to promote basic rights, defend grievances of the domestic workers, and provide feedback and support to ATABAL's efforts. In order to recruit new members and raise consciousness about the issues, La Esperanza organizes publicity drives, distributes invitations to events, and canvasses parks and other sites frequented by domestic workers. The group also utilizes the media by participating in radio and television programs, giving press interviews, and even joining in the Labor Day Independent March to show the flag for the domestic-service sector.

In terms of providing services, La Esperanza established a collective savings fund to provide financial assistance to members in case of emergency. Money for the organization's basic needs is raised through raffles held three times a year. The La Espanaza also established an employment exchange for domestic workers and a folk-dancing troupe, which provides entertainment for social events held at least three times a year. La Esperanza is also planning to establish a training and overall development center for domestic-service employees. In addition to the services already provided by the organization, the center will provide training in occupational skills, an open school, and a cultural and recreational center.

La Esperanza is also attempting to reform Chapter XIII of Mexico's Federal Labor Act of 1969 in terms of providing more protection to domestic workers in Mexico. In order to achieve international recognition by trade unions and the government, the group formed a confederation with women's trade unions and associations in 11 other Latin American and Caribbean countries in 1988. La Esperanza hopes that the government will pass legislation that recognizes them as workers and members of a trade union.

Partners/Opposition

From its inception until the latter halted operation in 1988, ATABAL collaborated with the Christian Union of Young Domestic Workers, a group designed to unite domestic workers in their otherwise lonely position in society through retreats, Bible readings, workshops, and nationwide meetings. Factors that hindered the initial organization of domestic workers include the women's suspicion of invitations to meet with strangers, apathy or lack of motivation to join due to lack of precedent or previous success, fear of losing their job, or irregular work hours not allowing them to attend meetings.

Employers of domestic workers were not supportive of the organizing of domestic servants and would sometimes threaten to fire those who did join.

Macro-environment

As Mexico City is the socioeconomic and political center of Mexico, many migrants move to Mexico City from the poverty-stricken areas of the country in hopes of improving their standard of living. For many single and uneducated countrywomen wanting to live in Mexico City, domestic labor is their only option. The fact that the middle class cannot afford to hire domestic workers, or can hire them only at a very low wage, makes for a greater supply and less demand for these domestic servants, 97% of whom are women. In addition, due to the economic crisis occurring in Mexico, many women from the country and the working-class districts of the city are being forced to contribute to the family income, often resorting to domestic work or other low-skilled jobs. Attempts to organize domestic servants originated in the 1920s, with several unions being established over the years in both cities and small towns, with varying success.

Impact and Remarks

The formation of La Esperanza as an outgrowth of ATABAL's efforts exemplifies the deep impact that organized leadership, motivation, and training can have on its members. With the continued support of ATABAL, La Esperanza self-organized in order to address the pressing concerns of domestic workers in terms of political, economic, and social needs. While educating themselves in matter of organizing, trade unions, and workers' rights, the women of La Esperanza persist in recruiting fellow domestic workers to their cause. During this process, they have realized the necessity of uniting themselves and their allies in the hopes of improving a situation that no one else cares to address.

CASE STUDY #17: BALTIMORE WORKING WOMEN (BWW), MARYLAND, 1978 (EQRT)

Problem

This case study falls within the domain of equal rights (EQRT). The main problem is that already existing organizations for working women did not address the specific issues of clerical workers. Baltimore Working Women's (BWW) goal was to gain rights and respect for working women.

Leadership Impetus

An informal group of women, most of whom were feminist professional workers in the city government, wanted to organize women office workers. Since few of the founders were clerical workers themselves, BWW was not necessarily formed for the founders' personal interests. However, the founders were affected by some of the same issues as the clerical workers in terms of women's role in society. The lack of political organization among clerical workers, a large segment of the women's work force, was also a major motivation for many of the founders (Goldberg, 1983).

While organized feminist movements justly demanded for equal pay and benefits for women and men holding similar positions, the vast majority of working women were employed in low paying jobs which ignored the especial needs of working women (e.g., paid maternity leaves and benefits, day care of children, sexual harassment). One scholar summed up the problem as:

> Title VII strategy championed by middle class feminists is of little use to women in female dominated occupations which required little or no skill. Most often the barriers to their competing with men are those of skill rather than sex discriminations. (Mason, 2002)

Even in top-level positions as scholars and professionals, women face the inescapable challenge of balancing the demands of personal life and professional work that often cause negative effects on their health and quality of life. The Nobel Prize winner Elizabeth Blackburn terms this as the *work–balance* challenge and eloquently describes its effects from her personal experience (Blackburn, 2008).

EMPOWER Methods Used

- Empowerment training and leadership development
- Media use
- Public education and participation
- Enabling service and assistance
- Rights protection and social action/reform

BWW provides an arena for gaining organizing skills for its members, including public speaking and participation in large public events, running a meeting, raising funds, attracting membership, and running a campaign. BWW gained media attention by holding press conferences. Through presentations at meetings and workshops, guest speakers, printed information, leafleting, public forums, and newsletters, BWW provided information about the history, present status, and legal rights of working women, particularly office workers. BWW also attempted to raise public awareness of the status of working women and the activities of the organization.

Enabling service and assistance was provided by BWW through fundraising for the organization and its members and outreach to potential BWW members. BWW also implemented direct social action to affect specific job areas. For example, BWW won job postings at a large city bank through various efforts, including leafleting, surveying, rallies, and public presentations.

Partners/Opposition

Working Women's Organizing Project served as a partner in terms of offering assistance in BWW's first questionnaire survey of working women in Baltimore. Funding for staff salaries and office space for BWW was provided by the Ms Foundation and the Women's Resource and Advocacy Center. BWW, as a local affiliate, works closely with the Working Women national organization to strive toward the general goal of garnering rights and respect for office workers.

Macro-environment

The working women's movement began during the mid-1970s when it seemed like affirmative action programs were being watered down during the Ford administration. BWW was one of the local affiliates of Working Women, a national organization sponsored by groups in San Francisco, Boston, and Cleveland.

Impact and Remarks

In 1983, there were 250 dues-paid members and approximately 2,000 people on the organization's mailing list. Two campaigns that the BWW developed addressed the working conditions of women employed in banks and age discrimination among all women office workers. An important impact of BWW was the personal development among organization members. Interviews of BWW participants revealed that increased public activism to improve working conditions was correlated with personal growth. Their self-confidence had increased in terms of public speaking and chairing meetings. An increased self-esteem allowed these women to be more assertive on the job during interactions with their employers. BWW has also led to increasing solidarity among the members (Goldberg, 1983).

CASE STUDY #15: COYOTE, UNITED STATES, 1973 (EQRT)

Problem

This case study falls within the domain of equal rights (EQRT). The main problem being addressed is violation of prostitutes' rights. Because COYOTE ("Call Off Your Old Tired Ethics") views the illegality of prostitution as the major cause of prostitutes' victimization, its overarching goal is the decriminalization of prostitution, which, they argue, would mean that prostitution would fall inside of the purview of the law. As it stands now, prostitutes have no legal recourse when they are abused or exploited.

Leadership Impetus

A self-proclaimed ex-prostitute named Margo St. James founded the COYOTE (the first organization of its kind) on Mother's Day in 1973 in San Francisco. COYOTE (Call Off Your Old Tired Ethics was formed with the help of a $5000 grant from the Point Foundation of the Glide Memorial Church in San Francisco. COYOTE emerged from another organization called WHO ("Whores, Housewives, and Others"). COYOTE's purpose was to serve as a coalition of housewives, lawyers, feminists, and prostitutes that would expose laws and law enforcement procedures that make prostitution problematic.

EMPOWER Methods Used

- ¤ Organizing partnerships
- ¤ Media use
- ¤ Public education and participation
- ¤ Enabling service and assistance
- ¤ Rights protection and social action/reform

St. James recruited 50 influential San Franciscans to form an informal advisory board and local sex workers to advocate reform. St. James' charisma, articulateness, openness, and overall likable personality drew media attention to the organization in newspapers and broadcast talk shows, and as a result she was widely known by local judges, district attorneys, detectives, police, pimps, prostitutes, lawyers, and bail bondsmen. Despite this media coverage, recruitment of working prostitutes was difficult because of prostitutes' fear of getting arrested as well as of being publicly identified. COYOTE also undertook protest campaigns focusing on prohibition of prostitution, discrimination against prostitutes such as police harassment and entrapment, discriminatory enforcement of prostitution laws, and the unjustifiable expenditure of tax revenue to control prostitutes COYOTE also attempted to educate the public in terms of debunking the stereotype of prostitutes as "disease-ridden and drug-addicted and to serve as support network for sex workers (personal interview). Another early effort of COYOTE was the citation campaign, which lobbied to change the law to punish prostitution as a victimless crime with both customer and prostitute being fined instead of the current arrest and incarceration process. Even though this campaign was not successful, it generated media attention, political controversy, and support from several government officials, which in turn gave COYOTE more visibility and legitimacy as an organization of prostitutes' rights. COYOTE sponsored a number of media events such as the Annual Hookers' Convention and the Annual Hookers' Ball, which generated as much as $93,000 in 1977.

During this time, COYOTE provided several services for prostitutes, including a hotline called SLIP (Survival Line for Independent Prostitutes), legal assistance after police arrest, suitable clothing for court appearances, and teaching of survival skills to use when in jail. COYOTE disseminated information, garnered media coverage, provided speakers, organized lawyers, and published a newsletter—*COYOTE Howls*—which was sold to women's centers, bookstores, university libraries, and other interested parties. To raise awareness of prostitutes' issues, COYOTE created a speakers' bureau to address legislatures, high schools, libraries, universities, barristers' clubs, women's groups, religious organizations, television and radio shows, and academic conferences. The speakers' bureau became COYOTE's main recruitment strategy. It provided a forum in which COYOTE could address discriminatory law enforcement practices such as the entrapment and quarantining of prostitutes, and violence against women. COYOTE itself instigated or sponsored at least 26 lawsuits on behalf of prostitutes.

> For example, with the support of the American Civil Liberties Union (ACLU) and the local Citizen Council for Criminal Justice, COYOTE filed numerous class action suits challenging the constitutionality of a California statute directed against anyone who solicits or engages in any act of solicitation.

Partners/Opposition

The Point Foundation of the Glide Memorial Church and the Playboy Foundation provided financial assistance during COYOTE's inception. COYOTE also received support from a number of lawyers and lawyers' groups such as the ACLU and Barristers' Club. With increased visibility, this grassroots organization based in San Francisco expanded their support base and legitimacy in the eyes of the mass media and in terms of government grants, foundation support, the academy, social science disciplines, and non-profit organizations.

Membership in COYOTE includes students, clients of prostitutes, politicians, media personnel, activists, and representatives from other advocacy organizations. COYOTE is an NGO and does not receive government funding. COYOTE has utilized private donations, honoraria, and governmental grants to finance its activities. Without paid staff or formal organization, volunteers are responsible for running the organization and providing services.

Macro-environment

Gender and racial discrimination in terms of selective enforcement of the law was also a major concern of COYOTE. Again, the press covered COYOTE's claims that law enforcement is biased in favor of the customers of prostitutes, or "johns." Also, a few local judges supported COYOTE's efforts. One judge charged the police with intentional and purposeful enforcement policy while dismissing charges against 37 prostitutes whose male customers were not arrested. In fact, merely organizing prostitutes could be considered an illegal act of conspiracy. Yet, within the first year of its existence, COYOTE had a membership of over 1,000, 10% of whom were working prostitutes.

Impact and Remarks

COYOTE was instrumental in removing the mandatory three-day venereal-disease quarantine imposed by the San Francisco Police Department. *The issuance of this temporary injunction was in effect an acknowledgement of the way in which such procedures constitute selective legal intervention.* Today, there are local chapters nationwide including COYOTE/Los Angeles and COYOTE/Seattle. In addition, COYOTE leaders and supporters helped form COYOTE affiliates such as the National Task Force on Prostitution (NTFP) in the United States, and the International Committee for Prostitutes' Rights (ICPR) in Amsterdam. COYOTE has had tremendous impact on the prostitutes' rights movement by challenging the traditional definitions of prostitutes as deviants and prostitution as a social problem. Several other national and international affiliates have also emerged through the years following the founding of COYOTE, such as PONY (Prostitutes of New York), HIRE (Hooking Is Real Employment) in Atlanta, Sex Workers Alliance of Vancouver, and the Australian Sex Industry Network (SIN). In 1998, Norma Jean Almodovar founded the International Sex Worker Foundation for Art, Culture and Education (ISWFACE)—a nonprofit foundation that is able to raise funds for COYOTE. It also showcases art done by and about sex workers from the 1800s in the Wild West in order to help break the stereotypes of sex workers (Almodovar, 2013; Jenness, 1991).

COYOTE and ISWFACE are still active and activism by sex-workers' organizations have emerged and have been established in several nations. The Sonagachi Darbar association in Kolkata, India, has emerged as a major model (supported by the UN agencies and Local Public Health Institute).

CASE STUDY #18: EXPORT PROCESSING ZONE (EPZ), SRI LANKA, 1979 (EQRT)

Problem

This case study falls within the domain of equal rights (EQRT). The major problem being addressed is the lack of organized support for the young women workers who suffer from exploitation and sexual harassment in the Sri Lankan export processing zones (EPZs).

Leadership Impetus

Since 1979, religious organizations, NGOs, feminists, and former women workers have provided community-based support to the women workers of the Sri Lanka EPZs in order to integrate the women into the village communities where they board. This case study represents an effort on behalf of EPZ women workers (Martens & Mitter, 1994).

EMPOWER Methods Used

- Enabling service and assistance
- Organizing partnership
- Rights protection and social action/reform
- Public education and participation

Religious organizations have established centers and organized social activities for the EPZ women workers. For example, seven Roman Catholic centers are located near the EPZ and provide a forum for meeting and socializing, boarding-house accommodations, library facilities, or counseling by the nuns. Former factory workers established a women's center that provides legal and medical assistance, library facilities, training in alternative skills, and seminars on women's rights. Another entity, called the Legal Advice Center (LAC), gives free professional advice and free or low-cost representation to EPZ workers. LAC also distributes legal pamphlets and organizes seminars and discussions in which the women are invited to participate.

One of the centers helped establish a food cooperative in response to the rising food prices in the area. Women workers bought shares to build up capital for the start of the cooperative. As a result of their solidarity, prices of food items went down and local shopkeepers were forced to lower their own prices. Other organizations helped the women workers organize protest campaigns against sexual harassment experienced when walking to and from work after dark. Because thieves and rapists would often prey on late-shift workers who were forced to travel along unlit areas at night, women formed groups to walk together. Later, they created posters and pamphlets, campaigned in the community both door-to-door and in churches and temples, and sent petitions to the local government requesting security and transportation for the women. Women workers also participated in the decision-making committees of the religious centers, although they did not control the operation of these centers. Key persons of the community also participated in these committees to guide discussion. An independent women's collective published and distributed an EPZ newspaper. It is sold to the public for a minimal fee, and in its pages, EPZ women are able to voice their opinions and share ideas with other workers. Not allowed inside the EPZ itself, the newspaper is often used as a tool of resistance by passing it along an assembly line or pinning it to a bulletin board. Managers have either found it useful to know their employees' views or have been suspicious of its real purpose.

Partners/Opposition

The community provided tremendous support in initiating programs and establishing centers for the EPZ women workers. Religious organizations, NGOs, and former factory workers have all intervened to improve the working and living conditions of these young women workers and motivate them to act on their own behalf. However, managerial opposition to organizing women workers continues to be widespread and strong.

Macro-environment

Between 1953 and 1971, women's participation in the industrial sector increased from 18.5% to 81.6% of the total Sri Lankan labor force. Self-employed and unpaid family workers decreased from 15% to 2.1%. In 1985, women constituted 28,414 of the total labor force of 35,786. Because the women workers live far from home, they lodge together in boarding houses. Most of the women are from traditionally conservative Asian cultural backgrounds in which women are submissive and obedient to male authority. They also have little or no experience with trade union representation and collective bargaining. In fact, in Sri Lanka, the EPZs discourage unions or organization of the women workers; and management often forbids talking among co-workers. There are also safety concerns about the women traveling to and from work after dark to attend meetings.

Impact and Remarks

The women workers of the Sri Lankan EPZ have empowered themselves in a seemingly hopeless working situation. They have gained confidence in their own ability to organize in the community and have demonstrated resistance on the factory floor. For instance, the women will use secret sign language or eye contact when talking is prohibited on the job, or will speak in a local language in front of foreign management to preserve their privacy. Another demonstration of solidarity and resistance was seen when the workers collectively lowered production targets when management pressured them to increase productivity, or when the group has helped those who are slow to reach their individual targets. Uniting against a common threat and successfully improving their plight has given these women a new sense of power never felt before.

CASE STUDY #19: GABRIELA, PHILIPPINES, 1984 (EQRT)

Problem

This case study falls within the domain of equal rights (EQRT). The major problem being addressed is the oppression of Filipino women living in cities, squatters' camps, and rural areas.

Leadership Impetus

In 1984, 42 women's organizations from different sectors established the national women's coalition known as GABRIELA (General Assembly Binding Women for Reforms, Integrity, Equality, Leadership, and Action). Its purpose was to join the struggle for liberation and the anti-dictatorship movement of the Philippines.

EMPOWER Methods Used

- Public education and participation
- Rights protection and social action/reform
- Work/job training and micro-enterprise
- Empowerment training and leadership development
- Organizing partnership

Serving as an umbrella body for all women in the Philippines, GABRIELA has regional branches throughout the country representing the interests of peasants, women workers, professionals, media, urban poor, and others. GABRIELA believes that in order for women to achieve freedom, the problems of foreign domination, landlessness, and political repression must be resolved in terms of the patriarchal value systems and structures in Philippine society. With this in mind, GABRIELA focuses on issues that affect women, including the effects of militarization and women's landlessness; the International Monetary Fund–World Bank and the debt crisis; the denial of women's reproductive rights; the neglect of healthcare for women; violence against children and women; development aid; and prostitution and the trafficking of women. Each GABRIELA group produces regular publications while also being active in organizing women around social and political issues, conducting programs on education, income-generating activities, and women's legal rights. The education and training department, for example, publishes resource and training materials and conference papers. The public information department produces newsletters such as the *GABRIELA Women's Update*—a quarterly publication featuring articles, news, artwork, and photographs from all member organizations about topics concerning Filipina women.

The highest policy-making body of GABRIELA is the National Assembly, composed of all member organizations. The National Council is composed of national and regional officers, national sectoral representatives, and GABRIELA Commission heads. GABRIELA has formed networks among local and international women's organizations in order to solve common problems together. GABRIELA also establishes collaborations with other agencies and organizations to promote equal opportunities for women and their development (Andrews, 1996).

Partners/Opposition

Founded in 1989, GABRIELA Network (GABNet) is a U.S.-based women's solidarity organization working with GABRIELA Philippines. GABRIELA Network has created education campaigns around such issues as the global traffic of women, world trade and the sex industry, the mail-order bride industry, First World and Third World perspectives on the women's movement, and gender relations in the Asian American community. GABNet operates a speakers' bureau, publishes a bimonthly newsletter called *kaWomenan* and trains Filipino women in leadership and activism skills. (*kaWomenan* combines *ka* from the Tagalog word *kasama* meaning "companion"; the English word "women" and the Tagalog suffix *an* meaning "reciprocity". Used together, *ka* and *an* mean collectiveness.)

Macro-environment

Filipino women have a long history of struggle against oppression, foreign control, and male domination. They have fought for equal opportunities in the workplace, for political rights, and for the right to education. In fact, the organization's moniker also refers to Gabriela Silang, the first Filipina general, who fought alongside her husband against the Spaniards in the 1700s. She continued her military involvement even when her husband died. She was also distinguished as leading the longest revolt against Spanish colonial rule. Gabriela Silang is revered among Filipino women as a symbol of courage and strength.

Impact and Remarks

Today, GABRIELA is an umbrella organization of over 100 women's groups, institutes, and programs that seek to liberate women from the repressive Filipino culture. It is the largest and only multisectoral women's assembly in the archipelago. Constituted primarily of middle-class women at its inception, GABRIELA now has a membership base of over 40,000 women of all socioeconomic statuses: peasants, workers and urban poor, women from religious institutions, and students across the country. GABRIELA has regional chapters in Metro Manila, Cordillera, and Mindanao; sub-regional chapters in Negros, Panay, and Samar; and provincial chapters in Bicol and Cebu. According to a documentary by Trix Betlam that profiles GABRIELA, this mass organization of nuns, students, professionals, and farm and factory workers proved important in the overthrow of the Marcos regime, and in subsequent Philippine politics.

GABRIELA (2008) is still active; in 2008 International Women's Day, it posted the following statement:

> On March 8, 2008, Filipino women once again call for a militant commemoration of the International Women's Day to honour the day of working women. The women's militancy to demand change and fight for their rights roots back from the historical condition of oppression and inequality of women. For working-class women, this meant inhuman and slave-like conditions in the form of feudal and capitalist exploitation.
>
> One hundred years ago, on 8 March 1908, 15,000 women marched through New York City to demand shorter work hours, just pay and the right to vote. In the same year in Europe women also set up strikes, protested against welfare cuts and campaigned for equal pay and unionization.
>
> In the Philippines, women's participation has always been significant in the people's historical struggle for sovereignty and against oppression and exploitation. Filipinas first commemorated International Women's Day in 1971 at the onset of the dictatorial rule of Ferdinand Marcos. With the establishment of GABRIELA in 1984, women under the alliance continued the militant tradition of commemoration IWD from then

on, recognizing the contribution of millions of working women's struggle in the past. (GABRIELA Philippines, 2008)

As late as in July 4, 2015, Dr. Judy Taguiwalo of the University of the Philippines, posted the following message on GABRIELA's Facebook demonstrating their active community outreach initiatives.

> Dr. Judy Taguiwalo, University of the Philippines professor, unionist, long-time women's rights advocate and member of the Free Sharon Cabusao, "Free Our Sisters, Free Ourselves" network, visits political prisoners Sharon Cabusao and Adel Silva at their jail in Camp Crame. Dr. Taguiwalo is also a former political prisoner during the time of the Marcos dictatorship. #FreeSharonCabusao #FreeAllPoliticalPrisoners. (GABRIELA, 2015).

CASE STUDY #23: INNABUYOG, PHILIPPINES, 1990 (EQRT)

Problem

This case study falls within the domain of equal rights (EQRT). The major problem being addressed is the rights violation of indigenous Filipino women—who are often poor, voiceless, and disempowered.

Leadership Impetus

The Cordillera Women's Education Action Research (CWEARC) was established in the Innabuyog region, a federation of indigenous women's community-based organizations in the Cordillera region of the Northern Philippines. It was founded in 1987 with the following mission: "WE empower indigenous women for the defense of land, food and rights and gain indigenous women's dignity" (CWEARC, 2015). Using the collective efforts of its members, Innabuyog strives towards justice, sustainable development, and the defense of their ancestral lands. Using the indigenous women's own initiative and resources, Innabuyog seeks to empower women so that they can improve their quality of life. Their programs are still active. Since 2006 CWEARC has adapted food sovereignty as its strategy in addressing the endangered, and consequently loss of, traditional food resources of indigenous women and their communities in the Cordillera region. This is particularly in the context of heightened mineral extraction particularly by mining corporations, intensifying commercial production in food and agriculture, and the persistent militarization of the region (CWEARC, 2014).

EMPOWER Methods Used

- ¤ Empowerment training and leadership development
- ¤ Public education and participation

- ◻ Work/job training and micro-enterprise
- ◻ Enabling services and assistance
- ◻ Rights protection and social action/reform
- ◻ Organizing partnership

Innabuyog covers the political, economic, social, cultural, and environmental issues important in the lives of indigenous women living in the Philippines. In order to enhance women's awareness of their basic rights as indigenous people and Filipina women, Innabuyog sends its members to human rights education seminars. To the extent possible, education is done in the villages with local resource persons. This type of forum allows the women to share their experiences, knowledge, concerns, and problems. For example, participants have heard personal testimonials of women whose rights have been violated. They have also learned how to handle encounters with military personnel who accuse them of being rebel supporters.

In addition, Innabuyog offers basic leadership training seminars. To raise public awareness, Innabuyog has documented rights violations committed against women in militarized areas in the journal of the Cordillera Women's Education and Resource Center (CWERC). Innabuyog has implemented small-scale socioeconomic initiatives and production activities in order to generate income for its members. Based on the principles of collectivism and mutual support, Innabuyog provides child-care services for working mothers. Many women had established their own daycare centers before asking for governmental assistance. In order to improve care-giving skills, Innabuyog organized three early childhood education seminars. It also gave books for the daycare centers and schools in the villages (CWEARC, 2015).

As community managers, Innabuyog organizations perform advocacy work at the village level on important issues concerning women. For example, drunkenness is considered one of the major problems encountered in the villages due to its negative consequences, namely increased domestic violence and wasting of money. As a result, Innabuyog lobbied for bans on liquor. Where regulations existed, Innabuyog lobbied to be given police powers that would enable them to patrol the village and arrest violators. As a result of the women's efforts, some village organizations have made domestic violence grounds for expulsion from the village. Innabuyog has also participated in rallies, forums, and other activities centered on peasant issues. For example, Innabuyog was instrumental in initiating a local anti-pesticide campaign in one province.

Partners/Opposition

Innabuyog serves as one of the hosts of the annual Asian Indigenous Conference. This gathering enables women to voice their concerns, aspirations, and efforts in addressing the issues of Asian indigenous women. Innabuyog also serves as the regional chapter of GABRIELA (Case #19) and is a member of the Philippine Organizing Committee (POC).

Macro-environment

Indigenous women play a vital role in ensuring the continuing existence of indigenous peoples and culture. They are often the main producers of food, family caregivers, and environmental protectors. Indigenous women have been active participants in the defense of their land and resources; they have actively opposed such potentially damaging activities as land surveys, mining prospecting, open-pit mining operations, and logging since the beginning of the twentieth century. Despite these crucial roles, indigenous women remain one of the most marginalized, discriminated, and oppressed sectors of society.

Asian indigenous people compose the majority of indigenous people all over the world. Yet they have not been able to voice the problems or issues that affect them. Neither governmental nor non-governmental organizations have addressed their concerns. Possible reasons include high rates of illiteracy among indigenous people (especially women), lack of organization, and lack of conference participation.

Impact and Remarks

Innabuyog has had many successes that have provided its members with valuable lessons and a source of strength and pride. For example, Innabuyog has responded to local needs by helping institute bans on liquor, illegal logging, and development aggression by foreign corporations.

After taking a basic leadership training seminar, one member organization of Innabuyog was able to negotiate with government agencies and officials in order to obtain a contract for a waterworks project in their villages. The organization implemented the project beyond the specifications defined by the government agency. Although the women eventually lost the project due to village politics (mainly the opposition of male village officials), the women gained an important learning experience.

Chosen by an international panel of advisors, Innabuyog was one of 50 exemplary organizations to be honored by the "We the Peoples: 50 Communities Awards." According to the awards panel, Innabuyog was an "example of citizens' initiatives [that] demonstrated success in ten categories of activity important to the United Nations." As one of the chosen communities, Innabuyog demonstrated positive and practical solutions to difficult problems [and offered] inspiring lessons to offer to other communities and to the United Nations (CWEARC websites, 2015).

CASE STUDY #25: NATIONAL ASIAN PACIFIC AMERICAN WOMEN'S
FORUM (NAPAWF), CALIFORNIA, 1996 (EQRT)

Problem

This case study falls within the domain of equal rights (EQRT). The major
problem being addressed is the marginalization of Asian and Pacific
American women and girls from the decision-making processes and structures that affect their daily lives.

Leadership Impetus

National Asian Pacific American Women's Forum (NAPAWF) was founded
in 1996 by a group of Asian American women who had met a year earlier at
the 1995 United Nations Fourth World Conference on Women in Beijing,
China. After a year of organizing and outreach across the United States,
over 150 Asian and Pacific Islander (API) women attended the founding
gathering of NAPAWF, held in Los Angeles, California. Their mission was
to organize a grassroots progressive movement for social and economic justice and the political empowerment of Asian and Pacific American women
and girls. At this first gathering, participants formed regional chapters,
committees, and an interim leadership body made up of regional representatives. They also identified the issues that NAPAWF would focus
on: (1) civil rights, (2) economic justice, (3) educational access, (4) ending
violence against women, (5) health, and (6) immigrant and refugee rights
for API women nationwide.

EMPOWER Methods Used

- Empowerment training and leadership development
- Public education and participation
- Enabling service and assistance
- Rights protection and social action/reform
- Organizing partnership
- Media use
- Work/job training and micro-enterprise

In order to move toward their mission, NAPAWF recruited underrepresented groups of API women and girls (lesbian, bisexual, transgendered, and immigrant) for NAPAWF membership and leadership.
NAPAWF compiled data about API women to educate the public and
inform the development of policies and advocacy strategies. NAPAWF
also developed a national clearinghouse to disseminate information in
several Asian languages. In order to increase knowledge of and understanding about the many issues affecting API women and girls, NAPAWF

provided and supported educational, advocacy, organizing, and outreach activities. NAPAWF also produced or sponsored programs and materials such as position papers, public workshops and events, speakers' bureaus, mentoring programs, labor organizing, and media campaigns. Specifically, NAPAWF wrote platform papers on the six major areas of focus, which are posted on NAPAWF's website. For the civil rights platform, NAPAWF promotes voter education and participation through a national resource and information network, as well as a progressive civil rights agenda that meets the needs of API women and girls.

In order to push certain legislation that protects civil rights for women and girls, NAPAWF testified before legislative and policy-making bodies and conducted letter-writing campaigns in addition to developing position papers. For the 2000 election, NAPAWF produced factsheets that outlined issues pertinent to Asian American and Pacific Islander women. Because of the lack of available data on the API population, NAPAWF advocated for more research on issues affecting APIs. In order to bolster support for issues pertinent to API women, NAPAWF supported and coordinated with the national network of shelters working with refugee women, and sponsored community workshops. Through investigation and development of national communications networks using computer technology, NAPAWF aimed to provide access to email and the Internet to low-income communities and local community-based organizations (CBOs). NAPAWF involved the women and girls in its advocacy efforts by providing leadership and education training. NAPAWF also developed a job training program for API immigrant women who are not familiar with the American employment system.

Partners/Opposition

NAPAWF collaborated with other Asian American organizations such as the Asian and Pacific Islander American Health Forum, the Association of Asian Pacific Community Health Organizations, the Asian Pacific Islanders for Reproductive Health, and the National Asian Women's Health Organization. NAPAWF's regional chapters collaborated with many local CBOs and activists to raise awareness about various issues concerning API women and girls. For example, the Seattle chapter was a member of Washington State APACE (Asian Pacific American Coalition for Equality), which focused on affirmative action. NAPAWF-DC co-sponsored a 2000 conference on API political participation with the Conference on Asian Pacific American Leadership (CAPAL) in Washington, DC. NAPAWF is funded primarily through foundation grants, and increasingly through membership support (donations and membership dues).

Macro-environment

Gender, race, class, age, and sexual discrimination both within and without the API population are major factors in the oppression of API women and girls. American culture perpetuates stereotypes about the immigration status and English-speaking ability of the API community. API women often are perceived as "exotic and erotic dragon women" or "dutiful daughters and wives."

Due to limited educational and employment opportunities, immigrant and non–English-speaking women and girls tend to be concentrated in industries characterized by long working hours, labor-intensive work, and low wages, such as garment "sweatshops," restaurants, and domestic service. According to NAPAWF's platform paper on health, the obstacles that most commonly limit access to primary and reproductive healthcare services for many API women and girls are: lack of insurance; lack of quality interpretation services, bilingual/bicultural providers, and translated materials about health plans and health education; patients' unfamiliarity with Western healthcare systems, particularly managed care; providers' unfamiliarity with or insensitivity to API health belief systems; transportation difficulties; and lack of affordable child-care services (HAN, 2015; NAPAWF, 2015). There is also a pervasive stereotype that members of a "model minority" do not experience social problems and therefore do not require any type of assistance.

Impact and Remarks

NAPAWF currently has 15 throughout the United States in

- Arizona
- Atlanta, GA
- Bay Area, CA
- Greater Boston, MA
- Chicago, IL
- Colorado
- Los Angeles, CA
- New York, NY
- Nashville, TN
- Orange County, CA
- San Diego, CA
- St. Cloud, MN
- Seattle, WA
- Twin Cities, MN
- Washington, DC

The founding sisters identified six issue areas to serve as the platform and foundation for NAPAWF's work:

1. Civil Rights
2. Economic Justice
3. Educational Access
4. Ending Violence Against Women
5. Health
6. Immigrant and Refugee Rights

NAPAWF unites our diverse communities through organizing, education, and advocacy, and works to connect state and local programs with a national vision of change (NAPAWF, 2015).

A rapid expansion of NAPAWH's recent geographic areas (e.g., increase in number of chapters) and scope of action (e.g., current focus on six action domains mentioned above) support its claim that it is an active and thriving organization.

CASE STUDY #13: NOW (NATIONAL ORGANIZATION FOR WOMEN), UNITED STATES, 1966 (EQRT)

Problem

This case study falls in the domain of equal rights (EQRT). The major problem addressed is the existence of sex discrimination adversely affecting women's rights and opportunities. In NOW's early history, the top issue for many activists was employment, specifically sex discrimination in job earnings, hiring and firing practices, and job advertisements (sex-segregated help wanted ads). Today, NOW is dedicated to making legal, political, social, and economic changes that will help to eliminate all gender-based discrimination.

Leadership Impetus

NOW was founded in 1966 in Washington, D.C., by a group of women attending the Third National Conference of the Commission on the Status of Women. They were frustrated with the Equal Employment Opportunity Commission's (EEOC) recent actions. Not only was the EEOC reluctant to advocate women's issues, it failed to pass a resolution demanding the enforcement of Title VII and calling for the reappointment of Richard Graham— the only male EEOC commissioner who was sympathetic to women's causes. This final decision by the EEOC sparked action by frustrated female activists to form NOW. The 28 founding members included Betty Friedan, author of *The Feminine Mystique;* as well as Catherine East and Mary Eastwood, key players in the feminist movement; and the Reverend Pauli Murray, an African-American woman and Episcopal minister.

EMPOWER Methods Used
- ¤ Media use
- ¤ Public education and participation
- ¤ Enabling service and assistance
- ¤ Rights protection and social action/reform
- ¤ Empowerment training and leadership development
- ¤ Organizing partnership

During NOW's first years, local chapter members were invited to sign up for a task force focused on various issues such as sex discrimination in employment or education, marriage and divorce laws, or the media's image of women. In fact, NOW leaders expected much of the action to occur locally. Members were encouraged to work on issues that they found personally interesting and that they believed in. Today, NOW focuses on such issues as sexual harassment, reproductive rights, violence against women, lesbian and gay rights, and gender equality. Through electoral and lobbying work, litigation, and mass actions (marches, rallies, pickets, counter-demonstrations, nonviolent civil disobedience), NOW makes its voice known to the public, press, and decision-makers. NOW's Political Action Committee, or NOW/PAC, supports candidates in congressional and presidential elections. NOW Equality PAC (NEP) supports candidates for state, county, and city offices, from governors to school board members. Many state and local NOW chapters have political action committees which can endorse candidates for governor, the state legislature, and local offices.

In an attempt to debunk the negative stereotypes of feminists, NOW launched a "Feminist Image Campaign" with the help of a Washington, D.C.–based advertising and public relations firm. Through print and television advertising now continues to depict the wide range of women who have contributed to NOW's efforts and success as a women's rights organization. Published quarterly, *The National NOW Times* informs members and interested parties of the latest issues and projects of NOW. On their official website, "Women-Friendly Workplace Campaign Speakout" allows women to vent their personal stories about discrimination at the workplace. The campaign is part of a larger effort to stop sexual harassment and other workplace abuses through protests, educational forums, and pledges made by employers and consumers to support a nondiscriminatory workplace.

Although NOW is a national organization led by four elected officials and has 50 state organizations, most of NOW's organizing and actions are performed by the local chapters. Past examples of local actions include protests against presidential candidate George W. Bush for his anti-abortion stance in Los Angeles and San Francisco; a candlelight vigil for hate-crimes victims; and local celebrations of Women's History Month. Each year, delegates of local chapters attend the national conference, during which policy is decided and proposals are voted upon. Through NOW's volunteer program, women can gain training and experience in public relations, computer science, or office support. The NOW internship program at the Washington, D.C., office offers college students comprehensive leadership training through empowerment workshops, weekly discussion groups, and direct participation in NOW's activities, including congressional and U.S. Supreme Court hearings, press conferences, demonstrations, and rallies.

Established in 1986 and affiliated with NOW, the NOW Foundation is a nonprofit organization dedicated to advocating for women's rights through education, litigation, networking, conferences, publications, training, and leadership development. Its projects have included a campaign that addresses anti-abortion terrorism, a summit for young activists about violence against women, a global feminism conference, and education for community activities about racial and ethnic diversity (Carabillo, 1993).

Partners/Opposition

NOW's early accomplishments could be attributed to the prestigious board of directors, who included best-selling author Betty Friedan, head of the Wisconsin Status-of-Women Commission Kathryn Clarenbach, vice-president of one of the top public relations agencies Muriel Fox, director of the Women's Departments of the United Auto Workers Caroline Davis, and former EEOC commissioners Aileen Hernandez and Richard Graham. Catherine East also explained NOW's early success by saying they "encourage[ed] the illusion that [NOW] was bigger and more powerful than it was" (Davis, 1991, p. 57). In the early years, their treasury rarely exceeded a few hundred dollars; board members paid for travel expenses out-of-pocket; NOW did not have a central office for its first three years; and they even exaggerated the size of its membership and power-base.

As a nonprofit organization, NOW receives all its operating funds from private donations and membership dues. In terms of opposition faced by NOW, various groups of misogynists discouraged NOW's organizing efforts and the feminist movement, in general. In addition, because sexism privileges all men as a class, in the same ways that white racism privileges all whites, sexism as a pervasive social system is the greatest barrier to NOW's struggles.

Macro-environment

In an environment where the liberals were in control at Washington and conditioned by the civil rights movement, a second wave of feminism took off

with the founding of NOW. There were several conditions that made the wom-
en's movement gain momentum at this particular point in history. Women's
lives had changed during the first half of the twentieth century in terms of
increased participation in the workforce and level of education, increased
life expectancy, and increased divorce rates. In turn, the American women's
movement revived feminism all over the Western world.

Impact and Remarks

"The purpose of NOW is to take action to bring women into full participation
in the mainstream of American society now, exercising all the privileges and
responsibilities thereof in truly equal partnership with men" (NOW, 1966).
During the first months of NOW's existence, its board of directors made
themselves very visible in Washington by meeting with the Attorney General,
Secretary of Labor, director of the EEOC, and chairman of the Civil Service
Commission, who was close to President Lyndon Johnson. Specifically, they
reminded Macy that Johnson had not yet appointed 50 women to top-level
government jobs as he had promised. NOW also asked for an executive order
to prohibit companies that conducted business with the federal government
from practicing sexual discrimination. In October of 1967, President Johnson
made this a reality by signing Executive Order #11375. In addition, NOW's
legal committee was instrumental in many landmark cases of job discrimination such as *Weeks vs Southern Bell*, which involved the protective labor laws
as well as cases in sexual bias in criminal law (*Weeks vs Bell,* 1967). NOW also
addressed the wage gap via the nationwide Equal Rights Amendment (ERA)
campaign, abortion rights via marches, harassment and violence via "Take
Back the Night" marches, hotlines and battered women shelters, as well as
racism and lesbian rights.

Today, NOW is the largest feminist organization in the country, with
more than half a million members and more than 550 chapters in all 50 states
and the District of Columbia (Goldberg, 1991). These ongoing efforts established NOW as a major force in national politics.

CASE STUDY #22: RURAL WORKERS' ORGANIZATIONS (RWOs), INDIA,
PHILIPPINES, SRI LANKA, 1987 (EQRT)

Problem

This case study falls within the domain of EQRT. The major problem being
addressed is discrimination against women in the workforce and the lack of
participation of women in RWOs.

Women waged agriculture workers account for 20–30 percent of
the waged workforce, rising to 40 percent in Latin America and the

Caribbean, and their numbers too are increasing in most regions (ILO, FAO, IUF, 2007). More often than men, women are likely to hold part-time, seasonal and/or low-paying jobs in the informal economy. However, differences exist across regions and sectors. For instance, women workers dominate many commercial value chains for high-value products such as fresh fruit, vegetables, flowers and livestock products, particularly in Africa and Latin America. In many cases, these modern chains provide better wages and working conditions for women than traditional agricultural employment.

Agricultural waged workers play already an important role in agricultural and rural development. Their contribution to sustainably increased food production and food security remains however virtually untapped. Their trade unions will need increased political, financial and technical support to play a greater role in the future and be empowered to strengthen links with producers' organizations in the interests of sustainable development and poverty eradication. (Saavedra, 2013)

Leadership Impetus

In order to encourage women's participation in rural workers' organizations (RWOs) in Asia, the Danish International Development Agency (DANIDA) funded a five-year joint project run by the International Labor Office (ILO) and the International Federation of Plantation, Agricultural and Allied Workers (IFPAAW) in 1987. The project was geared toward women members of RWOs and potential members of IFPAAW-affiliated organizations in the three Asian countries of India, the Philippines, and Sri Lanka.

EMPOWER Methods Used

- Empowerment training and leadership development
- Enabling service and assistance
- Work/job training and micro-enterprise
- Organizing partnership

Trade unions participating in the project nominated women to take part in a series of leadership training workshops who would eventually become liaison officers or organizers of the rural women. One-day workshops on general leadership principles were also offered to reach a larger number of women at one time. Select participants, often leaders in their villages or organizations, would later serve as the links between the community and the organizers from trade unions. These community women were instructed and encouraged to teach their new skills to their fellow community members in a variety of subjects identified as important by the women themselves. These included such areas as sanitation, personal hygiene, child-care, nutrition, adult education, literacy training, and skills-training for income-generating activities. All educational interventions focused on empowering the women in terms of raising awareness of trade unions and helping women develop of plan of action to alter the poor conditions in rural areas. Liaison officers also served as links between the rural community and the government, offering legal advice when needed. Liaison officers were also trained in developing audiovisual materials and in cross-cultural exchange.

Following an evaluation workshop with the project coordinator and liaison officers, it was decided that more focus should be placed on income-generation and socioeconomic activities and cooperatives. More than 150 activities were developed in order to raise the women's level of respect among the men in the villages, as well as to improve their immediate living standards. Activities included rope making, tailoring, rabbit-breeding, basket-weaving, and honey collection in India; pig-raising, poultry-keeping, knitting, vegetable-gardening, and fishing in the Philippines; and sewing, cattle-raising, and poultry-keeping in Sri Lanka.

Partners/Opposition

Due to the patriarchal nature of these three Asian nations, this type of change in the gender dynamics can be threatening to the privileged males. In fact, some of the participating women opted to withdraw from the project rather than upset the traditional power structures.

Macro-environment

Rural workers compose the majority of workers in developing countries. In Asia, a large proportion of the labor force is made up of women, who are also often responsible for running the household in addition to performing paid labor. Women's actual economic contribution to society is underestimated and unrecognized in terms of child-care in the informal sector and work in agriculture, handicrafts, marketing, and food processing and preparation, especially in rural areas.

Impact and Remarks

During the five-year project, a total of 53 women worker specialists were instructed in training other community women at the grassroots level. All participating women demonstrated increased awareness of their rights and responsibilities. Many of them even assumed decision-making roles in their unions. In addition, many unions formed women's committees at local, branch, and national levels; and constitutions were changed to include female representation on executive committees. As a result of the project, there was a multiplier effect in reaching rural women in order to empower them and increase participation in the RWOs.

The International Labor Organization (ILO) has been very active in coordinating and promoting women's employment related issues (ILO, 2015). Its strategic objectives include:

> Strategic Objective 2: a) Decent employment for women in India; b) Inter-Regional Programme to Support Self-Reliance of Indigenous and Tribal Communities through Cooperatives and other Self-Help Organizations (INDISCO); c) Pilot project on alternative employment opportunities for beedi workers in Karnataka and Tamil Nadu; d) Prevention of family indebtedness with micro-finance schemes and related services; e) Programme for entrepreneurship development and productivity improvement in Moradabad brassware industry; f) Preparatory assistance to the formulation and launching of an urban informal sector support programme in India; and g) A model programme for social and economic reconstruction in 10 villages in the state of Gujarat.
>
> Strategic Objective 3: a) Community wide drugs demand reduction in India; b) Community wide drugs demand reduction in the North-Eastern states of India; c) Developing a comprehensive strategy for alternative development in illicit opium poppy growing areas of Arunachal Pradesh; and d) HIV/AIDS prevention in the World of Work.
>
> Strategic Objective 4: a) Integration of rural women workers into mainstream trade unions of rural workers organisations; and b) South Asia and Vietnam Project on Tripartism and Social Dialogue in Action (SAVPOT).
>
> Pipeline activities include: an expanded programme for earthquake rehabilitation in Gujarat; a programme on core labour standards and the informal sector; and a project on rural reconstruction using employment-intensive methods in West Bengal. (ILO, 2015)

CASE STUDY #14: UNION OF WOMEN DOMESTIC EMPLOYEES (UWDE), RECIFE, BRAZIL, 1970 (EQRT)

Problem

This case study falls within the domain of equal rights (EQRT). The major problem being addressed is the rights violations of domestic workers in Recife, in northeast Brazil.

Recent data from the International Labour Organization (ILO) estimates that there are 52.6 million domestic workers worldwide, the vast majority of them women (83 %), of which nearly a third are excluded from national labor legislation and almost half of whom have no right to rest breaks and paid vacations. (MDG Fund, 2013)

Leadership Impetus

In the 1960s, domestic workers began to organize informally in the larger cities of Brazil with the assistance of the Young Catholic Workers (YCW). Associations in São Paulo and Rio de Janeiro officially registered in 1962 and 1963, respectively. In Recife, although UWDE was officially registered in 1970, the YCW movement had started to organize and collaborate with the working classes in 1964. When YCW discovered that domestic workers were often ashamed of their jobs and did not like to voice their opinions in front of the other workers, the YCW created a group specifically for them. Lenira Carvalho, who had joined the YCW in 1962, later became the UWDE president in Recife. In 1980, UWDE became a trade union.

EMPOWER Methods Used

- ¤ Rights protection and social action/reform
- ¤ Organizing partnership
- ¤ Empowerment training and leadership development
- ¤ Public education and participation
- ¤ Work/job training and micro-enterprise
- ¤ Enabling service and assistance

UWDE of Recife participated in many acts of social action to improve their working conditions. In 1963, domestic workers in Recife marched in a parade of workers for the first time. Following the return to democracy in Brazil in 1987, domestic employees actively lobbied members of the Constituent Assembly in the capital of Brasília where the new constitution was being prepared. In 1988, the National Council sent four representatives to the First Latin American and Caribbean Domestic Workers' Conference held in Bogotá, Colombia. UWDE also engaged in various types of collaborative efforts with similar bodies in Brazil. For example, in 1978, the National Council of Women Domestic Employees was formed, which served as a coordinating body of organizations of various cities, including the UWDE of Recife (Anderfuhren, 1994). A national congress of this body is held periodically. UWDE also participated in an advisory group along with representatives from six women's organizations from the northeast region. Advised by SOS CORPO (2015), this forum allowed members to share their problems and look for joint solutions. (SOS CORPO means a "Safe City for Women," which is the goal of a Feminist Institute for Democracy—in the city of Recife, in the Northeast of Brazil; ILO, 2002).

UWDE provides empowerment education activities, work training, and enabling services. There is an Education Group that imparts knowledge about trade union policies and the workings of political institutions through monthly meetings. In 1991, a set of courses on trade union activities was jointly administered by a UWDE organizer and two representatives from SOS CORPO. As a result of this program, a training manual was produced that would help standardize training elsewhere in the country. UWDE attempts to reach the general public, both employers and employees through the distribution of a bimonthly bulletin.

UWDE provides vocational training in all aspects of domestic work such as cooking, laundry, and even preparing food for deep-freezing. Acquiring additional skills can raise the prestige and income of the domestic worker. In order to break the isolation of the domestic workers' lives, UWDE organizes a number of leisure activities such as dancing festivals and a theater group. These enjoyable activities could also entice the young workers to join the union. Because employers do not have an established association of their own, UWDE counsels and informs employers about their employees' rights. Although this service takes away valuable time from their other functions, failure to do so would not be advantageous to the domestic workers when they are bargaining with their employers.

Partners/Opposition

In 1964, the military arrested all individuals who had collaborated with or assisted the domestic-service movement. Dedicated activists who continued to support the cause were forced to work in districts where they were unknown, to avoid persecution. During this time a Jesuit priest organized a group of workers that met immediately following Sunday mass. SOS CORPO offered its valuable assistance during the revision of the constitution to include domestic workers' rights; helped UWDE set up its bookkeeping system; gave advice for the Education and Training Group; and invited UWDE to collaborate on various projects. This close bond brought the feminists and domestic employees together in their respective struggles for equality.

In 1992, UWDE affiliated with the Workers' Central Union (CUT), the largest trade union confederation in Brazil. Affiliation with this confederation raises the credibility of UWDE among all workers and in the trade union arena. However, CUT itself may not be interested in UWDE as an affiliate, due the occupation's lack of status. Differences in education, hours of work, and the problem of sexual discrimination may also serve as barriers to UWDE's full integration into CUT.

Opposition to the growth of the union may stem from the perceptions held by the domestic workers themselves. Many view the union as a type of public service or form of social assistance run by the government. In particular, the young workers who are the least represented may feel that participation in any such activities is unnecessary. This may be true because young domestic employees hope to leave the sector in the near future; they feel the struggle is too difficult; and the union does not appeal to young workers in terms of their activities.

Macro-environment

Northeast Brazil is one of the poorest regions in Brazil, with the majority of the population precariously employed in domestic service, itinerant trading, small retail, and fishing. In 1985, there were approximately 3 million domestic workers in Brazil out of total labor force of 18 million. More women are employed as domestic servants than in any other occupation in Brazil; that number has more than doubled to 6.5 million by 2008 (MDG Funds, 2008). A 1991 study in Recife revealed that this occupation comprises equal numbers of migrants and local people, whereas in the recent past, the majority was composed of migrants.

Impact and Remarks

As a result of the domestic workers' lobbying efforts during the 1980s, many rights were secured, including the right to organize, a minimum wage, a "thirteenth month's wage," (annual bonus equivalent to one month's pay), a weekly time off with pay, annual holidays, maternity leave, notice of termination, and a retirement pension. These rights mark a significant increase in the value of domestic service. UWDE's success has helped raise the consciousness of the workers themselves, as well as their self-confidence.

> A study funded by the MDG-F on the economic impact of increased income to domestic workers showed that by enhancing traditionally marginalized job categories it is possible to improve the living conditions of low-income populations and thereby to improve the welfare of society as a whole. (MDG Funds, 2008)
>
> Oliveira, president of the Federation of Domestic Workers of Brazil (FENATRAD), was an active participant in the long process of negotiations that led, at the end of March, to the historic vote in the Brazilian Senate that for the first time protects nearby 6.5 million people working in domestic service.
>
> The law enshrines 16 new rights, ranging from a maximum workday of eight hours and a 44-hour work week, to overtime pay and a new provision requiring employers to pay the equivalent of 8 % of an employee's monthly salary to a fund to be used in case of dismissal, death or other contingencies. (MDG Funds, 2008)
>
> For later MDG Funds news and spotlights, see http://mdgfund.org/more/news.

During the last four decades, increased local and labor activism, involvement of international organizations in promoting health and well-being of people (e.g., UN, ILO, WHO, UNICEF, etc.), feminism movements, and minority rights have formed partnership among local and global initiatives globalization. Successful local initiatives soon become global (e.g., multiplications of SEWA and Grameen models). Our web-browsing reveals that the number of coalitions and alliances of workers' unions globally and the involvement of foreign donors and international organizations in multinational projects have increased sharply during the last four decades. As a result, it has become more difficult to evaluate and attribute impacts of isolated local organizations and programs. For instance, the merger of the UWDE and CUT means that they have grown much in scope and size of their operations, but this has also made it difficult to evaluate the exclusive impacts each in program or organization.

CASE STUDY #21: WOMEN LIVING UNDER MUSLIM LAWS (WLUML), MUSLIM COUNTRIES, 1986 (EQRT)

Problem

This case study falls within the domain of equal rights (EQRT). The major problem being addressed is the oppression faced by Muslim women. Due to the Islamization process or creation of Islamic states, "Family Codes," a set of personal laws regarding such issues as marriage, divorce, polygamy, and reproductive rights, are increasingly being adopted. These rigorous laws often serve to restrict further the lives of Muslim women. Furthermore, fundamentalists are advocating "separate development" for women, a policy comparable to South Africa's apartheid for blacks. "Women Living Under Muslim Laws is an international solidarity network that provides information, support and a collective space for women whose lives are shaped, conditioned or governed by laws and customs said to derive from Islam" (WLUML, 2015).

> On Wednesday, the U.N. Department of Economic and Social Affairs (DESA) released another major report, also dealing with the status of women around the world in 2010. The numerous indicators explored in the report include the rate of girls of primary school age enrolled in school, compared to that of boys.
>
> The seven countries with the biggest gaps are all Islamic countries—Chad (a 22 percent difference between boys and girls enrolled), Yemen (20), Pakistan (16), Guinea-Bissau (16), Mali (14), Iraq (13) and Niger (13).
>
> Two Islamic countries do break the pattern significantly—in Iran the percentage of girls enrolled in primary school is nine percent higher

than that of boys; Mauritania also has five percent more girls enrolled than boys.

When it comes to the difference between literacy rates in adult women and men, Islamic countries once again score worst for women.

Of the seven countries with the biggest literacy gaps, five are Islamic – Yemen (a 36 percent gender gap), Mozambique (30), Guinea-Bissau (29), Niger (28) and Pakistan (27). The non-Islamic two are Central African Republic (28) and Ethiopia (27). Of the 28 countries scoring worst for women when it comes to literacy, 20 are Islamic states. (Goodenough, 2010) Leadership Impetus.

The WLUML network was created in 1984 (headquarters in United Kingdom) in response to urgent human rights injustices committed against women in various Muslim areas in the 1980s. Although it is based in Muslim countries in Asia, Africa and the Arab world, WLUML also deals with women of Muslim descent living in Europe and the Americas, and non-Muslim women who are affected by Muslim laws through citizenship or marriage. In fact, this type of international network serves to link women from different Muslim countries and communities across the continents.

EMPOWER Methods Used

- ¤ Organizing partnership
- ¤ Enabling service and assistance
- ¤ Empowerment training and leadership development
- ¤ Rights protection and social action/reform

The WLUML network exchanges information regarding specific cases and the strategies employed to deal with them. An exchange program allows women to travel and interact with their counterparts from other Muslim countries. There is also a special meeting dedicated to discussing the various interpretations of the religious verses of Qur'an (Qur'anic Interpretation by Women meeting). Due to the diversity of economic, political, and cultural situations, the subordination of women is perceived in different ways. Because the Qur'an plays such a strong role in the lives of the Muslim women, an ongoing research group was established to answer any questions posed by WLUML activists. The Women and Law Program analyzes the laws in terms of their effect on the rights of women in Muslim society. The program is designed to increase the women's capacity to understand their circumstances and foster their participation in the development of their societies. Through these modes of sharing ideas, the women become aware of the general political trends, their legal and religious rights, and any different interpretations of Islamic thought

WLUML actively supports women's initiatives and defend women's rights. Requests from groups or individuals seeking assistance for legislative reform or protection from rights violations are circulated throughout the network. Furthermore, WLUML organizes collective projects that rely on cooperative efforts of the women in the network to address the concerns of the group:

> For more than two decades WLUML has linked individual women and organisations. It now extends to more than 70 countries ranging from South Africa to Uzbekistan, Senegal to Indonesia and Brazil to France. It links: women living in countries or states where Islam is the state religion, secular states with Muslim majorities as well as those from Muslim communities governed by minority religious laws; women in secular states where political groups are demanding religious laws; women in migrant Muslim communities in Europe, the Americas, and around the world; non-Muslim women who may have Muslim laws applied to them directly or through their children; women born into Muslim communities/families who are automatically categorized as Muslim but may not define themselves as such, either because they are not believers or because they choose not to identify themselves in religious terms, preferring to prioritise other aspects of their identity such as political ideology, profession, sexual orientation or others. Our name challenges the myth of one, homogenous "Muslim world." This deliberately created myth fails to reflect that: a) laws said to be Muslim vary from one context to another and, b) the laws that determine our lives are from diverse sources: religious, customary, colonial and secular. We are governed simultaneously by many different laws: laws recognised by the state (codified and uncodified) and informal laws such as customary practices which vary according to the cultural, social and political context. Its international priorities include: emergency relief; violence against women; microfinance; and water, sanitation, and health. (WLUML, 2015)

Partners/Opposition

An important issue raised by WLUML organizers is the lack of funding for women's networks. Similar to the lack of compensation for housework or child-care, women's work in networking is undervalued and may receive inadequate funding compared to NGOs headed by men. This serves as a significant constraint to WLUML. Because network efforts are difficult to monitor and evaluate, success of a program is hard to demonstrate quantitatively. WLUML stresses the qualitative importance of solidarity and reciprocity in aid and benefits, and the need for sustained effort to bring about social change.

Macro-environment

Women from Muslim countries and communities may be seen by the outside world as oppressed and helpless, a stereotype that WLUML wants to dispel.

Yet there is a disturbing tendency on the part of the international community to refrain from interfering in the private affairs, or to respect other cultures and/or religions when its practices pertain to the infringement of women's rights. This may be due to the fact that the infringement of women's rights often falls within the private sphere of society (such as domestic abuse) that is viewed as the personal business of the patriarchal family.

Impact and Remarks

The following two cases demonstrate the impact that WLUML can have on the Muslim community. In the first example, the Sri Lankan Muslim Women Research and Action Front (MWRAF) enlisted the assistance of WLUML when this governmental committee was asked to look into the issue of alimony for divorced women in 1989. Based on the information provided by the WLUML network, the MWRAF presented a memorandum and campaigned for local support, and later helped draft a reform proposal for the Muslim Marriage and Divorce Act. A similar situation occurred in Mauritius in 1989 when the Muvman Liberasyon Fam requested information to oppose the reintroduction of a Muslim law that dictates actions that would discriminate specifically against Muslim women.

The *World's Women Report 2016* shows that progress towards gender equality has been made in some areas, such as school enrolment, health and economic participation. At the same time the report shows that much more needs to be done to close the gender gap in critical areas such as power and decision-making and violence against women (UN, *The World's Women Report*, 2016).

A recent multinational survey by the PEW Research Center (2013) found that:

Overwhelming percentages of Muslims in many countries want Islamic law (sharia) to be the official law of the land, according to a worldwide survey by the Pew Research Center. But many supporters of sharia say it should apply only to their country's Muslim population.

Moreover, Muslims are not equally comfortable with all aspects of sharia: While most favor using religious law in family and property disputes, fewer support the application of severe punishments—such as whippings or cutting off hands—in criminal cases. (PEW Research Center, 2013)

Differences between those who want sharia to be the official law and those who do not are most pronounced when it comes to the role of wives. In 10 of the 23 countries where the question was asked, supporters of sharia as official law are more likely to say wives must always obey their husbands. Especially large gaps are found in Albania (+44 percentage points), Kosovo (+34), Bosnia-Herzegovina (+34) and Russia (+33).

Muslims who favor an official role for sharia also tend to be less supportive of granting specific rights to women. For instance, in six countries, those who want Islamic law as the official law are less likely to say women should have the right to divorce, including in Russia (–34 percentage points), Morocco (–19) and Albania (–19). However, the opposite is true in Bangladesh (+13) and Jordan (+12). (PEW Research Center, 2013)

It is clear that Muslim societies vary significantly in terms of their opinions and treatments of women in their respective societies. (This statement would be true for non-Muslim societies as well depending upon their levels of education and poverty.) At the same time our study has demonstrated that , women in many Muslim societies are not deterred from activism and self-organized movements that transform their lives for the better (e.g., Bangladesh, Iran, Turkey, and participants in WLUML's international initiatives.

As Ms. Saadia Zahidi, a senior Director of the World Economic Forum, sums up:

The oft-uttered phrase "the Muslim world" suggests a monolithic body. Yet the reality includes rich petro states at the cusp of dramatic change, such as Qatar, Saudi Arabia, and the United Arab Emirates, and countries such as Bangladesh, Egypt, Indonesia, Iran, Pakistan, and Turkey, which are part of what Goldman Sachs calls the Next 11, countries the investment bank says could rival the G7 over time. The world's 1.6 billion Muslims amount to nearly a quarter of the global population and contribute 16 percent of global GDP, a rate that is growing at 6 percent annually.

Some 800 million of these people are women—more than the combined populations of Brazil, Russia, and the United States. And an untold and still unfolding story exists in their lives, hidden in their classrooms, careers, and handbags. Changes that took half a century in the United States are being compressed into a decade in today's Muslim world, and they are only likely to accelerate. All of this underlines the conscious, often deeply personal and brave decision of millions of ordinary Muslim women and men to break family tradition and sometimes shun cultural pressures. (Zahidi, 2014)

While cultural practices are often the cause of the relative powerlessness of women, the good news is that, ordinary people do change cultural practices and the Muslim world is no exception. Professionals in human services may play a major role by accelerating the empowerment process. Concerned individuals and CBOs also play a major role in this process. Shaanaz Tapin-Chinoy, the board chair and cofounder of the Muslim Women's Fund is an excellent example of how one dedicated woman can lead a successful movement to promote Muslim women's empowerment (Tapin-Chinoy, 2015). Our meta-analysis reaffirms this conclusion over 80 times.

CASE STUDY #12: YWCA (YOUNG WOMEN'S CHRISTIAN ASSOCIATION), INTERNATIONAL, 1849 (EQRT)

Problem

This case study falls within the domain of equal rights (EQRT). The main problem being addressed is the lack of empowerment among women and girls. The original problem at the time of YWCA's founding was the need for guidance by to young girls earning their own income in urbanized areas. For more than 150 years, the YWCA has spoken out and taken action on behalf of women and girls. The YWCA is dedicated to eliminating racism, empowering women and promoting peace, justice, freedom and dignity for all. More than 2 million people participate each year in YWCA programs at more than 1,300 locations across the United States (YWCA, 2015a). Its stated mission and scope are:

> The World Young Women's Christian Association (World YWCA) is a global network of women leading social and economic change in over 120 countries worldwide. The World YWCA advocates for peace, justice, human rights and care for the environment and has been at the forefront of raising the status of women for more than a century. The World YWCA develops women's leadership to find local solutions to the global inequalities women face. Each year, it reaches more than 25 million women and girls through work in over 20,000 communities. Through advocacy, training and development the World YWCA empowers women, including young women, to lead social change. (YWCA, 2015b, Mission)

Leadership Impetus

The World YWCA was founded through the convergence of a social activist Lady Mary Jane Kinnaird and the committed Christian Emma Robarts. Mary Jane Kinnaird, born in 1816, was a philanthropist committed to young women's well being. Kinnaird was concerned about the safety of young women who moved to London city, often alone, to work or serve in the Crimean war. She raised funds and in 1855 set up housing for young single women in London. Equipped with a library, Bible classes and employment bureau, the housing provided a 'warm Christian atmosphere'. Kinnaird and her associates hoped to help young women cope with the pressures of work and believed it was important to care for the souls of young women along with their physical and mental health.

Emma Robarts, born around 1818, was also committed to young women. She set up a prayer circle in her hometown on the outskirts of London. In 1855, she brought together 23 women to hold intercession prayer for young women—they called themselves the Young Women's Christian Association. The group went beyond prayer and reached out to the young women they prayed for and involved them in activities to build the mind, body and spirit. (YWCA, 2015b)

In response to unhealthy social conditions in Great Britain's cities during the Industrial Revolution, Christian women first banded together in 1855 (Rice, 1947). (One source (Rice, 1947) states that France started the first Association group in 1849.) The early work of the YWCA movement aimed to provide young wage-earning girls and women new to the city with housing, recreation, and spiritual assistance. Several other countries in Europe, North America, Asia, and Africa later established their own associations. Although each organization catered to the unique needs of their young women citizens away from home for the first time, each organization was rooted in Christian ethics and values. In 1894, the World YWCA was founded by four national associations in Great Britain, Norway, Sweden, and the United States to establish a world fellowship of Christian women. YWCA has since expanded into a global movement worldwide that strives to empower women and girls and to eliminate racism and empower them. Although its work is still based on Christian ecumenical principles, YWCA welcomes women of all faiths.

EMPOWER Methods Used
- Rights protection and social action/reform
- Enabling service and assistance
- Empowerment training and leadership development
- Organizing partnership
- Work/job training and micro-enterprise

Although each local YWCA is an autonomous organization run and organized by women in the community, World YWCA members have a set of overall common goals. They are striving for gender equality and full integration of women locally, nationally, and internationally through training, advocacy, development, and strengthening the movement. In short, World YWCA strives "to improve women's lives, achieve social and economic justice, ensure human rights, and restore the integrity of the planet." World YWCA training programs teach leadership, management, and advocacy skills while focusing on development and other current issues affecting women. Members receive on-the-job training by assuming leadership positions in their local YWCAs. Women also benefit from mentoring relationships between women of different generations, ethnicities, and backgrounds. The training initiatives at national YWCAs are supported through the Leadership Training Fund.

World YWCA advocates for social and economic justice for women by lobbying governments and other decision-making bodies. For example, an international delegation of women attended major United Nations conferences and other non-governmental organization activities in New York, Geneva, and Vienna. Young members serve as consultants to the World Health Organization (WHO) on issues of young women's health. The World YWCA also has consultative status to the United Nations Economic and Social Council (ECOSOC) and United Nations Educational, Scientific, and Cultural Organization (UNESCO). World YWCA also mobilizes women around issues of women's rights, human rights, peace, and the environment.

The YWCA's stated priorities are:

> Our legislative priorities address three broad issue areas in which the YWCA offers programs: racial justice and civil rights, women's economic empowerment, and women's health and safety.
>
> As we move into the new year, we are eager to continue promoting the mission of the YWCA through strategic legislative advocacy and we look forward to working together with policymakers in Congress and the Obama Administration.
>
> Legislative Priorities for 114th Congress: The YWCA USA will focus its national advocacy efforts on legislation to:
>
> 1. End Racial Profiling
> 2. Work and Family Agenda
> 3. Domestic Violence and Gun Violence Prevention
> 4. Affordable Care Act
> 5. The Convention on the Elimination of All Forms of Discrimination Against Women (CEDAW). (YWCA, 2015a)

World YWCA provides technical and material assistance to national YWCAs that are conducting development projects. Through "development education," World YWCA visits each association in order to provide help with project planning, implementation, and follow-up. Designed to meet the needs of the community, past projects have included locating clean water sources, providing vocational training, and developing income-generating activities for members. YWCAs have also provided hostels for young women in need of housing, health programs, shelters for violence victims, preschools, youth leadership training, microcredit, and activities for elderly people.

National leaders attend consultations and training programs such as the International Training Institute, organized every three or four years for newly elected or appointed presidents and general secretaries or young women leaders. The World YWCA Resource Sharing Program allows YWCA associations to share human and material resources. Every four years, the World Council—the governing body of the World YWCA made of representatives from each national association—meets to set priorities for the future and write policy statements. World YWCA offers several publications available for purchase such as the quarterly magazine called *Common Concern Magazine*, books about YWCA's history, and prayer booklets.

Partners/Opposition

Each local YWCA is affiliated to the national YWCA of their country, which in turn is affiliated to World YWCA. YWCA is sensitive to the importance of local community priorities and the need for community participation in the formulation of its local advocacy strategy; its advocacy kit spells out steps though which it may serve local communities (see "Internal Policies to Support Local YWCA Advocacy"; YWCA, 2007). As a nonprofit membership association, each YWCA is run by and for women of the community and their families. YWCA organizations depend on monetary donations and gifts-in-kind from foundations, organizations, and individuals.

Macro-environment

During the time of YWCA's beginnings, the Industrial Revolution (roughly 1750 to 1850) forced men and women to migrate to cities to find employment. Due to a shift from handicraft to machinery, women were leaving their homes for the first time to earn a living. Without immediate support of family or community, the young girls had to cope with overcrowding, unsanitary living conditions, long working hours, and urban crime. During the same period, an evangelical movement in Great Britain was taking place that tried to spread the Christian faith in the face of new scientific discoveries and ways of thinking. Today, women continue to occupy relatively low positions in society both in industrialized and less industrialized nations. With limited opportunities for education, employment, and personal growth, women face considerable obstacles in taking care of their families and themselves.

Impact and Remarks

As one of the oldest and largest women's organizations, World YWCA has over 25 million women and girls from over 120 countries and 95 affiliated, autonomous national YWCAs. There are thousands of local YWCAs that provide for specific needs of the women in the community. For example, YWCA of the United States initiated a national campaign to help girls become familiar with technology in various aspects of their lives. YWCA of Australia launched an exercise support program for women who have had breast cancer surgery. YWCA of Egypt runs a project that helps mothers care for children with Downs syndrome. YWCA of Thailand promotes education and literacy among hill tribal women. With new YWCAs forming in Eastern and Central Europe, Latin America, and Africa, YWCA has become synonymous with empowering young women (Rice, 1947):

> The World YWCA Strategic Framework 2012–2015 is based on the ongoing work of the organisation. It builds on the programmatic content, lessons learnt and insights gained from member associations, including from the *Power to Change Fund*. The 4 year questionnaire, review of Constitution and the *Standards of Good Management and Accountability (SGMA)* have all provided the critical information on the health of the movement; the key areas of focus, trends and gaps. The outcomes of *Regional Training Institutes* and other interactions with the movement, as well as World YWCA board and staff sessions over 2010 contributed to this strategy development. (YWCA, 2012–2015)

"This Strategic Framework adopts a deliberate approach to partnerships which prioritizes the capacities and expertise of the YWCA within the context of the work undertaken by various stakeholders." They consider four types of partnerships are essential for the implementation of the partnerships. These are:

1. A cluster of rights-based partners (partners share same priorities)
2. Programmatic partners with whom YWCA will deliver the common outcomes
3. Partners for resourcing YWCA work. These are both the current and potential institutional and individual donors; and
4. Friends, volunteers and individuals within and outside of the movements work together. (YWCA, 2012–2015)

The YWC website posted nine success stories which exemplify the range of programs and outcomes (YWCA, 2015c, Success Stories).

9

Economic Development Case Studies

> We certainly noted that when given the opportunity, women
> handle money more efficiently. They have long term vision, they
> manage money more carefully. Men are more callous with money.
> Their first reflex is to blow it by getting drunk in a pub, or on
> prostitutes or gambling. Women, on the other hand, are endowed
> with a tremendous sense of self-sacrifice and try to get the best
> out of the money, for their children, but also for their husbands.
>
> —Muhammad Yunus, *Women Are Better with Money*

Summaries of Case Studies: Economic Development and Quality of Life

CASE STUDY #28: WORKING WOMEN'S FORUM (WWF),
INDIA, 1978 (ED)

Problem

This case study falls within the domain of economic development (ED). The
major problem being addressed is the high-interest loans supplied by moneylenders and the overall powerlessness and oppression experienced by low-
caste Indian women, who are often illiterate and living in slums. As a result,
these women have trouble feeding their families, poor health, and poor self-
image. The objectives of the WWF are:

> To improve their living and working conditions and create visibility to
> their various economic roles, To devise an innovative union structure
> aiming to reach out to large number of women workers at the grassroots
> within a short time span and ensure their participation at all levels from
> planning to implementation, To remain women intensive in nature and
> address the struggles of poor women workers against caste, class and gen-
> der oppression in the community and work place, To adopt effective and
> needs specific programme strategies, in the areas of credit, employment,

health, family welfare and support services: and To adopt participatory training strategies towards unionisation, conscientization and empowerment of women workers. To unionise women workers of the Informal sector on trade lines, providing a social platform. (WWF, 2015)

Leadership Impetus

Arunachalam, a well-known political activist and social worker, created the WWF as an experiment in Madras, India, after a flood in 1978. Realizing that poor women in the slums preferred to have access to credit rather than free rice and blankets, Arunachalam helped 30 women secure small loans in order to start or expand small businesses. Striving for participation, self-reliance, and sustainability among its members, WWF developed into a nonpolitical grassroots organization run by and benefiting poor women (Arunachalam, 1978).

EMPOWER Methods Used

- ¤ Empowerment training and leadership development
- ¤ Public education and participation
- ¤ Organizing partnership
- ¤ Enabling service and assistance
- ¤ Rights protection and social action/reform
- ¤ Work/job training and micro-enterprise

The following statement sums up WWF's strategy:

Entry point for members is credit. Provides members with access to funds as well as support services such as child care, education, health and family planning. When recruiting poor families are identified by field workers (organizers / internal cadres)—most are volunteers from same neighbourhood in which the poor women live and work. Build and maintain m/ship by word of mouth through existing members: area meetings in place where members/potential members live and explain ideology of organization. Field workers facilitate enrollment process—use of same class of organizers as potential members helps. Democratic methods of selection/training of working class women, which helps them take responsibility at all levels of the organisational structure: Continuous empowerment of all the members of the Forum which provides them a fair knowledge of legal, economic and human rights issues in addition to orientation in effective communication skills. Identification of their own pressing problems (i.e., gender, caste, class issues at the grassroots) and finding their own solutions to combat the same.

Key Services: trade union mobilisation, banking and access to credit, reproductive health care, skill training, & development of leadership qualities. Indian Cooperative Network for Women, a federally registered Cooperative, provides low interest loans to women enhancing their social and financial independence. Set up by WWF. (WWF, 2010)

WWF offers small loans or microcredit from national banks through neighborhood loan groups (NLGs), group leaders, area organizers, and WWF staff. The collateral for the micro-loans is the woman's own work and the group itself. Although the primary empowerment strategy is credit assistance, WWF strives to follow a holistic approach by offering a number of different services and programs that fall within our seven EMPOWER methods categories (see Chapter 6).

WWF began to offer leadership training upon realizing that further assistance was needed, even after loans were obtained. Three WWF leaders developed a curriculum around the themes of solidarity, the abolition of the dowry system, and self-awareness, and the dangers of superstition, child marriages, and sexual discrimination.

Select members can become forum leaders who head NLGs. This esteemed position entitles them to certain privileges, such as bigger loans, the respect of their peers, and enhanced status in the community. In return, leaders perform a set of relatively time-consuming duties such as collecting repayments, recruiting new members, and organizing political actions.

After 1990, WWF expanded itself into a global network called Grassroots Organizations Operating Together in Sisterhood (GROOTS) or Networking in Sisterhood. WWF publishes a newsletter that is sponsored by the United Nations' Development Fund for Women (UNIFEM). The publication is designed to share their experiences with other poor women in the developing and developed world.

Enabling services include the provision of daycare centers, nutrition education, hygiene and environmental sanitation; distribution of condoms; registration of common-law weddings; inter-caste weddings; and children's immunization.

In order to enhance their position in society, WWF has also become a powerful women's lobby through participation in such social action as nonviolent demonstrations against the dowry system, and a petition for civic amenities (Bangasser, 1994).

Partners/Opposition

WWF is affiliated with the International Federation of Plantation, Agricultural, and Allied Workers (IFPAAW). It is funded through its membership fees, development assistance from the Government of the Netherlands, and private contributions. UNIFEM sponsors the publication of the WWF newsletter through a special grant. In addition, WWF runs a health project in conjunction with the Government of India, the International Labor

Organization (ILO), and the United Nations Population Fund (UNFPA), formerly called United Nations Fund for Population Activities.

After a previous credit loan program failed to produce the intended result, the Food and Agriculture Organization of the United Nations (FAO), which had sponsored the unsuccessful program, offered to sponsor a leadership-training program for women receiving loans from WWF. However, some husbands of loanees may not be supportive of this alternative source of income or the empowerment and leadership training, and make trouble for the wives.

Macro-environment

Living in a patriarchal society, Indian women are often at the mercy of their husbands and perceived as second-class citizens both by cultural norms and in legislation. Valuable opportunities and resources such as credit, training, markets, and the political system are essentially inaccessible to women.

An Indian woman is expected to maintain the household and raise her family, yet at the same time she may be forced to earn an income if her husband does not provide enough money to feed her children. Many are also victims of physical abuse. Because divorce carries a stigma in Indian society, many women do not opt for this solution. Trapped in a desperate situation, poor Indian women have little voice or recourse to alter their circumstances (Bangasser, 1994).

Impact and Remarks

Currently, WWF owns its own cooperative bank and has more than 225,000 members in nine branches in the three southern Indian states of Tamil Nadu, Andhra Pradesh, and Karnataka. Members include urban petty traders, fisherwomen, landless laborers, weavers, ropemakers, and lace artisans, among others. Thirty-five percent of the women are urban, and 65% are rural, with ages ranging from 22 to 50 years old. Among them 56% are illiterate. In 2009, Dr. Arunachalam was awarded the Bharat Ratna, Rajiv Gandhi Mahila Shakti (Women's Power) award, and she was recognized for her leadership in promoting maternity benefits through the WWF which benefitted over 400,000 women (WWF, 2009).

Forum members often experience a "growing empowerment," which leads to a "strong psychological contract" between the Forum and its members in terms of developing an unwritten set of mutual expectations. WWF assists the women in focusing their resources on economic, political, and social enhancement, whereas the women are motivated to strive towards loan repayment, increased awareness, and continued expansion of the organization. WWF members are encouraged to also strive towards a sense of boldness *(dhairiyam)* and solidarity among themselves.

CASE STUDY #30: BANKURA WOMEN'S SAMITIES (SOCIETIES),
WEST BENGAL, INDIA, 1980 (ED)

Problem

This case study falls within the domain of ED. The major problem being
addressed is the vulnerability and exploitation of India's poorest rural workers, of whom women and adolescents constitute over half.

> Bankura is one of the most economically and industrially backward dis-
> tricts of West Bengal and within Bankura, Ranibandh block occupies
> the south-western corner touching the borders of Purulia and Medinipur
> districts. The entire block is hilly and forested and forms a part of the
> drought-prone region. Agriculture is dependent on rain and a single
> crop of paddy is taken from the undulating land if there is timely rain.
> Backyard cultivation of maize is undertaken by almost all households
> who have some land. On the high lands babui grass is cultivated in some
> areas mainly for rope making. The forest—which was once a source of
> food, fuel, fodder and occasionally of livelihood—still provides for fuel
> and some income from minor forest products. However collection of
> Kandu and Sal leaves, Mahua flower, Neem, Mahua, Zamun, Amlaki,
> Haritaki, Kusum and Sal fruits, and various kinds of medicinal herbs
> and barks still constitute a supplementary source of livelihood for the
> women. Ethnically the area is inhabited predominantly by tribal com-
> munities like Santal Bhumij, Kheria and Sabar. Other communities liv-
> ing in the area are Oriya Brahmins, a conglomerate of lower castes of
> Bengal who have embraced Baisnabism, other backward communities
> like Mahato, Deswali Majhi, Kora (Mudi), scheduled castes like Sunris,
> Kaira, Chamar, Dom etc. and a host of occupational and service castes
> like Kumbhakar, Karmakar, Teli, Napit, Dhobi etc. Of all the commu-
> nities, the Oriya Brahmins, Sunris and some Baisnabs are prosperous
> (obviously at the cost of Bhumij and Santal), and others largely belong to
> the group falling below the poverty line. (Banerjee, 1984)

Leadership Impetus

In May of 1980, the government of West Bengal held a Reorientation Camp
for migrant women agricultural laborers in Jhilmili, a small village in the
Bankura District of India. The meeting was attended by West Bengal's
Minister for Land Reform, the Land Reforms Commissioner, and the director of the Center for Women's Development Studies (CWDS). The main
grievance was the forest policy of the government—as explained by one
woman: "You think of a tree as a piece of dead wood. For us it is living. It gives
us fruit, fuelwood, fodder and shade. We care for a tree like our own child.
Only when our stomachs are empty would we think of cutting a tree" (Singh,

1991, p. 182). After hearing the needs and concerns of the peasant women, the Department of Land Revenue and Forests restored women's rights to the forests for minor forest produce such as fruits, flowers, and leaves; and directed local authorities to use local labor for all governmental projects. However, the rural women still needed a stable source of employment. Some of the women who attended this meeting formed a women's *samity* (society) in small villages in West Bengal. Within the year, two more groups formed in other villages. The Minister for Land Reform asked the CWDS director to assist the women's collective efforts.

EMPOWER Methods Used

- ¤ Organizing partnership
- ¤ Work/job training and micro-enterprise
- ¤ Empowerment training and leadership development
- ¤ Enabling service and assistance

After the samities were first formed, CWDS worked with the rural women, providing them with training in organizing and assistance in income-generation. The women had decided not to migrate for labor; therefore, work was necessary immediately. The women of Jhilmili village suggested that they collect *kendu* leaves and *sal* seeds and sell them to the government. *Kendu* leaves are used for making cigarettes.

With help from state officials and the chairman of the local *panchayat* (the block-level council), women from the samity received an agency from the local forest cooperative for the sale of leaves and seeds. This activity provided 200 women with a source of income for three months

In the samity of the Chendapathar village, the women produced *sal* leaf plates and cups with small machines. Private landowners (including poor landowning families) donated their degraded land to the women's samity in Bhurkura—the last of the original three samities. In three years, these samity members cultivated the wasteland, transforming the barren land into a forest of trees where tassar silkworms could be raised. Rearing tassar cocoons in the forests is a traditional occupation in rural areas of West Bengal. CWDS persuaded the local forest ranger to provide arjun and asan saplings, which the women planted (after the men had cleared the land). The Forestry Department from Birbhum also donated trees. At this time, Jhilmili and Chendapather samities also received land donations. In 1982, CWDS staff and a few samity members traveled to Calcutta to meet with the Chief Minister and the Minister for Land and Land Reforms to request government funding for the samities' plantation work. Government grants met labor and plantation costs and part of the maintenance costs. The Central Silk Board offered training in tassar rearing. The cocoons raised were sold to the Department of Sericulture, the samities' major client.

The samities later diversified their income-earning activities to include livestock rearing, ropemaking with native grass, storing *mahua* seeds and other projects that suited their needs and skills. *Mahua* fruits are used for food and brewing liquor. The samities buy the seeds from members who collect the berries and sell them back during off-season for a marginal profit.

To give all members a chance to work, most of the samities used a system of rotation for working on the plantations or with machines. Some of the samities also created an informal system of interest-free credit for members to undertake rice-processing or trading activities when direct employment was not available.

In addition to participation in economic activities, samity members participated in the local self-government of the village, the *panchayat,* as well as the National Commission on Self-employed Women and the West Bengal Tribal Development Co-operative Corporations, Ltd. Women of the original samities formed a spearhead or advisory team that counseled, motivated, and supported other women's groups just starting out in their own economic endeavors. Knowing that the CWDS would eventually withdraw their assistance, the four samities formed the Nari Bikash Sangha (Union for Women's Development) to provide a framework for joint action. One of its joint efforts included the creation of multipurpose childcare centers in five villages, which were to be supervised by members of the women's groups. CWDS provided continuous professional management training for samity members as well as vocational training in such activities as silk-rearing. CWDS also provided literacy classes, adult education classes, and childcare services for samity members.

Partners/Opposition

The CWDS (New Delhi; its director) attended the 1980 meeting in Jhilmili and ILO's Program for Rural Women (New Delhi) provided the samities with technical guidance and initial funding for samities' activities. CWDS also served as an advocate for the samities in dealing with the government agencies. The government was the major source of funding. Other local agencies, including the Forestry Department, donated materials for the samities' income-generating activities.

Macro-environment

The Santhal tribals who had previously occupied the land were displaced by settlers from the plains over the years. Forests, once thick and plentiful, were lost to traders, cultivators, and contractors who cleared the land for its timber and forest products. The clear patches were then used for agricultural produce, thereby destroying the tribals' source of food, fodder, and fuel. Because of limited opportunities for wage labor in parts of the Bankura district, individuals had to migrate to private farms in order to survive.

Migration is a grueling process that earns little money despite great risks to the migrants' health. Governmental employment programs only provided three weeks' worth of work. Most rural women in India are assetless, unemployed, illiterate, destitute, and overworked. Some women band together in collective Santhal tradition by making group ritual offerings to the forest, collecting minor forest products, and living close together in a cluster of hamlets.

Impact and Remarks

The success of the first samity in Bhurkura inspired and encouraged other women in neighboring villages to form their own samities in order to cultivate land donated by villagers in their respective communities. In 1991, 1,500 women in 36 villages were members of 13 such samities. Both landowning and landless women were permitted to join the collective. All 1,500 members reported benefits from the samities, which provided predictable employment in the local area with a women-controlled management system. The "Bankura experience" provided a demonstration model for nongovernmental organizations (NGOs) in states throughout India to emulate in terms of mobilizing rural women to participate in their own development. ILO's Rural Employment Policies Branch planned a program of wasteland development through rural women's organizations based on the original samities. Recognizing the benefits of empowering rural women, several government agencies expressed their support for developing similar programs (Singh, 1991).

As a result of their organizing efforts, samity members no longer need to migrate every four years to faraway districts to earn income for their families. Through their achievements, they have gained a new confidence that influences all aspects of their lives. Samity members have increased their bargaining power as workers and gained respect as members of their villages. As the central implementing unit in the village cluster, it plans activities, handles finances, maintains records of meetings, and meets with local government officials and village-level bodies. Samity leaders are trainers themselves, passing on the skills they learned to others, including government officers. In addition, nonproductive land has been reclaimed and used as an economic resource. Ecologically, erosion has been reversed, and groundwater has improved in quality. One samity member described the transformation that occurred as a result of the Bankura experience:

> We were like frogs in a dark well. No one had thought of extending our minds. Our idea of *we* meant the family, or at the most, the village, or the caste in the village. When we became members of a "multi-village, multi-caste organization," *we* suddenly expanded. Now it has become so much bigger—*we* are part of a network of organizations. This, plus the

knowledge that we have equal rights, has been like a shot of vitamins in our lives. We are stronger, and more determined today than ever before. (Mazumdar, 1989, p. 33)

Since the 1980s several self-organized rural and women's develop-ment cooperatives gained considerable experience in India and especially in the Kerala, Gujarat and West Bengal states where political activism and grass-roots movements were established social norms.

Large-Sized Multi-Purpose Co-operative Societies (LAMPS) were established by the West Bengal Government to rescue local workers from exploitation by private traders. But it was a structure imposed from above, not a development from below. Being organised as Co-operatives under bureaucratic control meant complicated procedures which were beyond the understanding of the illiterate or semi-illiterate workers. So, in spite of the provision for universal membership of persons belonging to the scheduled castes or tribes, membership and management remained con-fined to the elite groups of these communities. In 1981, they had virtually no woman as a member. By 1988, only 4% of the members were women. The partnership between LAMPS and the fledgling women's group at Jhilmili was forced by the district administration, which also informed the women of the actual price for Kendu leaves and Sal seeds that had been guaranteed by the State Government. The LAMPS management thus saw the women's group as a threat to their power, and refused to renew the partnership. Attempts were also made to break the growing solidarity of the women's groups, and to prevent their affiliation to the Tribal Development Co-operative Corporation. (CWDS, 2014)

Subsequently, Bankura projects joined similar projects in other districts including Purulia, as a coalition of several initiatives which local NGOs and West Bengal government initiatives.

CASE STUDY #29: BARRIO INDIO GUAYAS GUAYAQUIL, ECUADOR, 1979 (HPDP)

Problem

This case study falls within the domain of ED. The major problem being addressed is lack of basic infrastructure and inadequate state provision of housing and local services including education, sanitation, and health ser-vices in Guayaquil—Ecuador's largest city, chief port, and major center of trade and industry. Between 1940 and 1980, the low-income population settled in the tidal swampland areas of Guayaquil, also known as *subur-bios* (suburbs). In 1978, Indio Guayas (a 10-block area of swampland) was a "pioneer settlement" of young, upwardly mobile families, representative of the lower-income segment of unskilled, nonunionized labor who had moved from inner-city rental accommodations.

The main motivation in settling these (previously uninhabited) areas was to own a small piece of land, thereby avoiding high rent for inner-city housing. Landfills, elevated housing and pathways, and simple dams were required to maintain this marshy mangrove land. Thirty-five percent of Guayaquil dwellers did not have access to adequate and reliable water supplies, and the whole city suffered from water shortages and a collapsing sewerage system. Distance from the city center and lack of electricity, running water, sewerage, and roads not only increased the burden of domestic work, but also resulted in a dangerous and unhealthy environment for children.

Leadership Impetus

In their struggle to survive in such an adverse environment, women of the *suburbios* were forced to develop friendships with their neighbors, which gradually resulted in a collective desire to improve their situation. Out of desperation at their living conditions, women urged their neighbors (male and female) to form *barrio*-level (neighborhood) committees to petition for infrastructure (a common practice in Guayaquil). Since the 1940s, newly settled communities in Guayaquil have been forming *barrio*-level committees in order to petition for infrastructure. Under Guayaquil's political system, populist parties garnered votes from committee members by providing infrastructure. In the 1960s, President John F. Kennedy's Alliance for Progress program forced the Guayaquil Municipality to create the Department of Community Development in order to help poor communities "fight for infrastructure." The experience gained by local organizations during this time helped inhabitants gain community-organizing and leadership skills.

Although the majority of regularly participating members were women, they did not immediately assume leadership roles. Women moved into leadership positions after they became frustrated with the "corrupt management of the incumbent male presidents" (Moser, 1991, p. 145).

EMPOWER Methods Used

- ¤ Rights protection and social action/reform
- ¤ Organizing partnership
- ¤ Enabling service and assistance

Although both females and males belonged to the *barrio*-level committees, the women performed the day-to-day work, including the important function of petitioning for infrastructure, and implementing the community's plan when this infrastructure was provided. Politically pragmatic, the women would petition for the particular infrastructure they believed they would be most likely to get at any given time. Partnerships naturally formed between women neighbors working together out of a common preoccupation with their living conditions. The importance of these women in their community-managing roles is illustrated by the formation, organization, and success of the local-level protests challenging the government to provide the necessary infrastructure to improve the environment for their families.

Partners/Opposition

As mentioned above, political party leaders and government administrative officials provided infrastructure *only* in exchange for votes in elections. Therefore, the number, commitment, and support of committee members were critical to the success and long-term survival of the *barrio* committee. Although men joined local committees when they were formed, women were generally the only regular participants. Men's participation was neither regular nor reliable. In fact, men often had to be pressured by the committee and the women to participate at all.

Macro-environment

According to traditional sexual division of labor, Latin American women are responsible for taking care of the household, including the consumption needs of the family. Often, their responsibility will extend to the consumption needs of the entire community. Along with men and children, women are involved in community-organizing around issues of collective consumption and the lack of basic community services such as housing. Low-income women in Latin America have the additional burden of working in factories to earn income for the family. In Guayaquil, political party leaders, administrative officials, and *barrio* men believed that it was natural that women perform most of the participatory work, "because women have free time, while men are out at work" (Moser, 1991, p. 146). Of course, this was a myth; women were already burdened with the responsibilities of housekeeping, childcare, and outside paid work. In fact, in order to participate in community mobilization, these women made tremendous sacrifices in time and energy to improve their family's living conditions, which they themselves perceived to be one of their womanly duties.

Impact and Remarks

Since the late 1970s, the *barrio*-level committees have been especially concerned with basic infrastructural changes affecting potable water (States, 2014). Filling the swamp under the houses has been carried out by most families. Access roads surrounding the neighborhoods have replaced catwalks. Electricity has been installed. A piped water system has been built to reach the front of each house. All of these improvements have empowered participating women with the knowledge that they can take control of their environment and affect their surroundings through community organization. Women are no longer fearful about venturing outside because they have eliminated many of the dangers that existed in the past including assault, sexual violence, and robbery.

CASE STUDY #67: CHIPKO MOVEMENT, INDIA, 1973 (ED)

Problem

The Chipko

The major problems being addressed are the deforestation of the sub-Himalayan region in India, the destruction of its traditional ecological balance, and the threat to survival of the people living in the hill areas. As the historical event below shows, the Chipko movement was born initially nearly three centuries ago. "In India there is an ancient legend about a girl, Amrita Devi, who died trying to protect the trees that surrounded her village. The story recounts a time when the local Maharajah's tree cutters arrived to cut the villager's trees for wood for his new fortress. Amrita, with others, jumped in front of the trees and hugged them. In some versions of the tale their dramatic efforts prevented the forest's destruction; in others Amrita dies in her valiant attempt" (Chipko, 2015b). There were several Chipko (Tree Hugging) movements in India; the Chipko strategy was used for different goals in different geographical locations. This volume includes two separate Chipko movements; this case study is against massive deforestation by the timber industry. The second Chipko (# 69) movement focused on control of water supply.

In the 1960, accelerated industrial developments and rapid urbanization caused rapid deforestation in the Himalayan foothills. Export of timbers to foreign countries and rapidly expanding urban expansion threatened the livelihood of traditional villagers who depended on the forests for their livelihood.

Against these harmful deforestation policies a movement called Chipko was born. "Chipko" in Hindi means to cling, reflecting the protesters main technique of throwing their arms around the tree trunks designated to be cut, and refusing to move. Women's participation in the movement can be traced to a remote hill town where a contractor in 1973 had been given the right by the state to fell 3000 of trees for a sporting goods store. The area already was dangerously denuded. When the woodcutters were scheduled to appear, the men were enticed away from the village leaving the women at home busy with household chores. As soon as the woodcutters appeared, the alarm was sounded and the village's female leader, a widow in her 50s, collected twenty-seven women and rushed into the forest. The women pleaded with the woodcutter calling the forest their "maternal home," and explaining the consequences of felling the trees. The woodcutters, shouting and abusing the women, threatened them with guns. The women in turn threatened to hug the earmarked trees and die with them. And it worked! The unnerved laborers left, the contractor backed off. In 1974, women in a nearby area used the same tree hugging technique in order to protest the clearing of their forest lands. And in 1977, in another area, women tied a sacred threads around trees fated for death ... a symbolic gesture in Hindu custom confirming the bond of brother-sister relationships. They declared that their trees would be saved even if it cost them their lives. (Chipko, 2015c)

In 1987 Chipko was chosen for a "Right to Livelihood Award," known as the "alternate Nobel" prize honor. The honor was rightly deserved for this small movement dominated by women which had became a national call to save forests (Chipko, 2015c).

The Chipko protests in Uttar Pradesh achieved a major victory in 1980 with a 15-year ban on green felling in the Himalayan forests of that state by order of India's then Prime Minister, Indira Gandhi. Since then the movement has spread to Himachal Pradesh in the North, Kamataka in the South, Rajasthan in the West, Bihar in the East and to the Vindhyas in Central India. In addition to the 15-year ban in Uttar Pradesh, the movement has stopped clear felling in the Western Ghats and the Vindhyas and generated pressure for a natural resource policy which is more sensitive to people's needs and ecological requirements.

The Chipko Movement is the result of hundreds of decentralised and locally autonomous initiatives. Its leaders and activists are primarily village women, acting to save their means of subsistence and their communities. Men are involved too, however, and some of these have given wider leadership to the movement. Prominent Chipko figures include: Sunderlal Bahuguna, a Gandhian activist and philosopher, whose appeal to Mrs. Gandhi results in the green-felling ban and whose 5,000 kilometre trans-Himalaya footmarch in 1981–83 was crucial in spreading the Chipko message. Bahuguna coined the Chipko slogan: "ecology is permanent economy." (Chipko, 2015a)

The Chipko movement which began in 1973 and used Gandhian nonviolent civil disobedience movement has expanded to several other states in India. On 2014, India's President Pranab Mukherjee awarded the Gandhi Peace Prize to noted environmentalist leader of Chipko movement and

Gandhian from Uttarakhand, Chandi Prasad Bhatt. Although Bhatt is a man, it should be emphasized that it was the ordinary village women who have led and carried out the local Chipko movements across the nation (*The Pioneer*, 2014).

Leadership Impetus

In order to increase employment for local people, a group of male Sarvodaya workers at Mandal, Chamoli District, led by C. P. Bhatt, founded a workers' cooperative of unskilled and semiskilled construction workers in 1960. In 1964, the Dasholi Gram Swarajya Mandal (DGSM) cooperative was created, which would use forest resources to make farm tools in a small workshop. However, the Forestry Department refused to grant the ash trees needed by the cooperative and instead allotted 300 ash trees to a sporting-goods manufacturer for making tennis rackets. On April 24, 1973, approximately 100 DGSM workers and villagers from nearby areas marched to the site of the forest felling, while beating drums and singing traditional songs. After some negotiation, DGSM were granted the trees. However, a new set of ash trees was allotted to the manufacturer in another part of the district. But again the workers mobilized, protecting the trees for a period of six months.

The Forestry Department announced an auction of approximately 2,500 trees in the Reni forest overlooking the Alaknanda River. After realizing the connection between the recent landslides and floods and the clearing of forests, Bhatt suggested to the villagers that they hug the trees as a saving measure. *Chipko*, the Hindi word meaning "hugging," refers to the local village women who literally "hugged" trees in order to prevent the loggers from cutting them down. The very first use of the chipko strategy was recorded three centuries ago. Three hundred members of the Bishnoi community in Rajasthan, led by a woman named Amrita Devi, sacrificed their lives to rescue the trees by clinging to them. Gaura Devi organized the women of her village, Lata, to challenge the tree cutters. In the 1970s and 1980s, this resistance to the destruction of forests spread throughout India and became organized and known as the Chipko Movement (Shiva, 2013a).

EMPOWER Methods Used

- ¤ Rights protection and social action/reform
- ¤ Social Action Litigation (SAL)
- ¤ Media use

The first Chipko action took place spontaneously in April of 1973, and over the next five years spread to many districts of the Himalaya in Uttar Pradesh. The Chipko movement is composed of hundreds of decentralized and locally autonomous initiatives led primarily by village women. The women practiced

Satyagraha—nonviolent resistance and protecting the trees from the contractors' axes with their own bodies.

Partners/Opposition

Prominent Chipko figures include Sunderlal Bahuguna, a Gandhian activist and philosopher, whose appeal to the then Indian Prime Minister Indira Gandhi resulted in a green-felling ban, and whose 5,000-kilometer march across Himalaya in 1981–1983 helped spread the Chipko message. Bahuguna coined the Chipko slogan "Ecology is permanent economy." Chandi Prasad Bhatt, one of the earliest Chipko activists, fostered locally based industries founded on the conservation and sustainable use of forest wealth for local benefit. Another prominent Chipko figure was Dhoom Singh Negi, who with Bachni Devi and many village women, first saved trees by hugging them in the "Chipko embrace." They coined the slogan "What do the forests bear? soil, water and pure air." Arundhati Roy, Booker Prize–winning author and social activist, joined the movement and supported it with the royalties from her books. Dr. Vandana Shiva is one of the earliest activist to initiate the Chipko movement (Shiva, 1988, 2013a).

Macro-environment

The forests of India serve as a critical resource for the subsistence of rural peoples throughout the country, especially in hill and mountain areas. The forests provide food, fuel, and livestock fodder and serve to stabilize soil and water supplies. These vital resources are jeopardized due to the felling of trees for commerce and industry.

Impact and Remarks

Originating as a spontaneous protest against logging abuses in Uttar Pradesh in the Himalayas, the Chipko movement spawned much change. In 1980, the Chipko protests in Uttar Pradesh led to a 15-year ban on green-felling in the Himalayan forests of that state by order of India's then–prime minister, Indira Gandhi. Other results of the movement were the cessation of clear felling (clear-cutting) in the Western Ghats and the Vindhyas and political pressure for a natural resource policy that was more sensitive to people's needs and ecological requirements.

The Chipko movement has since expanded to Himachal Pradesh in the North, Karnataka in the South, Rajasthan in the West, Bihar in the East, and the Vindhyas in Central India. A feature published by the United Nations Environment Program described Chipko's impact in the following way: "In effect the Chipko people are working a socio-economic revolution by winning control of their forest resources from the hands of a distant bureaucracy which is concerned with selling the forest for making urban-oriented products" (International Institute of Sustainable Development [IISD] website, 1997).

In December of 1987, the women of the Chipko movement were awarded the Right Livelihood Award, also known as the "Alternative Nobel Prize." The honor is bestowed on persons for vision and work contributing to making life more whole, healing our planet and uplifting humanity (Shiva, 2013a, p. 218; Sontheimer, 1991). In 1972, Raturi's famous poem describing the Chipko efforts was written:

Embrace our trees,
save them from being felled
the property of our hills,
Save it from being looted.

—Raturi, 2015

CASE STUDY #69: "CHIPKO" MOVEMENT FOR WATER, DOON VALLEY, INDIA, 1986 (ED)

Problem

This case study falls within the domain of ED and in a part of expanded multi-site Chipko movement in India. The major problem being addressed is the destruction of the natural water-storage system in Doon Valley, India. Doon Valley is a major tourist attraction and hill resort in the Himalayan foothills (See Case No. 67 above for the history of Chipko movement). Due to mountain mining for chemical-grade limestone, forest uprooting, and the discarding of debris on the slopes, the natural system of water storage was destroyed. Twelve springs near the mines had gone dry, as well as the perennial waterfall (Mande-ka-Chhara).

Leadership Impetus

Beginning on September 16, 1986, rural women started a Chipko-inspired movement to blockade mining operations in the Nahi-Barkot area of Doon Valley. Adopting the strategy of the original women of the Chipko movement who protected the trees of the Himalayas region with their own bodies, the women of Doon Valley protested the destruction of the natural water-storage system. The internationally recognized scientist and activist Dr. Vandana Shiva eloquently describes the courage and wisdom of the village women of Chipko movement in the following quote:

The most dramatic turn in this new confrontation took place when Bachni Devi of Adwani village led a resistance against her own husband who had obtained a local contract to fell the forest. The forest officials arrived to browbeat and intimidate the women and Chipko activists, but found the women holding up lighted lanterns in broad daylight. Puzzled, the forester asked them their intention. The women replied:

"We came to teach you forestry."

He retorted: "You foolish women, how can you who prevent felling know the value of the forest? Do you know what forests bear? They produce profit, and resin, and timber."

The women immediately sang back in chorus:

"What do the forests bear?

Soil, water, and pure air.

Soil, water, and pure air, sustain the earth and all it bears."

—Shiva, 2002, pp. 76–77

EMPOWER Methods Used

- ¤ Rights protection and social action/reform
- ¤ Social Action Litigation (SAL) legal activism
- ¤ Media use

Using their internal *shakti*, the women of Chipko protested against the contractors who threatened their water supply through mining. Despite the contractors' bullying and sometimes life-threatening tactics, the women conducted peaceful protest through blockades of mining operations on the banks of a stream called Sinsyaru Khala. This stream served as the lifeline of the village and was full of fodder-producing bushes. A lawsuit was also filed that lasted a total of five years.

Partners/Opposition

The contractors served as the biggest obstacle to Chipko's efforts. On more than one occasion, the contractors stoned the women protestors and their children. They also struck the women's children with iron rods in order to stop the protests. On another occasion, a woman named Chamundeyi used her own body to prevent the trucks of the quarry men from advancing up the mountain. After dragging her along for a distance, the trucks retreated. The government was also an enabling factor in the destruction of the mountains' forests and streams. Despite the expiration of the mine's lease in 1982, the mine had yet to be closed as of late 1987. Decades of struggles of the Chipko movement was recognized by the President of India President presents Gandhi Peace Prize to Chandi Prasad Bhatt in 2014. "Bhatt has not only deepened our understanding of responsibility but also provided an object lesson to the world on the power of ahimsa," the Indian President added (*Z News*, July 15, 2014).

Macro-environment

The Doon Valley in the Himalayan foothills receives approximately 3,000 millimeters of rainfall over the three months of the monsoon. Its streams and springs provide water throughout the year. Some water is also stored in the rich humus of the oak forests in the higher reaches and at lower altitudes in the mixed natural forests. However, most of the water is stored in the cracks and fissures of the limestone rocks in the Himalayan range.

Impact and Remarks

The philosophy of the Chipko women's water-conservation movement dictates that the maintenance of nature's water cycle should be the focus of water management, not the construction of pipes and other modern technology. Traditionally, women have participated in nature's water cycle by treating water and making it potable. For centuries, women utilized the seven modes of purifying water listed in the *Sushruta Samhita*. For example, muddy water can be clarified using natural coagulants such as the nuts of the *nirmali* tree; *moringa* seeds inhibit the growth of bacteria and fungi. Even though women used locally available natural products and knowledge for water purification for centuries, women have been excluded from the process of modern water management and treatment. Due to the Chipko women's public protest and the five-year lawsuit, Doon Valley was saved from further limestone quarrying. The Supreme Court ruled that all quarrying must be terminated, except for three leases. This marked the first time in India's history that the subject of ecological conservation and development was scrutinized in such detail and in the context of a public-interest lawsuit.

CASE STUDY #31: COMMUNITY KITCHENS IN *PUEBLOS JOVENES*, PERU, 1980s (ED)

Problem

This case study falls within the domain of ED. The major problem being addressed is poverty in *pueblos jovenes* ("young towns")—the Peruvian term for squatter settlements in New Lima and other coastal cities where urban poor people reside.

Leadership Impetus

In response to the dire conditions and severely low income, women in *pueblos jovenes* began to organize community kitchens, or *comedores,* at the end of the 1970s in Lima. During this period, the economy in Peru was experiencing a severe depression. Fortunately, Western food aid had increased. There were massive popular protests and demonstrations by men and women.

The forerunner to the first kitchens was established following the 1978–1979 teacher's strikes organized by Sindicato Unitario de Trabajadores en la Educación del Perú (SUTEP)—the teachers' trade union. At the schools, the teachers prepared meals together for the strikers in a collective cooking pot— *olla común* (Graham, 1991; Lenten, 1993).

EMPOWER Methods Used

- ¤ Organizing partnership
- ¤ Enabling service and assistance
- ¤ Empowerment training and leadership development

The community kitchens were collectives of women who pooled their resources in order to purchase needed items in bulk. The women took turns preparing the meals for their families in a communal kitchen, usually the kitchen of one of the members. This economic efficiency allowed one meal per day for each of the group's members. The women were responsible for food transportation, distribution, and preparation.

As members of grassroots organizations, women successfully fed themselves and the community by seeking low-cost food items and sharing the work of preparing meals. The community kitchen reduced the cost of the meal relative to that prepared at home. The community kitchens served as ideal mechanisms to distribute food provided by international emergency food-donor agencies. The kitchens were an efficient way to feed many people at one time and to target the poor people who were in most need of the subsidized food. Participating in a community kitchen allowed the women to acquire skills in administration, bookkeeping, and organizing special activities, as well as to attend meetings and courses organized by development organizations. It provides a forum for the women in which to share their personal experiences and problems and to make new contacts both within and outside the neighborhood.

Partners/Opposition

Many of the community kitchens received food or other forms of assistance from development organizations such as Caritas (Caritas Internationalis), Centro de Estudios Cristianos y Capacitación Popular (CECYCAP), UNICEF and Obra Filantropica de Asistencia Social Adventista (OFASA) or a Catholic social service organization. Although the food aid was provided by these organizations, in some cases, development organizations interfered in the decisions made by the women, thereby threatening their autonomy. In general, however, the community kitchen was a humanitarian endeavor, so almost all political groups accepted the women's efforts.

The Shining Path Maoist guerilla organization, on the other hand, was antagonistic to the women leaders of the community kitchen movement.

Wanting to expand their political base to include the *pueblos jovenes*, the Shining Path targeted the women as well as other political opponents, through repression, intimidation, and assassination. Because the survival of their families depended on the continued existence of the community kitchens, the women did not retreat under the pressure, like other political groups did. As a result of the women's organized resistance against the Shining Path, the presence of this guerilla organization declined in the *pueblos jovenes*.

Many men were opposed to the community kitchen. Primarily, they objected to the associated activities in which the women participated, such as meetings or social gatherings that took the women out of the home during the evening, thereby reducing the amount of time they spent on housework and childcare. A woman's participation in the community kitchen could also threaten the man's expected role of breadwinner for the family. In fact, the very existence of the community kitchens demonstrated the men's inability to feed their families.

Macro-environment

Since the end of the reign of military government in 1980, Peru has experienced economic crises with each successive elected government. Peru has been plagued by high unemployment rates, declining wages, rising prices, and shortages of food and other resources. Population growth in the last three decades has been concentrated in the severely impoverished urban sector. In these squatter settlements or *pueblos jovenes*, there is sometimes no running water or electricity. A large proportion of the inhabitants of *pueblos jovenes* work in the informal sector, which is characterized by small-scale work, low productivity, and a low capital-to-labor ratio. Despite these disadvantages, their residents are highly cohesive and organized. The settlements themselves are often the result of a coordinated effort to take over a piece of land. In order to survive, the members often band together to ward off external threats such as dislocation efforts by the state, crime prevention in absence of municipal enforcement, as well as the need to obtain legal recognition and public services.

Impact and Remarks

The community kitchen movement has served as a survival strategy for the people living in the *pueblos jovenes*. It has led to increased awareness, self-esteem, independence, and general politicization of women. Not being able to feed one's family is now seen as a social problem that can be solved through collective means, rather than a personal one. Participation in community kitchens socializes the individual task of cooking for one's family. Participation in the community kitchen also enables the women to engage in paid work inside or outside of the home. Other types of community kitchens have developed over the years: one for children, one for the entire family in which meals are taken home to eat, and one formed by political parties. The National Committee of Comedores (CNC) was formed in 1986 following a national gathering of *comedores* from all over the country that was organized by the Episcopal Committee of Social Action. Since its founding, the CNC has organized many public actions and has talked personally with President Garcia to discuss their demands (Graham, 1991; Kusterer, 1993; Lenten, 1993).

Significant socio-political changes occurred after the Garcia regime:

> After a dozen years of military rule, Peru returned to democratic leadership in 1980, but experienced economic problems and the growth of a violent insurgency. President Alberto FUJIMORI's election in 1990 ushered in a decade that saw a dramatic turnaround in the economy and significant progress in curtailing guerrilla activity. Nevertheless, the president's increasing reliance on authoritarian measures and an economic slump in the late 1990s generated mounting dissatisfaction with his regime, which led to his ouster in 2000. A caretaker government oversaw new elections in the spring of 2001, which ushered in Alejandro TOLEDO as the new head of government—Peru's first democratically elected president of Native American ethnicity. The presidential election of 2006 saw the return of Alan GARCIA who, after a disappointing presidential term from 1985 to 1990, returned to the presidency with promises to improve social conditions and maintain fiscal responsibility. (World Facts, 2015, http://worldfacts.us/Peru.htm) (For more on recent Peruvian developments, see US Library of Congress: Foreign Relations, http://countrystudies.us/peru/96.htm.)

From the perspective of this volume, it is important to note that, in spite of major political and social changes that took place over the decades, the Peruvian Community Kitchen has demonstrated it as an important coping and empowering process for the poor. A recent news item in the *Christian Science Monitor* reports:

> The kitchens started in the 1970s and persisted through the '80s and '90s, through dictatorship, terrorism, and hyperinflation that brought Peru to its knees. And now that global food prices have put basic staples out of reach for families across the region, the kitchens that feed an estimated half million residents of metropolitan Lima every day are again providing a refuge. (CSM, 2008)

Interestingly community kitchen may also be used to empower women in other ways. On April 18, 2015, Megan Oteri writes the history of how her grandmother and mother established community kitchen in the US as early as in 1920:

> In the early 1920's Evanstonians could do just that for the modest price of only 85 cents per person. These meals were provided by the Evanston Community Kitchen, which originated as an experiment in cooperative housekeeping that drew nationwide attention to the city of Evanston, Illinois. At one time as many as 150 families relied on this centralized cooking facility to deliver dinner every night. The women who initiated it saw it as a way to liberate women from the kitchen. (Oteri, 2015; https://evanstoncommunitykitchen.wordpress.com/about/)

In this case, the Evanston community kitchen was not designed to fight hunger, but to liberate women from cooking everyday so that they may spend their time and energy on other empowering activities.

CASE STUDY #27: GRAMEEN BANK, BANGLADESH, 1976 (ED)

Problem

This case study falls within the domain of ED. The major problem being addressed is severe poverty among villagers in Bangladesh due to floods, droughts, and cyclones. The vast majority of Bangladeshis are malnourished, illiterate, and unemployed.

Leadership Impetus

Muhammad Yunus founded the Grameen Bank in 1976 while teaching at a university in southern Bangladesh. After meeting a village woman who was trying to earn a living by making bamboo stools, without money to buy materials, Yunus and his graduate student s designed an experimental credit program to assist such poor individuals. From his own pocket, Yunus lent the equivalent of $26 to a group of 42 workers. The experiment gradually developed into a million-dollar franchise run by Yunus (who had quit teaching), as well as a group of dedicated graduate students. Because the bank only catered to villagers, its name "Grameen," which comes from the Bangla word gram, or "village," is an accurate moniker. The percentage of women borrowers increased from 25%–40% between 1978 and 1983, which was understandable considering that the Grameen is a bank for the poor, and the poorest people in Bangladesh are landless women. Grameen Foundation helps the world's poorest people reach their full potential, connecting their determination and skills with the resources they need. We provide access to essential financial services and information on agriculture and health, assistance that can have wide-scale impact by addressing the specific needs of poor households and communities. We also develop tools to improve the effectiveness of poverty-focused organizations (Grameen web site: http://www.grameenfoundation.org/what-we-do). In 2006, Grameen Bank founder Yunus was awarded the Nobel Prize for his pioneering work for poverty reduction through collateral free microcredit innovation of giving collateral-free loans to poor women in Bangladesh; over 90 percent of the grateful women borrowers repaid their loans, a rate that far exceeded the repayment rates by more affluent borrowers in major banks in New York. The total amount of money loaned by the Grameen Bank in 1979 was 0.001 million US dollars; The Bank is based on the belief that credit is a basic human right, not the privilege of a fortunate few. By 2003 it provided over 2.5 billion dollars of micro-loans to more than two million families in rural Bangladesh. Ninety-four percent of Yunus's clients are women, and repayment rates are near 100 percent (Yunus, 2003).

EMPOWER Methods Used

- ¤ Organizing partnership
- ¤ Enabling service and assistance
- ¤ Work/job training and micro-enterprise

Grameen Bank lends mainly to women in small amounts of money for short periods of time. In order to qualify for a loan, a villager must prove that her familial assets fall below the bank's threshold. Although no collateral, credit history, or guarantor are required, the borrower must join a five-member group and a 40-member center, attend weekly meetings, and assume responsibility for the loans of her group members. Prompt payments of each of the five members guarantees credit for the group for the rest of their lives. At each meeting, borrowers make loan payments and critique each other's business plans. The interest rates are very high in order to encourage potential borrowers to consider seriously their decision to borrow money. The loans allow members to be self-employed in a variety of occupations, such as providing services, trading, processing, manufacturing, and shopkeeping. Fields in which villagers are working include agriculture, fisheries, weaving, and cellular phone networks and solar power.

Since 1980, Grameen has held workshops to promote social awareness in the style of *conscientization*. However, Yun believes these activities to be secondary because they are not "life-oriented." Once every two years, Grameen holds a five-day workshop for all center chiefs, called the National Workshop. At the first two meetings a document called "The Sixteen Decisions" was produced, which outlined the main philosophies and objectives of Grameen. It is recited at each center meeting. The Sixteen Decisions include rules on many aspects of their lives, such as keeping their houses in repair, growing and eating vegetables, keeping family size small, education, sanitation, clean water, prohibiting dowry, helping each other, performing physical exercise, and maintaining justice in the group. Yunus himself attended conferences on rural development and rural credit to share the results of his enterprise with other experts in the field. Grameen also finances sturdily built houses through mortgage payments by the borrowers. Under this agreement, the husband of the borrower must transfer land ownership to the wife. With land being the most important asset a Bangladeshi can own, and the cultural history of preventing women from owning land, this agreement was an innovation. The housing program has successfully financed over a quarter-million units (Yunus, 2003). For later developments, see *The Economist* (November 3, 2012).

Partners/Opposition

Yunus faced opposition to the Grameen Bank from politicians, academics, and development experts when he decided to make Grameen an independent bank. Some on the left believed Grameen to be "anti-revolutionary, throwing crumbs to the poor; credit turned villagers into mini-capitalists, drove agricultural wages up, and created an environment of intense competition that destroyed the chances of uniting the landless in revolt." Others thought that what Bangladesh really needed was integrated rural development, not just credit. Furthermore, large-scale replication was considered impossible because Grameen's success was thought to be due to one man—Yunus. The banking establishment was also opposed to opening another bank in Bangladesh.

Grameen received support from A. M. A. Mulith, Bangladesh's appointed Finance Secretary, who recommended the Grameen Bank project to General Hossain Mohammed Ershad, who had seized power of Bangladesh in 1982. The Grameen Bank Ordinance was passed in September of 1983. When Grameen became an independent bank, Yunus wanted to hire young and enthusiastic students who were willing to interact with the landless. He encouraged energy, vitality, and open communication among his staff. Branch managers were required to complete free-form narrative reports, which Yunus would read and use to incorporate changes in the operation of the bank. His managing style was innovative, to say the least. Yunus also received banking advice from two Chicago bankers recommended by the Ford Foundation. Ron Grzywinski and Mary Houghton, who had founded a community development bank, visited Yunus in Bangladesh. Several years later, the trio established the first Grameen replication in the United States. Grameen receives financial funding from International Fund for Agricultural Development (IFAD), the Ford Foundation, and the governments of Norway and Sweden.

Macro-environment

Bangladesh is a very poor country that has been dubbed "the Fifth World" and has been plagued with floods, droughts, and cyclones. Diplomats label Bangladesh "an international basket case." Each day, thousands of villagers, the majority of whom are malnourished and illiterate, come to the capital city of Dhaka to find employment, but with little success. Religious men would threaten women who joined groups. Yet, there is no Islamic (*Sharia*) law in Bangladesh, even though 85% of the people are Muslims.

Impact and Remarks

Over the past 20 years, Grameen Bank has extended micro-loans totaling over $1.5 billion for the purpose of self-employment of poor, landless villagers in Bangladesh. By the year 2000, there were more than 1,050 branch offices that served over 2 million clients, with 94 % being women. Each month, approximately $30–$40 million was loaned, and 97% of all loans were repaid. The high repayment rates were attributed to payments in weekly installments, monitoring of borrowers, and the bank's trusting relationship with the borrowers. Grameen, which now makes a profit, has a higher repayment rate than traditional banks. One-third of its borrowers have already crossed the poverty line. For a comprehensive assessment of Bangladesh and the role of rural development initiatives by NGOs, especially the Grameen Bank, please see "Bangladesh and Development" (in *The Economist*, November 3, 2012 issue). The excerpt below sums up:

"Most of the big improvements have taken place in rural areas, but Bangladesh is urbanising fast, which will bring a different suite of problems. Dhaka is one of the ten largest cities in the world, but has the infrastructure of a one-buffalo town:

> And as if all that were not enough, the government seems intent on killing one of the geese that lays the golden eggs. Incensed that the founder of Grameen Bank, Muhammad Yunus, should have had the temerity to start a political party, the prime minister, Sheikh Hasina, has hounded him from his position as the bank's managing director and is seeking to impose her own choice of boss on the bank, overriding the interests of the owner-borrowers. This is sending a chilling signal to other NGOs. (*The Economist*, 2012)

> But Bangladesh's record is, on balance, a good one. It shows that the benefits of *making women central to development are huge* (Italics ours). It suggests that migration is not just the result of a failure to provide jobs at home but can be an engine of economic growth. Indian's rural-development minister, Jairam Ramesh, said recently that "Bangladesh's experience shows…that we don't have to wait for…high economic growth to trigger social transformations. Robust grass-roots institutions can achieve much that money can't buy. (*The Economist*, November 3, 2012)

The Grameen movement has become a global phenomenon. Similar banks have been formed in Malaysia, the Philippines, Malawi, Africa, South America, and North America, in over 43 countries. One version has been implemented in inner cities like Chicago and Washington, serving 150,000 Americans. Prof. Yunus was awarded the Nobel Peace Prize in 2006 for his contributions and global leadership. (Yunus has started another multinational movement—he calls it " Social Business"—in which multinational corporations establish partnerships with poor people in commercial enterprises (e.g., Dannon yogurt, Nike footwear). The corporations save their production, marketing, and sales costs and sell the products for less to participating communities; they also split any profit by returning it for the benefits of participating poors in the community (Yunus, 2015).

As the number of women borrowers increased, Grameen staff noticed that the mothers would invest the money into their children or household expenses, whereas men would spend it on themselves. Women were also more likely to confront domestic troubles, whereas men worked away from the home, making food and a child's health higher priorities for the women. Grameen staff also asserted that women suffer from poverty more acutely than men. After becoming Grameen borrowers, women's self-perceptions also improved, from being shy and unsure of themselves to being assertive and self-confident.

Current Status

Active and expanded to additional countries. Prof. Yunus has diversified and initiated new movements called Social" Banking and "Social Business." These initiatives involve successful industries (e.g., Dannon yogurt and Nike shoe industries) to engage in philanthropy among poor communities in countries where they do business to promote goodwill and their own merchandise produced under endorsement of the Grameen project (Bornstein, 1996; Yunus, 2003).

CASE STUDY #26: SEWA (SELF-EMPLOYED WOMEN'S ASSOCIATION), AHMEDABAD, INDIA, 1972 (ED)

Problem

This case study falls within the domain of ED. The major problem being addressed is the lack of organization among self-employed women workers (mostly from the poor and working class) in order to fight for fair wages, decent working conditions, and health benefits, and against sexual harassment. Women workers, ranging from part-time factory workers, to vegetable vendors, to *bidi* (tobacco rolled in leaves) workers, to agricultural workers, gradually joined the SEWA cooperative, resulting in a diverse membership. According to one count:

> About 400 million workers constitute the working poor of India. They are mostly engaged in the informal economy, and do not have work and income security. They have no fixed employer–employee relations, and many are self-employed. They work long hours for very low wages or earn

very low income. They work in difficult and often hazardous conditions. Over 94% of the Indian workforce constitutes the informal economy. Women are a significant proportion of these workers. They work from dawn to dusk. Apart from little or no work security, they hardly have any social security. This means that they have no sick leave, no health or accident insurance, no maternity benefits nor child care. And in their old age, they have neither pension nor provident fund. Thus, most workers in our country are left to fend for themselves for survival. They are the most vulnerable of our citizens. They often have to face multiple and frequent risks which compound their poverty and vulnerability. (Mittal, 2013, p. 2)

It is in this context, SEWA began its mission and movement. In summing up the lessons learned by SEWA over four decades Mittal stated:

If the poor are to obtain their rightful place in the economy and in society, they must organize—unite and build their solidarity across caste, community, gender and geographic regions. Uniting and building their own membership-based, democratic, economic organizations is the first and essential building block in the struggle for justice. Whatever gains SEWA members might have made over the years is entirely due to their organizing, taking leadership and building their own movement. (Mittal, 2013, p. 16)

Leadership Impetus

On December 3, 1971, SEWA was formed to function as a union with the help of the Textile Labor Association (TLA)—the largest and oldest union of textile workers in India. Ela Bhatt, a lawyer and the leader of the TLA's Women's Wing, originated the idea of SEWA after developing services to improve the working conditions of all women workers.

There was initial opposition to SEWA's recognition as a trade union due to Indian labor laws mandating that unions be in a specific employer–employee relationship. With the support of TLA, SEWA successfully challenged the State Labor Department, and SEWA was registered on April 12, 1972, as a trade union of self-employed women workers, one of the first of its kind.

SEWA organizes women—who employ themselves in jobs such as small-scale sellers, home-based producers, casual laborers, and service workers—in order to regulate wages, strengthen the workers' production base, and improve working conditions. The union is open to all self-employed women over the age of 15.

EMPOWER Methods Used

- Organizing partnership
- Enabling service and assistance

¤ Work/job training and micro-enterprise
¤ Rights protection and social action/reform
¤ Empowerment training and leadership development
¤ Public education and participation

In order to assess the working and living conditions and the problems women faced, SEWA conducted a large-scale survey of women in Ahmedabad's slum areas. Based on their findings, SEWA realized that women were sorely lacking in protection in employment and were not generating enough income. SEWA's first intervention was to obtain access to institutional sources of credit for self-employed women. SEWA served as a mediator between the poor women and the banks by helping them fill out loan applications, telling them how the system worked and what was expected of them as borrowers. The Mahila SEWA Sahakari Bank was eventually established in July of 1974 to serve SEWA members exclusively.

SEWA established cooperatives of women such as dairy workers to pool resources and strengthen their bargaining power. SEWA attempts to procure raw materials, work, and training to develop their members' economic and social opportunities. SEWA provides a number of enabling services such as seminars that promote unity, cooperation, and community living among self-employed women; advice to the unmarried, widowed, neglected, and physically handicapped with their unique problems; literacy training; training in income-generation skills; grassroots organizers' training; daycare services; health training; and legal education. SEWA obtains help from the state and the central government for the social, economic, and political advancement of self-employed women and monitors laws pertaining to self-employed women for their proper administration. As SEWA leaders began to share their experiences in international forums, SEWA became a valuable resource in the women's movement. With this public visibility, SEWA placed pressure on the systems to change their exploitative ways.

Partners/Opposition

The TLA was instrumental to SEWA's founding and initial stages. However, when SEWA decide to engage in developmental activities in order to serve the needs of self-employed women workers (aside from organization), TLA disagreed. Due to this difference in opinion, SEWA became independent from TLA in May of 1985. Early financial aid SEWA received from the International Confederation of Free Trade Unions was used to construct a reception center and workshed in Ahmedabad; to fund a rural income-generation project on spinning, weaving, and milk production; and to purchase a rickshaw for transportation.

Other supporters include the Asian-American Free Labor Institute, Norway's International Development Agency, the Swedish International

Development Agency, Oxford Committee for Famine Relief (OXFAM), and the International Labor Organization (ILO). Since the International Women's Year (1975) and the launching of the International Decade for Women, SEWA also has collaborated with other women's groups worldwide, as well as with local rural women's associations. Bhatt was also awarded the prestigious Indira Gandhi Prize for Peace, Disarmament and Development in 2013 by President of India Pranab Mukherjee for her lifetime achievements in empowering women through grassroots entrepreneurship.

Macro-environment

At the time of its founding and in its initial stages, SEWA was centered at Ahmedabad, the largest city in the Indian state of Gujarat. Ahmedabad is an industrial city with over 60 textile mills, as well as a center for trade and commerce and home to educational research centers. According to a 1976 census, half of the state's population lived in slums and squatter settlements, most of whom worked in the informal sector—at home without regulations on hours of work or wages. According to survey conducted by SEWA, there were high health risks for rural women and children such as high female and infant mortality rates and poor nutrition of pregnant and nursing mothers. Banks were reluctant to advance loans to women who possessed no property of their own. Therefore, indebtedness to close relatives or private moneylenders was very high among self-employed women. Women earned less than men and were employed in the lowest-paid occupations. There was low literacy among rural women, and the educational levels of the children of self-employed women were low as well.

Impact and Remarks

SEWA's all-female membership provides a strong role model for women by uniting women from diverse educational, class, religious, and occupational backgrounds. Tremendous progress has been made in terms of awareness of rights and struggles against exploitation. SEWA has helped increase women's incomes and assets, access to services, range of job skills, and self-confidence. One of SEWA's early successes was the 1982 Indian Supreme Court decision that ordered the Municipal Corporation of Ahmedabad to provide a permanent site for women vegetable vendors' stalls on the terrace of the existing vegetable market. This was an important victory, considering the police harassment and difficulties in securing a suitable place to sell goods that were previously experienced by street vendors.

In 1977 Ela Bhatt was awarded the prestigious Ramon Magsaysay award which brought international recognition to SEWA. In 1980, the Indian government appointed Ela Bhatt as the Chairperson of the National Commission on Self-Employed Women, the first commission to study and document the problems of self-employed women. In 1989, Bhatt was appointed as the first female member of the central government's Planning Commission, a body that develops long-term economic and development plans for the country as well as makes decisions regarding program and policy development.

Current Status: Active and Diversified

Since the 1990s, SEWA has installed numerous programs and organizations, including the SEWA Bank cooperative, SEWA Bharat, and the HomeNet South Asia. SEWA Bharat is a federation of SEWA member organizations; presently, nine such SEWA member organizations are working in 35 districts of seven states in India, and together they account for a total membership around 1,200,000. Current membership exceeds 1,400,000 underprivileged women (SEWA, 2015).
According to SEWA:

> SEWA is both an organisation and a movement. The SEWA movement is enhanced by its being a sangam or confluence of three movements: the labour movement, the cooperative movement and the women's movement. But it is also a movement of self-employed workers: their own, home-grown movement with women as the leaders. Through their own movement women become strong and visible. Their tremendous economic and social contributions become recognised With globalization, liberalization and other economic changes, there are both new opportunities as well as threats to some traditional areas of employment.

Also there is much to be done in terms of strengthening women's leadership, their confidence, their bargaining power within and outside their homes and their representation in policy-making and decision-making fora. It is their issues, their priorities and needs which should guide and mould the development process in our country. Toward this end, SEWA has been supporting its members in capacity-building and in developing their own economic organizations (SEWA, 2015).
Another evaluation of SEWA by the WHO/SEARO states:

> Inequalities in health in a society are the outcome of unfair distribution of power between different groups within that society. Power relations within a society influence the Social and Economic Determinants of Health. This is why economic development and changes in the health care system by themselves have not been able to enhance the health status of marginalized groups to the extent desired. A case is now being made for using empowerment, together with economic development and health sector reforms, as a strategy for reducing persistent disparities in health and quality of life across gender and ethnic groups. It is believed that in the process of empowering itself, a group or community would tackle the underlying social, structural

and economic conditions that impact on its health. As a result, it would gain more control over the social determinants of health. Kar et al. justify the empowerment of women for better health for all on the following grounds: (i) In spite of longer lifespan, women suffer a greater burden of health risks and abuses; (ii) Women are the primary caregivers in almost all families; (iii) Women spend their discretionary money and time differently (from men), with priorities on better health and quality of life for children and family; and (iv) Compared to men, targeted education of women regarding health results in greater health benefits to children and families. (WHO/SEARO, 1995, pp. 7–8).

SEWA's initiatives are informed by changing priorities of its members. Even after four decades of direct rural development knowledge and experience, it is constantly responding changing priorities of its local members. The excerpt below illustrates SEWA's one of the recent priorities:

> Working in a country as vast and diverse as India is complex. SEWA listens to local communities and learns from their needs and experiences. The association aims to raise awareness, for example, of how to use more efficient and healthier cooking stoves; to determine availability, so the right sort of stove is delivered to the right people (i.e., the stove made for the South Indian population who mainly eat rice isn't suited to those who eat roti in North and Central India); and to guarantee affordability by working closely with local communities and financing partners.
>
> SEWA has also developed "Project Urja" (Shining) to provide solar lights to women's self-help groups across the impoverished Bihar-Mungar region, in cooperation with India's Ministry of Rural Development. By February 2013, the project provided 177 LED lights to seven villages, meaning that children can study after dark, women can cook better meals at night, and people can charge their mobile phones.
>
> For Bhatt, this is a shining example of how innovation and cooperation can transform lives and raise communities out of poverty. "At SEWA we are looking forward to a bright future where all our existing as well as new members make use of energy technology and improve their lives." (*Christian Science Monitor*, 2015)

Recently, after Ela Bhatt was awarded the prestigious Niwano World Peace Prize, she was asked how her work through SEWA contributed to world peace. Bhatt replied,

> Peace is not about a lack of activities of war. It is not just about general elections. Peace is substantive, lasting; it is about life. It is about the ordinariness of life, how we understand each other, share meals, and share

courtyards. And that is what women do ... And all these ordinary things are directly related to the health of nations. (Bhatt, 2010)

Emphasizing SEWA's goal on promoting ordinary women's self-reliance for fighting global poverty, Bhatt added:

So in reality individual peace and global peace are not separate. They are one and the same ... And poverty and violence go hand in hand. Violence cannot bring peace. Poverty is violence. And it happens with the consent of the society. Poverty and violence are not God made, they are man made. Poverty and peace cannot coexist. (Bhatt, 2010)

CASE STUDY #81: THE CHATRA LOKAHITA PROJECT, WEST BENGAL, INDIA (ED)

Problem

The small group "Lokahita" was initially formed to help farmers and their families' ED. The area of operation was in the villages Ghospur, Uttar, and Dakshin Chatra, in West Bengal. The villages are situated near the India and Bangladesh border. The village farmers were always dependent on farming, but as they did not own their own land, they were earning their livelihood as farm laborers, which could hardly sustain their families. With the introduction of tractors and other mechanized farming tools, the need for laborers was also reduced, and most of them did not have any regular income. To add to the Indian farmers' woes, the infiltration of Bangladesh refugees further reduced their employment rate and earning. Low income, less education, and poverty made them frustrated, and they started to take consolation in alcohol. They started ignoring their families, and conditions deteriorated every day.

With this social and economic background, the few educated and senior citizens of the locality formed the group known as Lokahita. They motivated other younger and educated members and formed a core committee. Their initial focus was to empower women members of the village and make them self-reliant so that they could sustain their children and families. They named the organization "Ghoshpur Lokahita Farmers' Welfare Samity" (Association), and it was registered on May 21, 1999, by the Government of West Bengal and supported by the National Bank of Agriculture and Rural Development (NABARD) and the United Bank of India.

Area of Operation

The association operated in about 104 villages in 470 small groups. Each group comprised ten members, all women. Altogether, more than 4,700 women were involved in different groups. The association assisted them financially and trained them in different professions according to their interests. Fifty percent of them were involved in the garment manufacturing and stitching business, 20% in the agricultural segment, 10% in rice-processing, and 10% in chicken and dairy farming. The association helped them in organizing workshops and marketing. The group members repaid loans from their new income. Apart from economic assistance, the association helped local society by educating women and children in evening classes, with a free supply of books and stationery and the like. Now they were able to keep records of their accounts, income, and expenditures.

Another gray area in villages was poor public health and bad road conditions. Lokahita organized programs for awareness of tuberculosis and medical help. They also conducted awareness programs for arsenic-free water and soil testing for cultivation. Women members repaired roads around their village before the rainy season. The association members organized various programs to celebrate national and regional occasions like Independence Day, Republic Day, the birthdays of national leaders, and so on. These events provided opportunities to women and children to organize events and exhibit their talent and skills at public forum.

Benefits

The income generated through these small group activities, supported by microfinance loans extended by banks through Lokahita, benefited the women (most members were women) and their families immensely. As it has been established that women do not waste money on alcohol and the like, they can offer their children a better life. They now understand the importance of education and are sending their children to school. The women of neighboring villages, who were initially skeptical about these group activities, are now inspired by the improvement of living standards and are forming new groups themselves, expanding the working area of Lokahita. Within less than a decade, Lokahita has become largest group in both North and South 24 Pargana districts. The association received many awards at state and national levels, including one from India's Finance Minister's office at New Delhi (Purnendu Kar, personal communication, November 2014).

CASE #86: BANCHTE SHEKHA ("LEARNING TO SURVIVE"), JESSORE, BANGLADESH

Problem

Angela Gomes (born in 1952) is the founder and director of *Banchte Shekha* ("Learning to Survive"), one of the most respected women's organizations in Bangladesh. Set up on a modest scale in 1981, the organization now accommodates 200 live-in trainees and also serves as a women's shelter. More than

25,000 women in 750 village-based organizations are active members of Banchte Shekha, and more than 200,000 indirectly benefit from its agenda. Gomes has been working on the issue of gender rights through social rights education and income-generation programs. Gomes was one of the five winners of the 1999 Ramon Magsaysay Award, Asia's most prestigious award. She was honored for community leadership. Her Banchte Shekha organization offers female-empowerment programs in nearly 430 Bangladeshi villages.

In the early days, Gomes used to borrow a bicycle and pedal alone through the dusty countryside near the Bangladeshi city of Jessore. She would talk to village women, listening to their problems, and offering what little help she could. Indignant at her interference in their traditional ways, the menfolk would sometimes hurl rocks at her as she passed. For all the effect they had, they might as well have been throwing ping-pong balls. "The oppression and insults merely made me more determined to achieve my goal," said Gomes.

Gomes runs one of the largest women's rural organizations in Bangladesh. Operating out of a 1.5-hectare training complex in Jessore, Banchte Shekha teaches rural women a vast range of income-generating skills, including handicrafts, raising crops, poultry and livestock raising, fish farming, beekeeping, and silk making (from the cocoon to the weaving loom, to the printing).

A Christian in a mainly Muslim country, Gomes recalled how, as a student at a mission school in Jessore, she would accompany one of the nuns on visits to local villages. The women spoke of mistreatment. The nun counseled patience. Gomes said, "I decided to talk to her. I said, 'If you can't bring any change, if you can't save these women, why do you keep telling them to be submissive? Why don't you help them to protest?'" (*Asiaweek*, 2000). The activist-to-be was expelled from school for "revolutionary" activities.

Known affectionately as *Bara Apa* ("Eldest Sister"), Gomes speaks Arabic and has studied the Koran. But when she was younger, even that was not enough to avoid suspicion about her motives and background. She says,

> I rubbed butter oil on my hair to make it gray, but it didn't work. I found my Christian name a great obstacle, so I changed it to Anju, which sounded more Muslim. I identified myself as a married woman whose husband had gone abroad to study. And I invented a son and a daughter.

Gradually she won the support of open-minded clerics who understood, as she did, that the Koran was not the source of local practices demeaning to women. For a while, Gomes was given shelter in a Muslim home. "The husband encouraged me to go on with my work," she said. "He assured me of every help and protection. I can't find the words to properly praise the goodness and affection he showed me" (*Asiaweek*, 2000).

Naming Gomes as the winner of the Ramon Magsaysay Award for Community Leadership, the board of trustees cited her role in "helping

Bangladeshi women assert their rights to better livelihoods and gender equality, under the law and in everyday life." Informed of the award, Gomes exclaimed: "It's just incredible" (Gomes, 2015b).

For several years, Gomes has been fighting ovarian cancer. It has slowed her down and but she still manages visits to Banchte Shekha villages to check on developments and meet the members she has come to know over the years.

CASE STUDY #82: KARMA KUTIR (HANDICRAFT HUT), KOLKATA, INDIA (ED)

Problem

The suburbs, slums, and pavements were crowded with bodies. People were raising families and trying to build a life between a drain and a sewer. And these were not Kolkata's ordinary poor, they were the results of two waves of refugee migration from Bangladesh. Rootless and unwanted, they had nowhere else to go (Mioitryee Basu, personal interview, December 16, 2014). If the men suffered, the women and children suffered more. Eminent social workers of the city came together to find a solution to this problem. *Karma Kutir* (Handicraft Hut) was the result. Karma Kutir chose to encourage women to revive traditional arts and earn themselves a living and supplement their family income (Karma Kutir, 2013).

Methods

Karma Kutir is a registered voluntary social welfare organization working relentlessly to generate self-employment opportunities for marginalized women and girls in rural as well as urban areas in India. Karma Kutir upholds the dignity of human life in all its activities. Since its inception in 1961, Karma Kutir has had the sole aim of helping the least privileged women and children. Its journey of helping people began with the rehabilitation of the uprooted people of erstwhile East Pakistan. Having full faith in the innate capacity of women, Karma Kutir has over the years dedicated itself to the empowerment of marginalized women through training in handicrafts, production, marketing, and self-employment.

Impacts

Karma Kutir runs a showroom in Kolkata where handicrafts made by the women at Karma Kutir are sold. The exhibitions organized by Karma Kutir are also great opportunities to showcase *kantha*, batik, and other products crafted by the women. Through all these activities, Karma Kutir not only provides a livelihood for needy women, but also preserves some heritage art forms of Bengal.

10

Health Promotion and Disease Prevention Case Studies

The primary goals of these movements are in the domain of health promotion and disease prevention (HPDP): these movements tend to be more focused on specific health threats in defined populations. Some of these are concerned with HPDP among demographic groups (e.g., women, ethnic minorities, infants); some are directed at prevention of specific health threats (e.g., HIV/ autoimmune deficiency syndrome [AIDS], auto accidents, tobacco abuse). The criteria for inclusion and methodology use are same for all the case studies in the four groups. These summaries give information on six dimensions of each movement and offer better glimpses of the dynamics of the movements that are not available in quantitative comparisons. These summaries, by themselves and without further commentaries on each, are important sources for learning how empowerment works in reality.

Health Promotion and Disease Prevention (HPDP) Cases

Each case has information on (1) case title, place, and domain; (2) the problems addressed; (3) leadership impetus; (4) EMPOWER methods used, (5) sources of support and opposition, (6) the macro-environment, and (7) impact and remarks.

CASE STUDY #41: ASIAN AND PACIFIC ISLANDERS
FOR REPRODUCTIVE HEALTH (APIRH), CALIFORNIA, 1989 (HPDP)

Problem

This case study falls within the domain of HPDP. The major problem being addressed was lack of representation of Asian and Pacific Islander (API) women on the local, county, state, and national public-policy levels about the issue of reproductive health.

Leadership Impetus

The precursor of the APIRH was created in 1989 in order to ensure access to safe abortions for all women. Established after the Supreme Court case of *Webster vs. Reproductive Health Services* (*Webster v. Reproductive Health*, 1989), Asians and Pacific Islanders for Choice (APIC) brought the voice of Asian communities to the policy debate over reproductive choice. In 1992, the organization changed its name to its current one in order to reflect an expanded mission of organizing women and girls around women's health and empowerment.

EMPOWER Methods Used

- Empowerment training and leadership development
- Rights protection and social action/reform
- Organizing partnerships and coalitions
- Enabling service and assistance

Through collaborations, outreach, education, community-based research, advocacy, and organizing, Asians and Pacific Islanders for Reproductive Health (APIRH, 2010), promotes the reproductive health and sexual well-being of Asian and Pacific Islander women and girls in California. APIRH provides technical assistance and training for youth programs and health clinics on popular education and teen reproductive health education. APIRH helps develop programs that enable young women to improve their communities. The HOPE (Health, Opportunities, Problem-Solving, and Empowerment) Curriculum for Girls Project develops leadership, mentoring, and organizing skills in adolescent girls. The HOPE for Women Project focuses on low-literacy immigrant and refugee women by using a popular education strategy. APIRH's national strategy is based on a long-term vision of building strong local and state grassroots leaders and organizing.

In 1995, APIRH held its landmark conference, "Opening Doors to Our Health and Well-Being," in the California state capitol, Sacramento. It was the first statewide effort to mobilize API women in California on issues of reproductive health and women's empowerment. Nearly half the 150 women participants were immigrants or refugees, representing more than 15 different ethnic groups and multiracial backgrounds; 30 adolescent girls took part in this gathering.

Through coalition work with reproductive freedom and abortion rights organizations, APIRH participates in campaigns with other reproductive freedom organizations to ensure reproductive choice and safe and affordable access to a full range of reproductive services, technologies, and procedures for women and girls. Through partnerships with Asian and Pacific Islander health organizations, APIRH works to promote policies and legislation at the local, state, and national levels, which address linguistic, cultural, and economic access to health care for everyone. APIRH works closely with other community organizations and clinics to learn about the needs of women and girls (APIRH, 2015).

APIRH conducts community-based research on reproductive health and other related health issues, in cooperation with the community. The Asian/Pacific Islander Reproductive Health Study was the first survey of API attitudes and knowledge about reproductive health and policies. Another APIRH study explored the attitudes, knowledge, and practices of API teenagers about sexuality and health. One 1995 APIRH report, called "The Health and Well-Being of Asian and Pacific Islander American Women," provided an analysis, summary, and bibliography of research and data on Asian and Pacific Islander women's health. It also described the process of organizing APIRH's "Opening Doors" conference.

Partners/Opposition

APIRH receives governmental and private foundation funding from such organizations as the Ms. Foundation, Ford Foundation, LA Women Foundation, National Institute of Environmental Health Sciences, and Packard Foundation, among others. APIRH is a progressive organization; it faces resistance from conservative groups such as pro-life or religious groups.

Macro-environment

As one of the most populous states, where 40% of Asians and Pacific Islanders in the United States reside, California is the home of some of the most controversial public policies. Policies like the 1989 *Webster* decision gave more power to the states to regulate abortions, thereby limiting reproductive choice for women. As more health and welfare policy decisions are given to states, advocacy groups like APRIH are responding to these changes in policy, budgets, and services through grassroots organizing efforts. Yet few data exist about API women living in the United States. According to the "model minority" myth, APIs are healthy individuals who need minimal health-related research and services. Among API women themselves, open discussion about sexuality, sexual practices, or orientation is not common. Due to this cultural barrier, some API women are ignorant of how their bodies work. This can have negative effects on their reproductive health (Marguerite, 2002).

Impact and Remarks

Since its founding, APIRH has built the capacity of Asian and Pacific Islander women and girls to advocate for reproductive rights and women's empowerment. Through such forums as its landmark "Opening Doors" conference,

APIRH has mobilized API women in California from different ethnicities and languages. APIRH has also increased the visibility of Asian and Pacific Islander perspectives in California and national pro-choice organizations and coalitions, as well as public-policy discussions at the local, county, state and national levels. For its work in reproductive health for Asian Pacific Islanders, APIRH has won the 1998 Association Child and Maternal Health Innovative Programs (AMCHP) Award and the Gloria Steinem Women's Achievement Award (Marguerite, 2002).

CASE STUDY #46: THE BOSTON WOMEN'S HEALTH BOOK COLLECTIVE, UNITED STATES, 1969 (HPDP)

Problem

This case study falls within the domain of HPDP. The major problem being addressed was the lack of information about women's health and lack of attention dedicated to women's specific health issues.

Leadership Impetus

In 1969, 12 women met at a women's liberation conference in Boston, one of the first of its kind. This group of women formed "The Doctor's Group," the forerunner to the Boston Women's Health Book Collective (BWHBC), to research and discuss women's unique health issues. In order to share valuable information and research, they created a course booklet and held classes for women. This booklet later evolved and became the national bestseller *Our Bodies, Ourselves*, first published in 1970.

EMPOWER Methods Used

- ¤ Public education and participation
- ¤ Media use
- ¤ Organizing partnership
- ¤ Rights protection and social action/reform
- ¤ Enabling service and assistance

The BWHBC mission is "to empower all women with knowledge of their bodies, health and sexuality." *Our Bodies, Ourselves (OBOS)*, first published in 1972 as book and updated since, is widely regarded as an essential resource on health and sexuality for women of diverse ethnic, racial, economic, geographical, and religious backgrounds. Over the years, it has been translated into almost 20 languages. A revised edition published in 1998, *Our Bodies, Ourselves for the New Century,* included a listing and critique of online health resources as well as chapters on how race, class, and gender-based oppressions affect the health of women. A Spanish-language adaptation called *Nuestros Cuerpos, Nuestras Vidas* was published early 2000 in the United States, Canada, and Mexico. *OBOS* has inspired similar books (not direct translations) about women's health in Denmark, India, and Egypt. "The Boston Women's Health Book Collective (also known as Our Bodies Ourselves) aims to empower women by providing information about health, sexuality, and reproduction. Advisory board members include Teresa Heinz Kerry, Susan Love, and Gloria Steinem." (To learn more, visit OBOS, 2015.)

The Women's Health Information Center (WHIC) serves as a non-lending library and resource center for BWHBC programs and the public. WHIC, one of the largest and oldest of its kind, offers data and documentation in 30 research areas. The *Women and Health Thesaurus* systematically organizes the huge volume of print materials housed at WHIC. Public Voice through opinions, letters, and meetings initiatives the BWHBC to amplify the voice of *OBOS* and the women's health movement contributing political critiques of current health issues, working with the media and speaking to the public. BWHBC leaders in particular areas of women's health are able to share their research with new audiences through opinion and editorial pieces and interviews with print and broadcast media. They have appeared on television news programs such as *The Today Show* and *Good Morning America*, as well as international women and health meetings such as the Beijing NGO Forum in 1995.

BWHBC has collaborated with many organizations to promote the health of women, including the Committee on Women, Population, and the Environment; Family Health International; International Reproductive Rights Research Action Group; National Black Women's Health Project; National Institutes of Health (NIH) Office of Research on Women's Health; and the World Health Organization (WHO). For the Spanish-language adaptation of *OBOS* (*Nuestros Cuerpos, Nuestras Vidas*), BWHBC collaborated with 19 women's health groups from 11 countries in Central, North, and South America and the Caribbean.

Latinas en Accion pro-Salud (ALAS) is BWHBC's Latina outreach project that forges partnerships with Latina community-based organizations, women's health organizations, and community health centers, both domestically and internationally.

Partners/Opposition

BWHBC collaborates with a wide community of individuals and organizations as described above. For the Beijing NGO Forum in 1995, BWHBC collaborated with the Women's Global Network for Reproductive Rights (Amsterdam), the International Reproductive Rights and Research Action Group (IRRRAG), and Women Health Philippines to sponsor a workshop series about the challenges faced by women in terms of their sexual and reproductive lives. Using the royalties from the sale of *OBOS,* BWHBC funded women's health projects, and advocacy work. The Boston Foundation and the Open Society Institute provide financial funding to support BWHBC's ALAS program (Latina Outreach Initiative). Other donors include the Educational Foundation of America, the Ford Foundation, the Kapoor Family Fund, the John D. and Catherine T. MacArthur Foundation, and the Mellon Foundation.

Macro-environment

During the first meetings attended by the founders of BWHBC, the women discovered that they shared common experiences in dealing with the medical establishment; namely, frustration and anger towards doctors who were condescending, paternalistic, judgmental, and uninformative. There was also a dearth of pertinent information about women's health. During the time *OBOS* was being written, the United States was in the midst of the second wave of feminism that emphasized reproductive health and sexuality.

Impact and Remarks

> Working together informally, the core group of women who would later form the Boston Women's Health Book Collective wrote a book that would become the bible of women's health, selling more than 4 million copies. They also created an organization that would carry their mission forward. From the first newsprint edition of Our Bodies, Ourselves, which became an underground sensation, to the brand new book, Our Bodies, Ourselves: Pregnancy and Birth, released in March 2008, the group has educated women and men, critiqued the medical system, examined inequalities based on gender, race, sexual orientation, class, and other categories, and urged readers to move from individual self-help to collective action promoting social policies that support the health of women and communities. (Stephenson and Zeldes, 2002)

Not only did these discoveries find their way into the various editions of *OBOS,* they informed many of their projects. Leaders in the women's movement and medical establishment have praised *OBOS* for the wealth of women's health information it offers. Their widely acclaimed book, *Our Bodies, Ourselves* (OBOS, 1972), is one of the most well-known contribution to the women's health movement. The BWHBC has become a vigorous advocate for women's health by challenging the institutions and systems that block women from full control over our bodies and devalue women's lives (OBOS, 1972, preface).

CASE STUDY #40: CENTRO DE INFORMACÍON Y DESARROLLO DE LA
MUJER (CIDEM) KUMAR WARMI, EL ALTO, BOLIVIA, 1985 (HPDP)

Problem

The major problem being addressed was the lack of medical services and
clinics for women, leading to poor reproductive health care in Bolivia for
women. Many El Alto residents were reluctant to visit clinics run by doctors
who had little knowledge of their cultural practices and beliefs. Major health
problems included maternal mortality, sexually transmitted diseases, and
complications from early pregnancies and unsafe abortions. Approximately
45% of mothers became pregnant as teenagers, which forced them to leave
school, work in poorly paying jobs, and engage in dependent relationships.

Leadership Impetus

The Centro de Informacíon y Desarrollo de la Mujer (CIDEM) is a nonprofit
organization that was formed in 1985 in El Alto, Bolivia. CIDEM's goal was
to educate women about health care, women's rights, and supporting women's
organizations. In 1986, CIDEM founded Kumar Warmi (Healthy Women)
Clinic—the first clinic in El Alto geared toward women—in response to
repeated requests for health services made by leaders of several women's
organizations.

EMPOWER Methods Used

- Enabling service and assistance
- Organizing partnership
- Public education and participation
- Rights protection and social action/reform

During its early beginnings, Kumar Warmi staff members visited mothers' clubs in El Alto to discuss health issues and to encourage individuals to
utilize the clinic. Participation widened from nearby residents to residents
of surrounding neighborhoods through a series of radio programs about
various health topics. In 1986, the Health Committee, comprising about 20
leaders of diverse women's groups, was created to serve as a liaison between
CIDEM and grassroots women's organizations. The committee also helped
design a HMO-like (health-maintenance organization) system of healthcare
in which members paid a small monthly fee in exchange for unlimited clinic
visits at no extra cost. Committee members benefited from training as health
outreach workers and were awarded with training certificates.

In the past few years, participation in the Health Committee has declined
due to the termination of food donations, which had sustained many of the
grassroots organizations. Women have turned to other groups who offer
monetary incentives to join (such as income-generating projects and credit

programs). However, a few groups are still together, bonded by friendship and sisterhood as well as cooperative activities such as buying ingredients wholesale to make Christmas cakes each year.

Currently, Kumar Warmi Clinic offers services that address the biological, legal, psychological, and sociocultural aspects of women's health including a special focus on traditional medicine. Educational programs provide information for pregnant women, family planning, adolescent sexuality, and prevention of cervical and uterine cancer (Paulson, 2000). CIDEM has also promoted several productive/economic projects, collaborated with local women's organizations, and advocated political and legal changes related to healthcare issues. In order to address and possibly prevent familial tension, CIDEM conducts family planning workshops for couples. By including men in the learning process, CIDEM hopes to alleviate some of the familial strain associated with the participating women's changed behaviors pertaining to reproductive health. CIDEM publishes a series of books, many of which share CIDEM's experiences and strategies relating to women's education and healthcare for the benefit of other organizations (Paulson, 2000, 2003).

Partners/Opposition

CIDEM collaborates with several women's health organizations in El Alto such as mothers' clubs and women's groups supported by Programs para la Mujer (PROMUJER), Organismo Nacional del Menor, Mujer y Familia or National Organization of Minors, Women and Family (ONAMFA), and the Center for Elementary Mathematics and Science Education (CEMSE) by providing workshops and training. The Center Inherited Disorders of Energy Metabolism (CIDEM) also works with the Inter-Institutional Women's Committee for El Alto. In the governmental sector, CIDEM collaborates with the Regional Secretary of Health; provides care to poor women who participate with public works projects through El Alto City Hall; and works with the government's Project for Improving Primary Care in planning and implementing training, research, and other health-related activities. In terms of direct patient care, CIDEM has developed agreements with several obstetrics clinics to insure that the medical personnel practice humane health care. In addition, the UN's MDG-F (Millennium Development Goals–Fund) has been experimenting with innovative poverty reduction experiments that benefit women in extreme poverty in areas including El Alto (MDG-F, 2013).

Macro-environment

The majority of El Alto's population is poor. Many families are migrants from the *altiplano* and bring with them rural aspects of their culture to the city. Often, migrants only speak Aymara or Quecha, are illiterate, and may have little contact with medical services. The migrant way of life also affects the stability of women's groups and continued participation in group activities.

In terms of health care, there is widespread resistance to and ignorance of modern medicine in El Alto. There is fear and suspicion of many medical procedures such as the insertion of foreign objects into the body. Access to health care differs by sex, class, and ethnicity. Many women do not have sufficient income to obtain health care; transportation to and from the health clinics; or adequate childcare to allow them to keep a doctor's appointment.

Impact and Remarks

CIDEM's integrated approach to health incorporates many facets of women's lives—from reproductive rights, to social conditions, to economic opportunities, to cultural norms. CIDEM tries to cultivate an interpersonal relationship with its clients as opposed to the strictly vertical relations of health professionals and patients. Participation in CIDEM's activities, such as the Health Committee, has bolstered the confidence of the women as leaders, counselors, and health outreach workers. The Health Committee has played a key role in the dissemination of healthcare information as well as CIDEM's unique approach to providing services (Paulson, 2000, 2003).

A disappointing aspect of the training program of local women is that their acquired knowledge and skills are often not marketable in the paid labor force outside of CIDEM. Kumar Warmi participants value their health and the knowledge accumulated through their efforts, however. They are confident in their ability to share this newly gained knowledge with other women through the organization and on an informal basis among relatives, friends, and neighbors. This, in turn, has increased the number of women who frequent the clinic.

In recognition of the fact that government and private institutions are increasingly providing reproductive health services, as well as the increased difficulty in securing funding, CIDEM has directed its efforts to training. Through books and workshops, CIDEM disseminates information about its methods of incorporating gender into health care service and delivery. CIDEM also has a contract for a training consultancy with the Centro de Investigación, Educación y Servicios (CIES). Specifically, CIDEM bases its methodology on continuous education and development of healthcare staff, grassroots participants, and group leaders; and the transformation of doctor–client relationships.

CASE #68: COMITE POR RESCATE DE NUESTRA SALUD (CPRNS), MAYAGÜEZ, PUERTO RICO, 1983 (HPDP)

Problem

This case study falls within the domain of HPDP. The major problem being addressed was the generation of hazardous industrial wastes (such as gas emissions) and associated health and ecological risks affecting mostly female employees at the Guanajibo-Castillo Industrial Park in Mayagüez, Puerto Rico. This 29-factory complex included a wastewater treatment plant and sewer plant as well as two pharmaceutical companies, six electronics plants, and nine clothing factories. Between 1983 and 1987, more than 60 incidents of gas emissions occurred at this complex, originating mostly from the pharmaceutical, electronics, and electrical-products industries.

Leadership Impetus

In 1983, a group of women workers headed by Cielo Martín and Santos Feliciano (garment factory employees) formed the *Comite Por Rescate de Nuestra Salud* ("Committee to Rescue Our Health") CPRNS, to protest several harmful incidents of gas emissions in their workplace in Puerto Rico. Both of the founders had previous organizing experience (as a labor organizer/political activist and as an active church leader). The main goals of the organization were to pressure the government into acknowledging the presence of toxic substances in the park, advise the harmful industries to implement pollution controls, and obtain appropriate medical care for the affected workers.

EMPOWER Methods Used

- Empowerment training and leadership development
- Media use
- Public education and participation
- Enabling service and assistance
- Rights protection and social action/reform
- Organizing partnership

When the gas emissions first affected workers, scientific advisors (medical doctors and psychologists) and neighbors of the industrial park tried to prove, through various scientific studies, that their health problems were directly related to exposure to chemical substances emitted from the industries. When their efforts were ignored, CPRNS organized demonstrations, rallies, marches, pickets, and public hearings. Monthly meetings, conferences and discussions at various universities, and a practicum for graduate students in community psychology were held in order to raise public awareness of the situation and garner further support for the cause.

As a result of their efforts, CPRNS was able to obtain extensive media coverage and disseminate information about their cause to the public. CPRNS stressed the importance of collective decision-making involving all stakeholders, empowering those affected, and representing all points of view. In keeping with this strategy, Martín, one of the CPRNS founders, encouraged the women's active participation in the monthly meetings by creating educational workshops about political organizing and environmental issues.

The workshops also suggested better ways to handle the situation such as asking questions and challenging the doctors' diagnoses.

Partners/Opposition

A group of scientists, lawyers, and consultants helped CPRNS gather and analyze information related to the gas emissions at Guanajibo-Castillo Industrial Park. CPRNS also enlisted the assistance of Misión Industrial, an environmental Community-Based Organizations (CBO); the Unión de Trabajadores de la Industria Eléctrica y Riego (UTIER), a trade union; and the Organización Puertorriqueña de Mujeres Trabajadoras (OPMT), a feminist organization. Despite the numerous studies correlating the exposure to occupational hazards with the workers' health problems, their employers and the Puerto Rican government believed that the levels of contamination were not sufficient to explain the employees' health problems. The workers' complaints were ignored, and the government and federal regulatory agencies failed to impose stricter regulations or penalties on the companies involved.

Macro-environment

In recent decades, Puerto Rico has become a manufacturing site for high and medium technologies such as garment-making, electronics, and electrical parts industries. Unfortunately, these industries have discharged hazardous wastes into the water, air, and soil, which have been shown to cause serious environmental and occupational health problems throughout the island. Despite the efforts of several environmental groups on the island, the Puerto Rican government has been unable to regulate the companies involved. In response to these environmental problems, affected workers and collaborating scientists of more than 90 communities have participated in protest efforts against the harmful industries, with various successes. In nearly all of these health struggles, women have distinguished themselves as spokespersons, coordinators, and members of committees. This is not surprising, considering the fact that due to occupational segregation by sex, women constitute the majority of workers in these potentially harmful industries.

Impact and Remarks

Through their efforts, CPRNS members gained credibility among the Mayagüez community some doctors. They also raised awareness of the potential health risks of polluting factories among many communities in Puerto Rico. CPRNS effectively challenged the powerful male industrialists, heads of government agencies, and the medical profession in their struggle to improve health conditions (Muñoz-Vázquez, 1996). As a result, the Puerto Rican government investigated the problems of gas emissions in the area and gathered scientific data about the health effects of organic solvent pollution. Furthermore, the CPRNS successfully induced the industries to replace some of the harmful substances used in their production processes with less dangerous ones. Among the CPRNS members, the women developed grassroots leadership skills, political knowledge, and a greater awareness of women's subordination in a patriarchal society.

CASE STUDY #44: GIRLS' POWER INITIATIVE (GPI), NIGERIA, 1993 (HPDP)

Problem

The major problem being addressed was teenage sexuality in Nigeria. Most adolescents received little or no sexuality education; and many knew very little about their bodies, reproduction, contraception, and disease prevention. Services designed for adolescents were extremely rare. Rates of pregnancy, sexually transmitted diseases (STDs) and AIDS among adolescents were high. Pregnant adolescents often got dangerous and illegal abortions that could result in illness, infertility, or death.

Leadership Impetus

A biologist and the head of the botany department at the University of Calabar in Nigeria, Dr. Bene Madunagu founded Girls' Power Initiative (GPI, 1993) in 1993 in partnership with Grace Osakue, a school administrator in Benin City. Osakue was, like Dr. Madunagu, a national and international advocate for women's health and rights. With the help of her colleagues, Madunagu gathered nine adolescent girls, including her own daughter, for the first Girls' Power Initiative meeting in July 1994 in Calabar. Word of mouth helped expand the group. In the southwest, Osakue started with seven girls in her group, which has since grown substantially. GPI is a non-governmental organization that works to promote self-esteem among young women and adolescent girls by giving them factual information about reproductive health and rights and by teaching them to voice their opinion in terms of their sexual needs and desires. GPI's goal is to help girls envision a more promising world for themselves (Madunagu, 1993).

EMPOWER Methods Used

- ¤ Enabling service and assistance
- ¤ Public education and participation
- ¤ Empowerment training
- ¤ Leadership development

The larger goal is for these young women to gain the self-confidence and self-knowledge to attain their potential in education, careers, motherhood, and relationships (GPI, 1993). By sharing information, GPI hopes to give the participants the power to shape their own lives. Topics such as true love, contraception, the definition of rape, rape prevention, and dealing with relationships are discussed. GPI facilitators employ inventive techniques such as interactive dialogues, games, and group work to draw shyer girls out and make them feel that their ideas and opinions are valuable. In order to allow poorer girls to participate, GPI provides a transport allowance. GPI holds public education events on violence against women, AIDS, women's rights, and staged a dramatic production called *Sex Is Not Love,* and provides the GPI curriculum in several schools in Calabar. GPI also operates a program in Benin City in the southwestern part of the country. As many as 500 young women, ages 8 to 19, are GPI members; hundreds more attend in GPI programs held in classrooms. GPI publishes a quarterly newsletter, *Girls' Power,* that is available at federal and state libraries and by local distribution. The newsletter reports on GPI's activities such as the empowerment education workshop, a Christmas show in Calabar, and a field trip to nearby villages. Also included in the newsletter are articles on the Nigerian women's movement, health education and upcoming events, pictures of past events, and a substantial section dedicated to the girls' opinions and personal stories written by the girls. Madunagu also responds to letters written by girls asking for advice.

Hearing the problems and opinions of the girls often spurs new GPI projects. For example, GPI collaborates with the Nigerian women lawyers' association to try to have rape hearings and trials moved to the privacy of judges' chambers instead of being held in open courts, which can bring blame and scorn to victims. GPI sponsored a national empowerment workshop, Skills Training Towards the Empowerment of Adolescent Girls.

Partners/Opposition

The International Women's Health Coalition (IWHC), based in New York, gave GPI its first seed grant and immediately furnished technical assistance. Andrea Irvin, IWHC's former Africa program officer, provided Dr. Madunagu with strategic advice on program design; just as important, she was the founder's sounding board, providing much encouragement and constructive criticism. IWHC also provided factual, scientific, and advocacy materials on women's health and rights—information that is not available in Nigeria and most other parts of Africa, and has been vital for both GPI facilitators and the girls who attend the gatherings and take part in the classroom curricula. The Ford Foundation awarded Girls Power Initiative (Nigeria) a $200,000 grant for Fiscal Year 1996.

GPI's candid discussions of sexual reproduction, women's health and rights, domestic violence, and male–female relationships can be controversial in traditional Nigerian society. GPI has occasionally been accused of "corrupting" young women, encouraging them to be sexually active, or making them "too bold" to find good husbands.

Macro-environment

In Nigeria, the vast majority of young women are trained to be subservient to their parents, their brothers, and their husbands. Although the number of Nigerian women professionals is increasing, and women have greater access to higher education and senior positions, the traditional Nigerian girl's upbringing of subordination persists, especially in the country's rural areas. In Nigeria, 72% of males and 82% of females have had sexual intercourse by the end of their teenage years. The mean age of marriage is 16.5 years; half of all Nigerian women have children by the age of 20.

Impact and Remarks

By educating the adolescents, the GPT Alumna Association (GPI) hopes to encourage them to alter the lives and perceived roles of women—and men—of the future generations of Nigeria. Madunagu eventually would like to make GPI a national program, but funding constraints and the difficulty of finding and training staff, including those who are not judgemental about adolescents, make this a long-term goal. Strongly encouraged by school officials and parents, GPI's school program is expanding to as many as 15 schools. Madunagu also plans to undertake a full-scale evaluation of the GPI program. (GAA, 2015)

Noteworthy is the fact that some GPI graduates have themselves commenced social action in their communities through groups they have put together for that purpose. Young Girls Foundation (YGF) is the latest of the seed groups founded by Lucy Isimeme Ejodamen, a 2004 graduate of GPI Benin. (GAA, 2015)

Since GPI's inception, many changes have taken place in the girls themselves. For example, many of the teenage girls speak with more confidence and have gained strength from the encouragement of their peers. Girls have expanded their vision of what they can be, not limiting themselves to being nurses or teachers. The words of the "Women's Decade" anthem, first sung at the Nairobi Women's Conference in 1985 and repeated at the close of each GPI meeting, echo GPI's mission (GPI, 1993):

All across the nation
All around the world
Women are longing to be free.
No longer in the shadows
Forced to stay behind
But side-by-side in true equality.
So sing a song for women everywhere

Let it ring around the world and never, ever cease
So sing a song for women everywhere
Equality, development and peace.

CASE STUDY #59: THE INTERNATIONAL NETWORK OF WOMEN
AGAINST TOBACCO (INWAT), 1990 (HPDP)

Problem

The major problem being addressed was the high rate of tobacco use among
women and young girls. More than 140,000 women die each year from
tobacco-related illnesses. Women who smoke also have an increased risk of
cervical cancer and osteoporosis. Smoking among girls in many societies is
increasing faster than among boys.

Leadership Impetus

The International Network of Women Against Tobacco (INWAT) was
founded in 1990 at an international conference on tobacco and health.
Despite the fact that many of the participants at the conference were women,
all of the speakers were men, and there were no workshops or sessions about
the effects of tobacco on women's health. In 1990, the International Network
of Women Against Tobacco was formed in Australia to develop women's
leadership, advocacy, and education on the issues of women and tobacco
(INWAT, 1990).

   Women tobacco-control leaders came together to address the complex
issues of tobacco use among women and young girls. INWAT believes that
"women, working together have the power to challenge the [tobacco] industry
and halt the epidemic." INWAT has members from all continents. It serves
as one of the specialized European networks of the European Network for
Smoking Prevention (ENSP)—an international nonprofit organization that
coordinates tobacco-control efforts throughout Europe. There are also local
INWAT organizations for individual countries.

EMPOWER Methods Used

   ¤ Public education and participation
   ¤ Organizing partnership
   ¤ Empowerment training and leadership development
   ¤ Rights protection and social action/reform

INWAT collaborates on the development of publications regarding women
and tobacco issues. INWAT publishes a newsletter, *The Net*, three times a
year for its international membership. INWAT Europe produces a newsletter

called *Network Europe*, which contains news updates about tobacco policy around the world and progress reports about the organization. INWAT also publishes an annual membership directory to enable members to network and share information. INWAT's website contains statistics about tobacco use around the world and other information relevant to the anti-tobacco movement. INWAT works with other organizations to promote anti-smoking messages. As part of the anti-tobacco community, INWAT supports the development of women-centered tobacco-use prevention and cessation programs and assists in the organization and planning of conferences on tobacco control. As a member of the ENSP, INWAT Europe representatives attend ENSP general meetings. ENSP and INWAT Europe organized a European conference on women and tobacco in November of 1998 that was attended by about 270 delegates from 25 countries. INWAT Europe also co-sponsored an expert seminar in London in July of 1999.

> INWAT promotes female leadership among its members and encourages other anti-tobacco organizations to do the same. At the World Conference on Tobacco or Health in the summer of 2000, INWAT presented its first award for excellence to help support women leadership in tobacco control. In 2015 for the first time more women will die from lung cancer than breast cancer. The second article is about the new Empower publication, a joint project in between WHO Europe and INWAT Europe. The last article is a tribute to Patti White our Board Member one of the 2015 Luther Terry Award winners. (INWAT, 2015)

> In 2015, the INWAT Lifetime Achievement Award has been presented to Professor Lorraine Greaves in recognition of the outstanding international contribution that she has made to tobacco control and women's health, through her work on tobacco and women (INWAT, 2015).

Partners/Opposition

INWAT receives grant funding from the U.S. Centers for Disease Control and Prevention (CDC), which is administered through the American Cancer Society, to maintain its office and distribute materials. INWAT Europe receives small contributions from the European Union as well as support from six participating countries. INWAT members provide their services and support for free.

Macro-environment

The tobacco industry has been targeting women to smoke since the late 1920s, associating women's smoking with freedom and liberation. Over the years, smoking advertisements enticed women and girls to smoke, with images of glamor, beauty, power, thinness, and independence. For example, advertising specifically targeted to young women in the late 1960s and early 1970s was correlated with smoking initiation by young women during the same period. In 1967, smoking initiation in girls under age 18 abruptly increased when tobacco advertising introduced specific brands of cigarettes for women. Some studies have shown that smoking the same number of cigarettes as men, women have higher rates of lung cancer. Girls and women are significantly more likely than boys and men to feel dependent on cigarettes and more likely to report being unable to cut down on smoking.

In the past, women's leadership in the tobacco-control movement was rare. Long-established organizations did not recognize that women's tobacco use was an increasing problem that might require some new approaches, or that women themselves had a serious role in tobacco-control leadership. There has been some progress, but still very few women are involved in tobacco control. This is especially true in continents like in Asia, Africa, and South America, where the smoking epidemic among women has just started.

Impact and Remarks

INWAT gave voice to the women working in the tobacco-control movement and is committed to repairing this problem. Today, women's issues are on the agenda at international conferences on tobacco and health. INWAT members joined committees and planning organizations to make this change happen. In 1998, INWAT had a total of 624 member organizations from 54 countries. INWAT Europe now has more than 20 member countries. By 2014, INWAT had more than doubled in membership to over 1,200 members; most are organizational members although individual membership is allowed (INWAT, 2014).

CASE STUDY #34: INTERNATIONAL PLANNED PARENTHOOD
FEDERATION (IPPF), 1952 (HPDP)

Problem

The major problem being addressed was lack of family planning, and the protection of
Reproductive and sexual rights.

IPPF works in 170 countries to empower the most vulnerable women, men and young people to access life-saving services and programmes, and to live with dignity. Supported by millions of volunteers and 30,000 staff, IPPF Member Associations provide sexual and reproductive health information, education and services through 65,000 service points. Those services include family planning, abortion, maternal and child health, and STI and HIV treatment, prevention and care. (IPPF, 2015a)

Leadership Impetus

Margaret Sanger, pioneer of family planning in the United States in 1921; she subsequently traveled to Bombay, India in 1952 where she and her mostly female colleagues founded the International Planned Parenthood Federation (IPPF). Her colleagues included volunteer leaders of national family planning associations in eight countries—India, Germany, Hong Kong, the Netherlands, Singapore, Sweden, the United Kingdom, and the United States of America. While there, they decided to administer a global program in six major regions of the world. In 1954, Margaret Sanger made a call to "organize the region of the Americas." The founders of the Western Hemisphere Region of the IPPF originated from the Planned Parenthood Federation of America, which was the major family planning organization in the United States. Since its inception, both its membership and financial resources have grown, enabling the IPPF to support its members in developing nations around the globe. The IIPF currently works in 170 countries to empower the most vulnerable women, men, and young people to access life-saving services and programmes, and to live with dignity. It was first formed in 1952 in Bombay, India, at the Third International Conference on Planned Parenthood and now consists of more than 149 Member Associations working in more than 189 countries. (The IPPF is highly developed and organized into six regions. As of 2014, it established 60,000 service points and continues to expand its services to most vulnerable women program; for instance, one of its latest initiative is prevention of mother-to-children transmission of HIV/AIDS in Bangalore, India (IPPF, 2015a).

EMPOWER Methods Used

- ¤ Public education
- ¤ Enabling service and assistance
- ¤ Right protection and social action/reform
- ¤ Organizing partnership

IPPF's member associations provide reproductive health services, including counseling, information, and a choice of family planning methods and providers. They seek to influence the policy-makers to improve national health services. Many work to prepare adolescents for responsible parenthood; others offer such services as infertility treatment, premarital counseling, pregnancy testing and breast and cervical cancer screening. Its stated mission is to improve the quality and reproductive health rights specially for poor and vulnerable people. (IPPF, 2015a)

Partners/Opposition

Because IPPF has "Category I consultative status" at the United Nations, IPPF collaborates with other voluntary, intergovernmental, and UN agencies that are concerned with reproductive health, the health and well-being of women and children, and the role of population in socioeconomic development. Collaborating organizations include the United Nations Population Fund (UNFPA), the United Nations Children's Fund (UNICEF), the WHO, and the World Bank, among many others.

Religious-political groups like Pat Robertson's Christian Coalition or Gary Bauer's Family Research Council want to outlaw abortion, cut public support of family planning, and stop sex education in schools. Abortion clinics and the doctors and staff who perform abortions have increasingly become the target of protest and physical threats.

> Its primary services include: contraception, women's health, sexual rights, youths and adolescents, humanitarian aids, HIV/AIDS, gender equality, and abortion. Within the range of policy analysis and services in these areas, as the excerpts below show, IPPF faces especial challenges in providing beyond health policies and clinical services; it is highly active in areas of promoting sexual rights, reproductive rights and services during humanitarian crises, and comprehensive response to HIV needs in poor and endangered communities education and empowerment supports.
>
> At global, regional and national levels, IPPF persuades governments and decision makers to promote sexual and reproductive health and rights, to change policy and to fund programmes and service delivery.
>
> All humanitarian crises present acute sexual and reproductive health challenges. Of countries worst affected by poor sexual and reproductive health, 9 out of the 10 are in a state of crisis.
>
> IPPF is at the forefront of efforts to ensure that a comprehensive response to HIV is situated within a larger sexual and reproductive health framework. (IPPF, *Our Work*)

Macro-environment

During the time period of the founding of the IPPF, the family planning movement was "an integral part of other movements for human freedom, linked as it was to the abolition of slavery, women's suffrage and attention to women's health" (IPPF Western Hemisphere Region, 1994, p. 9). The reproductive freedom of women made possible through family planning refuted the argument for the reduced position of females in society: that biology destines women to certain societal roles.

Impact and Remarks

> Supported by millions of volunteers and 30,000 staff, IPPF Member Associations provide sexual and reproductive health information, education and services through 65,000 service points. Those services include family planning, abortion, maternal and child health, and STI and HIV treatment, prevention and care. (IPPF, 2014–2015)

The IPPF's 2014–2015 performance report proudly announced:

> 2014 was our third year implementing IPPF's three Change Goals – Unite, Deliver and Perform. We have monitored the trajectory of our growth in performance to date, and are already seeing remarkable success in all three areas, as presented in our Annual Performance Report 2014–2015. Member Associations and collaborative partners in 55 countries contributed to 81 changes in policy or legislation that support or defend sexual and reproductive health and rights. At the regional and global levels, IPPF's advocacy contributed to 18 changes, of which 12 were advances in safeguarding sexual and reproductive health and rights in the post-2015 development framework. With the delivery of 149.3 million services in 2014, we are on track to achieve our ambitious target of doubling the number of sexual and reproductive health services provided between 2010 and 2015. Over eight in ten clients who accessed services were poor and vulnerable, while almost half of our services went to young people. IPPF's achievements in 2014 contribute to a strong performance culture where decisions are based on data, organizational learning happens at all levels, technical support is provided to increase effectiveness, and investments are made to support communities most in need. (IPPF, 2014–2015).

CASE STUDY #42: LA CASA DE LA MUJER, SANTA CRUZ, BOLIVIA, 1990 (HPDP)

Problem

The major problem being addressed was inadequate reproductive healthcare for women in Santa Cruz, Bolivia. Sixty percent of Santa Cruz residents live in poverty.

Leadership Impetus

La Casa de la Mujer was founded by three women in 1990 in order to advance women's health rights. They had been previously involved in a radio program, "Women of the Pueblo," to provide information and education for women and facilitate communication among different groups of women. Radio Santa

Cruz, a Jesuit organization that worked in grassroots education and literacy, sponsored the radio program. Also during this time, the founders were working with Guaraní Indian women to educate them in ecological practices and environmental protection. The organization would defend women's rights, strengthen other women's organizations, and provide opportunities for education and social activities. The Dutch organization HIV Humanistisch Instituut voor Ontwikkelingssamenwerking (HIVOS; International Humanist Institute for Cooperation with Developing Countries) funded the opening of La Casa de la Mujer as a social development organization. La Casa had an auspicious beginning on May 1, 1990 (the International Day of the Worker) when hundreds of women marched through the streets.

EMPOWER Methods Used

- ¤ Enabling service and assistance
- ¤ Public education and participation
- ¤ Media use
- ¤ Empowerment training and leadership development
- ¤ Rights protection and social action/reform
- ¤ Organizing partnership

La Casa focused on three issues: legal rights, sexual education, and labor training. La Casa provided gynecological care by a female doctor, an added incentive to women who were uncomfortable with disclosing female problems to a male doctor. The clinic offered services at hours and costs consistent with client demand. A psychological center offered counseling on family dynamics, depression, and worries or troubles concerning sexuality. La Casa focused on education, information, and empowerment of women, with an emphasis on building women's self-esteem as a foundation for making any behavioral changes. La Casa provided participatory education on reproductive health and sexuality. Games, skits, and other entertaining activities applied sexual issues to the daily lives of women. The activities brought together women of different backgrounds in an open and relaxed atmosphere and enabled the inclusion of men. They included men in educational programs as well. Health workshops conducted in poor neighborhoods targeted parents of children, and domestic workers and students on such topics as ovulation and menstruation, hormones, the female reproductive cycle, male sexual organs, and male hygiene and circumcision. La Casa also published health education materials that promoted participation and creativity on the part of the women and men. La Casa also provided health workers with training in effective communication strategies that put the client at ease when talking about reproductive health. Legal support was provided via La Casa's full-time legal center for women and men with legal problems such as domestic violence or child support. The legal center also ran the Training Center for Domestic Workers, which conducted workshops on legal issues, health, sexuality, and environmental management.

Through marches, petitions, and involvement with the La Casa's Departmental Forum on the law's, La Casa engaged in advocacy for the passage of a law against domestic violence. Through the Departmental Forum on the Environment, La Casa promoted the participation of poor sectors and women in marches and letter-writing campaigns. Through workshops, Pap smear campaigns, and pamphlet distribution, La Casa staff spread the word about the center. La Casa also supported and collaborated with other organizations such as neighborhood committees, parent–teacher associations, student organizations, and mothers' clubs in order to foster community involvement in their environmental program.

Partners/Opposition

Men often oppose sexual education for their wives and daughters because they are afraid the women will become promiscuous or gain a shameful reputation of being promiscuous. If men are resistant to the practices introduced by La Casa, adoption of a practice is less likely. Therefore, the inclusion of men in the learning process is vital to effective change in health behavior. La Casa collaborated with the Ecological Association of Eastern Bolivia (ASEO), the League for Environmental Defense (LIDEMA), and International Habitat.

Macro-environment

Compared to other Bolivian cities, Santa Cruz has the highest contraceptive prevalence rate, the lowest infant mortality rate, and one of the country's lowest maternal mortality ratios. In Santa Cruz, female sexuality tends to be controlled by family, the Roman Catholic Church, and other social institutions. This cultural norm affects the delivery of reproductive health services. Sex education and abortion have been publicly denounced, and reproductive health educators have been ousted from society; doctors and clients of abortion clinics are arrested. Women have expressed fear of seeking help due to these distorted images of reproductive health services as well as rumors that paint doctors as sexually abusive. Cultural norms also affect the practice of interventions. For example, one husband became violent when his wife obtained condoms to space her pregnancies; he assumed she was having sex with another man.

Impact and Remarks

Through its services and opportunities for reproductive health, La Casa built a broad participant base of women from many different sectors of society. Drawing from these women enriched the organization's own development and built relations among women of different social classes. La Casa staff learned to communicate with their clients through experimentation and experience and through the melding of folk-knowledge with academic approaches. By addressing women's short-term reproductive health needs,

La Casa developed empowering strategies for men and women to improve their lives.

CASE STUDY #35: LA LECHE LEAGUE INTERNATIONAL, 1956,
UNITED STATES (HPDP)

Problem

This case study falls within the domain of HPDP. The major problem being addressed was the lack of a support system and information source for breastfeeding mothers. There were many well documented scientific evidence of positive effects of breastfeeding (see Ember & Ember, 2003). And yet:

> At the end of World War II, most women bottle-fed their babies. By the time of La Leche League's founding, the breastfeeding initiation rate in the USA had dropped to 20% of babies. (LLLI, 2015)

Leadership Impetus

For a brief history of LLLI, see http://www.llli.org/lllihistory.html.

Leadership

In 1956, seven women founded La Leche League International (LLLI) after having their own experiences of nursing their own babies (https://en.wikipedia.org/wiki/La_Leche_League_International#History).

La Leche League International is an international, nonprofit, nonsectarian organization dedicated to providing education, information, support, and encouragement to women who want to breastfeed their babies.

EMPOWER Methods Used

- Public education
- Leadership participation
- Enabling services

"The LLLI Peer Counselor Program is designed to teach mothers how to help other mothers learn about breastfeeding. The peer counselors must have breast-fed at least one baby. They are trained to present breastfeeding information in clinics and provide telephone assistance and support to breastfeeding mothers" (LLLI, 2015). For more in-depth information about breastfeeding for health professionals, researchers, breastfeeding counselors, and medical students, La Leche League maintains the Center for Breastfeeding Information, which provides breastfeeding literature, current references, bibliographical lists, and general information. LLLI's Center for Breastfeeding Information (CBI) reports approximately 12,000 full-length studies and more than 200 categories of breastfeeding data; 100 new studies are added each month. LLLI also offers opportunities for both professional and lay instruction in breastfeeding management, lactation, and counseling. The Lactation Specialist Workshops provide Continuing Education Recognition Points (CERP) hours and continuing education credits for lactation consultants, nurses, LLL Leaders, and others who work with breastfeeding mothers. Co-sponsored by La Leche League International, the American Academy of Pediatrics, the American College of Obstetricians and Gynecologists, and the American Academy of Family Physicians, LLLI's Physician Seminars are offered throughout the world for physicians, lactation consultants, and other lactation professionals. LLLI's book *The Womanly Art of Breastfeeding* is published in eight languages and in Braille, and has sold over 2.5 million copies since the first edition was published in 1958. The telephone hotline 1-800-LA LECHE receives approximately 2,000 calls each month. This hotline provides telephone counseling 24 hours a day. LLLI holds an annual international conference which, in 1997, attracted more than 4,000 attendees from around the world. In 2016, LLLI will celebrate its 60th birthday. For historical developments and key events including conferences and the LLLI, visit its homepage: LLLI (2015).

Partners/Opposition

Macro-environment

In the United States, numerous states have enacted breastfeeding legislation, touching on the issues of nursing in public, working and breastfeeding, and jury duty while breastfeeding. Despite the health benefits that breastfeeding provides, some societies' attitudes toward breastfeeding are diverse and slow to change. Breastfeeding also provides economic benefits to society. For example, hundreds of millions of dollars continue to be spent by the U.S. government to purchase artificial baby milk. Yet studies show that millions of dollars could be saved if more women made this healthy choice—from healthcare savings to food packaging costs. In addition, employers have recognized the benefit of supporting breastfeeding among their employees due to the fact that a healthier baby results in the mother missing less time from work. In fact, over the past few years, more and more companies have installed breast pump rooms and looked at how the mother's schedule can be arranged to provide sufficient time to pump.

Impact and Remarks

Since its beginning LLLI has served a unique function through its lay volunteers who provide mother-to-mother information and support in breastfeeding and mothering. Through their dedicated work, the LLLI earned considerable credibility. LLLI is accredited by the U.S.'s Accreditation Council for Continuing Medical Education to sponsor continuing education for physicians. Soon its reputation and influence spread internationally:

> In 1981 LLLI was granted consultative status with the United Nations Children's Fund (UNICEF). In 1985 LLLI served on the International Board of Lactation Consultant Examiners, established to develop and

administer a voluntary certification program for lactation consultants. The first IBLCE exam was administered in July 1985.

Early in the organization's history, local newspapers rejected meeting notices that used the words breastfed and breastfeeding, calling them inappropriate for family publications. The name comes from the Spanish word, *leche* (pronounced "leh-cheh") meaning *milk*. It was inspired by a shrine in St. Augustine, Florida, dedicated to *Nuestra Señora de la Leche y Buen Parto*, meaning "Our Lady of Happy Delivery and Plentiful Milk."

In 1997, LLLI held its 25th Annual Seminar for Physicians, co-sponsored by the American Academy of Pediatrics and the American College of Obstetrics and Gynecologists. LLLI maintains consultative status with the United Nations Children's Fund (UNICEF), unofficial working relations with the WHO, acts as a registered Private Voluntary Organization (PVO) for the Agency of International Development (USAID), is an accredited member of the US Healthy Mothers/Healthy Babies Coalition, and is a founding member of the World.

Alliance for Breastfeeding Action (WABA). LLLI's board of directors has members from seven countries. The eight edition of this book **was** 2010 National Bestseller & 2012 Readers' Choice Award Winner. (LLLI, 2012, 2015)

These excerpts were taken from LLLI's website (LLLI, 2012).

CASE STUDY #57: MADD (MOTHERS AGAINST DRUNK DRIVING), UNITED STATES, 1980 (HPDP)

Problem

The major problem addressed was the high rate of fatalities and injuries caused by drunk drivers. Drunk driving is the United States' most frequently committed violent crime.

CAR CRASHES ARE THE LEADING CAUSE OF DEATH FOR TEENS, AND ABOUT A QUARTER OF THOSE CRASHES INVOLVE AN UNDERAGE DRINKING DRIVER.

National Highway Traffic Safety Administration. "Traffic Safety Facts 2011: Overview". Washington DC: National Highway Traffic Safety Administration, 2013. and National Highway Traffic Safety Administration. "Traffic Safety Facts 2011: Young Drivers". Washington DC: National Highway Traffic Safety Administration, 2013.

KIDS WHO START DRINKING YOUNG ARE SEVEN TIMES MORE LIKELY TO BE IN AN ALCOHOL- RELATED CRASH.

Hingson, Ralph, et al. "Age of Drinking Onset, Driving After Drinking, and Involvement in Alcohol- Related Motor Vehicle Crashes." DOT HS 809 188. Washington, DC: National Highway Traffic Safety Administration, January 2001.

Leadership Impetus

Mothers Against Drunk Driving (MADD) was founded in California in 1980 by Candy Lightner, the mother of 13-year-old girl who was killed by a repeat-offender drunk driver, along with seven of her concerned friends and mothers. Shortly thereafter, through California Assemblyman Robert Matsui, Lightner came into contact with Cindi Lamb. After her own daughter was paralyzed by a repeat drunk driver in 1979; Lamb and a few friends waged a "war" against drunk driving in Lamb's home state of Maryland. Together, Lightner and Lamb transformed MADD into the leading anti–drunk driving, nonprofit, grassroots organization in the nation and world. The major impetus was their outrage at the lax enforcement of laws on driving under the influence. In both women's cases, the accidents were caused by repeat offenders. In Lightner's case, the hit-and-run driver had three previous drunk driving arrests and two convictions. He plea-bargained to a charge of vehicular manslaughter and was sentenced to two years in prison, but was allowed by the judge to serve time in a work camp and later a halfway house (MADD35).

EMPOWER Methods Used

- ¤ Public education and participation
- ¤ Media use
- ¤ Enabling service and assistance
- ¤ Rights protection
- ¤ Social action for legal activism

In addition to activist efforts, MADD has provided support to victims of alcohol-related auto accidents and their families. For example, MADD started a victim hotline so that victims and families could speak to trained staff for information and emotional support. In addition, many chapters provided victim support groups and a range of victim support literature. Candlelight vigils were held each year to allow victims to share their pain with others. MADD also established youth programs at schools such as the MADD Poster Essay Contest, and raised public awareness through programs such as the "Designated Driver" program and "Project Red Ribbon" as well as through print and broadcast media such as the *MADD in Action* newsletter. In March 1983, a made-for-television film about MADD was produced by NBC, and its outpouring of responses from the audience led to the founding of 122 chapters in 35 states. Over 70,000 more members across the nation were attracted by a direct mail program.

Today, MADD's National Programs Department specializes in developing and maintaining public awareness programs at the chapter, state, and national levels, involving the community as a whole in supporting MADD's mission. MADD has several youth programs, including a student activist training program that increases knowledge about traffic safety issues and encourages high school students to become agents for social change in their local communities. At local chapters, victim advocates inform victims about criminal justice procedures and accompany them to court, help them apply for Crime Victims Compensation funds, or address other personal concerns of the victims. The MADD newsletter—*Driven*—informs the public of current activities, policy issues, and the latest statistics.

Partners/Opposition

MADD attributes its success to its name, timing, and extensive media coverage, beginning with television coverage of the congressional testimony by the victims' mothers. By the end of 1981, 11 chapters in four states were established and had raised an income of $500,000, a $65,000 grant from the National Highway Safety Administration for chapter development, a $100,000 grant from the Leavy Foundation (whose principal benefactor was an insurance company heiress whose daughter was slain by a drunk driver), as well as donations from the general public. By the fall of 1982, 70 chapters were established.

In collaboration with the National Endowment for Financial Education (NEFE), MADD prepared a series of brochures, *Picking Up the Financial Pieces*, which were also posted on the Internet. MADD also teamed up with corporate sponsors to develop anti–drunk-driving projects. For example, Allstate was a sponsor of MADD's "Tie One On For Safety" red ribbon campaign. The company provided assistance in advertising and public relations, distributed millions of red MADD ribbons, sponsored a public opinion survey on drunk driving, and helped raise awareness through speeches and media events.

Macro-environment

Alcohol-related crashes continue to be a major cause of total traffic fatalities. The National Highway Traffic Safety Administration (NHTSA) estimates that about three in every five Americans will be involved in an alcohol-related crash at some time in their lives. Economic costs of alcohol-related crashes are estimated to be $45 billion yearly. An additional $70.5 billion is lost in quality of life due to these crashes (MADD website). According to the NHTSA, during the period 1982 through 1997, approximately 333,586 persons lost their lives in alcohol-related traffic crashes (Lord, 1990).

Impact and Remarks

As the MADD organization grew, a new executive director, Dr. Phillips Roos, and 11 staff members were hired and the headquarters moved to its current location in Texas. By 1984, MADD had over 350 chapters; and today, there are more than 600 chapters and community action teams nationwide. Since the founding of MADD, many goals have been reached, including: providing victim assistance services, raising public awareness, as well as several legislative changes. For example, since 1980, more than 2,300 anti-drunk driving laws have been enacted nationwide, most notably the "Age 21 Law" that has been adopted in all 50 states, and the administrative license revocation laws that allow the suspension of licenses of drivers who fail a blood alcohol test. Today, MADD continues to focus on effective solutions for drunk driving and underage drinking as well as providing victim assistance (Lord, 1990).

> Over the years, MADD has been instrumental in getting drunk driving laws passed and the legal acceptable blood alcohol level reduced. By 1982, more stringent DUI laws were introduced in 35 states and passed by 24 states. A year later, 129 new DUI laws had passed, and the snowball effect continued. They also got the support of the federal government for raising the legal drinking age to 21, and in 1983 President Reagan signed the Uniform Drinking Age Act into law. In 2000, after years of lobbying, President Clinton signed legislation that would effectively lower the legal blood alcohol level in the US to .08. (MAAD, 2015)

In 2015, MADD continued its persistent and resilient movement against drunk driving repention movement.

> As a test of its resiliency and its commitment to its mission, MADD has dealt daily with vocal opponents, including individuals and industries unsupportive of the policies that MADD has pursued. When facing unrelenting opposition on the 21 drinking age and .08 laws, for example, MADD could have simply given up, buckling under the pressure. Instead, MADD fought hard and won. And the organization has been instrumental in passing policies that save thousands of lives every year. In the process, MADD has earned the well deserved reputation as an organization that would not be swayed from its goals. (MADD, 2015)

> By 1988, all states had set 21 as the minimum drinking age. Since that time, the 21 minimum drinking age law has saved about 900 lives per year as estimated by the National Traffic Highway Administration (NHTSA). In short, there are more than 25,000 people alive today because of the 21 minimum drinking age law in every state. Additionally, underage drinking rates also fell and continue to fall. From 1991 to the present, annual use of alcohol among 8th, 10th, and 12th graders has dropped 56%, 33%, and 18%, respectively. (MADD35).

CASE STUDY #36: FAMILY PLANNING MOTHERS' CLUBS,
SOUTH KOREA, 1968 (HPDP)

Problem

The major problem being addressed was lack of family planning practice in rural areas of South Korea.

Leadership Impetus

In 1968, the Planned Parenthood Federation of Korea (PPFK) organized Family Planning Mothers' Clubs in rural villages throughout the country. PPFK recruited 139 county field officers to work in county health centers to guide and promote the Mothers' Clubs in each county. In the first year, 12,650 Mothers' Clubs were organized. Membership was open to all married women in the village, aged 20 to 45 (Park, 1974; Park et al., 1976).

EMPOWER Methods Used

- ¤ Enabling service and assistance
- ¤ Public education and participation
- ¤ Work/job training and micro-enterprise
- ¤ Organizing partnership
- ¤ Empowerment training and leadership development

The Mothers' Clubs served as a source of information, education, and motivation for family planning among Korean villages. According to the PPFK's memorandum,

> the objectives of the Mothers' Club shall be to promote the practice of family planning for the improvement of motherhood and the planned family life; to spread family planning to become a normal part of everyday life; to develop a cooperative spirit among the members; and to urge active participation in community development to enhance productivity and to create optimal surroundings. (Park, 1974).

The chairperson of the club would also distribute pills and condoms to the members. Many of the clubs operated a Mothers' Bank that was financed by "rice savings" and income-generating projects. Club members would save a spoonful of rice from every meal to sell for profit. The money earned would then be deposited in the Mothers' Bank each month. The accumulated earnings were used to fund both club and community activities, including welfare programs for the villagers and community, and scholarships for students who wanted to pursue a higher education but could not afford it. Members also established cooperative stores where members could buy food, fuel, and other necessities at lower cost. PPFK conducted leadership and management training to improve the club leaders' skills. These training courses, which lasted from one day to one week, also provided the leaders with information on population and family planning as well as ideas for new community projects. Similar training sessions were offered to club members.

Partners/Opposition

The PPFK provided invaluable assistance in establishing and maintaining the Mothers' Clubs. It provided financial assistance to help cover the expenses of the monthly meetings. PPFK county field officers offered advice and technical assistance to club leaders in the management of the clubs, program development, and education of members. Health personnel and field workers of the local government also provided assistance to the Mothers' Clubs efforts. In order to acknowledge the hard work of the Mothers' Clubs, PPFK and government fieldworkers would annually assess their progress in areas of club management, family planning activities and practice rate, community development projects, mothers' banks, and income generation. Exemplary clubs were given awards from the Minister of Health and Social Affairs, provincial governors, and the PPFK president for outstanding work.

There was initial opposition to the Mothers' Clubs by men, especially village elders. However, as the Mothers' Clubs continued to demonstrate their dedication to improving the lives of women in particular and the village communities in general, the communities began to rally behind them. The members who were hostile to the club at the initial stage became sympathetic supporters. In some villages, men were proud of their wives' efforts in transforming the community.

Macro-environment

At the time of the Mothers' Clubs founding, open discussions of family matters were considered taboo. Abiding by a Confucian code of ethics, Korean society is male-dominated, with women having lower status. Women were traditionally limited to housekeeping and caring for children in their roles as wife and mother. The Korean family functioned as a way to pass down the family line from father to first-born son. The female was expected to marry early and bear at least one son to carry on the family name. As socioeconomic development continued, Korean women gained more responsibility and status within the family structure. The Mothers' Club movement helped advance women's position in society (Park, 1974).

Impact and Remarks

After its first year, about 2,000 clubs were organized each year following. Following the inception of Mothers' Clubs in Korea, the family planning practice rate increased from 25% in 1968 to 44.2% in 1976. The population growth rate dropped from 2.35% to 1.7% during that same period. In 1976, family planning Mothers' Clubs joined with other organizations at the village level to form the Saemaul Women's Associations. Since that time, the Mothers' Clubs have been formally known as the Family Planning Department of the Saemaul Women's Association.

Mothers' Clubs' community development work had a tremendous impact on many villages. Infrastructural changes included widening and straightening of village roads, planting of flowerbeds along roadsides, remodeling of public wells, installation of water supply systems, improvement of drainage systems, and planting of chestnut trees. Mothers' Clubs' efforts also had an economic impact on the villages. Cooperative shops were opened at village entrances. The mothers' banks enabled the villagers to carry out bigger projects such as the installation of electricity systems and the construction of bridges and village halls.

In addition to these objective measures of success, participants in the Mothers' Clubs reaped many personal or intangible benefits. Many of the cooperative activities performed by the Mothers' Clubs instilled a sense of solidarity and pride in the members. Club leaders gained valuable administrative skills, while members benefited from the various club programs. The Mothers' Clubs' success in their community development activities also earned them the respect and appreciation of the village people, which in turn boosted the morale of the village people to improve their way of living. Through all these successes, the Mothers' Clubs movement helped improve the status of women in Korean society by proving their worth and value within the village communities. Men who at first opposed women's participation in family planning activities and community development were now acknowledging the efforts of women and their role in improving the quality of life of their villages.

CASE STUDY #74: MOTHERS' VOICES UNITED TO END AIDS (GEORGIA)

Problem

The major problems being addressed were the lack of AIDS research, funding, and prevention education, and the lack of opportunities for mothers of HIV-infected individuals to participate in AIDS prevention-advocacy efforts. Several mothers' groups organized to raise their voices to prevent HIV/ADS and more humane treatment of those inflicted with HIV/AIDS; in addition, groups of concerned and distinguished citizens also raised their voice against inadequate and often misleading information given out to victims and high-risk populations (McCaffey, 1999).

Leadership Impetus

In 1991, five individuals united to provide information about the AIDS crisis to the public and to provide mutual support to each other as mothers and relatives of HIV-infected individuals. The founders designed a Mother's Day card and distributed it to hundreds of organizations. The card read: "On this Mother's Day help us fight for what we care most about in our lives, the health and well-being of our children. ... It's time to find a cure!" After receiving letters and unsolicited financial support from thousands of individuals all over the country, Mothers' Voices was launched in a restaurant in lower Manhattan. Over 200 women vowed to establish a constituency of mothers to work for increased government funding for AIDS education, research, prevention, treatment, and a cure.

EMPOWER Methods Used

- ¤ Rights protection and social action/reform
- ¤ Public education and participation
- ¤ Empowerment training and leadership development
- ¤ Media use
- ¤ Enabling service and assistance
- ¤ Organizing partnership

Mothers' Voices, the only national, grassroots, nonprofit organization that mobilized mothers as educators and advocates for sexual health and HIV prevention, was created in 1991. The organization's intent was to "[harness] the power of mothers to stop the AIDS epidemic" (MVG).

Other award-winning programs include:

- ¤ For RealYouth
- ¤ HIV/STD public advocacy and health literacy.
- ¤ Women of the Village, a talent pool of dynamic, innovative skilled women professionals who donate a portion of their proceeds to the vision, mission and work of MV-Georgia. Visit our powerful circle of women (http://www.mvgeorgia.org/)

Mothers' Voices provided critical resources to help mothers educate their children about sexuality, drug use, and HIV prevention. *Listen to Mothers' Voices* was the Mothers' Voices national newsletter that was published two times a year. It provided the latest information to 40,000 individuals and organizations about HIV-prevention strategies, AIDS research, and education and policy initiatives. Suggested actions to press elected officials for increased funding were also provided in the newsletter. The Mothers' Voices Website gave access to information on the organization's missions, programs, HIV/AIDS facts, and links to other HIV-related sites. Mothers' Voices' messages were carried in the *New York Times, Good Housekeeping, Redbook,*

Prevention, the *New York Daily News, POZ Magazine, AIDS Treatment News,* the *Oprah Winfrey Show, CBS This Morning,* the *Sally Jesse Raphael Show, Atlanta Journal-Courier,* and the *Miami Herald.*

Partners/Opposition

Mothers' Voices participated in such AIDS organizations as the AIDS Research Task Force of National Organizations Responding to AIDS (NORA); the National Coalition to Support Sexuality Education (NCSSE); and the National Coalition to Save Lives Now.

Mothers' Voices also provided grants for research and education to the Pediatric AIDS Foundation, Cold Spring Harbor Laboratory; North Shore University Hospital's Peer to Peer Education Programs, and other AIDS/ HIV-related activities.

Macro-environment

Social stigma, ignorance about HIV/AIDS, and lack of availability of affordable of HIV/AIDS treatment required open discussion and dissemination of information and treatment services. Mothers' Voices became a powerful advocate and source of education.

Impact and Remarks

Mothers' Voices currently has five chapters in Atlanta, Miami, Houston, Los Angeles, and Chicago; 12 advocacy districts; and over 40,000 mothers and supporters from around the nation. In 1994, the Mothers' Day card campaign garnered 250,000 individual signatures that were delivered in a petition to Congress, calling for greater federal commitment. In 1995, the campaign reached 95% of the congressional districts. The first luncheon grew to an annual awards event that was attended by approximately 1,000 mothers and supporters in the spring of 1996. Mothers' Voices received special recognition from the American Foundation for AIDS Research, the AIDS Action Council, and City of San Francisco. Mothers' Voices expanded the scope of their organization to include all parents or guardians as educators and advocates for HIV prevention. While this movement began primarily with mothers, their supporters grew to include fathers, guardians, grandparents, aunts, uncles, etc. Campaigns designed to involve mothers against various threats including HIV/AIDS continue to gain momentum (Engle, 2002). In 2002, Engle describes Mother's Voice outreach and educational program at length; the quotation below:

> Mothers' Voices publishes a 36-page handbook, available in English and Spanish, designed to help parents communicate with their children about their sexual health in developmentally appropriate stages. The content is similar to that contained in the one-hour seminars. Through self-administered quizzes, parents are encouraged to examine their own values

and their own preconceptions and prejudices, and are helped to recognize opportunities to talk with their children in age-appropriate ways about delicate subjects. The developmental stages of childhood are outlined in simple terms, with an emphasis on what to expect of infants, toddlers, preschoolers, early school-age children, preteens, and teenagers and beyond. (Engle, 2002)

CASE STUDY #78: NATIONAL ALLIANCE FOR THE MENTALLY ILL (NAMI), UNITED STATES, 1979 (HPDP)

Problem

The major problem being addressed was the lack of advocacy and support for care givers and families of mentally ill individuals.

Leadership Impetus

Two mothers of mentally ill sons, Harriet Shetler and Bev Young, founded NAMI (the National Alliance for the Mentally Ill) in 1979 in Madison, Wisconsin. The women had met for lunch in 1977 after being introduced by a church acquaintance. After discovering that they shared similar fears and experiences in dealing with the stigma of mental illness, Shetler and Young forged a grassroots, family mental health advocacy movement that challenged public policy and popular awareness. NAMI's official inception began with a meeting of 254 persons in Madison, Wisconsin, who began to consider how to help themselves and their mentally ill relatives. Although there were a number of concerned and caring professionals and providers in attendance, the founders were determined to make NAMI an organization governed for and by families and healthcare professionals.

EMPOWER Methods Used

- ¤ Public education and participation
- ¤ Enabling service and assistance
- ¤ Organizing partnership
- ¤ Media use and advocacy.

NAMI is a grassroots, self-help support and advocacy organization of families and friends of people with serious mental illness, and those persons themselves. NAMI's mission is to eradicate mental illness and to improve the quality of life for those who suffer from "no-fault" brain diseases such as schizophrenia, depression and manic depression, schizoaffective disorder, panic disorder, obsessive-compulsive disorder, and borderline personality disorder. In order to achieve NAMI's mission, the organization is built on four cornerstones: support, education, advocacy, and research. Shetler and Young's first efforts were dedicated to connecting the existing independent parent groups throughout the country that had formed to provide solace and basic information to relatives of individuals with severe mental illness. By 1980, NAMI had achieved incorporation, received nonprofit tax-exempt status, and elected an initial board of directors. NAMI's board of directors consists only of family members and consumers. However, mental health professionals may become associate members. NAMI also runs a hotline for people with questions about mental illness. Callers have included consumers, parents, spouses, siblings, or children of persons with mental illness; professionals; students; and teachers. Approximately 50 trained volunteers monitor the phone lines, answer questions, and provide phone numbers of the nearest NAMI affiliate. Celebrities such as Diana Ross and Larry King; magazines such as *Parade, U.S. News and World Report, Time, Reader's Digest, Ladies Home Journal, Essence, Family Circle, Self, YM,* and *Sassy*; television programs; and other media sources recommend the NAMI hotline to those in need of information.

In 1982, NAMI opened its first office in Washington, DC, in 1982 in order to focus its efforts on influencing Congress, the president, and key decision-makers. NAMI provided the previously absent voice of the caring families and consumers in a field long dominated by physicians and other professionals and service providers. NAMI demanded accountability from the government, which was not making a significant investment in either research or services focused on mental illnesses. NAMI also enlisted politicians, some with mentally ill relatives in their own families, to herald NAMI's cause. The "Campaign to End Discrimination" was a five-year, nationwide effort to end discrimination against people with severe mental illnesses. NAMI also conducted the Program of Assertive Community Treatment (PACT) Across America initiative. Although 25 years of research support PACT's superior effectiveness over office-based traditional mental health care, few persons with the most devastating and chronic mental illness can access this type of community-based care.

> Despite the documented treatment success of PACT, only a fraction of those with the greatest needs have access to this uniquely effective program. Only six states (DE, FL, MI, NJ, RI, TX) and the District of Columbia currently have statewide PACT programs. Many more states have at least one or more PACT programs in some parts of their state. In the United States, adults with severe and persistent mental illnesses constitute one-half to one percent of the adult population. It is estimated that 10 percent to 20 percent of this group could be helped by the PACT model if it were available. (NAMI, 2012).

NAMI has its own communications services department that is available to the news media around the clock. It provides expert analysis on a wide range of issues related to severe mental illnesses; current data on research, treatments, and rates of prevalence; interviews with national spokespersons, technical experts, and persons with serious mental illness and their families;

and comments on breaking news. NAMI regularly produces press releases and maintains a Press Room site on their web page.

Partners/Opposition

NAMI affiliates work jointly with members of the American Psychiatric Association to mount Mental Illness Awareness Week. In 1998, the executive directors of NAMI and the National Association of Social Workers (NASW) formed an agreement to increase professional membership in NAMI from members of the social work community. NAMI is supported financially primarily through contributions of members. Less than 2% of NAMI funding comes from the government. Some critics believe NAMI has a narrow focus, in terms of advocating for expanded insurance coverage, on severe brain-based disorders and excluding other diseases with strong environmental components, such as post-traumatic stress disorder. However since narrower insurance coverage is less expensive and more palatable from a political perspective, NAMI continue to limit their efforts to severe biological illnesses in adult patients.

Macro-environment

In the United States, there are about 8 million people afflicted with severe mental illnesses. Schizophrenia strikes over 1% of the total population; depressive illness disables 5%–7%. Mental illness is more common than multiple sclerosis, muscular dystrophy, cystic fibrosis, Alzheimer's disease, leukemia, and many other more widely known and supported illnesses. Although, severe mental illnesses can strike anyone at any time, most often severe mental illnesses are diagnosed in young people between the ages of 16 and 25. From the beginning, NAMI was focused on the unmet needs of people suffering from the severest and most disabling forms of mental illness—schizophrenia and manic-depressive illness and severe depression. These individuals are most in need of long-term help and support. Severe mental illnesses were highly stigmatized in most societies; for decades parents were blamed as the cause of their relatives' mental disorder. One-third of the homeless population is composed of mentally ill persons who do not have adequate resources for mental health care. Between 40% and 60% of all persons with a severe mental illness are living at home with their families, often without adequate services. Caregivers and family members need support needed to care for the mentally ill.

Impact and Remarks

As of 2012, a total of 116 VA hospitals and medical centers in 46 states were hosting NAMI education classes for families of veterans in just the second year of this rapidly increasing initiative. In 2011, over 135,000 people walked in 84 "NAMIwalks" events across the country; it trained and certified over 1,500 volunteer teachers who educated over 12,500 new families and individuals through peer-led programs; family-to-family became an evidence-based program. Under their family-to-family program, a family with experience in giving care to mentally ill person/s acts as a "peer" counselor/educator assigned to a family without such experience. In 2011, it trained over 2,000 new volunteers and distributed more than 500,000 brochures for mental illness education of the public. NAMI families find courage and hope in "Family to Family" education and support programs. NAMI has over 1,000 state and local affiliates and over 185,000 members. NAMI also has affiliates in Puerto Rico and Canada and has helped Australia, Japan, and the Ukraine to start sister organizations. Most notably, the American Institute of Philanthropy (AIP), the nations' leading charity watchdog, awarded NAMI with an A-plus rating for its cost-effective charitable spending and fund-raising practices. According to Dr. Steven Hyman, director of the National Institute of Mental Health, NAMI is the "greatest single advocacy force [in mental health] and in some ways, [they] have greater moral authority than the professional societies" (http:www.schizophrenia.com/; NAMI, 2012).

CASE STUDY #64: NARIKA, BERKELEY, CALIFORNIA, 1992

Problem

Narika addressed domestic abuse of South Asian women and children in the San Francisco Bay area. Mainstream shelters did not always take into account the cultural and language barriers faced by South Asian women. Its website says:

> Narika's toll-free Helpline (1-800-215-7308) enables any individual who has been a victim of domestic violence to call in and speak to any one of our sensitive and knowledgeable advocates. (http://www.narika.org/)

Leadership Impetus

In 1992, a group of six women founded Narika to establish a helpline for abused women of South Asian origin (India, Pakistan, Bangladesh, Sri Lanka, Nepal, Sikkim, and Bhutan). Because of the many battered women were seeking help in informal ways, the founders decided to direct their energies into setting up a structure for serving domestic violence victims. These included women who were battered by their husband or partner; who were being harassed or stalked by an ex-husband or ex-partner; who witnessed domestic violence between their parents; who grew up in violent, abusive homes; who were abused by their parents and/or siblings; who were abused by their in-laws or being pressured into arranged marriages; who were abandoned, divorced, or widowed; whose children had witnessed maternal abuse; who were victims of rape or date rape; and women dealing issues of cultural identity, sexual identity, and intergenerational conflicts.

EMPOWER Methods Used

- ¤ Enabling service and assistance
- ¤ Public education and participation
- ¤ Organizing partnership

Narika provided advocacy, support, information, help, and referrals to women and children in abusive situations through its toll-free helpline. The multilingual/-cultural volunteers and staff did not give professional advice but offered "a sisterly ear," providing the information women needed to make their own decisions. They spoke Hindi, Tamil, Malayalam, Gujarati, Konkani, Kannada, Telegu, Sinhala, Bengali, Urdu, and Punjabi. The helpline advocates offered an opportunity for women to talk about their situation, express their feelings, and discuss their options without fear of shame or criticism. Narika offered referrals to shelters, medical clinics, legal services, counseling services, and agencies offering immigration advice to victims of domestic violence. It also provided advocacy and assistance to abused women dealing with social service and legal agencies, and help with translation and/or interpretation services.

Narika provided community education on domestic violence targeting schools or factories where there was a concentration of South Asian women workers. Speakers spoke on the issue of domestic violence and resources available. Narika also provided consultations and training to police, probation officers, legal agencies, and medical and mental health professionals about domestic violence issues in the South Asian community so that these service providers were better able to serve South Asian women. Narika also had a youth outreach program that targeted South Asian youth, both male and female.

Partners/Opposition

Narika collaborated regularly with three other agencies in the San Francisco Bay Area: the Asian Women's Shelter, Nihonmachi Legal Outreach, and Cameron House. Narika would often refer their callers to seek refuge at the Asian Women's Shelter or seek legal aid at the Nihonmachi Legal Outreach. In collaboration with these three agencies, Narika held the first-ever conference on Asians and domestic violence. These four agencies also collaborated on the youth risk prevention (adolescents and youths involved in problems that require health or legal help) program and public education. Narika also worked with religious leaders and other community leaders to enlist their support in educating the public about domestic violence. The Department of Health Services, California Endowment, Bank of America Foundation, Cirrus Logic, Vanguard Foundation, Raj Kaur Rekhi Memorial Fund, Kisknan-Shah Family Foundation, Jain Foundation, and numerous individual donors provided financial support for Narika. At the time of Narika's inception, there was the usual divide in the South Asian community with the progressives (both men and women) supporting the organization and the traditional members of the community (men and women) opposing its existence. The detractors were not organized or active; opponents would not take the organization seriously, viewing it as a group formed by Americanized women. Narika focused its efforts to work and collaborate with allies rather than identify its "enemies."

Macro-environment

South Asian women face language and cultural barriers in attempting to use the resources available to them in mainstream domestic violence shelters. Aside from the obvious barrier of speaking a different language, a woman may feel more comfortable speaking in her native language on such emotional and personal issues as domestic abuse even if she speaks English fluently. On the other hand, a South Asian woman may feel reluctant to disclose personal matters to a member of her own (often close-knit) community for fear of gossip, rumors, or shunning. The threats or type of abuse perpetrated may also differ for South Asian women than for American-born women. For example, a husband may threaten the women with deportation or shaming her within the (often close-knit) ethnic community or cutting her off from financial resources.

Impact and Remarks

Approximately 200 new individuals would call Narika each year, in addition to the women seeking continued support from Narika. There was increased awareness of domestic violence and the resources available to its victims, and increased exposure to anti–domestic violence messages within the South Asian community. Narika had a positive impact on its target population. They conducted outreach in rural areas in order to encourage and assist community members set up their own services for domestic violence victims. Its groundbreaking conference on domestic violence in 2009 in Asian communities was attended by approximately 350 people and covered by the media (Narika, 2009). Narika's policy and philosophy was based on the empowerment of women. Advocates encouraged women to make their own decisions based on the information and resources available to them. Narika provided that sense of permission to do what was best for them.

CASE STUDY #48: NATIONAL BLACK WOMEN'S HEALTH PROJECT, UNITED STATES, 1981 (HPDP)

Problem

The major problem being addressed was the lack of public discussion, organization, and advocacy around such issues as domestic violence, breast cancer, abortion, and class division within the black community.

Black Women's Health Imperative, previously the National Black Women's Health Project', was formed in 1984 in Atlanta, Georgia out of a need to address the health and reproductive rights of African American women. NBWHP was principally founded by Byllye Avery. Avery was involved in reproductive healthcare work in Gainesville, Florida in the 1970s and was particularly influenced by the impact that policy had on women of color and poor women. Additionally Avery was also concerned with healthcare choices and wanted "to provide an environment where women could feel comfortable and take control of their own health. (NBWHP, 2015)

Leadership Impetus

In 1981, health activist Byllye Avery founded the National Black Women's Health Project (NBWHP) as a pilot program of the National Women's Health Network. The mission of this organization was to improve the health of black women through education and advocacy. The organization provided a forum for black women to discuss domestic violence, incest, breast cancer, abortion, obesity, and class division—issues that were not commonly talked about among black women at that time. Avery developed self-help groups as a way to help women address their own personal issues. In 1984, NBWHP was incorporated as a nonprofit organization.

EMPOWER Methods Used

- Enabling service and assistance
- Public education and participation
- Rights protection and social action/reform
- Empowerment training and leadership development
- Organizing partnership

The work of the NBWHP was at three levels: individual and group; community (by influencing local health policies); and national (by influencing policy-makers and the public). In 1990, NBWHP established the Public Education and Public Policy Program office in Washington, D.C., to ensure that black women were represented in federal policy decisions. This office also provided technical assistance and support to local activists on health and reproductive rights. It also served as an information clearinghouse on black women's health issues. The Walking for Wellness Program, created in 1992, was a "walking and talking" exercise program for black women and their families. Walks took place at parks, malls, or recreation centers. Through this program, NBWHP collaborated with the American Heart Association, the National Council of Black Mayors, *Prevention Magazine,* *Essence Magazine,* and the Black Nurses Association. The Walking for

Wellness Program was featured in several magazines, such as *Heart and Soul, Essence, Prevention,* the *New Age Journal, Walking,* and *Runner's World.* In 1995, NBWHP published and distributed an orientation and training manual for new participants. An Annual Walk for Wellness was held at the NBWHP's Annual Conference in 2014 (http://lifebalanceconference.com/).

In 1989, NBWHP created SisteReach—an international program that worked with black women's organizations in Nigeria, Cameroon, Brazil, and the Caribbean. The program provided technical assistance to women in developing countries who were trying to improve women's lives. It also promoted awareness of the health status of women of African descent and strove to link groups in the United States with those abroad. The Substance Abuse Prevention program developed self-help and policy advocacy groups in seven historically black colleges and universities in Tennessee, Louisiana, Maryland, and North Carolina. African-American college women were trained on drug and alcohol abuse prevention issues. The program also developed a monitoring program for at-risk community youth as well as linkages between the college students and community women in order to mobilize advocacy for substance abuse prevention.

After 1983, NBWHP convened national conferences for the improvement of the health of black women both nationally and internationally. The First National Conference on Black Women's Health Issues in 1983 brought together more than 1,500 women from throughout the United States and the Caribbean and from various socioeconomic backgrounds.

The Self-Help Group and Chapter Development program was the primary organizing tool of NBWHP activities. It gave members a forum to deal with their personal health issues with the help of other members. The facilitators of the self-help groups and chapters met each year at the Annual Self-Help Developers Meeting/Leadership Development Institute. NBWHP developed audiovisual and other written materials in order to raise awareness among NBWHP members and the general public of the major health challenges facing black women. For example, there was a self-help developer's manual, a video on gynecological self-examinations for mothers and daughters, and a black women's guide to physical and emotional health. Membership in NBWHP was open to individuals and organization that supported NBWHP's mission. Members received policy updates and newsletters focusing on health issues affecting black women, and NBWHP activities.

Partners/Opposition

NBWHP received financial support from a number of progressive foundations and funders. For example, NBWHP worked with local and national agencies on some of their program activities, such as the Walking for Wellness collaboration with the American Heart Association (mentioned above). In order to tackle the problem of poor health outcomes among black women, NBWHP built coalitions with like-minded organizations.

Macro-environment

Poverty, racism, fragmented health and social delivery systems, overcrowded schools, drug abuse, crime, and other social ills plagued the black community and other people of color. Yet, at the time of NBWHP's inception, such issues as domestic violence, abortions, and breast cancer as they affected black women's were not widely discussed.

Impact and Remarks

In 1988, NBWHP established the first Center for Black Women's Wellness in the Atlanta housing projects. The center provided health, social, vocational, and educational services. In 1993, NBWHP implemented the Annie E. Casey Fund's Plain Talk Initiative, which developed strategies to help sexually active teens to prevent unintended pregnancies and the contraction of AIDS and other STDs. In 1994, NBWHP opened its first state office, The Well, California Black Women's Health Project, in Los Angeles, California. In 1996, NBWHP moved its national headquarters from Atlanta, Georgia, to Washington, D.C. In 1998, NBWHP released *Our Bodies, Our Voices, Our Choices: A Black Woman's Primer on Reproductive Health and Rights.*

Today, local chapters, self-help groups, and Walking for Wellness groups operate in cities throughout the United States. NBWHP's nationwide constituency consists of more than 10,000 members and supporters of varying incomes, sexual orientations, religious beliefs and health concerns. NBWHP has provided information and built the skills of countless black women. It has established itself as a critical voice on black women's perspectives. Policymakers, media, funders, and other organizations frequently call upon NBWHP to represent black women.

CASE STUDY #51: NATIONAL LATINA HEALTH ORGANIZATION (NLHO; ORGANIZACION NACIONAL DE LA SALUD DE LA MUJER LATINA), OAKLAND, CALIFORNIA, 1986 (HPDP)

Problem

The major problem being addressed was the lack of public awareness about the health problems of Latina women and the lack of bilingual and bicultural medical and mental health services.

> Given that Hispanics are one in six people in the United States, the findings in the CDC report are a major step in the arsenal of facts documenting that

we need to rethink health for everyone. For the past 30 years, data have accumulated that the health of Hispanics did not fit the standard model. Today we see the urgency and the need to create new models of health and wellness to achieve the best health outcomes for all,' said Jane L. Delgado, PhD, MS, President and CEO of the National Alliance for Hispanic Health, the nation's leading Hispanic health advocacy group. (CDC, 2015)

Leadership Impetus

The National Latina Health Organization was formed on March 8, 1986, when a group of Latina women (Puerto Rican, Chicana, Mexican, Cuban, South American, and Central American) came together on International Women's Day. They decided that the organization would use a new approach for providing good health care to Latina women: Latinas helping Latinas. Its mission was to raise consciousness among Latina women from all walks of life about their physical, emotional, and spiritual health.

EMPOWER Methods Used

- Enabling service and assistance
- Empowerment training and leadership development
- Media use
- Rights protection and social action/reform
- Public education and participation
- Organizing partnership

NLHO offered a series of bilingual classes and workshops called "Latina Health Issues ... Better Health through Self-Empowerment." This educational program provided important health information as well as a source of support for the participants who wanted to make healthful changes in their life. NLHO trained some of its members to become self-help facilitators.

Beginning in January of 1994, NHLO worked with San Francisco youth on a tobacco prevention and intervention program called the "Girls Against Tobacco Campaign." NLHO developed an educational curriculum for middle-school students that covered physiology, tactics used by the tobacco industry to promote smoking, second-hand smoke, health hazards, and the tobacco-control movement. At the end of each unit, peer-support groups facilitated by the girls themselves and supervised by the teachers were held. During the spring semester, 15 girls considered at risk to drop out of school, experiment with drugs or sex, or join gangs were chosen to participate in a special program that helped them deal with the pressures of living in a multicultural city. At the end of the program, a tobacco education event was held. At this time, because the city and state were trying to introduce legislative action to control the tobacco industry, there was a lot of local and national media coverage about the girls' work. The girls were also honored by city and state political figures. Due to the program's success, the program was given enough funding to continue for another six weeks. During that time, the girls discovered that there was a disproportionate number of alcohol and tobacco billboards in the areas adolescents frequented. NLHO presented the results to youth-serving community leaders and initiated a letter campaign to billboard companies and the Board of Supervisors' president.

NLHO was also a founding member and sponsor for the California Intergenerational Women's Health Coalition, which helped underrepresented women and girls lobby state governments for equal health coverage for all women. Made possible by a Ms. Foundation grant, the coalition celebrated "Lobby Day" on March 8, 1994 (International Women's Day). Over 50 NLHO members (mostly women of color; 75% were Latina) traveled to Sacramento to present personal testimonies and participate in a press conference.

NHLO's publishing house, Latina Press, printed and distributed books about the health-related issues concerning Latina women. NLHO convened and co-sponsored national conferences and forums; NLHO leaders were represented on state and national boards and advisory councils across the nation and participated in radio and television interviews and other public forums. NLHO collaborated with several agencies on projects serving Latina women such as a series of Spanish-language welfare reform forums, a guide to breast cancer resources for Latinas in the Bay area, and a coalition report on Latinas, health, immigration, and violence. In addition, NHLO served as a fiscal agent for the Women and Cancer Walk, a benefit event for Bay Area community-based organizations that tried to raise consciousness about women's cancers.

Partners/Opposition

NLHO received funding from several organizations and foundations, including the State of California Health Department, San Francisco Foundation, the Goldman Fund, the Ford Foundation, Pacific Bell, the California Wellness Foundation, San Francisco AIDS Foundation, and the California State Office of AIDS, among others. In addition, NLHO received grant funding for specific projects such as the grant from the Ms. Foundation for "Lobby Day" mentioned above. Proposition 99, a 1988 state tobacco tax that provided money to health education programs, provided funding for the Girls Against Tobacco Campaign.

Macro-environment

According the U.S. Census Bureau, in the 1990s, the Latino or Hispanic-origin population in the United States was approximately 31 million, or approximately 12% of the total population, with the majority in California.

Latinas were 11.3 % of the total female population in the United States. They were one of the fastest-growing and most diverse groups in the country. According to the 2010 Census, 308.7 million people resided in the United States on April 1, 2010, of which 50.5 million (or 16 percent) were of Hispanic or Latino origin. The Hispanic-origin population is projected to make up 25% of the total U.S. population by the year 2050. Although there are more Latinos in the labor force than any other ethnic group, they are over-represented in the numbers of the uninsured and the medically under-served. Nationally, 32.4% of Latinos were uninsured in 1990, compared with 12.9% for whites and 19.7% for blacks. As of the December 2013 report, nearly 60% of the state's uninsured population is Latino (http://www.census.gov/prod/cen2010/briefs/c2010br-04.pdf).

> California had the greatest number of uninsured residents of any state, seven million, and the seventh largest percentage of uninsured under 65 in the country. Many of the state's uninsured are employed; however, the percentage of residents who receive coverage through their jobs has declined dramatically, dropping from 63% in 1988 to 54% in 2012. (http://www.chcf.org/publications/2013/12/californias-uninsured)

In California in 2000 more than 6 million uninsured; over half of those were Latino. Latinos often face discrimination because of the stereotype that all Latinos are illegal aliens. They may be denied or delayed medical treatment due to suspicion of being undocumented. Emergency-room care is one of the few sources of health care available for many poor and undocumented Latinos.

Impact and Remarks

NLHO established itself as a voice of the national Latina women population for health and reproductive issues. The organization was granted NGO status for the 1995 United Nations Fourth International Women's Conference in Beijing, China, and was chosen to represent the U.S. Latina perspective to the U.S. official delegates. Its youth program trained over 150 adolescent girls in facilitator and self-empowerment skills. Some of the participants won an award from the president of the San Francisco Board of Supervisors for their work in removing tobacco billboards from the area surrounding their school. Three of the most active girls in the anti-tobacco campaign continued to participate on panels, television talk shows, and City Council meetings presenting their facts, sharing their feelings, and educating the public about the dangers of alcohol and tobacco access in their environments. NLHO co-founder and executive director Luz Alvarez Martinez received several awards for her efforts in empowering Latina women—including the Fabulous Feminist Award from the San Francisco chapter of National Organization for Women (NOW).

CASE STUDY #52: NATIVE AMERICAN WOMEN'S HEALTH EDUCATION
RESOURCE CENTER, LAKE ANDES, SOUTH DAKOTA, 1988 (HPDP)

Problem

The major problem being addressed was the lack of public health programs
and services that are geared toward Native American women. The center was
established in 1985 as a nonprofit organization:

> In 2013, the states with the highest percentage of American Indian and
> Alaska Native population were Alaska (14.3%), followed by Oklahoma
> (7.5%), New Mexico (9.1%), South Dakota (8.5%), and Montana (6.8%).
> The percentage of American Indians and Alaska Natives who lacked
> health insurance in 2013 was 26.9%. (http://www.cdc.gov/minorityhealth/
> populations/REMP/)

Leadership Impetus

Native American Women's Health Education Resource Center (The Resource
Center) is a reservation-based organization (the first of its kind) that was created by the Native American Community Board (NACB) in February of 1988.
The NACB was formed in 1985 by a group of Native Americans living on or
near the Yankton Sioux Reservation in South Dakota in order to address issues
of health, education, land and water rights, and economic development of
Native American people. NACB's first effort was a fetal alcohol syndrome pro-
gram called "Women and Children in Alcohol." In 1986, the Native American
Community Board was incorporated as a nonprofit tax-exempt organization
(NACB, 1993).

EMPOWER Methods Used

- Public education and participation
- Enabling service and assistance
- Work/job training and micro-enterprise
- Rights protection and social action/reform
- Organizing partnership

The Resource Center offers a number of health educational programs as
well as social services for the Native American population. The Domestic
Violence Program of the Resource Center runs a battered-women's shelter—a
four-bedroom home available to women and children who have experienced
domestic violence and sexual assault. Other services provided include rape
advocacy, support groups, court advocacy, referrals to other service agencies,
housing referrals, and assistance in getting reestablished in the community
after leaving abusive partners.

The Resource Center was the first organization in South Dakota to provide AIDS education. This program offers workshops catering to high school students, spiritual leaders, and families; trains trainers (including high school peer counselors); provides pre- and post-test counseling; and assists with problem-solving for people with AIDS and their families. The Resource Center sponsors cancer awareness programs focusing on such topics as breast self-examination, colon and uterine cancer, and the dangers of smoking and chewing tobacco. In light of the fact that approximately 70% of people above the age of 40 on this reservation are diabetics, the Resource Center provides classes and other activities to empower diabetics with information about proper diet and exercise. Native American Women's Health Education Resource Center serves as a clearinghouse of educational materials for distribution to Native American audiences. Tribes and agencies throughout the United States and Canada have requested materials such as reports, posters, pamphlets, and videos on several topics, including AIDS, fetal alcohol syndrome, environmental issues, and Native women's reproductive health.

The *Wicozanni Wowapi* newsletter provides updates on the work of the Center as well as new information regarding AIDS, environmental issues, diabetes, Native women's reproductive health, and other pertinent information. The newsletter is available for a minimal fee upon request. Through the "Green Thumb" Project, the Resource Center provides vegetable seeds and rototills gardens for members of the community. The purpose of this project is to encourage healthy eating and economical alternatives to processed foods. The Resource Center also operates a food pantry that gives emergency assistance to people who are in need of food.

The Child Development Program focuses on children in the community with special needs, providing them with many of the cultural opportunities not offered in school. Through their adult learning program, the Resource Center prepares adults for entrance into the job market by teaching computer skills, typing and job readiness skills, and preparation for the General Educational Development (GED) examination. The Resource Center offers scholarships of $300 and $150 to two qualified Native American women each semester (as of 2011, students enrolled in less than six hours or receiving a tuition waiver from the institution will receive $150; students enrolled in six hours or more will receive $300). The Dakota Cultural Institute, a project of the Resource Center, produced an audiotape in order to teach and preserve the Dakota language and culture.

Native Shop is an economic development project of the Native American Women's Health Education Resource Center that market products to raise funds for the Resource Center's programs. The merchandise sold at the Native Shop includes T-shirts, mugs, postcards, tote bags, language and culture tapes, and books, CDs, and tapes featuring American Indian artists; each item conveys a positive health message on topics ranging from fetal alcohol syndrome, to violence against women, HIV/AIDS prevention, and environmental protection.

The Resource Center organizes Native women in their communities locally and nationally to become involved in social change, policy development, and advocacy for better community health. The Dakota Roundtable is a forum that brings together representatives from several tribal nations from the four states of North Dakota, South Dakota, Nebraska, and Iowa in the first of a series of Roundtables to address community health issues.

Partners/Opposition

Cangleska, Inc., an organization that addresses domestic violence through outreach and direct service, gave two educational grants that kicked off Domestic Violence Prevention Month on the Yankton Sioux Reservation (for more information, see website: http://cangleskainc.ourorganizationtoolbar.com/).

The local police training session and youth workshop on domestic violence were sponsored by the Resource Center. Organizing on the Pine Ridge Reservation, Cangleska expanded to address domestic violence issues throughout the Native American community. Two of the founding members of Cangleska received the Marshall's Domestic Peace Prize for their efforts. Bradley Angel, Greenpeace's Southwest toxics coordinator, assisted the Dakota People of the Yankton Sioux Reservation in ongoing efforts to stop a major landfill project from moving forward Self-motivated environmentalists join Greenpeace to work on prevention/control of environmental toxins and hazards (http://www.greenpeace.org/international/en/press/releases/greenpeace-toxics-campaigner-w/o).

Macro-environment

A 1993 Health Survey for Yankton Sioux Reservation Community revealed that there was major distrust and discontent with health care provided by the government's Indian Health Service, a lack of preventive and early detection measures for cancer, and a disturbingly low rate of condom use (NACB, 1993). In addition, alcohol-related deaths were particularly high, while the practice of breastfeeding was uncommon. The rate of diabetes in the Native American community was much higher than the average of the general U.S. population; diabetes mellitus affected 70% of those over 40 on the Yankton Sioux Reservation.

> Reported in the December, 2000 issue of Diabetes Care: Diabetes has been growing in prevalence among Native Americans and Alaskan Natives, according to a recent study by the federal Centers for Disease Control and Prevention. The study found a nearly 30 percent increase

in diabetes diagnoses among these populations between 1990 and 1997. During this time period prevalence among women was higher than among men, but the rate of increase was higher among men than women (37 percent v. 25 percent). The increase in prevalence was highest in Alaska, where it rose 76 percent during the 1990s, and lowest in the Northern Plains region of the United States, where it rose by 16 percent during this time period.

The *Lakota Sioux* made national news when NPR's *Lost Children, Shattered Families* investigative story aired. It exposed what many critics consider to be the "kidnapping" of Lakota children from their homes by the state of South Dakota's Department of Social Services (D.S.S.). Lakota activists such as Madonna Thunder Hawk and *Chase Iron Eyes*, along with the *People's Law Project*, have alleged that Lakota grandmothers are illegally denied the right to foster their own grandchildren. They are currently working to redirect federal funding away from the state of South Dakota's D.S.S. to new tribal foster care programs. This would be an historic shift away from the state's traditional control over Lakota foster children.

In early 2014 a Lakota group launched *Mazacoin*, a digital currency that is claimed to be the "national currency of the traditional Lakota Nation." (http://www.theatlantic.com/politics/archive/2014/03/lakota-nation-thinks-cryptocurrencies-could-be-new-buffalo/358844/. Accessed on January 20, 2017)

Impact and Remarks

A community survey conducted by the Resource Center during September and October of 1997 revealed that the majority of respondents (those who had used the Center's programs and services since the Center opened in 1988) reported increases in skills and knowledge learned, positive lifestyle changes, and positive community changes. Seventy-two percent of respondents felt that they had learned ways to make healthier choices, and 76% reported that they felt better about themselves because of the Center's programs and services. Respondents also commented that the services taught the children about their culture and language and skills necessary for personal growth and provided a much-needed haven for abused women.

In response to local activism including those by the NABC, following US Senators took an initiative for better policy and services for Native Indians. They are U.S. Senators Barbara Boxer (D-CA), Patty Murray (D-WA), Jon Tester (D-MT), Richard Blumenthal (D-CT), Tammy Baldwin (D-WI) and Maria Cantwell (D-WA) today sent a letter to Secretary of Health and Human Services Sylvia Burwell urging the Department to improve emergency contraception access at Indian Health Services (IHS) facilities.

Emergency contraception is a crucial element of women's health care and can safely prevent pregnancy, including after sexual assault [the Senators wrote.] It is estimated that one in three Native American women is a survivor of rape or attempted rape—nearly twice the national average. These numbers make it all the more important that women who depend on IHS for their health care have timely over-the-counter access to emergency contraception.

Following the Food and Drug Administration's (FDA) approval of Plan B One-Step as an over-the-counter drug, several of the senators in May 2013 urged former Health and Human Services Secretary Kathleen Sebelius to implement a long-term solution—such as national policy guidance to all IHS facilities—to ensure that Native American women are receiving timely access to emergency contraception. At the time, the department responded that an update of the IHS pharmacy policy was in progress, but almost two years later the senators said they had seen no such written directive or policy to ensure that IHS pharmacies are complying with FDA standards.

A recent survey completed by Senator Boxer's staff revealed inconsistencies in how IHS pharmacies are providing emergency contraception. The senator's staff spoke directly with pharmacists at more than 20 IHS facilities and found that some IHS locations do not offer emergency contraception at all and, of those that do, many imposed age restrictions varying from 14 to 18, which are contrary to FDA approval and product labeling.

The senators continued,

We request that you share the steps your Department has taken towards updating its policy and provide a clear timeline for when that process will be completed. Further, we ask that you share with us data from surveys of pharmacies the IHS has undertaken in order to assess access to emergency contraception and the steps that the Department and IHS plan to take to monitor patient access moving forward. (Boxer et al., 2015)

CASE STUDY #45: DE MADRES A MADRES, HOUSTON, TEXAS, 1990s (HPDP)

Problem

The main problem being addressed was the inadequate prenatal care received by Latina women.

Leadership Impetus

To increase the number of women receiving prenatal care, a program called *De Madres a Madres* ("From Mothers to Mothers") was started in a

Hispanic community in Houston, Texas, in the 1990s (McFarlane & Fehir, 1994). This program was unusual in that it attempted to target women before they entered the healthcare system. According to the mothers' mission statement, *De Madres a Madres* was an organization of volunteers, promoting mother-to-mother support for at-risk pregnant Hispanic women through caring, sharing information, and developing a safety network for a healthier community.

EMPOWER Methods Used

- Empowerment training and leadership development
- Enabling service and assistance
- Rights protection and social action/reform
- Organizing partnership

The program began with a community assessment designed to identify leaders in the community and potential volunteer mothers. Fourteen volunteer mothers, all of whom were long-term residents of the community, were identified and trained by a community health nurse. Each mother approached pregnant women and inquired about their pregnancies. The volunteer would then offer the women community resource information and a follow-up call or home visit. During these home visits, the volunteer would often learn of other pressing issues facing the mother, such as pending eviction, sick children, or lack of health insurance. This program was driven by the idea that information is power and that the pregnant women, if given culturally relevant information, would effectively use it. In addition, the pregnant women also passed on the community resource information to their friends and family. At the end of the third year, the center formed a coalition in order to address the inaccessibility of eligibility cards for health care. Volunteers assisted pregnant women in filling out the necessary paperwork. As more and more women shared their positive experiences with their family and friends, the center became a virtual hub of activity with husbands and children coming in to help as well.

Partners/Opposition

Emotional and financial support, from family and friends as well as the community, is an essential factor in enabling the success of the program. Particularly because De Madres a Madres is a volunteer-based organization, garnering support from loved ones and friends helps keep the program functional.

Macro-environment

Early access to prenatal care is essential to the health of both women and their infants, yet one-third of all pregnant women do not receive adequate care. Latina women are more likely than either Anglo- or African-American women to receive inadequate care. Barriers to receiving care include fear and denial as well as lack of health insurance and difficulty in getting transportation or child care.

Impact and Remarks

The theoretical basis for the De Madres a Madres program was Freire's concept of empowerment education and Wheeler and Chin's feminist theory. The practical application of these theories are demonstrated in the program by the concepts of voluntarism, empowerment of indigenous women through unity, validation of women as key health promoters, and the recognition of a community's ability to identify and address its health needs.

Continued expansion of this prenatal care program resulted in greater diversity of clients and volunteers. But despite the resultant initial tension, the women managed to connect over matters of child care, food preparation, and family concerns. By the end of the fifth year, paid staff members from the community were hired, and the program had expanded their mission to include the entire family unit. Empowerment of the women occurred from involving the women in every level of decision-making, developing their leadership skills, and giving them a sense of ownership in the center and the community.

CASE STUDY #53: NATIONAL ASIAN WOMEN'S HEALTH ORGANIZATION (NAWHO), SAN FRANCISCO, CALIFORNIA, 1993 (HPDP)

Problem

The major problems being addressed are the underutilization of health care services by Asian Americans, the lack of health advocacy organizations for Asian Americans and the absence of Asian American women's health issues on the national agenda.

Leadership Impetus

Founded and incorporated in September of 1993 by Mary Chung, president and CEO, the National Asian Women's Health Organization (NAWHO) sought to fill a void in public health advocacy for Asian Americans as well as to empower Asian American women beyond accessing existing opportunities. Chung's vision was to increase the access of Asian women and families in the United States to quality healthcare and information, and to involve them directly in the development of the public policies that affected their daily lives. NAWHO began with a start-up grant from the Jessie Smith Noyes Foundation to conduct reproductive health work in the Asian American community, and received 501(c)3 status as a non-profit organization in February 1993. It was established by Mary Chung (Ross, 2006). NAWHO was the first national organization dedicated to improving the health status of Asian Pacific Islander women in the United States. NAWHO conducts surveys, generates data, and fosters women's leadership as advocates for Asian and Pacific Islander Americans (Ross, 2006, p. 1).

Join Us Support Us

The National Council of Women's Organizations is the leading coalition that makes fighting for women's rights more effective by working together. Every day, NCWO highlights and promotes the diverse work of our more than 200 member organizations representing 12 million women through our list serve, briefings, conferences and policy work. (NCWO, 2015)

It carries out its key functions through seven task forces:

Task Forces:

1. Domestic Priorities Task Force
2. Women's Health Task Force
3. Global Women's Issues Task Force
4. Corporate Accountability Task Force
5. Media and Technology Task Force
6. Older Women's Economic Security Task Force
7. ERA Task Force. (NCWO, 2015)

EMPOWER Methods Used

- Public education and participation
- Rights protection and social action/reform
- Empowerment training and leadership development
- Enabling service and assistance
- Media use
- Organizing partnership

NAWHO conducted the first national Asian women's health conference for health professionals and community advocates. The first National Asian American Breast Cancer Summit was held in New York, and its follow-up meeting in Napa, California, in 1996. Participants, who included community advocates, private industries, and representatives from government health programs, formulated the National Plan of Action on Asian American Women and Breast Cancer. NAWHO presented the plan at a congressional briefing co-sponsored by the national office of the American Cancer Society in Washington, D.C., and attended by several members of Congress. The briefing was the first educational forum on improving breast cancer public policy for Asian American women (A. Hirohama and C. Pascual, personal communication, December 10, 1998).

The 1995 South Asian Women's Health Project attempted to raise awareness about the health needs of the South Asian women's community. Over 150 South Asian women, a majority of whom did not have health insurance, participated in the health assessment that featured the first South Asian Women's Health Day. In collaboration with Planned Parenthood of Golden Gate and other San Francisco Asian organizations, NAWHO established the Youth Leadership Project in 1998. Five adolescent girls were trained in public speaking, community activism, and media in preparation for a special educational briefing with the San Francisco mayor. Other past education programs have focused on diabetes and breast and cervical cancer. NAWHO conducts training sessions for health care professionals in eight states to improve outreach efforts in early detection and screening programs. NAWHO also provides training to those enrolled in their Leadership Network in tobacco-control public education and policy (NAWHO, 2013).

In conjunction with the health care professionals training, NAWHO established a national toll-free information and referral number (the first of its kind) to provide Asian American women with breast and cervical cancer information in English and four Asian languages—Laotian, Korean, Vietnamese, and Cantonese.

NAWHO created the NAWHO Leadership Network to expand the leadership base of Asian American women, improving their skills in order to better organize their own communities around health issues. NAWHO sponsors skills-building training sessions, provides technical assistance, and organizes speaking engagements. NAWHO has garnered extensive media coverage on its programs by generating publicity and discussion about the health of Asian women and families. On its reproductive health project alone, NAWHO was featured in over 50 articles in both ethnic and mainstream newspapers; two television interviews with network affiliates in Los Angeles; and radio coverage on over 15 stations in the Bay area and in Los Angeles. NAWHO has been featured in *Newsweek,* the *Los Angeles Times, Ms. Magazine, Journal of the National Cancer Institute, San Jose Mercury News, The Record (New Jersey), Rafu Shimpo, A. Magazine, AsianWeek,* and the *Orange County Register.*

Partners/Opposition

NAWHO has received financial support from a number of different foundations and organizations, including the California Wellness Foundation, the Ford Foundation, the National Institutes of Health, and the National Center for Chronic Disease Prevention and Health Promotion at the Centers for Disease Control and Prevention (CDC). NAWHO also collaborates with various community organizations and agencies on specific projects such as the American Cancer Society, the Korean Immigrant Workers Association, and the Los Angeles County Commission for Women. Several prominent politicians support NAWHO through participation in the annual National Leadership Training Conference. Several congressional members including Barbara Boxer gave special presentations at the conference (Boxer, 2011).

Macro-environment

Health programs and public policy consistently overlooked the "model minority" of Asian Americans. There were major gaps in research, information, and knowledge about Asian Americans' healthcare needs. Asian Americans are most diverse ethnic group and face language and cultural barriers as well as racial discrimination from the public and health care providers. While Asian Americans have the highest level of education and income, they also tend to have lower health insurance coverage and they underutilize health care services than several ethnic groups. As of 2011, the percentages of uninsured population by ethnicity are as follows: whites 13%, Asian Americans 28%, Blacks 21%, Hispanics 32%, and Native Americans 27% (see Henry J. Kiser Family Foundation, 2013).

Impact and Remarks

NAWHO is recognized for its expertise as a leading health organization by the community, medical, media, and government sectors. With offices in San Francisco and Washington, NAWHO has a general membership of over 3,200 individuals and 150 organizations from 25 states and the District of Columbia. NAWHO has accomplished many "firsts" since its founding in 1993, initiating health campaigns at the community and policy level involving Asian American women and girls from different ethnic communities and class backgrounds. For example, NAWHO's national leadership training was the first to be specifically geared for Asian American women and girls and their work to improve community and public health. In San Francisco in 1995, NAWHO organized the first national Asian women's health conference, which mobilized 530 participants to discuss the critical health issues affecting Asian American women and girls. As a result of this conference, the San Francisco Board of Supervisors declared November 17th, 18th, and 19th "Asian Women's Health Days" for the City and County of San Francisco. Supervisor Mabel Teng presented a commendation to NAWHO in recognition of this achievement. In 1997, NAWHO was invited to a White House meeting with President Bill Clinton and Vice President Al Gore. Later, President Clinton recognized Asian American women as a top priority population during the announcement of his new "Race and Health Initiative" on February 21, 1998.

CASE STUDY #77: NATIONAL EATING DISORDERS ASSOCIATIONS
(NEDA), UNITED STATES, 1977

Problem

The major problem being addressed was the high rate of eating disorders.

> NEDA was formed in 2001, when Eating Disorders Awareness & Prevention
> (EDAP) joined forces with the American Anorexia Bulimia Association
> (AABA)—merging the largest and longest standing eating disorders pre-
> vention and advocacy organizations in the world. The merger was the most
> recent in a series of alliances that has also included the National Eating
> Disorder Organization (NEDO) and the Anorexia Nervosa & Related
> Disorders (ANRED). (NEDA, 2015)

Leadership Impetus

The National Eating Disorders Organization (NEDA) is one of the oldest eating disorder organizations in the United States.

EMPOWER Methods Used

- ¤ Public education and participation
- ¤ Organizing partnership
- ¤ Enabling service and assistance
- ¤ Media use

NEDA offers a wide variety of information sources about eating disorders. The information phone line provides basic eating-disorders
information and treatment resources without charge. The treatment
resource directory provides access to over 900 resources for eating disorder treatment internationally. The eating disorders information packet
contains detailed written material, including an overview of the types
of eating disorders, warning signs, guidelines to approaching someone
who has (or you suspect might have) an eating disorder, a reading and
resource list, and a copy of the current NEDA newsletter. The Eating
Disorders Support Group Information Packet provides step-by-step
instructions for starting a local eating disorders support group. NEDA
also has a complete library of audiotapes of the presentations made by
eating disorders specialists, educators, and medical researchers at their
annual conferences. NEDA created a five-day lesson plan for teachers
that provides material and information to be used in the classroom for
students in grades seven through 12 (ages 12–18). Topics include the cultural basis for body dissatisfaction and the drive for thinness, set point
theory of body weight regulation, nature and identification of eating disorders, and prevention of eating disorders. *Skin Deep* is a video produced

by Disney Educational Productions in collaboration with the National Eating Disorders Organization support groups.

Partners/Opposition

The Laureate International (a consortium of international universities), a private, not-for-profit, free-standing universities and hospitals—has supported the development of the field of eating disorders through its innovative treatment programs, the sponsorship of the initial meetings that launched the Academy of Eating Disorders, and its funding of numerous research projects. The Laureate network of more than 80 campus-based and online universities offers undergraduate and graduate degree programs to over 950,000 students around the world. The students are part of an international, academic community that spans 29 countries throughout the Americas, Europe, Africa, Asia, and the Middle East.

Macro-environment

Eating disorders are based on a complex interaction of feelings, attitudes, and behaviors. They can be influenced by a response to the problems of adolescence, low self-esteem, depression, and stress. Some common risk factors of eating disorders include: adolescent or young adult females from a middle- to upper-socioeconomic group in Westernized cultures; working or aspiring to work in a field that places high emphasis on thinness, such as acting, modeling, ballet, or gymnastics; and a previous history of being overweight or teased about weight that results in dieting behavior.

Impact and Remarks

The eating disorders prevention video, produced by Disney Educational Productions, in collaboration with the NEDA, won two first place awards. *Skin Deep* by Blake Edwards received a Golden Eagle (first place) in 1989 at CINE (Counsel for International Non-theatrical Events) in Washington, D.C. The video was also a finalist at the New York Festival for films and videos and won gold at the 1995 International CINDY Competition and Festivals. CINDY describes itself as:

> **CINDY**, an acronym for "Cinema in Industry," began in 1959 as an industrial film awards event. It was created by the Industry Film Producers Association (IFPA), an American non-profit industrial film organization based in Los Angeles. They currently present 14 different CINDY Award events each year honoring the theatrical, broadcast, non broadcast and interactive media professionals around the globe. (http://cindys.com/about/)

Its recent accomplishments include sustained partnerships with established educational and research universities, production and use of innovative educational media, and community and professional education programs. Latest examples include the "EATING DISORDERS AND PARENTING IN 2015" program and book directed and authored by professors Daniel le Grange and Sara Buckelew of the University of California at San Francisco Medical School (Psychiatry Department; <http://www.edcatalogue.com/eating-disorders-parenting-2015/>.

CASE STUDY #47: OVER SIXTY HEALTH CENTER (OSHC), CALIFORNIA, 1976 (HPDP)

Problem

The major problem being addressed is the lack of health facilities designed to maintain and improve the health of elders, particularly those without adequate access to care.

Leadership Impetus

The Over Sixty Health Center (OSHC), the first geriatric care clinic in the nation, was founded by six elderly members of the East Bay Gray Panthers in 1976 out of a need to provide quality care to the community's seniors. Lillian Rabinowitz in particular was a key player in making OSHC a reality; its mission is to provide high-quality health and social services in the San Francisco Bay Area East Bay community. Its services include primary health, dental care, pediatric, chronic disease, and HIV/AIDS treatment (OSHC, 2015). When Rabinowitz was 60 years old, she retired and took a one-day-a-week social work job providing services to the elderly. Her experiences helped to raise her consciousness about elder care, as did her 1973 introduction to Maggie Kuhn— the founder of the original elder rights organization, the Gray Panthers. As a result of their efforts, programs were established that brought young people and elders together and expanded graduate programs in gerontology and health-care facilities. In 1976, Rabinowitz wrote a proposal requesting funding for a geriatric clinic in Berkeley, California, for which she received $29,000 to build the OSHC with the help of six other East Bay Gray Panthers (Sanjek, 2009).

EMPOWER Methods Used

  ¤ Public education and participation
  ¤ Enabling service and assistance

In 1980, after visiting adult day healthcare centers in Great Britain, Rabinowitz resolved to establish similar centers in her own community of Alameda County to replace the existing nursing homes that provided inadequate care and even subjected their residents to neglect, mistreatment, and physical or emotional abuse. In 1982, the first of four adult day healthcare centers opened at Oakland Highland General Hospital as an alternative to institutionalizing the elderly.

OSHC also offers social services such as home assessments; arranging for home support services, transportation, and other needed services; applying for benefits; and consultation to patients and families. Dental services such as dental exams, hygiene, fillings and crowns, partial and complete dentures, and extraction are also provided. OSHC also publishes a biannual newsletter entitled *Health and Aging.* Each issue focuses on a particular topic such as mental health and the elderly, and the articles are written by physicians, public health professors, and other public health professionals.

Partners/Opposition

Its current executive director is Martin Lynch who met the Panthers while protesting county cuts to health and social services under Proposition 13. Impressed by the OSHC founders and their innovative work that involved cooperation among the young and the elderly, he told the Panthers to call if they needed his help. He was offered the executive directorship in 1982. Since then, the clinic has moved from a tiny storefront on San Pablo Avenue to an old post office on Alcatraz Avenue and a second branch office at East Oakland Senior Center. In 1995, Lynch received the Robert Wood Johnson Community Health Leadership award, a $100,000 prize that recognizes outstanding contributions to health care in communities that are not traditionally served by the system. Its LifeLong Medical Care services expanded and continued and earned the winner of the 2012 East Bay Express Reader's Choice Award for best non-profit. Readers were asked to submit nominations for several categories. LifeLong Medical Care received the highest number of nominations as best nonprofit organization (LLMC, 2015). Its initiatives under "LifeLong Medical Care is the winner of the 2012 East Bay Express Reader's Choice Award for best non-profit. Readers were asked to submit nominations for several categories. LifeLong Medical Care received the highest number of nominations as best non-profit organization (LLMC, 2015).

Macro-environment

In addition to being the first geriatric care clinic in the nation, OSHC was the first to integrate health care and social services in order to provide assistance to low-income elders for health and independent living. In order to recruit seniors to visit the clinic as well as attract initially skeptical community members, Leatha Phillips, one of the other founders as well as a board member, would do outreach in the streets.

Impact and Remarks

The Life Long Health Center is recognized nationally as a model of geriatric care in a community-based setting. A recent news posting in Berkeleyside online news in 2014 sums up OSHC and its quality of care in these words:

> Hundreds of people gathered Sunday afternoon to celebrate the grand opening of Lifelong Medical Care's new West Berkeley clinic, and for many of the dignitaries, it was a reunion of sorts. Amid speeches about the glorious new building and the patient-centric care it will foster, came memories of Berkeley in the 1970s and the push to revolutionize health care. Congresswoman Barbara Lee, State Senator Loni Hancock, Assemblywoman Nancy Skinner, Arnold Perkins, the former director of the Alameda County Public Health Department, and Lifelong CEO Marty Lynch all referred to the period 40 years ago when there were multiple pushes to bring medical services to various underserved communities.
>
> The Berkeley Free Health Clinic had been founded in 1969, followed by the Suitcase Clinic, the Over 60 Health Center, Berkeley Primary Care Clinic at Herrick Hospital, the West Berkeley Health Center and others. Many of the clinics merged over the years (others are thriving independently) to form Lifelong Medical Care, which now serves more than 50,000 clients a year in three counties. Many of those dignitaries had worked in the health care reform movement. (Over 60 Health Center, 2014)
>
> "The new $13 million, three-story clinic at 2031 Sixth St. is designed to treat the whole patient, not just his or her specific ailment. On each floor there is a "pod" (really an elongated office) with long counters, multiple computers and chairs. Exam rooms are right nearby. The ideas is that all the people who treat patients are in close contact so they can easily confer on the best treatment. For example, if a doctor determines a patient has diabetes, she can immediately put that client in touch with the person who runs diabetes or healthy cooking classes. If the patient needs a blood test, the doctor can send him to the blood lab—right down hall. (Over 60 Health Center, 2014)

CASE STUDY #54: PACIFIC INSTITUTE FOR WOMEN'S HEALTH (PIWH), LOS ANGELES, CALIFORNIA (HPDP)

Problem

The major problem being addressed was the lack of research on women's health and lack of collaborative partnerships among local, national, and international agencies to reach women and homeless needing health care.

Leadership Impetus

Pacific Institute for Women's Health (PIWH) is a nonprofit organization that was founded in 1993 by Prof. Joanne Leslie, Francine Coeytaux, S. Marie Harvey, Barbara Pillsbury, Jane Rubin-Kurtzman, and Carole Browner at UCLA. The founders were new acquaintances who had monthly lunch meetings to discuss their common concerns about women's health and women's lives. With many years of cumulative experience working with the major institutions addressing international women's health, they decided to take advantage of this research and practical expertise by founding PIWH. Its mission is to improve women's health and well-being locally and globally through applied research, advocacy, community involvement, consultation, and training. The Western Consortium for Public Health originally funded the founders' efforts as a feasibility study.

EMPOWER Methods Used

- ¤ Organizing partnership
- ¤ Enabling service and assistance
- ¤ Rights protection and social action/reform
- ¤ Empowerment training and leadership development

One of PIWH's primary goals is to create partnerships with community groups, policy-makers, researchers, service providers, and clients (both local and international) in order to share lessons learned and plan for future actions. PIWH has four program areas: adolescent health and well-being; reproductive and sexual health; women's rights and empowerment; and health promotion, prevention, and access to health services.

With an emphasis on building community partnerships to improve adolescent health, PIWH provided technical assistance to youth-serving organization in several African countries. In order to share information among researchers and service providers, PIWH coordinated bi-national (U.S. and Mexico) symposia on adolescent reproductive health as well as a collaborative initiative with service groups in the United States and developing countries. In the area of reproductive and sexual health, several research studies were conducted in partnership with local, national, and international agencies such as Kaiser Permanente of Southern California and People Assisting the Homeless (PATH). Working with NGOs in Latin America, PIWH developed materials, conducted workshops, and initiated advocacy for emergency contraception as a woman's right. In the program area of women's rights and empowerment, PIWH is conducted a 3-year initiative called "People connect." Funded by the William H. Gates Foundation, this project trained women's NGOs in developing countries in communication and technology skills. The "Women Linking" project collaborated with a Kampala-based women's NGO to improve the status and lives of women in Uganda. *Jagriti—The Awakening* is a video project that documents the efforts of grassroots women's organization and the oppressed lives of women in Nepal. The Women's Health Leadership Program is a five-year initiative to empower women and build leadership skills in ethnic and under-served communities through training, mentoring, peer learning, and networking opportunities. The *2013 Greater Los Angeles Homeless Count* determined that there are 58,423 individuals experiencing homelessness in Los Angeles on any given night, 74% (43,410) of whom go unsheltered—they literally live on the street. This program has expanded to several nations and programs that focus on women's leadership development in nonprofit organizations (ICA, 2015). The ICA has been working with several organizations including the PATH in several countries; its most recent work after the earthquake in Nepal (2015) is one example:

> After the massive 7.8 earthquake in Nepal on April 25, 2015, which killed nearly 8,000 people and destroyed 300,000 dwellings, people need to start rebuilding. There is an urgent need to provide emergency shelter, food, clean water and blankets, as well as restore lost livelihoods and rebuilding of houses with earthquake resistant technology. ICA is working with International Development Exchange (IDEX) who is in Nepal on the field. (http://www.idex.org/)

Partners/Opposition

PIWH has a small core staff and a multidisciplinary group of over 50 associates, the majority of whom are affiliated with other academic or community-based organizations throughout the West Coast, including the UCLA School of Public Health, the Global Fund for Women, and the Rand Corporation. PIWH in 2010 received over $8 million in funding for their research studies and projects from various foundations, including the CDC, the Educational Foundation of America, and the John Merck Fund, to name a few.

Macro-environment

Despite decades of human and capital investment in developing countries for the benefit of women and children's health, few models have been applied to similarly needy communities in the United States. In terms of health care and empowerment, women face the issues of gender-based violence, access to health care and contraception, and certain traditional cultural practices.

Impact and Remarks

By focusing on all conditions affecting women's lives and utilizing a diverse group of participants, views, and opinions, PIWH has improved women's health and well-being locally, nationally, and internationally. Through collaboration with researchers, activists and policy-makers in partner agencies, PIWH has formulated solutions and strategies for empowering women and mobilizing needy communities. In order to share the lessons learned through its various projects and initiatives, PIWH has released a series of publications that are available to the public, and publishes a biannual newsletter called *Soundings*. With more than 40 programs operating in 24 countries, PIWH has touched the lives of countless women throughout the world.

CASE STUDY #38: WOMEN'S CENTER OF JAMAICA FOUNDATION (WCJF) PROGRAM FOR ADOLESCENT MOTHERS, JAMAICA, 1978 (HPDP)

Problem

The major problem being addressed was the high adolescent pregnancy rates in Jamaica, which are among the highest in the Caribbean. An early, unplanned pregnancy puts the adolescent mother at an economic disadvantage in terms of the potential loss of job skills and education.

Leadership Impetus

With initial financial support from the Pathfinder Fund, the IPPF, and the Jamaican government, the Program for Adolescent Mothers began in 1978 with 17 students as a pilot project of the Women's Center of Jamaica Foundation (WCJF) in Kingston, which was directed by Pamela McNeil. The Program's objectives were to help adolescent mothers (ages 12–16) to complete their education and prevent a second pregnancy in their adolescent years (Barnett et al., 1999).

EMPOWER Methods Used

- Enabling service and assistance
- Public education and participation
- Work/job training and micro-enterprise

The program offered a variety of services to adolescent mothers during and after their pregnancies. Enabling mothers to continue their education during their pregnancy, the program offered academic instruction for the adolescent mothers. In order to ease the transition into motherhood, the program offered daycare for infants, classes in parenting and child nutrition and health, information about women's and children's legal rights, jobs skills training, and personal and group counseling. The program also provided information about family planning, decision-making, and STD prevention. The program worked with local health clinics and hospitals, thereby ensuring access to contraception, reproductive health services, and prenatal care. The program offered counseling for the girls' parents. Parents were invited to attend initial counseling sessions with the girls. The teenage fathers were also invited to attend counseling sessions and participate in other programs of the WCJF, where they learned about contraceptive use and the importance of continuing their education (Barnett et al., 1999).

Partners/Opposition

A variety of organizations collaborated with and supported the WCJF, such as schools, churches, the legal system, and health centers. These groups often referred pregnant teens to the program. In turn, the program referred its participants to appropriate community programs. Funding for the WCJF was provided by the Jamaican government, the UNICEF, the United Nations Population Fund, the U.S. Agency for International Development, Association for Voluntary Surgical Contraception (AVSC), the Christian Children's Fund of Canada, and local chapters of international service organizations, such as the Rotary and Kiwanis clubs.

During its inception, community members were very skeptical about the program. However, these negative and even hostile views gradually changed to acceptance among school officials, religious and civic leaders, and teens themselves. In order to raise awareness of the problems as well as to establish a working relationship with school officials, national WCJF director Pamela McNeil spoke at Parent–Teacher Association meetings. Impacts were significant on the teens who were not able to finish their education and on adult women with multiple children and did not have any employable skills. Due to the success of the program and the efforts of its staff, all schools in the Kingston area were accepting students from the WCJF and referring pregnant students to it.

Macro-environment

The mean age of first sexual intercourse in Jamaica is 15.9 years for women and 13.9 years for men. Although young people are aware of contraception, fewer than half used a birth control method during their first sexual encounter. Myths about contraception side-effects such as infertility, infections, vaginal bleeding, brain damage, and memory loss, and ineffective methods to prevent pregnancy such as drinking boiled Pepsi or papaya juice, explained the non-use of family planning. Due to social and cultural taboos, pregnant girls found it difficult to remain in school during their pregnancy. However, the Ministry of Education's (of Jamaica) public education policy ensured that teens whose education was interrupted by pregnancy could return to the regular school system. Because abortion is illegal in Jamaica, it is rarely an option for adolescent girls. As of now:

> In Jamaica, Sections 72 and 73 of the Offences Against the Persons Act (1861) reads: Criminalise women who chose to terminate a pregnancy, who, if convicted "shall be liable to be imprisoned for life with or without hard labour."
>
> Criminalise medical professionals who facilitate a woman's exercise of choice to have her pregnancy terminated, and the parents and guardians who facilitate termination of pregnancies of girls under the age of 18. If convicted, they "shall be liable to be imprisoned for a term not exceeding three years with or without hard labour." (JO, 2014)

Impact and Remarks

More than 16,500 girls participated in the program from 1978 through 1994, and most returned to school after their pregnancies. The program expanded to seven main centers and 13 outreach stations across Jamaica. It also served as a model to other organizations in Caribbean and African nations. Final evaluation of the program confirmed that several socioeconomic confounding factors in addition to unplanned pregnancy led to school dropouts and that a valid impact evaluation at the end of a program is unable to determine the key reasons and relative importance of these on school completion and dropouts (Bourne et al., 2009).

CASE STUDY #58: PROTOTYPES: A CENTER FOR INNOVATION IN HEALTH, MENTAL HEALTH, AND SOCIAL SERVICES, CALIFORNIA, 1986 (HPDP)

Problem

The major problem being addressed was the limited resources for women who have multiple problems such as drug addiction, mental illness, trauma, HIV/AIDS, unemployment, lack of insurance, and homelessness.

Leadership Impetus

To meet the needs of women with multiple problems in a rapidly changing community, the late Dr. Vivian Barnett Brown founded Prototypes, "A Center for Innovation in Health, Mental Health and Social Services," in 1986. Brown was a clinical psychologist and pioneer in substance abuse and mental health treatment and prevention. Brown provided the initial funding of Prototypes by taking out an equity loan on her house as well as through her income from her training and consultant work. In less than two years, Los Angeles County awarded Prototypes a contract to establish a residential treatment center for women and children.

EMPOWER Methods Used

- ¤ Enabling service and assistance
- ¤ Work/job training and micro-enterprise
- ¤ Media use
- ¤ Public education and participation

Prototypes offered a number of enabling services to women who have alcohol or drug addiction, mental illness, and were living with HIV/AIDS, at 15 program sites, often integrating services for the convenience of the client. Prototypes' residential treatment services began in 1988 at the Women's Center in Pomona thanks to an award from the L.A. County Drug Abuse Program Office. The Women's Center had a perinatal program that served drug and/or alcohol-addicted pregnant, postpartum, and parenting women and their children that was funded by the Drug Program of L.A. County. In order to encourage the women to accumulate marketable job skills, Prototypes also established a nonprofit business—the Word Processing Center, which offered vocational training to recovering drug abusers. Funds generated supported the drug rehabilitation services. Prototypes also encouraged the women to cultivate other inherent skills or talents and suggested profitable ways to use them. In 1989, Prototypes established an AIDS prevention and outreach program for high-risk women known as Prototypes/WARN (Women and AIDS Risk Network). Funded by the L.A. County Department of Health,
the center provides community-based mental health services and employable skill development programs.

Partners/Opposition

Most Prototypes programs involved collaborations with other agencies. For example, the Women Helping to Empower and Enhance Lives (WHEEL) Project was funded by the National Institute on Drug Abuse. The project among other initiatives studied the relationship between child/adolescent sexual abuse and crack cocaine abuse. It found that:

> About 64% of sample women had ever used crack; 56% had been sexually abused by age 18. In logistic regression analyses, any sexual abuse in childhood, penetrative sexual abuse in childhood, and sexual abuse by a family member in childhood were significantly associated with lifetime crack use. Sexual abuse in adolescence was indirectly associated with lifetime crack use through running away from home and rape in adulthood. (Freeman et al., 2015)

Macro-environment

With little resources available to women with multiple health problems (such as drug addiction, sexually transmitted diseases, mental health problems etc.), these individuals would often accumulate other problems as they tried to cope with the day-to-day details of life—taking care of their children, earning a living, maintaining a home. Other drug rehabilitation programs often did not allow the woman's children to accompany them. Because there was no one to care for their children, many mothers would not enter treatment. Allowing the women to bring their children with them not only enhanced the women's treatment but also allowed important services to be given to the children.

Impact and Remarks

Currently, there are 14 program sites throughout L.A. County and two centers in Washington, D.C. Prototypes' efforts have been recognized by all levels of government with contracts from federal, state, county, and city agencies, as well as private-sector grants. The founder, Dr. Brown, received many honors due to her work, including the American Psychological Association's McNeil Award; an appointment to the Federal Advisory Committee for Women's Services, which advises the federal Substance Abuse and Mental Health Services Administration; and an appointment to the L.A. County Narcotics and Dangerous Drugs Commission. Members of Prototypes were invited to meet President Bill Clinton's transition team to discuss the impact of AIDS on women, youth, and people of color. In 1996, Prototypes Women's Center was featured as a model residential treatment program for women with multiple diagnoses by the nationally broadcast *News Hour with Jim Lehrer.* As of 2013, it served 12,000 individuals annually and have served more than 100,000 individuals since it was established. Youth who have been able to gain control of their lives and a steady income are available at Prototypes recent web posting (Prototype, 2015).

CASE STUDY #62: RAPE CRISIS, CAPE TOWN, SOUTH AFRICA, 1975 (HPDP)

Problem

The major problem being addressed was the lack of resources for rape survivors in South Africa and light punishment of sex offenders.

Leadership Impetus

Anne Mayne and four other women (Ann Levett; an Indian doctor; a medical receptionist; and an accountant) founded Rape Crisis shortly after Mayne attended the United Nations International Year of the Women Conference in Mexico City in 1975, and made a subsequent trip to the United States. Both of these events helped shape her as a political being. Herself a rape survivor, Mayne's involvement in the anti-rape cause helped her heal from her traumatic experiences and take action in curbing the crime.

The first Rape Crisis center in South Africa was established following the publication of an article in *Cape Times* newspaper, which stated that a group of women (including Mayne and her colleagues) were interested in speaking to women who had been raped (Mayne, 1989). There was an overwhelming response, with women calling continuously for three consecutive days.

EMPOWER Methods Used

- Enabling service and assistance
- Media use
- Public education and participation
- Rights protection and social action/reform

Mayne's first public speaking engagement took place at a Rotarian luncheon. The Rotary Club showed their support for her efforts by paying for the printing costs of 4,000 information leaflets; a pharmacist later donated a beeper (pager) so Mayne and her colleagues could answer calls immediately. Different service organizations frequently invited Rape Crisis to give talks at their meetings. Rape Crisis periodically holds a national conference in one of the cities that have a rape center to share information and update one another on progress or changes. During the early days of Rape Crisis, Mayne appeared on national television with the director of the National Institute of Crime Prevention, the wife of a Parliament member, and a law professor to debate the issue of rape in South Africa. The public responded to this appearance with support and encouragement.

Rape Crisis offers moral support to rape victims, assistance in obtaining medical treatment and abortion if necessary, and legal help in the courts. In 1985, Rape Crisis developed a training section on battered women. Due to the overwhelming response, Rape Crisis launched a public campaign to build a battered women's shelter. The shelter is a much-valued resource for abused women that provides a safe and caring environment free of violence, drugs, alcohol, and abusing men.

Partners/Opposition

The director of the National Institute for Crime Prevention openly supported Rape Crisis and confirmed that the statistics used by Rape Crisis (which had been gleaned from U. S. studies) could be applied to South Africa. Volunteers from the community of various ethnicities, many of whom were rape survivors themselves, were also a valued source of support.

Macro-environment

In South Africa, the police do not take rape crimes seriously, letting even the most violent men out on bail. Violent gangs who commit a lot of the rapes are common in the townships. Fearful of being the next target of the gangs, neighbors are unwilling to help or support a rape victim. Very few black women reported incidences of rape committed by white men due to the blatant disregard on the part of the police. Stereotypes existed that black men were more inclined to be rapists, yet one police station's records showed that rapes by white men of black women were six times higher that rapes by black men of white women. Domestic workers were often targets of white rapists who took advantage of the domestic workers' lack of power and social standing.

Impact and Remarks

The founding of Rape Crisis was essentially the very beginning of the anti-rape movement launched in South Africa. Approximately 60% of the clients were colored (i.e., neither white nor black) women, the rest being white. Despite outreach at various nurses' associations and teachers' association in the black townships, few black women sought the help of Rape Crisis. Due to long work hours and long traveling distances from their jobs to their homes, setting up Rape Crisis services in their own communities proved very difficult as well. According to one report, murder and rape rates in South Africa have been significantly higher than other African nations (Blow the Whistle, 2014). According to one report on prevalence of rape titled "South Africa's Rape Crisis", in the Time Magazine, "one-in four men in South Africa say they have done it" (Lindow, 2009).

Another report, claims that rate of rape in South Africa: "has stabilised, with a slight decrease of 3%, since 2008/9 from 47,588 to 46,253 in 2013/14.The Medical Research Council has estimated that only one in nine rapes are reported to the police. Thus the actual numbers of rapes in South Africa is much higher than numbers recorded by the police" (Africa Check, 2014).

CASE STUDY #63: SAKHI, NEW YORK, 1989 (HPDP)

Problem

The major problem being addressed was the oppression and domestic violence perpetrated against South Asian women in New York or the tri-state area (New York, New Jersey, and Connecticut), which has the largest concentration of South Asians in the country.

Leadership Impetus

Founded in June 1989 by five women professionals, Sakhi (means a "woman friend") for South Asian Women is a nonprofit community-based organization committed to ending violence against women of South Asian. Sakhi serves women originally from India, Bangladesh, Pakistan, Sri Lanka, and Nepal, as well as the larger South Asian diaspora, including parts of Africa and the Caribbean.

> Founded in 1989 by a group of five South Asian women—Anannya Bhattacharjee, Mallika Dutt, Tula Goenka, Geetanjali Misra, and Romita Shetty—who were from diverse professional fields such as banking, film, law, and public health, Sakhi, meaning "woman friend," was created to fill a critical need—in spite of an abundance of religious and cultural centers, professional associations, and ethnic-specific groups within New York's large South Asian immigrant population, there was no place for women to address the silenced subject of domestic violence. (Sakhi, 2015)

EMPOWER Methods Used

- ¤ Public education and participation
- ¤ Media use
- ¤ Work/job training and micro-enterprise
- ¤ Empowerment training and leadership development
- ¤ Organizing partnership
- ¤ Rights protection and social action/reform

Sakhi's Domestic Violence Project served an average of 50 South Asian battered women a month who were or had been in abusive relationships. Sakhi conducted regular support groups meetings, monthly immigration and matrimonial clinics, and provided referrals for job training and attorneys. It also helped women access public assistance, safe housing, and other social services, accompanied women to court, advocated for legislation to help battered immigrant women, informed women about their rights and options, talked to community members and the media, and provided free, semester-long English classes for South Asian women.

In order to provide educational information to its members and the South Asian community in general, Sakhi distributed and screened the groundbreaking video *A Life Without Fear*, which chronicled the life of one immigrant abused woman and her attempts at breaking free of violence. This video, the only one targeting the South Asian community in the United States, has been used by women's studies departments, domestic violence shelters and organizations, and community groups throughout the country.

Sakhi also published a quarterly newsletter called *Voices of Sakhi* that was mailed to over 2,000 members of the community.

The South Asian Women's Health Initiative was created in order to educate and inform South Asian women about violence, health, and accessing health care; to raise awareness of violence against women among physicians and healthcare providers; and to develop a core of South Asian physicians and mental healthcare providers sensitive to the needs of South Asian battered women.

In addition to the variety of services provided to domestic violence survivors, Sakhi provided organizational training to volunteers and encouraged women to actively participate in the organization. Sakhi enabled volunteers and survivors of violence to develop their leadership potential and to speak out against abuse, when they were ready to "come out" as survivors of violence. Several efforts initiated by survivors proved to be great opportunities to voice their opinions about domestic violence. For example, five battered women in 1989 organized a leafleting session in Jackson Heights, Queens; ten marched in the India and Pakistan Day Parades, four gave media interviews, three participated in the biannual volunteer training, and 15 participated in the March Against Violence, held on March 8th, 1998.

Partners/Opposition

Private grants, community fund-raisers, and individual donations support Sakhi's mission of providing services to survivors of domestic violence. Sakhi has received grants from the Ford Foundation, the Asian American Federation of New York, and the Chicago Resource Center. Sakhi works in solidarity with other domestic violence groups, immigrant rights coalitions, and South Asian organizations both locally and nationally who believe in its mission. Sakhi is also a member of the Asian Domestic Violence Institute, a group of individuals and organizations from around the country that serve Asian survivors of violence.

Macro-environment

Many of the women in need of Sakhi's assistance had no other place to turn; they may avoid mainstream social service agencies and shelters due to barriers of language, culture, and immigration status (P. Vora, personal communication, 1999). Not only were there few South Asian language interpreters, but those who did such work were mostly men who were neither trained on domestic violence, nor monitored, nor held accountable for their actions in any systematic way.

Impact and Remarks

Starting with five volunteers in 1989, Sakhi has since grown to two full-time staff members, 60 volunteers, and a base of 2,000 supporters. On average, Sakhi receives between 10 and 25 new calls per month from abused women; annually, about 250 survivors of violence are helped. Sakhi helps South Asian battered women overcome their struggles in leaving the abuser(s) and in leading a decent, independent, violence-free life. Often the same women who have sought help from Sakhi play an active part in the organization by giving other South Asian women the support they need. Like many grassroots organizations, SAKHI is rich in their dedication and efforts for their chosen causes; but relatively less concerned with quantitative evaluation of impacts. On January 30, 2015, its Executive Director wrote the following in her farewell message after five years as the ED:

> We've launched four new programs since I began—Youth Empowerment, Women's Health Initiative (which was a re-launch), Deferred Action for Childhood Arrivals (providing immigration support) and most recently Sexual Assault Services. Our staff has doubled. Our finances are strong and secure, and our mission, vision and impact are clear and innovative. (http://www.sakhi.org/2015/01/30/farewell/)

CASE STUDY #71: THE SALTA PROJECT, SAN DIEGO, CALIFORNIA, 1995 (HPDP)

Problem

SALTA stands for Salud Ambiental Lideres Tomando Accion or Environmental Health, Leaders Taking Action. The major problem being addressed was environmental racism. In San Diego, the hazardous waste facilities and the operation of polluting companies caused disproportionate levels of toxic pollution in communities of color.

Leadership Impetus

Created in 1995, the project tried to strengthen San Diego's Latino communities. Although the *promotora* model had been successfully used to promote health in communities and schools, SALTA was the first application of the *promotora* model for social change and community organizing.

EMPOWER Methods Used

- Empowerment training and leadership development
- Public education and participation
- Rights protection and social action/reform
- Media use

The SALTA project consisted of a two-tiered training program (SALTA, 2015). First, women from the community were recruited and trained to be *promotoras de salud ambiental* ("environmental health promoters"). They received education on lead poisoning, pest control, household cleaning products, and toxic chemicals. They were trained in community organizing, empowerment, and policy advocacy. After this 12-week training period, each *promotora* recruited and trained her own group of women, while continuing to assist the community on environmental issues. For example, in 1993, the San Diego Port District began importing fruits and other products that required fumigation with methyl bromide—a highly toxic pesticide, potent ozone depletory, and reproductive toxin. The *promotoras* organized candlelight vigils, attended Port Commission meetings, and brought up the issue at community meetings. The *promotoras'* efforts led to media coverage in the *San Diego Union-Tribune* and increased community participation (Barraza-Roppe et al., 1998).

Partners/Opposition

The SALTA program received a seed grant from the U.S. Environmental Protection Agency's (EPA) Environmental Equity Grant Program. The James Irving Foundation provided funding for the development and testing of the SALTA training. A grant from the California Endowment allowed the Environmental Health Coalition (EHC) to hire five SALTA *promotoras* as part-time community organizers. Other funders of the program included the Association for Community Organization for Reform Now (ACORN) Foundation, Campaign for Human Development, McKay Foundation, Peace Development Fund, and San Diego Foundation for Change. SALTA's major opposition came from the major companies that generate hazardous waste in the communities of San Diego. In 1996, the San Diego Port District filed a lawsuit (later dismissed) against EHC and the school district seeking an injunction to stop any protest about the facility. In the end, the lawsuit only drew more media attention to the issue and sparked further efforts by the whole community. The district's city councilman even joined the struggle.

Macro-environment

The SALTA *promotora* model capitalized on the strengths and resources of the Latino/Mexican community in San Diego. Latinas traditionally are the family and community health gatekeepers. Latino men in this low-income community are often under-employed or working two jobs to support the family. Time was a barrier for men. Because SALTA meetings were held in safe, family-centered locations such as a school or community center, women were less reluctant to attend an activity outside of the home. In San Diego, communities of color are often older neighborhoods that have dangerous toxic environments next to homes and schools. For example, Barrio Logan, which is over 90% Latino, ranks third in the volume of hazardous waste generated and second in the volume of hazardous materials stored onsite for all of San Diego County.

Impact and Remarks

During its first year, EHC trained 18 *promotoras*, who in turn trained more than 200 Latinas from the most affected communities in San Diego. One of the SALTA *promotoras'* greatest successes involved their fight to end methyl bromide fumigation at a Port District facility next to Barrio Logan (described above). Their efforts, combined with the media coverage and increased community participation, led to a victory for the EHC. In July 1997, the Port Commission adopted a fumigation use policy that banned the importation of commodities requiring use of methyl bromide. This was the first policy of its kind to be enacted in the country.

CASE STUDY #72: SOUTH CAROLINA AIDS EDUCATION NETWORK (SCAEN), SOUTH CAROLINA, 1987 (HPDP)

Problem

The primary problem being addressed was the lack of AIDS educational programs that catered to the specific needs of women in a culturally diverse community.

Leadership Impetus

The South Carolina AIDS Education Network (SCAEN) was founded in January of 1987 (and incorporated in November, 1987) by DiAna DiAna, who became its president and executive director (DiAna, 1990). DiAna began as an informal AIDS educator by distributing condoms to her mostly African-American clients in her hair salon in Columbia, South Carolina, after she became aware of AIDS and its effects on the community after seeing AIDS educational videos on TV while styling their hair (DiAna, 1990, p. 219; Sumpter, 1990). Subsequently, DiAna met Bambi Sumpter, who had a doctorate in public health from the University of South Carolina in human sexuality and family life education (Sumpter, 1990).

EMPOWER Methods Used

- Enabling service and assistance
- Public education and participation
- Media use
- Support and advocacy

SCAEN operated primarily out of DiAna's Hair Ego hair salon and provided a variety of educational and informational materials and programs such as AIDS pamphlets, mini-seminars, follow-up services, and educational groups, as well as AIDS presentations in schools, churches, civic groups, and women's groups. DiAna and Sumpter developed special AIDS educational materials for children and adolescents (coloring books, a $50 poster contest), a booklet for poor readers or non-readers, and "AIDS plays" that were performed by students of a local university for other students. The major focus of SCAEN activities is to create opportunities in which members of the community can actively participate in educating themselves about AIDS.

DiAna also created a support group for parents called Mothers Against AIDS (MAA) that provided an opportunity to exchange information, learn coping skills, and learn more about the disease, as well as to raise consciousness. In addition, SCAEN wrote a weekly column in a local community newspaper that discussed AIDS-related issues and ways readers could relate the given information to their own lives.

Partners/Opposition

The Women's Caucus of the AIDS Coalition to Unleash Power (ACT UP) and the Lesbian and Gay Community Services Center in New York City provided support to SCAEN by producing a book describing the activities of SCAEN as well as other research and program efforts concerning the AIDS crisis.

Macro-environment

Women with HIV-positive status have relatively fewer resources (economic, institutional) and fewer support networks than their male counterparts. Women are more vulnerable to rape, battering, and other acts of sexual violence that can increase the chance of contracting HIV. Due to women's subordinate position in heterosexual relationships, women as a group are more often uninformed, undercounted and misdiagnosed than men (Sumpter, 1990).

Impact and Remarks

In its first three years in existence, SCAEN gave one-to-one information to over 9,000 individuals in South Carolina and received requests from organizations nationwide and worldwide for information regarding AIDS. Funding for SCAEN came from the salon's client tips and donations from the community as well as the founders' own pockets. Government funding was denied to SCAEN because agencies claimed that SCAEN lacked grant-writing expertise and possessed inadequate management procedures. An NIH website in 2012 wrote this about the SCAEN initiative:

> The fledgling organization initiated a full-scale campaign to use popular culture to entice people to think about AIDS prevention. They wrote plays, sponsored talent shows, and held Tupperware-style parties with prizes that could be used to make sex safe. Always lighthearted in approach but conveying a powerful message, SCAEN insisted that southerners, particularly African Americans, needed to understand the pleasurable benefits of safer sex and the risks of being unprotected. Despite the good work of this grass roots campaign, in 2012 South Carolina was

one of the top three states in the nation with the highest numbers of HIV diagnoses in teens. (NIH, 2012)

CASE STUDY #55: SISTERS NETWORK, INC., HOUSTON, TEXAS, 1994 (HPDP)

Problem

According to a reliable source, "Black patients were nearly twice as likely as white patients to have died from breast cancer. The researchers also found that black patients were less likely than white patients to be diagnosed with either the luminal A or luminal B breast cancer subtypes" (Medicinenet, 2013).

It continues

> African-Americans were more likely to have the hard-to-treat triple-negative breast cancer subtype and had a lower likelihood of having the luminal A subtype, which tends to be the most treatable subtype of breast cancer and has the best prognosis, study author Candyce Kroenke, a research scientist at Kaiser Permanente, said in an association news release. (http://www.medicinenet.com/script/main/art.asp?articlekey=169013)

Clearly they are at greater risk and need useful information, education, and services to protect them from this fatal risk.

Leadership Impetus

Sisters Network, Inc. (1994) is the first national African American breast cancer survivors' support and education group. It is "committed to increasing local and national attention to the devastating impact that breast cancer has in the African American community (Sisters Network, 1994). Three African American breast cancer survivors, among them Karen Eubanks Jackson, who became the national president of the Sisters Network, founded the organization in 1994. Before its founding and after her lumpectomy in November 1993, Jackson pursued her personal mission of reaching out to as many black women as possible and warning them about the dangers of breast cancer. With her daughter, Caleen Burton Allen—a media-relations manager for the Port of Houston—by her side, Jackson approached African American women in malls, churches, and neighborhood walkways to ask if they, or anyone they knew, had dealt with breast cancer. She would then share information with those women.

EMPOWER Methods Used

- Enabling service and assistance
- Public education and participation
- Media use
- Organizing partnership

Sisters Network is committed to increasing local and national attention to the devastating impact that breast cancer had in the African American community. These women saw the need to unite survivors, the community, and health professionals for the sole purpose of fighting the breast cancer epidemic. The main foci of the organization were education, prevention, emotional support, and heightening the awareness of breast cancer, particularly in the African American community. Sisters' Network aimed to provide emotional and psychological support and to educate the community about cancer. Sisters Network provided a speakers bureau (which had experts on mastectomy and other topics related to breast cancer), in-home support, a national newsletter and a website. The network held outreach campaigns in churches and youth groups, coordinated a service to match pairs of survivors no matter where they live in the United States, and conducted an annual Gift for Life Block Walk. During this walk hundreds of volunteers fan out across a black community, handing out brochures and pinning pink ribbons on women to increase awareness of the dangers of breast cancer.

Partners/Opposition

Sisters Network addresses the breast health needs of African American women, through its local chapters and partnerships with existing service providers. Breast cancer survivors who are committed to establishing the much-needed community breast health services organized approximately 25 chapters nationwide. Chapters utilize funds raised and donations in order to provide education, resources, and referral opportunities to thousands of women. Sisters Network is a member of the National Coalition for Cancer Survivorship (NCCS), and it has grown into a nationwide grassroots network of independent organizations and individuals working in the area of cancer support and information.

Macro-environment

Historically, society and culture strongly associate a woman's femininity with her female body parts, and many women associate breast cancer with losing a breast. Due to this fear associated with breast cancer, many women are reluctant to acknowledge the risk of breast cancer or the benefits of breast cancer screening. Although the fear of losing a breast is prevalent with all women, members of the Sisters Network feel that black women are more spiritually oriented. They may choose to deal with the situation through deep prayer or willpower rather than face the possibility of a cancer diagnosis. There also is a belief within black neighborhoods that breast cancer is a disease that afflicts white women. According to the Office of Special Population at the National Cancer Institute in Washington, poor women do not receive as optimal a treatment as non-poor women of all races do. There is also a greater tendency for black women to receive radical mastectomies rather than lumpectomies.

Impact and Remarks

Two of the chapters were founded by women whom Jackson met at medical conferences. Sisters Network created the camaraderie among black women that was lacking before. It is made up of African-American breast cancer survivors who have bonded together to raise awareness about the disease within black neighborhoods. "Membership is 3,000, which includes more than 40 affiliate survivor run chapters nationwide. The organization's purpose is to save lives and provide a broader scope of knowledge that addresses the breast cancer survivorship crisis affecting African American women around the country" (Jackson, 2015).

On December 15, 2008, Sisters Network Inc. (SNI) announced:

> I am so humbled that the vision of opening the Sister House, a warm, inviting and informative facility to educate/empower the African American community about the importance of breast health and to provide accommodations for all breast cancer survivors has become a reality. Sisters Network has made a major impact nationally and locally on the issue of breast cancer, but there is much more work to be done. The Sister House provides a wonderful foundation for our organization reach the next level. We have accomplished Phase One of a three phase vision—we are blessed. (Jackson, 2015)

Due to Jackson's leadership, Sisters Network has experienced phenomenal growth resulting in over 42 survivor-run affiliate chapters, serving more than 3000 members and associate members nationwide. Sisters Network® Inc. has become the leading voice in the African American women's fight against breast cancer. In addition, Jackson developed several national outreach initiatives, including: The Gift for Life Block Walk® and the Pink Ribbon Awareness Project.

Jackson is a widely recognized minority breast health advocate, promoting legislation on the state and federal level. A highly sought after speaker and expert on the African American women's breast cancer experience, Jackson has traveled nationally and internationally, bringing her message to the U.S. Army's Comprehensive Breast Cancer Center in Germany, the National Congressional Black Caucus and the Centers for Disease Control and Prevention (CDC), as well as other organizations. Jackson has been featured in numerous national newspapers, magazines, television, radio programs, and Internet media outlets, inclusive of the U.S. News & World Report, the Health Network, HBO special: Cancer: Evolution to Revolution, Essence, MAMM, Jet, and Web MD Health. (Jackson, 2015)

CASE STUDY #49: SUPPORTIVE OLDER WOMEN'S NETWORK (SOWN), PHILADELPHIA, PENNSYLVANIA, 1982

Problem

The major problem being addressed was lack of support groups for women aged 60 years and older to cope with the many challenges of the aging process.

Leadership Impetus

Inspired by her grandmother and other older women she was working with, Merle Drake (at the age of 26) founded the Supportive Older Women's Network (SOWN) in 1982. Her own 82-year-old grandmother had survived several deaths in her family without having adequate support to cope with these drastic changes in her life. Subsequently, Drake started nine older women's support groups in senior centers throughout Philadelphia and sought funding for groups in subsidized housing and long-term care facilities.

EMPOWER Methods Used

- Enabling service and assistance
- Empowerment training and leadership development
- Media use
- Public education and participation

SOWN support groups offer their members a stable network to help older women cope with problems; share experiences, information, and resources; overcome stereotypes of aging; and empower themselves. SOWN staff are part-time working women. Media coverage in newspapers, word of mouth among the elderly population, presentations at local, regional, and national conferences, and speeches given at senior centers, churches, synagogues, and housing residences helped motivate the creation of new groups for interested older women. SOWN published a comprehensive manual and designed a technical assistance program to provide guidance to start similar organizations outside of Philadelphia.

Partners/Opposition

SOWN developed collaborations with the public housing authority, women's organizations, senior center networks, long-term care facilities, mental health agencies, and volunteer associations. SOWN garnered support from many private foundations such as the Pew Charitable Trust, the William Penn Foundation, and the Fannie Rippel Foundation. In 1987, SOWN became a member of Women's Way, a Philadelphia-based women's fund-raising coalition. SOWN also provides contracted services to local Area Agencies on Aging (AAA) and residential facilities (Kaye, 1997; N. A. Morrow, personal communication, 2000).

Macro-environment

Due to several factors, women are disproportionately affected by the challenging issues of aging. Women are more likely than men to suffer significant stress as they get older. Negative images of older women portrayed in the media and popular culture can weaken women's self-esteem.

Impact and Remarks

SOWN's success lies in its ability to build long-term informal support networks for older women. Over 40% of SOWN Groups meet for longer than ten years. Over a thousand women participate in local chapters of SOWN. Although members represent a variety of life experiences and racial, ethnic, and educational backgrounds, they find commonality in their journey through old age. In urban Philadelphia, SOWN members are 70% African-American, 70% poor, 90% widowed and living alone, and 61% frail or handicapped.

The distinguishing feature is its emphasis on self-help and empowerment among older women. By training leaders and giving back the reins of the group to the participating members, women are taking control of their own lives.

CASE STUDY #79: STEP UP ON SECOND: A CENTER FOR RECOVERING MENTALLY ILL ADULTS, SANTA MONICA, CALIFORNIA, 1984 (HPDP)

Problem

Santa Monica lacked services for homeless and housed adults recovering from mental illnesses such as schizophrenia, bipolar disorder (manic depression), and severe depression. There was a lack of opportunities for individuals with severe and mental illness to reintegrate into the community (Abrams, 1986; T. E. Carey, personal interview, *LA Times*, 1993).

Leadership Impetus

Step Up on Second was founded by Susan Dempsay and other concerned members of the Westside Alliance for the Mentally Ill (AMI) in 1984 with the organizing help of the Mental Health Association (MHA) of Los Angeles County, a private, nonprofit agency. With $50,000 in seed money contributed by concerned families, the founding group rented a 7,000-square-foot warehouse in downtown Santa Monica. The founders envisioned a program that would serve mentally ill clients in a community-based environment as well as transform the stigmatized public image of the mentally ill. Dempsay became involved in working with the mentally ill when her 18-year-old son was diagnosed with schizophrenia. After several years, Dempsay also organized a seven-member board for the center that allowed Step Up to establish its own organizational identity separate from the MHA (Abrams, 1986).

EMPOWER Methods Used

- Enabling service and assistance
- Work/job training and micro-enterprise
- Public education and participation
- Media use
- Empowerment training and leadership development
- Rights protection and social action/reform

Step Up's Vocational Department helped members with job training, job searches, interview skills, resume-writing, and ongoing job coaching. For example, members could train at *Fresh Start,* a mini-market located in front of the Step Up center. Once they acquired basic skills, many trainees found jobs in the community. Step Up had a contract with the State Department of Rehabilitation that was dedicated to working with mentally ill clients. Through collaboration with Step Up's vocational counselors, permanent placements were secured at travel agencies, Frye's Electronics, the Veterans' Administration, Daniel Freeman Hospital, Young Men's Christian Associations (YMCAs), the City of Santa Monica, the L.A. Unified School District, and several retail organizations.

Services for homeless participants included showers, laundry, mail service, shelter placements, and outreach. In 1994, Step Up opened a new building with housing for 36 handicapped persons in accessible, furnished single apartments that included private bathrooms and kitchenettes. The facility also expanded classroom space, the vocational training department, private areas for case management, and a convenience store located adjacent to the program area.

Step Up was also committed to increase public understanding and acceptance of mental illness. At the Fresh Start convenience store, clients were able to interact with the community. Clients also participated on Step Up's advisory committee and board of directors. Step Up participated in newspaper and radio interviews. Dempsay herself was a very charismatic leader and had ties with the entertainment world. Step Up collaborated in the production of several educational videos, public service announcements, and major motion pictures (*Step Up on 2nd* newsletter, 2014).

Partners/Opposition

In the summer of 1986, financial problems threatened to push Step Up out of their building headquarters. However, the nonprofit Los Angeles MHA purchased the building. With the assistance of an anonymous donor, the building was leased to Step Up for a nominal amount. Step Up received financial support from the Los Angeles County Department of Mental Health, the State Department of Rehabilitation, the City of Santa Monica, and the federal government, as well as grants from local businesses, foundations, and private donations (Abrams, 1986; L. Mansouri, personal communication, 1998).

The Santa Monica community voiced strong opposition to the establishment of Step Up. Businesses were concerned that Step Up members would loiter in the town's business district, making the city more dangerous and less pleasant. The police, fire department, and paramedics were occasionally called to deal with crises or medical emergencies. Stigmatization of the mentally ill and homeless individuals hindered the community's acceptance of the program. However, after 15 years, there was recognition of the value of the program. Other critics said that treatment and housing programs should be separate and not run as a joint program like Step Up.

Macro-environment

Family members of the mentally ill are often shamed into silence due to the stigma attached to mental illness. In part due to the federal policy that deinstitutionalized the mentally ill in the 1960s, community programs for the mentally ill were scarce. A report by Ralph Nader in the 1980s noted the deplorable state of support for mental health in California and praised Step Up for its cost-effectiveness and therapeutic value.

Impact and Remarks

Step Up was praised by local police and city officials as a benefit to the community (Rojas, 1997; *Step Up on 2nd* newsletter, 2014). The Santa Monica Police Department even took people to Step Up for services. Dempsay received awards on the national, state, and local levels for her contributions. Step Up proved itself to be a user-friendly and accessible mental health program. By empowering the mental health consumer, Step Up debunked the stereotypes associated with the mentally ill. It was also a very cost-effective program for treatment and support for mentally ill.

CASE STUDY #37: TRADITIONAL CHILDBEARING GROUP, BOSTON, MASSACHUSETTS, 1978 (HPDP)

Problem

The ICTC established the Traditional ChildBearing Group (TCB) which focused on traditional childbirth and midwifery among African-American women. The major problem being addressed was the lack of quality prenatal health care among Boston's African-American women.

The formation of the International Center for Traditional Childbearing (ICTC) was inspired by the Childbirth Providers of African Descent (CPAD), a national Black midwife support group founded by midwife Sister Ayanna Ade in 1981. When CPAD dissolved in 1988, Sister Shafia Monroe (founder of ICTC), felt an obligation to create something similar for generations of the community of Black midwives. In August 1991, with support of a national group of midwives and healers, Sr. Shafia Monroe founded the International Center for Traditional Childbearing (ICTC) in Portland, OR. (ICTC, 1991)

Leadership Impetus

A practicing midwife, Shafia Monroe, and her colleagues founded the Traditional Childbearing Group, Inc. (TCB) on Mother's Day in Boston, Massachusetts. It stressed the tradition of nurturance and support throughout the childbearing period and beyond by providing comprehensive services ranging from nutrition to parenting guidelines.

EMPOWER Methods Used

- Empowerment training and leadership development
- Media use
- Public education and participation
- Enabling service and assistance

The TCB staff members built skills by getting involved in the policy issues and social problems of the community. TCB also wrote proposals for grants to raise money to maintain services and rent office space for informative meetings, to centralize services, and have a reading room for staff and community, as well as to hire administrative staff. TCB held annual all-women symposia featuring lectures and demonstrations by African-American women healers on such topics as massage, chiropractic, nutrition, sisterhood, herbal medicines, the technique of wrapping babies on the back, and the history of African-American women healers. Overall, these symposia had an empowering effect on participants and observers through the sharing of valuable information.

TCB also garnered extensive media coverage in local Boston newspapers and other media. In terms of public education, TCB attempted to reach the community through pamphlet distribution; sexuality education classes for teens at juvenile detention centers and in summer work programs; and prenatal and breastfeeding workshops at the women's state prison, ghetto high schools, and the municipal hospital. TCB developed videotapes for the nurse-midwifery services at Boston City Hospital and trained future midwives. TCB carried out projects for the urban African-American community such as promoting and providing information on parenting, nutrition, and other non-maternal healthcare issues. TCB also advocated home birth or delivery as opposed to medicalized childbirth in hospitals. Finally, TCB offered much-needed health care services such as individual prenatal care visits, childbirth classes, and comprehensive maternity services for fees ranging from $5 to $600. For those who could not afford to pay, fees were waived.

Partners/Opposition

Within Boston's black community, it was a respected grassroots organization that was viewed as providing tremendous benefit to its members. The newspaper media also covered TCB extensively. However, elected officials, physicians, and health officials did not recognize or lend support to the issue of home birth due to safety concerns.

Macro-environment

In the 1970s, the number and percentage of out-of-hospital births increased across the nation. Some reasons for turning from hospital delivery to planned home birthing included the desire to have a natural birthing experience that the mothers could control; dissatisfaction with the fragmented, impersonal, often insulting and unnecessarily medicalized hospital and clinic services; and preference for a low-cost home birth.

Impact and Remarks

TCB's effect on the community was reflected in the following statistic: the childbirth education classes reached over 1,000 adults and teens annually, and an estimated 1,800 callers received information, advice, and referrals on the 24-hour phone line. Up to 300 clients attended the breastfeeding workshops, and about 45 teenage girls attended the parenting classes each year. TCB held all-women's symposia each year that were attended by African-American women of diverse backgrounds. At theses symposia, the participants heard lectures and demonstrations about women healers, sisterhood, and alternative medicine, among other topics (Waite, 1993). The ICTC actively collaborates with a local radio station KBOO to reach Oregon communities (website: http://kboo.fm/program).

In 2007, ICTC launched their official website (www.ictcmidwives.org), which became the official web site for black midwives (www.blackmidwives. org), which remains linked to ICTC. It also started the *Black Midwives and Healers Review* newsletter. The ICTC also led the efforts to prepare the HB 2211 report which provided credible evidence showing the *Doulas* (a Greek word for women who serve and help other women and also means the traditional birth attendants/midwives) as an effective and affordable option for childbirths and care for poor women. The Oregon Health Authority passed HB 3311 in 2011, and ICTC was the first approved Doula credentialing organization (Doula, 2011). In 2012 the ICTC hosted the Eighth International Black Midwives and Healers Conference in Miami, Florida. During October 9 to 11, 2015, the ICTC hosted the Ninth International Black Midwives (Doula) and Healers Conference in Portland, Oregon (Doula, 2011).

CASE STUDY #70: TRI-VALLEY CITIZENS AGAINST A RADIOACTIVE ENVIRONMENT (CAREs), CALIFORNIA, 1980s (HPDP)

Problem

The major problem being addressed was health risks that were both occupational (a fourfold increase in two types of malignant cancer in employees) and ecological (well water contamination and air pollution) associated with the operation of a nuclear weapons facility, Lawrence Livermore National Laboratory (LLNL) managed by the University of California (CARE, 2015).

Leadership Impetus

Marylea Kelley founded the Tri-Valley Citizens Against a Radioactive Environment (CAREs), holding its first meeting in her apartment in the mid-1980s. The Tri-Valley CAREs' main objective was "to transform the nuclear weapons mission of LLNL to peacetime goals."

EMPOWER Methods Used

- Rights protection and social action litigation
- Organizing partnership
- Media use
- Public education and participation
- "Tri-Valley CAREs was founded in 1983 in Livermore, California, by concerned neighbors living around the Lawrence Livermore National Laboratory, one of two locations where all US nuclear weapons are designed. Tri-Valley CAREs monitors nuclear weapons and environmental clean-up activities throughout the US nuclear weapons complex, with a special focus on Livermore Lab and the surrounding communities" (http://www.trivalleycares.org/new/aboutus.html)

In order to locate sources of information about health and safety standard violations committed by the laboratory and the legal procedures required for verification of environmental impacts, the CAREs group members talked to their neighbors, canvassed door to door, disseminated informational leaflets, and held organizational meetings. The group also contacted the Department of Health, the EPA, and the Department of Energy (DOE), asking these agencies to heed their own statutes pertaining to public safety. The Tri-Valley CAREs joined the Livermore Environment and Peace Alliance, a coalition composed of representatives from about 20 local Bay area peace and environmental groups that exchanged information. The coalition also prepared a coordinated strategy for important forums such as EPA hearings, DOE stakeholders' meetings, University of California Regents meetings, congressional visits, and press conferences. These forums provided an opportunity for public solidarity, media coverage, and voicing the group's position on the issues.

Partners/Opposition

Members of the Livermore Environment and Peace Alliance and the Western States Legal Foundation spearheaded a major lawsuit on behalf of the Tri-Valley CAREs and the Southern California Federation of Scientists Against the University of California. The Tri-Valley CAREs were also members of and received support from a national coalition that offered policy information, and an international group of nuclear weapons survivors from Kazakhstan to islands of the South Pacific.

Macro-environment

LLNL and Los Alamos are the two main centers controlling the design and development of all nuclear weapons under the management of the University of California. Due to the secrecy shrouding nuclear weapons in the past, the complex that is responsible for the production of nuclear weapons has been able to bypass public oversight or review of their dealings with some of the most hazardous materials known to man. Each of the 18 sites of the complex, CAREs alleged, had concealed dire health consequences to their workers and the ecology of the surrounding communities. Furthermore, LLNL, along with the corporate contractors, was a powerful supporter for continued development of new nuclear bombs.

Impact and Remarks

During the ten years of its existence, the Tri-Valley CAREs achieved many successes in its struggles, including delaying or canceling major nuclear weapons–related projects at the LLN (Pilisuk et al., 1996). As a result of the group's efforts, the Livermore facility instituted additional monitoring for safety, discontinued the incineration of radioactive wastes, and publicized its cleanup. The Tri-Valley CAREs served as a model of what grassroots communities could accomplish in the face of both a local problem and a large-scale or global nuclear dilemma.

CASE STUDY #66: WOMEN AGAINST GUN VIOLENCE (WAGV),
CALIFORNIA, 1994 (HPDP)

Problem

This case study falls within the domain of HPDP. The major problem being addressed was the proliferation of guns on the streets, the high rate of gun-related deaths of adults and children, and the gun manufacturing industry's exploitation of women's fear by encouraging women to buy guns for self-protection.

> In 1993, in response to the gun industry's expansive marketing campaign toward women, the surging handgun homicide rates, and believing that women are agents of social change, then 64 year old Los Angeles Police Commissioner *Ann Reiss Lane* co-coordinated with Betty Friedan, leader of the feminist movement and author of The Feminine Mystique, a national conference that articulated guns and gun violence as a women's issue and a public health concern. This coalition of women and their families hoped to profoundly change the climate of the gun violence debate by working with elected officials, survivors, and communities. Out of this conference *Women Against Gun Violence (WAGV)* was born. Now, in 2013, both women and men make up WAGV's Board of Directors as it educates the public, policymakers and the media about the human, financial and public health consequences of gun violence. (WAGV, 2013).

Leadership Impetus

The idea was sparked by reporters who had asked feminist Betty Friedan to respond to the gun manufacturing industry's claim that gun ownership was a women's equality issue. This marketing strategy also claimed that women had an obligation to own a gun to protect themselves and their families. Coordinated by then–Los Angeles Police Commissioner Ann Reiss Lane, a symposium entitled "The Betty Friedan Symposium: Articulating Guns and Violence as a Women's Issue" was held in Los Angeles in 1993. From this forum developed the activist group Women Against Gun Violence (WAGV), a coalition of organizations and individuals dedicated to operating a state-wide campaign to educate, organize, and mobilize California women to try to put a stop to gun violence by reducing the availability of guns in California. Launched in January of 1994, WAGV was a project that was funded by the California Wellness Foundation.

EMPOWER Methods Used

- ¤ Enabling service and assistance
- ¤ Rights protection and social action/reform

¤ Media use
¤ Public education and participation
¤ Organizing partnership

The WAGV fought to tighten standards for gun manufacturing, eliminate "kitchen table" gun dealers (private sales) from residential neighborhoods, and persuade the law enforcement agencies to track the history of each gun used in a homicide. WAGV had an all-women Leadership Council chaired by Ann Reiss Lane, which set policy and fund-raising goals as well as made organization plans.

The WAGV participated in public protest including vigils and pickets by women and children (such as the annual "Stop the Violence" March in downtown Los Angeles; the "silent march of the shoes" in which thousands of pairs of shoes representing murdered children were collected and displayed in public places; and a public memorial for murdered children). WAGV served as a source of data on gun violence for the print and electronic media, locally and nationally. WAGV also tried to focus public attention on gun violence and the need for citizen action through community outreach. An annual "Education for Action" luncheon helped coalition member organizations understand the problem of gun violence and motivated them to action.

The Victim Remembrance Project drew the attention of public officials to the victims of homicide, suicide, or accidental shootings by notifying elected officials representing the residential area of the victims. WAGV offered condolences to the families of the victims, referrals to grief counselors, and training and advocacy around gun-related issues. The victims' families could also submit pictures and a brief story about the victim, which were then posted on the WAGV website. WAGV heavily relied on collaboration, and participated in several groups that bought together representatives from several fields. WAGV's Municipal Policy Study Group united elected officials from the all cities and towns of Los Angeles County to support consistent gun laws in each of the cities and towns in cooperation with members of the L.A. City Council. Some of the ordinances included the banning of "Saturday night specials" (which was realized in Los Angeles and passed as state law, effective January 2000); gross receipts on tax on businesses that sell guns; banning private gun sales from homes; mandatory trigger locks; and banning gun shows on public property.

Partners/Opposition

The WAGV has ties with more than 100 organizations and individual members, including YWCA, Drive-By Agony, Church Women United, the Junior League, the Mexican American Legal Defense and Education Fund, NOW, and the Southwest Ecumenical Council. The National Rifle Association and the California Shooting and Sports Council represent the opposing views when gun safety laws are under consideration (T. Perrina, personal communication, 1997).

Macro-environment

California is the national leader in the number of gun deaths and the number of handguns manufactured. Nearly 10% of all children killed in industrialized countries are killed in California, 90% by guns. More Californians died from gunshot wounds than from car crashes. In 2014, 126 law enforcement officers were killed nationwide in the line of duty—a 24% jump over 2013. Of those, 14 were in California. Recently MSNBC reported that:

> "In the early 1990s, California's gun laws were weak and full of gaps, and the toll of gun violence across the state rose to unprecedented levels—at one point 15 percent higher than the national average," reads the study by the San Francisco based Law Center to Prevent gun Violence. San Francisco-Now California's gun laws are the strongest in the nation and "the state's gun death rate has plummeted" (MSNBC, 2013). According to the San Francisco based Law Center for to Prevent Gun Violence (LCTPGV, 2014) "Every year, more than 30,000 Americans die from gun violence."

Impact and Remarks

Gun control is a complex issue that extend beyond gun violence. A recent PEW Research Center (PRC, 2015) survey noted that: "For the first time in more than two decades of Pew Research Center surveys, there is more support for gun rights than gun control. Currently, 52% say it is more important to protect the right of Americans to own guns, while 46% say it is more important to control gun ownership (PRC, 2015). That does not mean that Gun Control is not in public interest.

The Law Center to Prevent Gun Violence in San Francisco has been fighting for smart gun laws for over 20 years; they have noticed a trend: the states with stronger gun regulation have lower gun death rates, and the states with weaker regulation have higher gun death rates" (LCTPGV, 2014). The public and groups like MAGV have been very active in gun control in California. According to Robyn Thomas, executive director of the Law Center to Prevent Gun Violence, we could be doing much better; "Among all the industrialized nations, 80% of all firearms deaths occur in the United States" (MSNBC, 2013).

The city of West Hollywood passed California's first ordinance banning the sale of "Saturday night specials"—small, cheap guns used most often by criminals and youth due their easy availability and disposability. When Los Angeles followed suit, Councilmember Jackie Goldberg, sponsor of the measure, distinguished WAGV (Perrina, 1997) and the city of West Hollywood for their significant leadership. This ordinance is now a state law. California, the most populous state in the nation, led the country, according to the report from the National Law Enforcement Officers Memorial Fund (http://www.latimes.com/local/lanow/la-me-ln-california-law-enforcement-fatalities-20141230-story.html):

In 2014 the Law Center to Prevent Gun Violence (LCTPGV) stated:

> Every year, more than 30,000 Americans die from gun violence. But there's more to the story. The Law Center to Prevent Gun Violence has been fighting for smart gun laws for over 20 years, and we've noticed a trend: *the states with stronger gun regulation have lower gun death rates, and the states with weaker regulation have higher gun death rates.*"

The LCPGV further notes:

> "The good news is that there's been tremendous progress. Since the horrific tragedy at Sandy Hook in 2012, *37 states have passed an unprecedented 99 laws strengthening gun regulation.* Ten states have enacted major overhauls.

CASE STUDY #56: WOMEN FOR SOBRIETY (WFS), UNITED STATES, 1975, (HPDP)

Problem

The major problem being addressed was the lack of women-centered support groups for alcoholics. Existing groups such as Alcoholics Anonymous (AA) historically included mostly male alcoholics; they did not involve women's issues specifically. The WFS was designed to help women in need of help (WFS, 2011).

Leadership Impetus

Based on her own alcoholic experience, her recovery attempts with AA, and her study of sociology, Jean Kirkpatrick formulated a plan of recovery called "New Life" in 1973. In 1975, Kirkpatrick formed Women For Sobriety, Inc. (WFS), the first mutual self-help organization for women alcoholics only, which used the New Life philosophy. Kirkpatrick, who has a Ph.D. in sociology, believes that a woman's experience as an alcoholic is a distinct phenomenon. In order for women to have lasting sobriety, she believed, programs for them must address their special needs, especially the building of self-esteem.

EMPOWER Methods Used

- ¤ Media use
- ¤ Enabling service and assistance

◘ Public education and participation
◘ Empowerment training and leadership development

A 1976 newspaper article about Kirkpatrick and WFS written by Patricia McCormack of United Press attracted attention from alcoholic women across the nation. A story in the October 1976 issue of *Women's Day* describing a woman's drinking problem and how she overcame her problem with WFS's help generated thousands of letters. As a result of the nationwide attention, Kirkpatrick wrote a book, *Turnabout: Help for a New Life* (Doubleday), which described her struggles with alcoholism and recovery. Recognized as an expert on alcoholism in women, Kirkpatrick was regularly interviewed for radio and television. She spoke at alcoholism conferences and other public speaking events, which generated interest for WFS. She also testified before the Senate regarding the special needs of women alcoholics.

The WFS "New Life" Program promotes behavioral changes through positive reinforcement (approval and encouragement); positive thinking; and metaphysical methods (relaxation techniques, meditation, diet, and physical exercise). During WFS meetings, women talk about positive things that had happened in the past week, not about their past drinking experiences. All women get a chance to speak during each meeting, which is led by a certified moderator. In this all-women forum, members receive nurturing and support in a safe environment. Improving self-esteem, taking responsibility for their actions, and learning not to dwell on negative thoughts make up the core philosophy of WFS. The "13 WFS Affirmations" reflect the "four themes of abstinence": positive thinking; belief in one's own competency; spirituality; and emotional growth. The program motto is read at the end of each WFS meeting: "We are capable and competent, caring and compassionate, always willing to help another, bonded together in overcoming our addictions." WFS also has online chat groups that enable women to join an open forum led by a certified group moderator to discuss WFS's philosophy of recovery. A pen pal program gives women who cannot attend regular group meetings the opportunity to correspond with current members. The WFS newsletter, *Sobering Thoughts*, includes inspirational essays by Kirkpatrick and other relevant WFS information for members.

The annual conference allows WFS to display the literature about women and alcoholism that it produces (brochures, books, and audio/video tapes). The conference also sponsors workshops on alcoholism issues, WFS group meetings, and a fund-raising auction.

Partners/Opposition

WFS obtains its operational money from group donations, sale of literature, speaking engagements, workshops, and outside donations.

Macro-environment

> An estimated 7,500,000 women alcoholics live in the United States alone. Prior to the 1970s, there was very limited research on women alcoholics and their treatment needs. Women alcoholics were likely to be referred to AA, a support group created largely by male alcoholics. In all-women AA groups, women are more likely to be spontaneous and more open to discussing sensitive issues. Some argue that women alcoholics suffer from triple stigmatization: as an individual with an addiction, as a woman who has failed to fulfill her gender role in society, and as a sexually promiscuous woman (promiscuity is often associated with women alcoholics).

Impact and Remarks

There are more than 300 self-help groups using the WFS philosophy in the United States, Canada, England, New Zealand, Australia, Ireland, and Finland; several treatment facilities, hospitals, and women centers are also using the WFS program as their recovery program for women. WFS has received over 60,000 letters from women and their families who have achieved sobriety (Kaskutas, 1996).

One study of WFS reports:

> The organization's current data base is over 100,000 strong and growing, with the overwhelming majority of contacts made via email. In 1997, WFS averaged 25 to 30 new email inquiries per week. By comparison, in 2012 WFS receives between 100-150 new email inquiries per week and responds almost exclusively by email now, roughly ninety percent of the time. Direct contact by phone accounts for most of the remaining ten percent of inquiries. WFS Web Site At the end of 1995, WFS created its first web site, and by 1997 the site averaged 1,000 page views per month. Consistent with the internet explosion over the next 20 years, the newly revised and updated web site has become the organization's electronic trump card for future success, currently averaging over 30,000 views per month. (Fenner & Gifford, 2012)

Since WFS's inception in 1976, the "New Life" Program has been adapted for other addictions. In addition, a growing interest in the program among men has spawned Men For Sobriety groups in the United States and Canada (Kaskutas, 1994). WFS provides a supportive and safe environment for women alcoholics. It offers a self-help choice for women who need help in getting over their alcohol addictions. Not only did WFS members achieve sobriety, they improved their self-esteem.

On June 19, 2000, WFS's founder Dr. Jean Kirkpatrick passed away at the age of 77. Her life experiences and recovery journey, expressed so well in her books and the WFS Program, have had such a personal and positive impact on many women alcoholics. Her greatest heart's desire was to see that WFS continue after her passing so that not one single woman would have to take the journey to recovery alone (http://www.womenforsobriety.org/wfs_jean.html).

A recent paper on the 35 years of WFS accomplishments since its inception reports (Fenner & Gifford, 2012):

The organization's current data base is over 100,000 strong and growing, with the overwhelming majority of contacts made via email. In 1997, WFS averaged 25 to 30 new email inquiries per week. By comparison, in 2012 WFS receives between 100–150 new email inquiries per week and responds almost exclusively by email now, roughly ninety percent of the time. Direct contact by phone accounts for most of the remaining ten percent of inquiries. WFS Web Site At the end of 1995, WFS created its first web site, and by 1997 the site averaged 1,000 page views per month. Consistent with the internet explosion over the next 20 years, the newly revised and updated web site has become the organization's electronic trump card for future success, currently averaging over 30,000 views per month. (Fenner & Gifford, 2012, p. 6).

The study continues:

Since its inception in 1998, when it had only one chat meeting and 25 participants, the online forum has expanded to offer multiple message boards as well as 14 formal chat meetings per week across many time zones, led by chat leaders who are certified based on the same competencies that WFS requires for face to face group moderators. The WFS online community continues to grow, showing in 2011 a thirty-one percent increase in forum membership and participation over the previous year. Additional statistics for 2011 reveal a total of 291,529 posts on the message boards and 49,000 private messages among the members. (Fenner & Gifford, 2012, p. 7)

CASE STUDY #39: WOMEN'S HEALTH CARE FOUNDATION, QUEZON CITY, PHILIPPINES, 1980

Problem

There was a lack of opportunities for women in the Philippines to obtain modern health care beyond maternal health care or public health services offered during their childbearing years.

Leadership Impetus

The Women's Health Care Foundation (WHCF) was founded in 1980 by a group of physicians, lawyers, business people, and researchers who were dissatisfied with existing health services for women that focused primarily on maternal and child health and family planning. The founders of the WHCF believed that health services should address all of women's needs through infancy to old age, and that gender perspectives should be incorporated into program and service delivery. WHCF also wanted to provide women with accurate information so that they could make proper decisions about their own health care.

EMPOWER Methods Used

- ¤ Enabling service and assistance
- ¤ Rights protection and social action/reform
- ¤ Work/job training and micro-enterprise
- ¤ Organizing partnership
- ¤ Public education and participation
- ¤ Media use

The WHCF operates three fixed-site clinics in the metropolitan Manila area and an outreach program that traveled to poor communities. Both the WHCF clinics and outreach program provided physical examinations and basic laboratory services, such as pregnancy tests, semen analysis, and blood tests. Client fees were kept low, and staff were trained to perform multiple tasks due to limited resources. Services took into account the multiple societal roles of women and men. For example, the WHCF offered counseling in family planning and infertility; STD prevention education and treatment; information on cancer screening and domestic violence; and prenatal and postnatal care. One of the clinics had facilities for births, and clinic staff attended home births as well. Women were referred to other social service agencies for problems that fell outside the domain of WHCF. Because women often put their family's health needs before their own needs, services were also offered for men and for children (such as immunizations).

Staff members visited homes to promote clinic services and to conduct seminars on responsible parenthood, family planning, STDs, and other topics. An important component of the WHCF outreach program was the training of local women as community health workers. As part of a UNFPA-funded project launched in 1991, the field staff conducted small group discussions during which women and youth (male and female) talked about their reproductive health needs and problems. The contraceptives were sold to distributors at cost, and Community Health Workers (CHWs) were allowed to add on a few pesos for profit. Because the vendors worked in the same areas as sex industry workers (prostitutes, etc.) and it was part of their job description to be persuasive salespeople, they were also trained as safe-sex motivators and sources of information on fertility and prevention of STDs.

In order to continue monitoring government policy on women's health issues, Woman Health Philippines was created. This new organization promoted the Filipino woman's right to health and reproductive freedom and served as secretariat during the First National Convention of Health NGOs. To help meet women's need for accurate health information, the WHCF established the Institute for Social Studies and Action (ISSA) in 1983.

Partners/Opposition

The WHCF nurtured alliances with family planning organizations, women's health advocates, legislative lobbying groups, and HIV/AIDS support networks. Several organizations emerged from collaborative efforts between WHCF and other NGOs, including the Philippine NGO Council for Health and Welfare; KALAKASAN (means "Working for the Safety and Dignity of Women & Girls") organized to counter domestic violence; the Alliance for Women's Health, Bukluran Para Sa Kalusugan ng Sambayanan (BUKAS) which serve as Training Centers / Social Halls with Lodging, Library Resource Center, and Women's Vote for Family Planning. WHCF built an international network of supporters and allies, including US Agency for International Development (USAID), United Nations Funds for Population Activities (UNFPA), United Nations International Children's Emergency Fund (UNICEF), the Ford Foundation, Margaret Sanger International, Johns Hopkins Center for Communication Programs and Family Health International (FHI) a nonprofit organization and government agencies, such as the Department of Health, the Department of Science and Technology, the Department of Social Welfare, and the Department of Labor and Employment, which used WHCF staff as resource speakers and consultants. The conservative elements in the Catholic Church launched attacks on reproductive rights. Unfortunately, these proponents wielded a disproportionate influence over policy-makers and program implementers. The FHI describes its mission and scope of work as:

> At Family Health International we bring research and public health programs together to improve people's lives. Our researchers increase understanding of the technologies and health care systems best suited to people in need. Our public health professionals combine this scientific information with best practices from the field—and our experience of 35 years—to deliver evidence-based health programs that have real impact. We give hope and build futures for poor and disadvantaged people throughout the developing world by: ... working with communities to provide public health services. ... investigating new drugs and devices to prevent pregnancy—as well as to prevent and treat disease. ... bringing partners together to mitigate the impact of illness and death. Most of all

we are about people. The following pages provide a glimpse of our work through their stories." (FHI, 2007)

Macro-environment

The Philippine health situation offered two choices to people in need of treatment: (1) free or very-low-cost services from government-run centers and hospitals (often with shortages of staff and high patient volume); and (2) expensive private services, often from tertiary institutions that were not geared to women's health needs. Women's health concerns were thought to be adequately served by maternal and child health (MCH) programs. Increasingly, however, women's advocates have emphasized that MCH programs do not meet women's total health needs.

Impact and Remarks

WHCF became not only a point for delivery of a wide array of health services, but a source of healthcare expertise in the Philippines. WHCF played a pivotal role in emphasizing health rights as an important component of women's rights. Through WHCF and ISSA's efforts, women found a voice and expressed their viewpoints in this debate. In addition, advocacy efforts raised awareness of women's health issues among policy-makers, government officials, and NGOs.

CASE STUDY #60: WOMEN IN NEW RECOVERY (WINR), UNITED STATES, 1994 (HPDP)

Problem

There was a lack of residential recovery facilities and services for alcoholic and drug-addicted women and their children. The majority of the women in the program faced a variety of social problems, including abuse, a lack of family support, and low self-esteem.

Leadership Impetus

Patricia Henderson, a recovering drug addict and alcoholic, founded Women in New Recovery (WINR) in 1994 as a way to share her experiences of addiction and sobriety with other women. After nine years of sobriety, she left her job as a paralegal to set up a 12-bed house in Mesa, Arizona. In the very beginning, WINR was a one-woman operation, financed with Henderson's own money. Eventually, she would teach residents of the program to do some of the work. Former residents now make up the entire WINR staff (http://www.winr.org/). The program does charge the women for its services, with two different fee schedules.

EMPOWER Methods Used

- ◘ Enabling service and assistance
- ◘ Empowerment training and leadership development
- ◘ Work/job training and micro-enterprise
- ◘ WINR believes that:
- ◘ "Since women abuse drugs and alcohol for different reasons than men, finding a program that recognizes these differences, and strategizes specifically how women handle addiction and relapse, ensure the maximum effectiveness of treatment. Gender-specific treatment also eliminates distractions from the opposite sex. All too often mixed gender treatment allows women to seek other ways to fill the void and escape from dealing with their feelings. In the simplicity and safety of an all-female setting she's able to fully self-disclose personal experiences, without fearing judgment, as the female addict often suffers from chronic low self-esteem." (http://www.winr.org/)

WINR is open to any alcoholic and drug-addicted women who need a place to recover from their addictions. During the first six months of the program, women are expected to get a job and work with a sponsor. They attend daily 12-Step meetings and in-house peer group meetings led by certified professionals in the relapse prevention field. Residents can learn a variety of living and employment skills such as money-management instruction, onsite computer training, and communication skills classes. One of the facilities offers GED and college course work. After this intense period of learning self-discipline and self-control, the women begin to direct their own recovery during a transitional phase. The third phase of the program allows responsible residents to be reunited with their small children while still living in a safe environment, namely the WINRs and Kids House. (One of the single mothers in the main program was instrumental in establishing this program, which is currently helping seven families.) WINR residents are involved in community activities such as Neighborhood Watch, cleanup campaigns, weekly AA Big Book study, and AA and Narcotics Anonymous (NA) 12-Step meetings in Mesa and surrounding communities. This allows residents to reintegrate into society as useful and productive members (http://www.winr.org/).

Partners/Opposition

The communities in which WINR facilities are located have been supportive of the program. Volunteers from the professional community run seminars that teach valuable living and employment skills. The program receives referrals from a variety of agencies, including treatment centers, hospitals, detoxification units, probation, and parole. Several local businesses donate computers and services to the center.

Macro-environment

One of the biggest barriers women face in seeking treatment for substance abuse is the stigma attached to women's chemical dependency. For this reason, women often delay treatment until they reach a more debilitated point in their illness than men. Furthermore, most treatment programs ignore women's unique problems of child care, physical and sexual abuse, parenting, pregnancy, sexually transmitted disease, lack of education and employment, and higher rates of poverty.

Impact and Remarks

WINR has grown from one small house to nine houses and two apartment buildings located in Las Vegas and three Arizona cities offering primary houses for single women, primary houses for mothers with kids, and transitional houses for women who wish to extend their stay. Program participants achieve sobriety and a set of skills that help them to reintegrate into their communities. They learn to prioritize their social, emotional, physical, and family concerns with the help of WINR and other community resources. Many former residents have found employment at WINR facilities, thereby providing new residents with support, empathy, and expertise, as well as an example to follow. Having these role models in the program not only guides current residents to recovery but reinforces in the staff members a sense of accomplishment.

CASE STUDY #75: WOMEN ALIVE COALITION, INC., LOS ANGELES, CALIFORNIA, 1991 (HPDP)

Problem

The major problem addressed was the lack of support and treatment services for women living with HIV/AIDS (http://www.women-alive.org/).

Leadership Impetus

Women Alive is a coalition of, by, and for women living with HIV/AIDS. It was founded in 1991 by four HIV-positive female members of Being Alive (People with HIV/AIDS Action Coalition). The founders envisioned a support network for women with HIV that helps HIV-infected women connect with each other, bring others out of isolation, exchange information about HIV treatments, and take charge of their lives.

EMPOWER Methods Used

- ¤ Enabling service and assistance
- ¤ Public education and participation
- ¤ Empowerment training and leadership development
- ¤ Rights protection and social action/reform

Women Alive operated a drop-in center—a small two-bedroom house in Los Angeles. Walk-in clients could obtain referrals to women-specific social services or professional psychological assistance, or access a specialized library that contained information about HIV, AIDS, and treatment. Women Alive's peer counseling program offered both one-on-one counseling and weekly support groups such as a Spanish-speaking group for HIV-positive women and their families; a group for heterosexual, HIV-positive men and women; a group for HIV-positive lesbians; and a completely anonymous support group (Positive Images) that brought HIV-positive women together through a toll-free, party-line telephone call. HIV-positive female volunteers operated the Women Alive hotline—a national toll-free peer-support hotline that offered emotional support and HIV treatment information to women callers from across the nation. Not only did this service help women with AIDS who wanted to remain anonymous, the volunteers also gained a sense of accomplishment and build self-esteem. Treatment advocates answered questions about medical care, treatments, or lab work. A monthly legal clinic offered one-on-one consultations with a female attorney. In addition to these support services, Women Alive offered weekly yoga classes and massages. Women Alive attempted to make HIV information "reachable and understandable to every woman throughout the world." To keep members apprised of the latest news on treatment as well as the organization's events and activities, Women Alive published a quarterly newsletter called *Awareness Is Life –Involvement in Power.* In addition to informative articles, the newsletter included personal stories of women with HIV and a list of resources where they could access services or participate in clinical studies. Women Alive also published a biannual Spanish-language newsletter called *Ecos Femeninos.* Women Alive published and distributed the first-ever HIV treatment guide for women, called "Knowledge, Action, Health: A Woman's Guide to HIV Treatments." This free 83-page booklet included detailed information about various medications for HIV and their costs, how to become involved in clinical trials, and understanding the nature of AIDS. Women Alive distributed more than 40,000 copies in eight months.

Women Alive provided community leadership and mentors other women to become effective advocates. In 1995, Women Alive sponsored 27 women to attend the "National Women and HIV" conference in Washington D.C. In 1997, Women Alive launched a national advocacy campaign entitled "Who's the 'cure' for? Do research to save women's lives!" All peer counselors, including support group facilitators and hotline operators, would complete a six-week training program to gain the necessary leadership skills. Through efforts like these, Women Alive helped empower women with HIV.

Partners/Opposition

Women Alive is funded primarily through private foundations. Women Alive works collaboratively with Being Alive as a sister organization:

> Being Alive is a nonprofit membership organization created and operated by and for people living with HIV/AIDS that engenders a sense of independence and self-determination in its members and builds a healthier and more powerful community of HIV-positive people. Being Alive accomplishes its mission through a comprehensive array of emotional support, treatment education, prevention, advocacy, wellness and social services." (http://beingalivela.org/ and http://www.avert.org/women-and-hiv-aids.htm)

Macro-environment

According to CDC, "Women account for one in four people living with HIV in the United States; African American women and Latinas are disproportionately affected at all stages of HIV infection" (CDC website accessed February 16, 2015; http://www.cdc.gov/hiv/risk/gender/women/index.html).

At the end of 2012 it was estimated that 52 percent of people living with HIV and AIDS in low- and middle-income countries are women. Every minute one young woman becomes infected with HIV, with sub-Saharan Africa reporting the percentage of young women aged 15–24 living with HIV being twice that of young men. (See more at: http://www.avert.org/women-and-hiv-aids.htm#sthash.lPLUfdH1.dpuf.)

Yet women benefit less than men from the new therapies. Women with AIDS/HIV are disproportionately non-white and poor. They tend to get diagnosed later in their disease progression, and they must deal with a host of issues, from childcare to transportation, that often make receiving early and high-quality healthcare difficult if not impossible. Long waits in public clinics are often impractical for women with young children and no childcare or babysitters. Furthermore, women with AIDS seldom have the community support, financial resources, and institutions available to homosexual men. Because of these and other obstacles, women with HIV-related symptoms receive delayed treatment.

Impact and Remarks

As an advocate for women with HIV, Women Alive fought to increase the percentage of females in AIDS clinical trials. Its treatment advocacy campaign raised awareness among pharmaceutical companies and researchers about the need to study the effects of HIV drugs on the bodies of women. Women Alive–sponsored activities created a mechanism for HIV-infected women to empower themselves through meaningful activity, participation in a community of people affected by AIDS, and accessibility to cutting-edge treatments and life-prolonging treatment information.

CASE STUDY #76: WOMEN AT RISK, CALIFORNIA, 1991 (HPDP)

Problem

The major problem being addressed was the lack of support groups for HIV-positive women.

Leadership Impetus

In 1991, Ann Copeland (who contracted HIV from a bisexual boyfriend) and Linda Luschei (who was infected by her husband) formed Women at Risk. Linda and Ann realized how crucial the support group would be to their emotional, psychological, and physical well-being, and decided to help bring other HIV-positive women together. Both founders were from an upper-middle-class neighborhood (Manhattan Beach, California) and college-educated.

EMPOWER Methods Used

- ¤ Enabling service and assistance
- ¤ Public education and participation
- ¤ Rights protection and social action/reform
- ¤ Media use

Women at Risk had four programs: starting and maintaining support groups for women; One-on-One peer companion program; education and prevention through their Speaker's Bureau; and a "Should I Be Tested?" workshop. Women at Risk had five support groups, located in Hermosa Beach, Santa Monica, San Luis Obispo, Torrance, and South Central Los Angeles. Two of the groups were ethnically oriented; Torrance was monolingual Spanish-speaking, South Central was for women of color. Each group was co-facilitated by a licensed therapist and an HIV-positive woman. The groups provided psycho-social support and helped HIV-infected women get out of their isolation and despair by talking with other individuals suffering the same plight (*Women at Risk* by Pat Rolands, 1999).

Partners/Opposition

Public and private attitudes towards sexuality may hinder an effective response to the AIDS crisis and threaten progress in the fight against AIDS. Due to the stigma attached to being HIV-positive, infected individuals are often shunned by society and pushed into isolation. Shortly after the time of Women at Risk's founding, basketball star Magic Johnson revealed that he was infected with HIV. His high-profile image helped jolt the nation into acknowledging the AIDS epidemic. At that time, many residents in the South Bay area of California, especially in the more affluent beach communities, were slow to realize that AIDS could touch their lives. Women at Risk collaborates with several organizations, including Women Alive (Case No. 75).

Macro-environment

Women with HIV face other unique problems. Women tend to be less aware of the risk of HIV. In many cases, they are infected by men who they do not know are bisexual or IV-drug users. Moreover, women with HIV are more likely to be black or Latina, have modest incomes, and no health insurance. For all of these reasons, women often miss out on the advantages of early treatment, and when they do receive care, it is often of lower quality than that available to men. An HIV-positive status carries tremendous stigma in society. The fear of being ostracized by one's own community keeps many HIV-infected women from seeking help.

CASE STUDY #65: MOTHERS AGAINST VIOLENCE IN AMERICA (MAVIA), UNITED STATES, 1993

Problem

The major problem being addressed was violence perpetrated by and against children. According to the National Center for Health Statistics and Children's Defense Fund, three children will die from child abuse every day.

Leadership Impetus

Pamela Eakes founded Mothers Against Violence In America (MAVIA) in Seattle in December of 1993 to combat the problem of youth violence. Eakes, who served as Tipper Gore's Deputy Chief of Staff during the 1992 presidential election, had 20 years of experience in advertising, marketing, and public relations. MAVIA was a grassroots, community mobilization organization committed to reducing violence by and against children through preventive education and grassroots advocacy.

EMPOWER Methods Used

- ¤ Public education and participation
- ¤ Rights protection and social action/reform
- ¤ Media use
- ¤ Organizing partnership

The educational outreach program reached students and parents through a grassroots network of supporters and volunteers. Speakers' bureaus, annual conferences, special events, and outreach materials were utilized to spread the word about MAVIA's cause. The speakers bureau presentations included topics on youth violence prevention; victim awareness; media literacy (learning skills of critical viewing and how each of us, collectively and individually, takes and makes meaning from our media experiences); gun violence prevention; community organizing; options, choices, consequences curriculum; men and violence prevention (learning the men's role to promote nonviolence); and public policy. Over 30,000 students and parents were reached each year through MAVIA speakers' bureaus.

MAVIA also raised consciousness of violence in the community. For example, it held an annual "Solutions to Violence in Our Lives" conference for middle school and high school students and parents. It sponsored a year-long gun safety campaign in Seattle and Boston that featured brochures, billboards, and video public service announcements encouraging the use of safety devices for firearms. MAVIA also sponsored a commemorative quilt called "Chain of Remembrance" that honored the lives of children who had died violently. Finally, MAVIA produced a resource handbook informing parents how to respond to media violence. The Public Policy program advocated at federal and state levels for legislation that promoted MAVIA's goal of creating a safer environment for all children. For example, MAVIA successfully advocated for passage of the federal "assault weapons ban" and legislation raising the age of possession of firearms in Washington State from 14 to 18.

MAVIA sponsored the student-initiated Students Against Violence Everywhere (SAVE) program in elementary, middle, and high schools, honored in 1997 by the Washington Council on Crime and Delinquency for Outstanding Achievement by a Community Organization. One of the SAVE programs consisted of a two-year elementary school public service performance partnership with KCPQ-13, Seattle's Fox Network television affiliate. This Emmy-nominated program reached over 25,000 students. The Youth Recognition Program awarded annual Youth Peacemaker awards and Legacy of Caring scholarships to students who exhibited extraordinary commitment to reducing violence in their schools and communities. MAVIA formed an advisory board of leading authorities in the fields of law enforcement, justice, medicine, education, government and business, community leaders, respected authorities, and survivors of violence.

Partners/Opposition

MAVIA received funding and in-kind support from members, businesses, and foundations such as the Boeing Company, Microsoft, PriceCostco, Group Health Cooperative, Public Employees Mutual Insurance Company

(PEMCO), Washington Mutual, Weyerhaeuser, General Telephone & Electronics (GTE), the Geffen Foundation, and the Seattle Foundation. MAVIA was also in partnership with Coinstar, Inc., as a charitable beneficiary of Coinstar's "Coins That Count" program. Jars of coins could be donated to MAVIA by visiting the Coinstar machines at the entrances to local supermarkets in Western Washington.

Macro-environment

American culture and media is saturated with violent messages that the vast majority of our population view as being inevitable. Children are exposed to violence through cartoon shows, films, and even their own families. There is growing apathy among the country that this type of exposure to violence is unpreventable. When child murderers catch the headlines across the nation, the problem of youth violence became more evident.

Impact and Remarks

MAVIA established more than 100 MAVIA and SAVE (Students Against Violence Everywhere) chapters in 27 states. MAVIA had a member/supporter network of more than 4,000 advocates. As a national network of mothers, fathers, students, and concerned people, MAVIA established itself as a leader in the grassroots movement to create a violence-free America. Founder Eakes received numerous awards for her efforts with the organization, including the 1995 YWCA Isabel Coleman Pierce Community Service award, a 1995 City of Seattle and Providence Medical Center Violence Prevention award, and four KOMO-TV Hometown Hero awards. MAVIA was commended by the United States Department of Justice for violence prevention efforts, and was selected to participate in the White House Leadership Conference on Youth, Drug Use, and Violence.

CASE STUDY #43: WOMEN'S REPRODUCTIVE HEALTH AND DEVELOPMENT PROGRAM (WRHDP), YUNNAN, CHINA, 1991 (HPDP)

Problem

The main problem being addressed was the set of reproductive health risks faced by rural Chinese women. These risks were rooted in a lifetime of inadequate diet, illness burdens, heavy workloads, poor educational opportunities, gender-discriminatory feeding, and other social practices.

Leadership Impetus

The Women's Reproductive Health and Development Program (WRHDP) was created in 1992, as a project funded by the Ford Foundation, through meetings among policy-makers from the Province of Yunnan's health, social, and development sectors (Li & Wang, 1998). During these initial visits, Ford Foundation program officers realized that they needed to take into account the concerns of local leaders in order to create a successful program. The rural women were best qualified to determine what changes were needed and to identify the best methods to achieve those changes.

EMPOWER Methods Used

- ¤ Organizing partnership
- ¤ Enabling service and assistance
- ¤ Work/job training and micro-enterprise
- ¤ Empowerment training and leadership development

In the initial stages of the project, working groups composed of local community members and organizations were formed to assess the reproductive health needs of women. In addition to the conventional assessment methods of focus groups and household surveys, village women used photography to identify and articulate their needs to policy-makers.

The community and outside agencies collaborated in the planning of several projects based on this needs assessment. For example, the women started reform projects for biogas tanks, silage pits, potable water projects, and nurseries in order to improve their living conditions. In partnership with local organizations, the women worked to provide scholarships for girls from poor families to stay in school, and literacy classes for village women. They developed and conducted family planning classes for men and women and participated in classes on nutrition and reproductive health. The village women participated in income-generating activities, such as pig raising, handicrafts, and mulberry tree cultivation. The women of Yunnan and the participating organizations also collaborated with national and international experts in the development of community-based indicators for reproductive health program planning and evaluation. Through training in capacity-building, the women leaders were able to take control of the program and their living conditions and become aware of the influences they could exert on larger organizations.

Partners/Opposition

Working groups composed of leaders from local women's organizations, county and provincial and academic institutions, and national and international experts collaborated and supported WRHDP. Some of the government and community organizations included the County Bureau of Public Health, the Country Women's Federation, the Family Planning Commission, the Education Commission, and the Office of Poverty Alleviation.

Macro-environment

Yunnan Province is located in a remote region of China and is China's third-poorest province. As in the rest of the People's Republic of China, Yunnan's healthcare delivery system changed drastically in the early 1980s when rural economic reforms dismantled the collective agricultural economy. The cooperative medical system, through which communal funds were pooled to support health clinics and "barefoot doctors," was also dismantled. Rising healthcare costs forced many rural residents to pay their medical expenses out-of-pocket. With little incentive for health workers to carry out environmental sanitation and disease prevention work, they tended to focus on expensive curative treatment and drug sales.

Village women's health reproductive health is not only affected by health-related activities. Education, housing, and agriculture also play a part. For example, WRHDP recognized that a woman's health during pregnancy, childbirth, and lactation is profoundly influenced by the broader social, economic, cultural, and environmental aspects of her life.

Impact and Remarks

The WRHDP helped women and women's organizations in poor communities to understand, articulate, and act on their health needs. The program institutionalized a planning process that involved communities and women in these communities in decision-making and program design. In turn, reproductive health policies reflected the needs defined by the community.

Both health workers and women leaders became more aware of the influence they could exert on organizations. The WRHDP affected the way activities and projects were carried out. The village women's daily activities were also been affected. For example, the women set up a daycare nursery in order to protect their children from the dangerous environmental conditions of their work sites. The women's participation in WRHDP led to increased self-reliance, self-efficacy, self-confidence, and a sense of local ownership. This participatory approach empowered the women in Yunnan by giving them skills that they continue to build on.

CASE STUDY #61: ARRAK BAN (ANTI-ALCOHOL CAMPAIGN), INDIA, 1996 (HPDP)

Problem

The main problem addressed was excessive drinking by men in Indian villages that often led to the beating of their wives and children and the wasting of the family income on alcohol (AAM, 1991; Frese, 2012).

Arrak is low cost liquor that is generally consumed by poor people. The anti-arrak movement started as a spontaneous movement in a remote village in Dubagunta in the southern state of Andhra Pradesh in India. It was a women's movement which saw the articulation of the issue of family violence in a public forum. The movement questioned notions about the political apathy of suffering masses and inability of women to take initiatives on their own without men's help. It is through this movement that rural women in the state of Andhra Pradesh created history.

The tax revenue from alcohol sales was Rs 390 million in 1970–71; by 1991–92 had that had increased to Rs 8.12 billion. Consequently government was not motivated to ban sales of alcohol which the village women demanded. (AAM, 1991)

Leadership Impetus

In the Indian state of Andhra Pradesh, a revolt against Arrak (alcohol) began in response to the excessive drinking by the village men:

In 1991–92, the average family income in the state of Andhra Pradesh was Rs 1,840 per annum. Of this, Rs 830 was spent on liquor. Men were spending nearly 75 percent of their income on drinking. This figure itself indicates how much expenditure of a household was on arrak.

—AAM, 1991

EMPOWER Methods Used

¤ Public participation
¤ Rights protection and social action litigation

Frustrated women raided liquor shops in their villages in Andhra Pradesh, piled liquor bottles and set fire to them, broke bottles of alcohol, and shouted anti-alcohol slogans that stunned spectators. The village women demanded removal of Arrak (local liquor) shops and threated politicians that they would vote against them if they did not ban liquor shops In 1991–92, the average family income in the state of Andhra Pradesh was Rs 1,840 per annum. Of this, Rs 830 was spent on liquor. Men were spending nearly 75 percent of their income on drinking. This figure itself indicates how much expenditure of a household was on arrak (UK Essays, 1991). This movement had the characteristics of a social movement as it mobilized the women involved in it to struggle for a specific goal and objective. Here the goal to be achieved was the ban on sale of arrak and women as a whole participated for the cause.

The women involved in the Arrak ban used the methods of rights protection, political activism, and social action/legal reform. They rampaged in local liquor stores and confiscated alcohol. They also staged strikes by with-holding cooking, laundry, and sex from their husbands. In 1991, a literacy drive began in the village had as its lesson a tale of an angry wife forcing the closing of an Arrak shop. This inspired women readers in Doobagunta to set fire to their village's Arrak outlet. They later ambushed the delivery trucks sent to replenish the supply and emptied the bottles onto the road. Without a designated leaders or coordination, a mass movement swept across the countryside, with women in towns like Kakinada, Mothkur, Sayipeta, and Raghunathapuram following the example of the first angry women. Women from every social class and political party joined the movement.

Partners/Opposition

The Indian government considers drinking to be a very dangerous vice among its citizens. In fact, India's Constitution calls upon states to exercise prohibition, and many attempts have been made, such as "dry" areas, edu-cational campaigns, and consumption taxes. Some states have strict anti-alcohol laws (e.g., Gujarat). The women's rights organizations and the leftist/communist parties support the poor women's struggle to ban alcohol shops and sales. The alcohol shop owners, suppliers, and some politicians oppose prohibition.

Macro-environment

Consuming alcohol to the point of inebriation after a day's labor is common-place in many rural areas of India. It is estimated that 40% of the Andhra Pradesh's rural men are alcoholics. Ironically, the high taxes placed on liquor have proved very profitable to some Indian states. In Andhra Pradesh, Chief Minister Rama Rao allowed the manufacturing of state-approved alcohol and selling it in state-approved stores prior to the beginning of the campaign. In Indian society, women are seen as second-class citizens and are tradition-ally not expected to voice their opinions against men.

Impact and Remarks

Although a ban on alcohol has been declared in some Indian states such as Andhra Pradesh and Haryana, and temperance has become a national issue, men's drinking behavior has not changed. Bootlegging emerged as a lucra-tive business catering to Arrak-loving men. Even when women turned in Arrak dealers to the authorities, the men were released without punishment. Needless to say, enforcement of the alcohol bans is not strict, with bootleg-ging earning an estimated $285 million a year. As a result of the ban on alco-hol, one of the largest government revenue sources (taxes on liquor) has been eliminated, and spending cuts were made in health care and schools.

CASE STUDY #1: THE RESCATA NDO SALUD: PROMOTORA EMPOWER
MODEL (SEE DISCUSSION OF THIS CASE IN THE TEXT IN PP. 150–151 IN
CHAPTER 5 AND CHAPTER 11).

Note: This case has been discussed in depth in several pages; in addition we
have added a website where readers can view a 14 minute video on the project.

CASE #33: MAHILA MILAN, BOMBAY, INDIA, 1988 (D)

Problem

This case study falls within the domain of development (D). The major problem being addressed is the conditions of pavement dwellers in Bombay, India.
For example, there is severe poverty, a lack of housing and jobs as well as
harassment and property thefts by the local police.

Leadership Impetus

Mahila Milan is a women's organization that was formed in 1988 by SPARC
(Society for the Promotion of Area Resource Centres) to empower women of
the "E Ward" slum in Bombay, India. SPARC is a self-made group that was
formed in 1985 after the Supreme Court made it legal to demolish pavement
huts. SPARC was the community's response that helped to organize slum and
pavement dwellers as well as to fight for their rights. Wanting to be more than
a charity organization, SPARC attempted to chart out their specific needs by
surveying 6,000 households and nearly 27,000 individuals about background,
income, family structure etc. Because government and voluntary agency programs often overlook women, SPARC specifically targeted the female portion of the slum dweller population.

EMPOWER Methods Used

- Empowerment training and leadership development
- Enabling service and assistance
- Rights protection and social action/reform
- Organizing partnership
- Work/job training and micro-enterprise

This collective of women pavement and slum dwellers has formulated survival
strategies, established democratic decision-making vehicles and used its own
resources to improve the living conditions of the urban poor. They have negotiated with the state for shelter planning both in terms of design and location.

SPARC instructed the members of *Mahila Milan* in dealing with day-
to-day problems such as admitting a sick child to the hospital; talking to the
municipal authorities; filling out forms for ration cards (which is needed to

get subsidized foodgrain, establish identity and place of residence) and filling out forms for bank loans and electricity connections.

Mahila Milan has also used the method of social action in order to fulfill their needs. In one instance, Mahila Milan led a group of forty women to the ration office to convince officials to give cards to families whom they had originally refused. In the second instance, 500 members of the Mahila Milan successfully filed suit against the Bombay Municipal Corporation (BMC) for stealing the pavement dwellers' belongings and destroying the unauthorized pavement huts where many slum women reside. In large part because the women had noted the license plate number of the BMC van and made detailed lists of what was stolen, the women won their case against BMC and received compensation for the stolen items.

Mahila Milan has established a collective savings fund for housing of $25,000 in four years and $2222 for daily emergencies. The latter is used for loans with nominal interest (2 rupees/month) for buying medicine, school-books or clothes. Seventy-four percent of slum-dwellers earn less than the minimum daily wage of Rs 18 (equivalent to $1).

With assistance from SPARC, Mahila Milan has also initiated income generation projects for women (teaching them to stitch, make files, folders and decorative items) and offered adult education classes. There are now Mahila Milan branches in 5 areas of Bombay (Dharavi, Wadala, Goregaon, Mankhurd and Chmbur) and 2 southern cities (Madras and Bangalore) that are actively participating in their local communities. The local Mahila Milan branch in Dindoshi created a cooperative society, built 50 houses, a community hall, a park and public toilets on a plot of land (18,000 sq. ft) that SPARC had acquired to build permanent and legal housing.

Partners/Opposition

In addition, SPARC and Mahila Milan have worked in conjunction with the National Slum Dwellers' Federation (NSDF) in areas of research, negotiation and other activities. The national group compensates for the local groups' limitations in completing formalities at the same time helping slum dwellers participate in policy and implementation decisions that directly affect them. For example, the NSDF took part in World Bank meetings for housing for the poor. As a result, SPARC helped 10,000 people apply for the program. In turn, the NSDF has benefited from this collaboration with Mahila Milan in terms of encouraging women leadership. Rather than overlooking women as potential leaders as in the past, the NSDF now has the example of the Mahila Milan to follow (p. 141).

Macro-environment

In urban areas of India such as the west coast metropolis of Bombay, there exists extreme poverty for some of its citizens. A lack of housing, jobs and welfare agencies contribute to dire conditions. In addition the local authorities seem to have little sympathy for the plight of those individuals forced to live in slums without suitable housing. Harassment and property theft of pavement dwellers is not uncommon.

Impact and Remarks

Following the initial assistance from SPARC, Mahila Milan is now run by local women like Rehmat Sheikh, Leela Naidu, Sona Pujari and Shehnaaz Sheikh. These women were previously employed in the low-paying domestic sector and who have now made strides in redefining their environment and empowering themselves. As a result of the formation of the Mahila Milan, its members, mostly uneducated migrants from rural areas, are now confident and respected participants of the community and are recognized for the important strides they have made. No longer afraid of the police or organizations such as the BMC, they can take comfort in the fact that they are able to make a positive difference in their environment. Mahila Milan's united action has effected changes in relationships within their families and communities. For the first time in Bombay, women have emerged as community leaders.

References

Gahlot, Deepa. "A SPARC of Hope for Slum-dwellers" in: Women's Feature Service *The Power to Change: Women in the Third World Redefine their Environment*. New Delhi, India: Zed Books Ltd., 1993, pp. 138–143.
We the Peoples: 50 Communities, website: http://iisd1.iisd.ca/50comm/commdb/list/c16. htm

CASE STUDY #50: DISABLED WOMEN'S NETWORK (DAWN) CANADA, 1985 (HPDP)

Problem

The major problem being addressed is the lack of health and social services organizations for disabled women. Support and services for disabled mothers are almost totally inaccessible or do not exist. According to the Health and Activity Limitation Survey by Statistics Canada, 16% of all Canadian women are disabled.

Leadership Impetus

Seventeen women with disabilities founded DAWN Canada in June 1985. These women gathered together from across Canada to discuss issues of personal concern. Since the founding meeting disabled women organized across the country, keeping in touch by mail and phone. Eventually, DAWN Canada received funding from the Secretary of State for some special projects. DAWN groups continue to be organized on a local, provincial, and national level. In 1992, DAWN Ontario was formed, a province-wide organization for women with all types of disabilities that is controlled by women with disabilities.

DAWN members include women with disabilities and non-disabled women, lesbians, bisexual women, aboriginal women, Franco-Ontarian women, women from many ethnic, racial, cultural, and religious backgrounds and women of all ages, from teens to seniors.

EMPOWER Methods Used

- ¤ Enabling service and assistance
- ¤ Public education and participation
- ¤ Rights protection and social action/reform
- ¤ Media use
- ¤ Organizing partnership

DAWN Canada is a feminist organization that supports disabled women in their struggles to control their own lives. DAWN produces resources about health care for women with disabilities; lobbies the government on issues affecting women with disabilities such as employment, advocacy, training, education, transportation, housing and health care.

As a service to their members, DAWN Ontario produces brochures on disabled mothers, sexuality, and how to talk to your doctor. DAWN also publishes an access checklist, a guide for health care professionals and a newsletter called Violence against Women with Disabilities. DAWN Ontario provides role models for girls with disabilities and develops resources for girls with disabilities.

DAWN speaks for the rights of women with disabilities to make sure we can take part in women's groups, activities, events and services, such as women's shelters, rape crisis centers and feminist counseling, and works with other women's and disability groups. For example, women with disabilities speak about violence at conferences, seminars, and events such as "Take Back the Night" marches.

DAWN Ontario was featured on the local TV station and local newspaper in December 1996 when its office moved to Sudbury, Ontario to better the northern area.

Partners/Opposition

DAWN works with others who share the concern for social justice, such as the Employment Equity Coalition; the Coalition Against Depo Provera; and the Coalition Against Extra Billing in Ontario.

DAWN is also involved in a research project with the University of Toronto and Women's College Hospital. Through focus groups, the research focuses on the health care needs and difficulties in trying to get reasonable services of women with disabilities.

DAWN received funding from the Ministry of Citizenship, Culture and Recreation to develop an annotated bibliography and research report on disabled women and violence. The Trillium Foundation provided funding for a three year Internet Access Grant and for an Equipment Grant.

Macro-environment

Over one million women in Canada have a disability. Over two-thirds of these women—about 670,000—have been physically or sexually assaulted before they reach puberty. This figure is twice as high as it is for women without disabilities. One out of three women with disabilities in Canada—about 330,000—experience physical and sexual assault as adults. This compares to about one out of four women without disabilities.

Poverty, isolation and dependence on attendant services make women with disabilities far more vulnerable to violence. Although they need a supportive and safe environment more than anybody, lack of accessible transportation and communication effectively shuts them out. The vast majority of women's shelters and rape crisis centers are inaccessible. Staff and volunteers know little or nothing of disability issues. If a woman with a disability does manage to reach a center or shelter, she may be turned away and she may suffer further abuse. A 1986 DAWN Toronto Survey found that disabled girls are twice as likely to be sexually assaulted.

When a woman with a disability seeks justice through the courts, lawyers and judges may not be sympathetic and many may not even believe her testimony. Even if the courts accept her testimony, rarely will she find retribution. In fact, it may work against her. Many judges consider a woman with a disability less capable of parenting than her abusive husband, and they may give the husband full custody of their children. If a woman with a disability reports assault by an attendant, she may lose essential services. If she reports assault by a spouse, she may lose financial support or stability.

The unemployment rate for women with disabilities is 74%. The median employment income for a disabled woman is $8,360 (Canadian). The median employment income for a disabled man is $19,250. (Health and Activity Limitation Survey, Statistics Canada.)

Impact and Remarks

DAWN is a leading edge organization of women by women and for women with disabilities. DAWN is inclusive and supportive of each other for future generations. DAWN members support each other to be more powerful, better informed, aware of our issues, and our unique and inventive solutions.

DAWN serves as an inspiration, known to fight together for the rights of disabled women. DAWN is a well-recognized and respected organization throughout not only Ontario, but North America.

Reference

Dawn Ontario, website: http://www3.sympatico.ca/odell/dawnpage.htm

CASE STUDY #73: WORLD (WOMEN ORGANIZED TO RESPOND TO LIFE-THREATENING DISEASES): OAKLAND, CALIFORNIA, USA, 1990 (HPDP)

Problem

This case study falls within the domain of health promotion/disease prevention (HPDP). The major problem being addressed was the lack of support groups specifically designed for HIV-positive women in 1990. The groups that did exist were only open to women with full-blown, symptomatic AIDS.

Leadership Impetus

After testing positive for the HIV virus in 1990, Rebecca Denison was not able to find a women's HIV support group. After much frustration and searching at various AIDS conferences and other AIDS events, and with the moral support from her friends in ACT-UP (AIDS Coalition to Unleash Power), WORLD (Women Organized to Respond to Life-threatening Diseases) was formed.

EMPOWER Methods Used

- ¤ Public education and participation
- ¤ Enabling service and assistance
- ¤ Rights protection and social action/reform
- ¤ Media use
- ¤ Empowerment training and leadership development

WORLD's very first function was to talk with the Surgeon General in order to voice their needs and exchange information. This original delegation to see the Surgeon General included an Asian women in her early twenties, a white lesbian activist, an African-American mother of two, an Anglo wife of a hemophiliac, an African-American grandmother and the author, and an Anglo woman with no previous organizational leadership experience.

Denison continued to attend meetings such as the AIDS Clinical Trials Group (ACTG) in Washington, D. C. in March of 1991 and to talk with researchers about the impact of certain medications on women. Yet, Denison was still dissatisfied with the lack of organization of HIV women. With the help of her husband, she created the first issue of the WORLD newsletter called *A Bay Area Newsletter by, for and About Women Facing HIV Disease* in May of 1991. It contained information about the gynecological manifestations of HIV in women, two observational studies that women could join, a list of support groups and a Latina HIV-positive grandmother's testimonial.

After copies were distributed to 200 agencies, activists and HIV-positive women, the *San Francisco Examiner* ran an article about it in the weekly AIDSWEEK column which itself prompted over thirty calls statewide. Today, this monthly newsletter has over 12,000 subscribers in every state of the US and around the world.

WORLD's "HIV University" provides members with HIV treatment education. Doctors, nurses, pharmacists, therapists and activists from the community volunteer their time to teach women about concepts and terms related to HIV treatment. This program is being replicated in 18 cities around the nation. Weekend retreats allow members to experience spiritual healing and a source of inspiration to reach out to other women in their communities. Women are able to exchange information on treatment, disclosure, relationships and other important issues.

WORLD holds social and educational activities for the public and HIV-positive women; and has a speakers' bureau of WORLD members who perform outreach and talk in schools, universities, conferences and churches. Through funding from Ryan White Title IV, WORLD was able to hire HIV-positive peer advocates to do counseling, education, and referrals at AIDS clinics.

WORLD's board of directors, staff and clients reflect the AIDS epidemic among women. The majority of women are HIV-positive and women of color.

Partners/Opposition

During its inception, WORLD received moral support from members of ACT UP, an already established grassroots AIDS organization and her family. WORLD has also garnered needed media attention to publicize its existence and win further support from the community.

Macro-environment

An HIV-positive status often brings to the bearer discrimination, despair and a sense of loneliness. Due to the stigma attached to the condition and a general fear and ignorance of the disease, co-workers, neighbors, friends and even family will often react negatively rather than sympathetically in the face of the contraction of the AIDS virus. Those individuals testing positive for HIV are often discriminated against in terms of employment, housing, schools and even medical care.

Impact and Remarks

As a self-empowered group, WORLD faces many difficulties including lack of funding, serious health problems and the deaths of members, economic disaster and unsupportive or even abusive partners. In addition, due to their inexperience in running an organization, many practical aspects had to be learned. Nevertheless, the WORLD organization is a success, offering a forum in which women are free to be themselves, admit their illness and yet survive, be proud and even flourish in spite of it. They welcome and embrace a diverse group of women who share their fears and problems at the same time that they recognize and respect their differences.

Through WORLD's programs, more than 100 women have graduated from HIV University. More than 200 women, children and families have been served by peer advocates. More than 250 presentations have been given in 20 states and 8 countries. More than 300 HIV-positive women have written personal testimonial for the WORLD newsletter. And more than 90,000 telephone calls from across the nation have been received by people wanting support information or referrals.

By organizing themselves, HIV-positive women may begin to build their self-esteem and self-reliance, give voice to their problems, end their own personal victimization, and leave a legacy for the future community of HIV-positive women.

References

Denison, Rebecca. Call Us Survivors! Women Organized to Respond to Life-threatening Diseases (WORLD) in Schneider, Beth E. & Nancy E. Stoller (eds.) *Women Resisting AIDS: Feminist Strategies of Empowerment*, p. 195–207, Temple University Press, Philadelphia, 1995.
WORLD (1999) *WORLD Newsletter*. Number 104, December 1999.

11

Summing Up

KEY ISSUES AND IMPLICATIONS

This concluding chapter highlights the key issues that have emerged from the information and analyses presented in the previous chapters and discusses the implications of these key issues for policy, research, and action, in three sections:

1. Progress made in the human development approach (HDA) related to women's empowerment and global public health (GPH);
2. Lessons learned from the EMPOWER model used for our meta-analysis of women-led movements; and
3. Application of the EMPOWER model for designing and implementing the Rescatando Salud project for promoting childhood immunizations through empowering *promotoras* in poor and under-served communities in Los Angeles.

Implications for Research and Empowerment of Women for GPH

The primary focus of this volume has been on the importance of empowering ordinary women to promote the health and well-being of powerless and marginalized populations. "Ordinary women" are those who do not occupy an office or position that makes them more influential in their communities than an ordinary citizen. At the outset, it must be emphasized that empowering women, as a strategy as well as a goal of development, must not be used to justify shifting the onus of development efforts onto the poor and the victims. The poor do not create poverty; they are the unfortunate victims of it. Nor do the poor command the power and the resources necessary for social development. If they had sufficient resources and capacities to remove poverty and powerlessness from their lives solely by their own efforts, they would not be poor and powerless. The poor are motivated to seek for a better life and work diligently when they have a chance; our meta-analysis of the

80 case studies and numerous grassroots empowerment movements across the world have clearly established this fact. However, the evidence presented in this book also shows that the poor and the powerless need instrumental support. Collectively they may create a fairer social system that reduces, if not eliminates, damaging disparities, sectarian conflicts, and violence that are often fueled by prolonged marginalization of the poor and exploitation of the fear and mistrust of the people by the leaders in power. It should also be noted that while an individual poor person may not have much power to make a difference, when many poor and powerless are organized for a just cause, and are joined in their struggle by credible community leaders and professionals, powerful movements are born. Rather than absolving the powerful and privileged from the burden of developing a more just and equitable society for all, the rich and the affluent should acknowledge their legitimate obligation to society. A just society is more than a moral imperative for us; it is a utilitarian necessity without which we cannot have fair and sustainable development. Indeed, increasing inequalities can hinder further development and endanger recent achievements. Analyses by Paul Kennedy (1989), Paul Collier (2007), Daron Acemoglu and James Robinson (2012), and Thomas Piketty (2014) confirm growing inequalities and the threat they pose for sustainable human development. In a review of Piketty's 2014 book *Capital in the Twenty-first Century*, Lawrence Summers, a distinguished economist in his own right (Summers is not known for bestowing unwarranted praise), writes:

> Piketty, in collaboration with others, has spent more than a decade mining huge quantities of data spanning centuries and many countries to document, absolutely conclusively, that the share of income and wealth going to those at the very top—the top 1%, 0.1%, and 0.01% of the population—has risen sharply over the last generation, marking a return to a pattern that prevailed before World War I. There can now be no doubt that the phenomenon of inequality is not dominantly about the inadequacy of the skills of lagging workers.... Even if none of Piketty's theories stands up, the establishment of this fact has transformed political discourse and is a Nobel Prize–worthy contribution. (Summers, 2014b)

The debates between two eminent development economists, Amartya Sen and Jagdish Bhagwati, on "economic growth" versus "human development" approaches warn us that the future of human development in many economically less developed nations (including India) is at great risk unless governments step in now by adopting a global tax and fair redistribution of wealth, to prevent soaring inequality from contributing to economic or political instability down the road (Kumar, 2013). Angus Deaton was awarded the Nobel Prize in 2015 for his pioneering research on the origins of health, wealth, and inequality as described in his book *The Great Escape* (Kahneman & Deaton,

2010). He claims that governmental efficiency is the primary driver of human development; he further argues that foreign aid is wasteful because it promotes corruption among those in power and dependency of the people on foreign. He strongly advocates supporting local nongovernmental initiatives in addition to eliminating corruption and improving governmental efficiency. While Deaton's emphasis on helping local initiatives does not single out self-organized women's movements, it most certainly includes all local movements and strongly supports the central premise of this book; that is, women's empowerment is a major path for health and human development. The lessons learned from our literature review and meta-analysis will hopefully inspire human service professionals, scholars, and activists to support self-organized movements that serve as an additional effective force for reducing human sufferings and inequalities in our societies.

Progress in the Human Development Approach

As the deadline for the UN Millennium Development Goals (MDGs) for 2015 approached, the UNDP, WHO, and the World Bank undertook several comprehensive reviews of the progress made by the HDA since its inception in 1990 (a 20-year review) and the progress made in MDGs since they were adopted in 2000 (a 10–12-year review). Our review is based on four recent in-depth review reports cited below. Detailed descriptions of all findings of these reports would take too much space, and most readers may not be interested in the full reports. This section presents highlights of the findings of these four reports that are directly relevant to women's empowerment for GPH.

THE *ICPD BEYOND 2014 GLOBAL REPORT*

The *ICPD Beyond 2014 Global Report* (ICPD, 2014a) is a landmark United Nations review of progress, gaps, challenges, and emerging issues in relation to the International Conference on Population and Development (ICPD) Program of Action led by the UN. It gathers data from 176 Member states, alongside inputs from civil society and comprehensive related research. The report concludes that development gains from the past 20 years cannot be sustained unless governments tackle the inequalities that hurt the poorest and most marginalized (ICPD, 2014b).

GLOBAL HEALTH 2035: A GRAND CONVERGENCE—THE LANCET COMMISSION ON INVESTING IN HEALTH

The Lancet Commission focused on a 20-year reprise of the World Bank's 1993 *World Development Report*—the World Bank's first and only annual report that was solely dedicated to examining why health should be included in development agendas (Jameson et al., 2013, *Lancet*). The central conclusion of the Lancet Commission's analysis was that a "grand convergence" of health risks and priorities of the poor and rich can be accomplished within one generation, i.e., by 2035, provided that the heads of state throughout the world make appropriate levels of investments in health and developed efficient organizations and instruments for investing the resources for health development. According to the World Bank:

> The inability to manage risk properly leads to crises and missed opportunities. This poses significant obstacles to attaining the World Bank Group's two main goals: ending extreme poverty by the year 2030 and boosting shared prosperity of the bottom 40% of the population in developing countries. Managing risk effectively is, therefore, central to the World Bank's mission. The WDR 2014 concludes that effective risk management can be a powerful instrument for development—it can save lives, avert economic shocks, and help people build better, more secure futures. These two goals of the World Bank are shared by the UN MDGs. (WDR, 2014)

In 2013, The United Nations released a report: *The World's Women 2010: Trends and Statistics*, a one-of-a-kind compilation of the latest data documenting progress for women worldwide in eight key areas: population and families, health, education, work, power and decision-making, violence against women, the environment, and poverty. In the book's introduction, United Nations Secretary-General Ban Ki-moon stated that:

> progress in ensuring the equal status of women and men has been made in many areas, including school enrolment, health and economic participation. At the same time, it makes clear that much more needs to be done, in particular to closing the gender gap in public life and to prevent the many forms of violence to which women are subjected. (*The World's Women*, 2010)

HUMAN DEVELOPMENTS: 2014–2015

Progress in a Diverse World

The *ICPD Beyond 2014 Global Report* (UN, 2014a) is the culmination of a landmark UN review of progress, challenges, and emerging issues in relation to the ICPD Program of Action. The document also underlines that the number of people living in extreme poverty in developing countries has fallen dramatically, from 47% in 1990 to 22% in 2010, but many of the estimated 1 billion people living in the 50–60 poorest countries will stagnate as the rest of the world gets richer. The report concludes: "Nearly 1 billion people have escaped extreme poverty. Child and maternal mortality have been cut by nearly one-half. There are more laws to protect and uphold human rights." This report also concludes "that development gains from the past 20 years cannot be sustained unless governments tackle the inequalities that hurt the poorest and most marginalized." In short, the results of the past two decades of efforts have been mixed (https://unstats.un.org/unsd/demographic/products/Worldswomen/WW2010pub.htms).

ICPD Beyond 2014 Global Report also finds that growing inequalities will undo significant gains in health and longevity made over the past 20 years. To sustain these gains, the report, which was launched on February 12, 2014, in New York by the UN Secretary-General Ban Ki-moon and the UN Population Fund (UNFPA) Executive Director Dr. Babatunde Osotimehin, argues that governments must pass and enforce laws to protect the poorest and most marginalized, including adolescent girls and women affected by violence as well as rural populations.

> The just released HDR (2015) concludes: Gender inequality remains a major barrier to human development. Girls and women have made major strides since 1990, but they have not yet gained gender equity. The disadvantages facing women and girls are a major source of inequality. All too often, women and girls are discriminated against in health, education, political representation, labour market, etc — with negative repercussions for development of their capabilities and their freedom of choice. The GII measures gender inequalities in three important aspects of human development—reproductive health measured by maternal mortality ratio and adolescent birth rates; empowerment, measured by proportion of parliamentary seats occupied by females and proportion of adult females and males aged 25 years and older with at least some secondary education; and economic status expressed as labour market participation and measured by labour force participation rate of female and male populations aged 15 years and older. (UNDP HDR, 2015)

Paradigm Shifts: From Germs to Gender Equality and Empowerment (GEE)

Social change is inevitable but is a slow process. This volume presents a review of the major paradigm shifts in public health that began with pre-scientific and metaphysical causal beliefs about major diseases to vertical interventions (top-down and disease-specific) for prevention and control of deadly infectious diseases. Subsequently, with the introduction of the germ theory, the biomedical paradigm of disease prevention thrived and dominated the public health profession through most of the twentieth century. By that time, many deadly and perennial epidemics of infectious diseases that had killed and disabled hundreds of millions of people across the globe were either eradicated (e.g., smallpox) or significantly controlled (e.g., cholera, malaria, tuberculosis) in industrialized and affluent societies. However, the old killers did not totally disappear from the globe; they continued to cause heavy destructions among the poor and powerless segments of world communities. The major reason of this health disparity was not the absence of effective biomedical technology: it was *behavioral*. Often the simplest technologies that save lives do not get adopted soon enough by the poor and powerless communities. For instance, according to UNICEF, global experience shows that 6 million of the almost 11 million children who die each year could be saved by low-tech, evidence-based, cost-effective measures such as vaccines, antibiotics, micronutrient supplementation, insecticide-treated bed nets improved family care and breastfeeding practice (UNICEF, 2014). Oral rehydration therapy (ORT), which involves mixing water, salt, and sugar and administering the solution to infants with severe diarrhea, alone may prevent between 2 and 3 million infant deaths per year globally (UNICEF, 2014). Yet millions of children die per year in poor communities because ORT is not used when needed.

Another powerful example of an effective intervention is Dr. Scrimshaw's (2013) pioneering work, promoting the availability of affordable food for starving poor children:

> To help protein-starved children in Central America, Dr. [Nevin] Scrimshaw created a gruel made of corn, sorghum and cottonseed flour that was nutritionally equivalent to milk. In India, he adapted the same principle to peanut flour and wheat. He then brought both products to market, where they sold for only pennies. Working in Central America, Dr. Scrimshaw also helped eliminate endemic goiter in children—a swelling of the thyroid gland that can lead to mental retardation, deafness, and dwarfism. The ailment is caused by a mother's iodine deficiency. (Scrimshaw, 2013)

In recognition of Nevin Scrimshaw's pioneering research and visionary leadership in promoting the nutritional status of the world's poor, the International Nutrition Foundation wrote:

> World-renowned nutrition researcher Nevin S. Scrimshaw dedicated his career of almost seven decades towards the alleviation of hunger and malnutrition. His work substantially improved the lives of millions of people in dozens of countries around the globe—efforts for which he was recognized with the 1991 World Food Prize. In its citation that year, the prize committee cited Scrimshaw "for his revolutionary accomplishments over six decades, in fighting protein, iodide, and iron deficiencies, developing nutritional supplements, educating generations of experts, and building support for continued advances in food quality around the world." (INF, 1991)

UNICEF declared that more than 70% of almost 11 million child deaths every year are attributable to six causes: diarrhea, malaria, neonatal infection, pneumonia, preterm delivery, or lack of oxygen at birth. Most of these are preventable. "Recent estimates suggest that malnutrition (measured as poor anthropometric status) is associated with about 50% of all deaths among children" (Rice et al., 2000). With wider and rapid adoption of these and similar innovations, our world in the twenty-first century should be able to eliminate the deaths of millions of children every year. Malnutrition is the underlying cause of death for at least 3.1 million children, accounting for 45% of all deaths among children under the age of five and stunting growth among a further 165 million.

On the other extreme of the economic disparity scale, affluent people indulge in health-damaging behavior such as tobacco use, poor nutrition, alcohol abuse, and a sedentary lifestyle. The Centers for Disease Control and Prevention (CDC) and the Institute of Medicine (IOM) estimated that more than half of deaths in the United States were attributable to unhealthy behaviors or lifestyles (McGinnis & Foege, 1993). This transition of major causes of deaths from infectious diseases caused by germs to chronic diseases caused by human behavior is widely known as "the epidemiological transition", that is, a major shift in the paradigm of causes of deaths from germs to human behavior and lifestyle.

The examples above and numerous others confirm that the modern science-based health promotion and disease prevention field has undergone several paradigm shifts from *fighting germs to promoting gender equality and empowerment* (from Germs to GEE). It began with confronting germs that cause specific infectious diseases; it subsequently expanded to include individual health-related lifestyle behaviors (e.g., smoking, diet, unprotected sex) that endanger health (e.g., CVD, cancer), and finally more recently global health has emerged as the strategy to address sociocultural factors that promote gender equality and empowerment. Some old infectious diseases still exist, but global health is increasing its focus on social inequalities and cultural factors that damage our health and QOL.

Fifty Years of the Anti-Tobacco Movement

In 1964, the US Surgeon General released a landmark report on deaths and disabilities due to tobacco smoking in the United States (Terry, 1964). This report concluded that tobacco smoking is:

- ¤ Associated with 70% higher all-cause mortality rates among men
- ¤ A cause of lung cancer and laryngeal cancer in men
- ¤ A probable cause of lung cancer in women
- ¤ The most important cause of chronic bronchitis

In 2014, the Surgeon General released a 50-year follow-up of developments in tobacco smoking since the 1964 report. The Executive Summary of the 2014 follow-up report states:

> In the United States, successes in tobacco control have more than halved smoking rates since the 1964 landmark Surgeon General's report came out. "Americans" collective view of smoking has been transformed from an accepted national pastime to a discouraged threat to individual and public health. Strong policies have largely driven cigarette smoking out of public view and public air space. Thanks to smoke free laws, no longer is smoking allowed on airplanes or in a growing number of restaurants, bars, college campuses and government buildings. (Sibelius, 2014)

The Assistant Secretary of Health, Howard Koh, noted (in the 2014 *SG Report* Foreword):

> Of all the accomplishments of the 20th century, historians rank the 1964 Surgeon General's Report as one of the seminal public health achievements of our time. Armed with both science and resolve, we can continue to honor the legacy of the report by completing the work it began in the last century. The current 2014 Surgeon General's report represents a national vision for getting the job done. With strategy, commitment, and action, our nation can leave the crossroads and move forward to end the tobacco epidemic once and for all. (Koh, 2014).

Most health professionals would concur. This and the eradication or drastic reduction of other major diseases that killed and disabled hundreds of millions of people (e.g., small pox, tuberculosis, malaria, respiratory illnesses) established the population-based public health intervention as a valid and effective health promotion and disease prevention (HPDP) model.

Case for a Second Look

While at first glance, per several aggregate measures, progress may look impressive, it also tends to conceal important variations and trends that deserve further attention and action. The decline in the rate of tobacco smoking in the United States is a case in point. We are thrilled by the phenomenal reduction of the overall prevalence of tobacco smoking in the United States by nearly half since the first Surgeon General's report in 1964, but we must also take a second look beyond the aggregate data to identify threats and developments that may be concealed behind a success story told by those data that still require serious attention. Let us point out two such examples from the tobacco-smoking trend. First, Figure 11.1 shows that the aggregate smoking rate in the United States has declined by 25% in 46 years (from 43% in 1965 to 18% in 2011); that is a 0.54% decline per year. This happened as a result of the growing national concern about the problem and massive involvement of the communities, health professionals, and anti-smoking activists and non-smokers over a period of 50 years, against the strong opposition of the tobacco industry and their enormous investments in media and misinformation campaigns. However, we must learn the central lesson from this mass movement of over one-half century: that even when the majority of the public may support a just cause, change is often very slow. Idealists, donors, and uninformed activists tend to set their goals too high or too soon, which may ensure failure because changing health behaviors that are rooted in cultures and lifestyles takes much longer than they can imagine. A 25% decline in smoking in 50 years may be too slow to the campaigners, but that is what it took to reduce tobacco use prevalence in the United States.

   Also, the Surgeon General's follow-up report of 2014 noted that, while overall tobacco use had declined sharply, the diseases and risks from smoking by women had risen sharply over the previous 50 years and were now equal to those for men—for lung cancer, chronic obstructive pulmonary disease, and cardiovascular diseases. Aggregate rates do not reveal the pockets of high-risk groups. According to the theory of "diffusion of

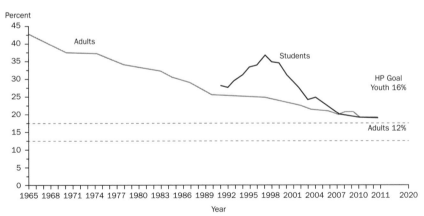

*Percentage of high school students who smoked cigarettes on 1 or more of the 30 days preceding the survey. Data first collected in 1991 (Youth Risk Behavior Survey, 1991–2011).

**Percentage of adults who are current cigarette smokers (National Health Interview Survey, 1965–2011).

FIGURE 11.1 Trends in Cigarette Smoking in the United States: 1965–2011 (Centers for Disease Control and Prevention).

innovation," the late adopters and opponents of a change in communities are different types of people than are the early and majority of adopters, and they are driven by different sets of beliefs and motives (Coleman et al., 1957; Rogers et al., 1973). Conversion of these population segments to non-smokers would often require different change strategies than those that were effective with the majority in the communities. Tobacco companies are increasingly focusing on younger people, especially women, and smokers in poorer countries where smoking laws are less stringent and local governments welcome the tax revenue from tobacco products to enrich their treasuries.

We present a second body of evidence to show that a major change in health-related behaviors that are rooted in our culture and lifestyle takes much longer than we would like. The total fertility rate (TFR) represents the total number of children born to a woman through her reproductive life. The data in Figure 11.2 show that

> U.S. fertility rates fell to low levels during the periods of economic hardships; there were sharp declines in TFR during the Great Depression in 1930s and early '40s around the time of the energy crisis in 1970s or "oil shock"; and since the onset of the recent recession in 2008. The U.S. total fertility rate (TFR) stood at 2.0 births per woman in 2009, but preliminary data from the National Center for Health Statistics show that the TFR dropped to 1.9 in 2010, well below the replacement level of 2.1. A similar decline of fertility rates has been reported in Ireland, Italy, Spain, Sweden, and several other European countries. (PRB, 2012)

Between 1955 and 2010, the U.S. TFR had the greatest decline, from 3.7 to 1.9; a decline of 1.8 children in 55 years (or an unremarkable decline of

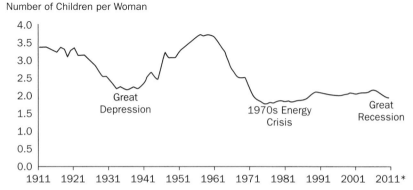

FIGURE 11.2 Total Fertility Rates in the United States: 1911–2011 (Centers for Disease Control and Prevention).

Source: National Center for Health Statistics.

0.037 children per year). More important, most of this decline occurred during the economic hardships due to the energy crisis and the recent great recession; in other words, due to micro-economic causes and financial hardships. Both smoking prevalence and the TFR rate declines in the United States were very slow processes and are functions of major macrosystemic changes rather than due to a single bold intervention to change a specific health-related behavior.

COST-EFFECTIVENESS ANALYSIS (CEA) OF PUBLIC HEALTH INTERVENTION

While a slow rate of decline in health risks, especially when it involves changing human behavior and cultural practices, is the norm rather than an exception, it would be a big mistake to conclude that investments in prevention interventions are not cost-effective. Putting a price on averting suffering and the untimely death of a patient and her or his family is not an easy task. Yet responsible healthcare planning demands some justification for financial investment for preventable deaths and disabilities. The goal of a cost-effectiveness analysis (CEA) is not to find the ideal solution at the lowest cost, but rather to identify the most cost-effective strategies in a set of options that have similar results. This would be a topic for a full book. Health economists have been struggling with this very complex issue of costs–benefits of effective public health interventions, and the CDC has been estimating costs–benefits of disease prevention. We present here a few examples to illustrate how cost–benefit ratios are determined, as well as the return on investment (ROI) in HPDP.

The **CHOICE (CHO**osing **I**nterventions that are **C**ost-**E**ffective) project is a WHO initiative developed in 1998. Value for money and efficiency are fundamental considerations guiding investment in health, and WHO-CHOICE provides a way to measure them. This is true in settings where lack of finance is no longer the greatest barrier to achieving better health outcomes; it is also true in less well-resourced settings, where inefficiency is measured in lives lost and human suffering. Cost-effectiveness analysis supports priority setting by defining areas of action where the greatest health gains can be achieved. As such, it is directly related to Universal Health Coverage. It is moreover an important prerequisite to achieving universal coverage, since shifting from a less to a more cost-effective set of health activities is equivalent to raising new finance. Generalized cost-effectiveness analysis (WHO-CHOICE) also allows the definition of an optimal set of interventions, taking into account setting-specific factors such as the burden of disease, health system practice, and economic conditions. Tools to facilitate country-level cost-effectiveness analysis of a wide range of health activities are available. In parallel, WHO-CHOICE publishes and disseminates an online knowledge base of regional-level cost-effectiveness information (WHO:CHOICE, 1998).

The WHO alerts us of the likelihood of increasing costs for future prevention efforts because of the changing nature of the health threats we face:

> However, we're shifting away from an era of "magic bullets," i.e., the model of disease elimination by single-dose vaccines conferring lifelong immunity. The HPV vaccine and the malaria vaccine won't provide lifelong immunity. Much of the "low-hanging fruit" and quick fixes are gone, so the easy victories in global public health might be over. We seem to be heading now to the next frontier of progress, one that involves more complex methods and doesn't have any magic bullets. But the huge progress that is possible to make at this next stage, in cancers and cardiovascular disease and a whole host of non-communicable diseases, not to mention the unfinished battle against HIV/AIDS, TB [tuberculosis] and malaria, this still could be an exciting message if it were conveyed effectively. (WHO:CHOICE, 1998)

Estimating "costs" and "benefits" is contextually defined and requires in-depth analysis that is beyond the scope of this volume. We cite some examples of the cost–benefit logic of investing in public health departments in California. UC Berkeley professor Timothy Brown (2014) estimated the causal impact of variation in the expenditures of California county departments of public health on all-cause mortality rates and the associated value of lives saved. His findings show that

> an additional $10 per capita expenditures in public health reduces all-cause mortality by 9.1 deaths per 100,000 population. At current funding levels, the long-run annual number of lives saved by the presence of county departments of public health in California is estimated to be approximately 27,000 (26,937 lives, 95% confidence interval). The annual value of these lives is estimated to be worth $212.8 billion using inflation-adjusted standard U.S. government estimates of the value of a statistical life ($7.9 million). (Brown, 2014)

Brown concludes that California would save an average of 26,937 lives each year, for a total cost of $2.95 billion. However, the total value of these lives saved is $212.8 billion. Industries often consider the financial benefits (ROI) of investing in workers' health in terms of increased productivity and costs saved by preventing injuries and illness. Here is one example, from William C. Weldon, Chairman and CEO of Johnson & Johnson:

> We dedicate resources to prevention because, like any successful investment we've made, it yields steady returns. Those returns take two forms: a healthier, more productive, more committed workforce and significantly lower overall healthcare costs. For every dollar we invest in our workers'

health, we see a return of more than $4 in reduced health care costs, lower absenteeism, and improved productivity. Our health care spending averages 4% below benchmarks for our industry. From 2001 through 2009, we avoided more than $21 million in health care expenditures. (Weldon, 2011)

The Human Development Approach (HDA)

As discussed in the first two chapters of this book, a major paradigm shift took place in health-related sciences and professions in the mid-twentieth century. We may identify two seminal changes; first, the *"globalization"* of public health, including the establishment of global health organizations (e.g., WHO, UNICEF); global consensus development and declarations; and the emergence of primary health care (PHC; Alma-Ata declaration) as a comprehensive strategy for health for all, rather than disease-based, separate, vertical programs. The second change is the integration of issues that extend *"beyond health"* but affect population health under the rubric of the HDA. The HDA emphasized that "human development" cannot be measured by any single, aggregate, objective criterion such as "life expectancy" or gross domestic product (GDP) per capita income, or literacy rate, and that "human development" includes improvements in several important dimensions of human life—freedom, equality, justice, and overall quality of life including health. The HDA was adopted by the UN System in 1990; it developed a composite Human Development Index (HDI), which initially included measures of life expectancy at birth (as a measure of health status), literacy (as a measure of human capacity), and income (as a measure of economic autonomy). Subsequently, the HDI included two additional measures: the Gender Development Index (GDI) and Gender Equality Measures (GEM) as indicators of women's positions in decision-making processes, and the level of gender equality. Dr. Mahbub ul Haq, the then-director of the UNDP who led the development of the HDA, and Prof. Amartya Sen, whose theory and research provided a major intellectual foundation for the UNDP's HDA framework, both strongly felt that human development should be measured in terms of advancements in the basic freedom, capacities, and well-being of the people. In the words of the two founders of this approach: "The objective of development is to create an enabling environment for people to enjoy long, healthy and creative lives" (Mahbub ul Haq, 1934–1998). According to Sen, human development is concerned with advancing the richness of human life, rather than the richness of the economy in which human beings live (Sen, 1999).

Helen Clark (2010), the Administrator of the UNDP, assessed the impact of the HDA in these words:

> The premise of the HDI, considered radical at the time, was elegantly simple: national development should be measured not simply by national income, as had long been the practice, but also by life expectancy and literacy. The new HDI had its shortcomings, as the Report's authors forthrightly acknowledged, including a reliance on national averages, which concealed skewed distribution, and the absence of "a quantitative measure of human freedom." Yet it successfully advanced the Report's central thesis, stated succinctly in its first sentence: "People are the real wealth of a nation." Twenty years later the conceptual brilliance and continuing relevance of that original human development paradigm are indisputable. It is now almost universally accepted that a country's success or an individual's well-being cannot be evaluated by money alone. Income is of course crucial: without resources, any progress is difficult. Yet we must also gauge whether people can lead long and healthy lives, whether they have the opportunity to be educated and whether they are free to use their knowledge and talents to shape their own destinies. That was the original vision and remains the great achievement of the creators of the Human Development Reports, Mahbub ul-Haq of Pakistan and his close friend and collaborator, Amartya Sen of India, working with other leading development thinkers. Their concept has guided not just 20 years of global Human Development Reports, but more than 600 National Human Development Reports—all researched, written and published in their respective countries—as well as the many provocative regionally focused reports supported by UNDP's regional bureaus. (Clark, 2010)

Gender equality and the empowerment of women occupied a central place in the HDA and ranking of the world's nations using the HDI.

> Achievements over the ensuing 20 years have been remarkable, including gains in women's status, population health and life expectancy, educational attainment, and human rights protection systems, with an estimated 1 billion people moving out of extreme poverty. Fears of population growth that were already abating in 1994 have continued to ease, and the expansion of human capability and opportunity, especially for women, which has led to economic development, has been accompanied by continued decline in the population growth rate from 1.52% per year in 1990–1995 to 1.15 in 2010–2015. Today, national demographic trajectories are more diverse than in 1994, as wealthy countries of Europe, Asia and the Americas face rapid population ageing, while Africa and some countries in Asia prepare for the largest cohort of young people the world has ever seen, and the 49 poorest countries, particularly in sub-Saharan Africa, continue to face

premature mortality and high fertility. Our greatest shared challenge is that our very accomplishments, reflected in ever greater human consumption and extraction of the earth's resources, are increasingly inequitably distributed, threatening inclusive development, the environment and our common future. (UNDP, 2014)

The major finding of world economic developments during the past five decades is that economic gains are not distributed equitably across nations; the richest countries get richer and the poorest get poorer. This unequal income distribution is true across the rich and poor nations and between the rich and the poor within each nation. It is true that millions of people have been lifted from abject poverty during the last two decades (most of them are in two rapidly developing large countries: China and India); at the same time we have more than 1 billion people in the world living in countries that are hopelessly stuck in poverty, and most are getting worse.

Paul Collier, former Director of Research at the World Bank, summed up the situation in his book *The Bottom Billion: Why the Poorest Countries Are Failing and What Can Be Done About It* (Collier, 2007). He concludes:

Most of the five billion, about 80%, live in countries that are indeed developing, often at amazing speed. The countries at the bottom coexist with the twenty-first century, but their reality is the fourteenth century: civil war, plague, ignorance. (Collier, 2007, p. 3)

Collier added that even during the "golden decade" (in 1990s) when the world prospered, the income of the people in the bottom billion declined by 5%. Finally, he added that, as time passed, the disparities between the bottom billion and those above them would become more divergent; consequently their integration would become harder, not easier (Collier, 2007, p. 4). When Collier wrote his book, the world population was 6 billion; he estimated that 1 billion out of 6 were in abject poverty and misery. According to the World Population Clock (see: http://www.census.gov/popclock/), at the time of this writing (on July 28, 2015) the world population is 7.25 billion; one-sixth of that would be 1.20 billion people in abject poverty). He counted 58 countries that fall into this group. The 2014 UN Human Development Report estimated that 2.2 billion people were under or near poverty level and were highly vulnerable (UNDP HDR, July 24, 2014).

PROGRESS IN MDGS RELATED TO WOMEN: PROMOTE GENDER EQUALITY AND EMPOWER WOMEN (MDG #3), AND IMPROVE MATERNAL HEALTH (MDG #5)

The *World's Women Report* released in 2012 (UN Women, 2012) presented a 20-year overview of progress related to women's empowerment and maternal health (MDGs #3 and #5) between 1990 and 2010. The overall records have been very mixed, and based upon the latest data made available, the targets on several MDGs for 2015 have not been reached. Here are some of the highlights.

In 2010, there were about 57 million more men than women alive in the world. This number should be a cause of concern because the level of "excess" men in a society represents a cumulative measure of the number of "missing women" due to neglect, abuse, and violence experienced by women (including selective abortion of female fetuses) in these societies. In societies where women have access to optimal levels of education, employment, health care, and gender parity, there would be more women alive than men. This is true for almost all modern and economically advanced societies, including the Northern and Western European nations, the United Kingdom, the United States, Japan, and the cities of Singapore and Hong Kong. Conversely, even in nations with high levels of income, greater gender inequality and power-lessness lead to more deaths and disabilities among women; consequently the gender ratio in these countries would show more men per 100 women. Therefore, more men alive per 100 women are a good measure of the degree of gender inequality experienced by women. The size of variation in the gender ratio across the world is shocking. For instance, for every 100 women alive, Norway has 100 men (a perfect ratio); Denmark has 99; Japan has 95 men; the United States and the United Kingdom have 97 men each; Hong Kong, 88; the Russian Federation, 86. Conversely, China has 108 men per 100 women; India, 107; Pakistan, 106; Bangladesh, 102; and Indonesia, 101. The picture is very different in several economically affluent nations in the Middle East; Qatar has 326 men per 100 women; the United Arab Republic has 234; Oman has 175; Bahrain has 164; Kuwait has 146; and Saudi Arabia has 135 (UNFPA, 2013).

Some positive changes include: people are marrying at older ages; global fertility has declined to 2.5 (TFR) children per women—but where early marriage dominates, a TFR of five or more is common. Globally, women live longer than men; but in poor countries, women's risk related to childbearing and pregnancy wipe out the advantage they may otherwise have for living longer. In sub-Saharan Africa, North Africa, and the Middle East, women account for more than 50% of those living with HIV/AIDS. In rich countries, on the other hand, women are smoking tobacco and drinking alcohol more, and that compromises their life expectancy. Problems of malnutrition are increasingly affecting both rich and poor nations; the poor because of poverty, and the rich because of poor food habits. Fast food and obesity are ubiquitous (UNDP, 2013).

There has been a significant reduction in infant mortality rates (IMR) globally, but IMR remains very high in many sub-Saharan countries. While life expectancy at birth has increased significantly, the disparities are still too high. For instance, a Japanese baby born in Japan has a life expectancy at birth of 86 years (both genders combined for 2009–2013); for a person born in Sierra Leone, the life expectancy is 45 years only; or 41 years less than a

Japanese citizen. It is relevant to point out that in large, multicultural metropolitan areas, which are increasing rapidly across the world, significant disparities in life expectancies exist among ethnic populations living within the same geographic locations.

TRENDS IN MATERNAL MORTALITY: 1990 TO 2010

The fifth MDG aims to improve maternal health, with a target of reducing the maternal mortality rate (MMR) by 75% between 1990 and 2015 (UNDP, 2013).

> Globally, an estimated 287,000 maternal deaths occurred in 2010, a decline of 47% from levels in 1990. The global MMR in 2010 was 210 maternal deaths per 100,000 live births, down from 400 maternal deaths per 100,000 live births in 1990. The MMR in developing regions (240) was 15 times higher than in developed regions (16). Sub-Saharan Africa had the highest MMR at 500 maternal deaths per 100,000 live births; while Eastern Asia had the lowest among MDG developing regions, at 37 maternal deaths per 100,000 live births. Ten countries have already achieved this target (between 76% to 95% reduction); 50 countries are "making progress"; 14 countries have made "insufficient progress," 11 are characterized as having made "no progress" and are likely to miss the MDG target unless accelerated interventions are put in place. (UNFPA, 2012)

SEXUAL AND REPRODUCTIVE HEALTH (SRH)

> New estimates for show that sexual and reproductive health services fall well short of needs in developing regions. An estimated 225 million women who want to avoid a pregnancy are not using an effective contraceptive method.

The final MDG report by the UNDP (2015) documents the progress made in MDGs and highlights the persistent challenges in these words:

> Despite this progress, every day hundreds of women die during pregnancy or from childbirth-related complications. In 2013, most of these deaths were in the developing regions, where the maternal mortality ratio is about 14 times higher than in the developed regions. Globally, there were an estimated 289,000 maternal deaths in 2013, equivalent to about 800 women dying each day. Maternal deaths are concentrated in sub-Saharan Africa and Southern Asia, which together accounted for 86 per cent of such deaths globally in 2013. (UNDP 2015: The Millennium Development Goals Report 2015, p.39).

The report presents key problems confronting SRH:

Of the 125 million women who give birth each year,

- ◘ 54 million make fewer than the minimum of four antenatal visits recommended by the World Health Organization (WHO); and
- ◘ 43 million do not deliver their babies in a health facility.

GENDER PARITY IN EDUCATION AND EMPLOYMENT

The MDG goal number 3 was to "Eliminate gender disparity in primary and secondary education, preferably by 2005, and in all levels of education no later than 2015" (UNDP, 2015). Overall, considerable gains have been made in gender parity in primary school level education; however, unacceptable levels of gender disparity remain at higher levels of school education. The latest MDG evaluation report concludes:

> The largest gender disparities in enrollment ratios are found in tertiary education, with only one developing region, Western Asia, achieving the target. The most extreme disparities are those at the expense of women in sub-Saharan Africa and Southern Asia and at the expense of men in Eastern Asia, Northern Africa and Latin America and the Caribbean. Only 4 per cent of countries with available data in the developing regions had achieved the target for tertiary education in 2012. (UNDP 2015: The Millennium Development Goals Report 2015, p. 29)

These findings mean that far lower proportions of women are enrolled in upper grades in schools, in advanced academic and professional specialties (exceptions include nurses, school teachers, social workers, outreach primary health workers, and hospitality workers). It is estimated that two-thirds of the 774 million adult illiterates are women. Interestingly, men's dominance in the tertiary level of education has reversed globally, except in sub-Saharan Africa and South and West Asia. However, women tend to study "soft" subjects, including education, humanities, health and social sciences, more often than men; men more often study sciences, engineering, and medicine.

Employment

The final MDG report on progress in women's employment and work concludes:

> Despite notable gains by women, significant gaps remain between women and men in the labour market. Women are still less likely to participate in the labour force than men. As of 2015, about 50 per cent of all working-age women (aged 15 and above) are in the labour force, compared to

77 per cent of men (UNDP, 2015, p. 32). Globally women earn 24 per cent less than men, with the largest disparities found in Southern Asia (33 per cent) and sub-Saharan Africa (30 per cent). Of 92 countries with data on unemployment rates by level of education for 2012–2013, in 78 countries women with advanced education have higher rates of unemployment than men with similar levels of education (UNDP, 2015, p. 32).

Finally, working women still bear their traditional responsibilities for household activities even when they work outside the home, which places them under a triple burden: work at home, work outside for long hours, and suffer gender discrimination and violence. In spite of increased social awareness of women's rights and the importance of women's participation in elected offices, across the world only about 17% of women occupy elected positions in government. Some Nordic nations and India have reserved a quota for women legislators; still, the level of women legislators tends to be less than 30% (UN: MDG Progress, 2015).

Globally, in spite of the past several decades of global development aids and loans, the income disparities between nations and between the rich and poor within most nations are increasing. On aggregate measures (e.g., GDP per capita) using nations as the unit of analysis, the progress made may look impressive; but on measures of disparities between the rich and the poor, the gap is increasing. Based upon a recent analysis, Goda (2013) concludes that:

> The results of this study indicate that (i) non-population adjusted inequality between countries (inter-country inequality) increased between 1820 and the late 1990s but then decreased thereafter, while there was a steady decrease after the 1950s when population weights are taken into account; (ii) income inequality between "global citizens" (global inequality) increased significantly between 1820 and 1950, while there was no clear trend thereafter; (iii) contemporary relative income inequality within countries (intra-country inequality) registered a clear upward trend on a global level since the 1980s. (Goda, 2013)

The World Bank and other multinational financial institutions use the Gini index to measure income disparities within and between nations. It is defined thus:

> Gini index (a standard economic measure for income inequality), varies significantly across the globe. Developed economies tend to have lower income inequality; developing countries have greater disparities between regions, genders, ethnicities and education. In 2011, Norway had the lowest Gini coefficient of 25.6% in the world, while South Africa had the most unequal income distribution, at 63.6%. (World Bank, 2015)

Among developed economies, the United States has one of the highest income inequality levels, with its Gini coefficient reaching 47.4% in 2011, compared to only 34.4% in Germany. Countries with the most unequal income distribution are clustered in southern Africa and Latin America. Because of its history of racial inequality under the apartheid regime during 1948 to 1994, South Africa has the highest income inequality in the world, with a Gini coefficient of 63.6% in 2011. In most developing countries, income inequality remains relatively high due to the existing income gap between gender, ethnicity, regions, and educational/skills levels. Other countries with very high 2011 Gini indices include Ecuador (59.2%) and Colombia (58.3%). In 2011, China's Gini coefficient stood at 51.6%, significantly higher than India's 39.9%, but slightly lower than Brazil's 51.7%. In many countries, the lack of adequate government policy and resources, combined with inefficiency and corruption, also contribute to poor distributions of income.

In the private sector, women are present on most boards of directors of large companies, but their number remains low compared to men. This is especially notable in the largest corporations, which remain male-dominated. Of the 500 largest corporations in the world, only 13 have a female CEO.

INCOME AND HAPPINESS

Women also earn significantly less than men working in comparable positions (e.g., in the U.S., women earn 77% of what men earn in the same positions). These and other evidence of gender discrimination and violence against women and minorities cited throughout the text of this book indicate that aggregate and overall economic development alone is not a good measure of progress; more equitable distributions of opportunities, income, and resources, especially greater investment at the bottom of the economic pyramid, is more important for overall progress in human development and quality of life. Heymann (2010), through her in-depth analyses of case studies across the world, has demonstrated that investments (better wages, benefits, and working conditions) at the bottom of the ladder (BOL) of employees mean greater profits for the company as well as better benefits for all workers. Prahalad (2006) has demonstrated that building business partnerships with the poor at the bottom of the pyramid (BOP) ensures a win-win arrangement for both partners; when poor people participate as business partners, not as targets of marketing. While these two strategies (BOL and BOP) are not directed exclusively at women, it is important to note that women are paid less and are more powerless and poorer than men (70% of the poor are women). These two models (BOL and BOP), along with various microfinance initiatives (MFI) such as Self-Employed Women's Association (SEWA), the Grameen Bank, and our EMPOWER and similar models, constitute a new genre of methodology that empowers women through enhancing their economic emancipation and income-generating capabilities, and removing cultural barriers to health and quality of life (HQOL) (per Sen's "capabilities paradigm," which includes both basic freedom and personal competencies).

A key related question is: "Does having more money make people happier?." The following summary by Chamorro-Premuzic (2014) addresses this question.

The authors reviewed 120 years of research to synthesize the findings from 92 quantitative studies. The combined dataset included more than 15,000 individuals and 115 correlation coefficients. The results indicate that the association between salary and job satisfaction is very weak. The reported correlation (r = .14) indicates that there is less than 2% overlap between pay and job satisfaction levels. Furthermore, the correlation between pay and pay satisfaction was only marginally higher (r = .22 or 4.8% overlap), indicating that people's satisfaction with their salary is mostly independent of their actual salary. A similar pattern of results emerged when the authors carried out group-level (or between-sample) comparisons. In their words: Employees earning salaries in the top half of our data range reported similar levels of job satisfaction to those employees earning salaries in the bottom half of our data range" (p. 162). This is consistent with Gallup's engagement research, which reports no significant difference in employee engagement by pay level. Gallup's findings are based on 1.4 million employees from 192 organizations across 49 industries and 34 nations (Judge et al., 2010).

Nobel Laureate psychologist Daniel Kahneman and his colleague Angus Deaton (Kahneman & Deaton, 2010) thus described their study on money and happiness:

Recent research has begun to distinguish two aspects of subjective well-being. Emotional well-being refers to the emotional quality of an individual's everyday experience—the frequency and intensity of experiences of joy, stress, sadness, anger, and affection that make one's life pleasant or unpleasant. Life evaluation refers to the thoughts that people have about their life when they think about it. We raise the question of whether money buys happiness, separately for these two aspects of well-being. We report an analysis of more than 450,000 responses to the Gallup-Healthways Well-Being Index, a daily survey of 1,000 US residents conducted by the Gallup Organization. We find that emotional well-being (measured by questions about emotional experiences yesterday) and life evaluation measured by Cantril's Self-Anchoring Striving Scale (Cantril, 1965) have different correlates. Income and education are more closely related to life evaluation, but health, care giving, loneliness, and smoking are relatively stronger predictors of daily emotions. When plotted against log income, life evaluation rises steadily. Emotional well-being also rises with log income, but there is no further progress beyond an annual income of $75,000. Low income exacerbates the emotional pain associated with such misfortunes as divorce, ill health, and being alone. We conclude that high income buys life satisfaction but not happiness, and that low income is associated both with low life evaluation and low emotional well-being. (Short, 2014)

These and related studies show that more money, above a certain level, does not have a linear relationship with happiness; incomes at or below the poverty line clearly have negative effects on quality of life.

THE KERALA MODEL: GROWTH VERSUS DEVELOPMENT

The global adoption by the UN Member nations of the various UN and WHO charters and declarations on the HDA and initiatives confirm this consensus. However, while most economists agree that both growth and development are necessary, how best to remove the barriers to freedom and accelerate human development has been an issue of much debate especially among development economists. The recent debate between two world-renowned development economists, Sen and Bhagwati (Bhattacharya, 2013), on how to promote India's future socioeconomic development captured global attention. The key issues at the heart of this debate are relevant to all developing nations; especially for this book, as it concerns itself with empowerment within the context of HDA. For this reason, it would be appropriate to review the issues and implications of this debate at some length.

For this discussion, development economists may be divided into two schools:

1. *The pro-growth school*, which argues that increasing national wealth, usually measured by the GDP or the market value of all goods and services produced by a country/state in a given year and per capita GDP at PPP (purchase power parity), is the first priority for national progress; and
2. *The pro-development school*, which argues that progress in key aspects of human development (e.g., education, health, social equality) or overall quality of life is the primary goal of human development, and that economic growth requires a healthy and capable workforce.

The HDA of course includes economic progress, but it goes beyond economic progress for the country as a whole; they use a composite measure of HDI, including life expectancy (as a proxy measure of health), literacy (as an indicator of human capacity required for progress), per capita GDP (as an indicator of economic growth), GEM, GDI, and the level of poverty (as a measure of human deprivation).

The central argument of the HDA advocated by the UN is that human progress or development cannot be measured by a single objective indicator such as GDP or measures of national wealth or economic growth alone. The growth-advocates, on the other hand, hold that a poor country like India should first focus on the economic growth of the nation. Once the economic pie has enlarged sufficiently, then the country will have the funds required to invest in human development (eminent Columbia University economist Jagdish Bhagwati and others advocate the growth approach). They concede that exclusive focus on economic growth in Step One (Track-1 as they call it) and reducing investments in human development (e.g., education, health, social reforms) may increase inequality initially. But they argue that eventually the country will have more funds from the growth approach in Track-1 to invest in human development initiatives in the second phase (Track-2) from a larger economic pie from successful economic growth. In short, the poorest, who need help most, must wait until the country has enough money for human development investments. It is important to note that both schools agree that economic growth and human development are both required; the debate is about which comes first and how to achieve both goals most efficiently. Unfortunately, many journalists who try to simplify complex issues in their media coverages are passionate but not always well-informed followers of the two schools; and the protagonists' impetuous pronouncements have degraded the Sen–Bhagwati intellectual debate on a profound issue into a media sensation. Growth and development issues are both at the center of all human progress. Most of the eminent economists who are concerned with the issues of human development, for understandable reasons, do not wish to take sides on this debate in the public media. Some scholars believe that the debate has become an "uninteresting" event (e.g., Nussbaum), and many believe that the split between the two adversaries has been much exaggerated. An eminent economist, Sir Partha Dasgupta (2015) of Cambridge University, who has made pioneering contributions in the fields of nutrition and natural resource economics and has spent a lifetime analyzing poverty, reviewed the books written by Sen-Dreze and Bhagwati-Panagariya, and holds that both Sen and Bhagwati have failed to take a holistic view of the Indian growth experience. He believes that the consequences of depleting natural resources due to high population growth and ecological degradation are missing from the worldview of both camps of economists. Dasgupta argues that "Our world is heading toward a population of nine billion, with everyone aspiring to the lifestyle of a resident of a high-middle-income country. But environmental requirements of that scenario on a sustainable basis would require more than two Earths" (Dasgupta, 2015). He believes that a noisy media debate between the "growth" versus "development" cannot bypass the central issues of ecological and environmental imperatives for sustainable human development.

In short, the pro-growth group's thesis that a trickle-down economic growth from the rich to the poor would take care of the poverty and disparities just does not happen (Collier, 2007; Piketty, 2014). Most of the beneficiaries of growth have been the rich and the middle class. In addition, most of the growth happened due to recent unusual economic growth in two developing countries: China and India. Most of the other developing countries were not as fortunate as these two countries. Furthermore, the poorest in India did not get any better either; the country now ranks lower than Bangladesh on gender development measures and life expectancy at birth. While many escaped poverty, at the same time it is also true that the disparities between rich and poor nations and between the rich and poor within nations increased significantly. High levels of farmers' suicide in India are one example. A recent study of farmers' suicide in India found that:

> The liberalization of the Indian economy is most often associated with near double digit growth, the rise of India as an economic powerhouse and the emergence of wealthy urban middle classes. But it is often forgotten that over 833 million people—almost 70% of the Indian population still live in rural areas. (Sinha, 2014)

Most of the victims are poorer farmers with small pieces of land who chose to cultivate cash crops and had to borrow money for their cash-intensive crops (e.g., coffee, cotton). They were vulnerable to market price fluctuations and had no cash to sustain them in hard times. The key findings from Collier's book (*The Bottom Billion*), cited earlier, confirm that during the high economic growth period of the 1990s, the income of the people at the bottom billion actually decreased more than 5%. The second important fact to remember is that governments have an important responsibility to create conditions that promote growth—which includes better education and human capability development, a healthy workforce, and fair wages and working conditions. Another important factor is the role of the government in designing and implementing fair and effective redistributions of the benefits of economic growth to all people. Available evidence shows that a strategy of growth that makes it easier for the rich to get richer, and a laissez-faire economic policy that counts on the rich people's conscience to develop an equitable system of distribution of benefits of growth to all, allows the current level of disparities to get worse. The issue of human development is much too complex to be resolved by focusing on economic "growth" singularly; or just sequencing them differently. Like an expert juggler in a circus who manages to keep several balls in the air simultaneously, our national planners must be able to balance the State's responsibilities for growth, development, equality and justice, ecological imperatives, and peace and safety of all citizens. A society cannot be fair or empowered until it eliminates abuses of the poor and powerless; therefore, empowerment of the powerless is not a political slogan. It is an imperative for human progress for all.

Since the debate on "growth" versus "development" goes beyond women's empowerment and concerns all people, especially the poor and the powerless people around the world, it would be appropriate to examine how a nation-state may make progress in human development before it becomes affluent. One of the effective ways to do this is to understand the "Kerala Model," as it is widely known. The Kerala model is essentially this: Kerala is clearly not among the rich states of India, and yet on human development indicators, including health status, literacy, and women's empowerment measures, it ranks at the top of all Indian states, including the five richest. The State of Gujarat (the state of India's current Prime Minister Narendra Modi who is credited for rapid economic growth in that state), on the other hand, which opted for the growth option under Modi, does have higher income but lags behind Kerala on all other indicators of human development. Why? The development advocates, including the leadership of Kerala, argue that human development or quality of life cannot be limited to and measured by economic growth alone. People must have basic education, good health, basic freedom, gender equality, social protection, and opportunities to enhance their capabilities to improve their quality of life. The economic growth approach does not address or measure these important aspects of our overall progress toward a better quality of life. Progress is a multidimensional concept and requires a broader approach rather than an exclusive focus on economic growth or any one domain of human life. Development advocates further argue that no nation-state consisting of a population that is primarily illiterate, sick, poor, and exploited is likely to compete with other nations in the global market and become financially self-reliant to address its human development needs.

The records of the last 50 years show that the wealth disparities between rich and poor nations and between the rich and the poor within nations have become greater, not smaller. "Taken together, the bottom half of the global population own less than 1% of total wealth. In sharp contrast, the richest 10% hold 86% of the world's wealth, and the top 1% alone account for 46% of global assets (Credit Suisse Global Wealth Report, 2013, p. 10).

Within this context, a review of the Kerala model is particularly relevant. It presents a unique case for understanding what would be a better pathway for progress for poorer societies. Historically, some development economists and scholars of modernization (Inglehart et al. of the World Values Survey) have argued that the poor and agrarian societies must achieve a threshold of economic growth and modernity before they can accomplish the preconditions for modernization, specifically in terms of transformation of traditional and survival values to self-expressive and emancipative values (e.g., economic prosperity, freedom, empowerment, and egalitarian values). The pro-poor position represented by the UNDP holds that expansion of choice, freedom, education, good health, and equality of opportunities are the preconditions for human development.

The data in the first four rows of Table 11.1 show that on economic indicators, Kerala is significantly behind Gujarat (item #3: GDP per capita in *crores* of rupees [1 *crore* of rupees = 10 million rupees], and item #4 indicates ranks among all Indian states); yet on the overall HDI (item #1), Kerala scores much higher than Gujarat (HDI scores of 0.789 and 0.527, respectively). Indeed, Kerala ranks at the top of all Indian states on human development

TABLE 11.1

Comparison of Kerala and Gujarat on Key Indicators

INDICATORS		INDIA	KERALA	GUJARAT
1. HDI (March 2014)***		.467	.790	.527
2. GDP in crore Rs. (1 crore = 10 million rupees (2011–2012)*			315,206	611,767
3. Per capita income in rupees (2011–2012)*			80,924	89,668
4. Economic rank among Indian states*			18	2
5. Women per 1,000 men (2011 census)		940	1,084#	918
6. Birth rate per 1,000 pop.***		29	17	16
7. Literacy***	Female	65.4%	92%	70%
	Male	82.7%	96%	87%
8. Life expectancy at birth***		63.5	74	64.1
9. Percent below poverty level***		21.9%	7.5%	16.3%
10. Infant mortality***	Female	46	11	51
per 1,000 births	Male	49	12	44
11. Babies delivered in hospitals***		41%	100%	55%
12. Homes without latrines***		53%	4.8%	42.7%
13. Underweight persons***		26.1% M/ 31% W	9.9% M/ 10.5% W	26.0% M/ 30.3% W
14. HIV awareness***		80% M/ 57% W	99% M/ 95% W	80% M/ 49% W
15. Population vaccinated (NFHS-3)		51.2%	79%	44%
16. TFR per woman in 2012**		2.4	1.8	2.3

*Annexure State-wise Per Capita Income and Gross Domestic Products
http://pib.nic.in/archieve/others/2013/dec/d2013121703.pdf.

#The only state in India where women outnumber men.

**Estimate of Total Fertility Rates from the *SRS Report* (2012), Census Commission of India.

***Source of data List of Indian States by GDP

National Family Health Survey-3: http://www.indiahealthstat.com/health/16/nationalfamilyhealthsurveysnfhs/633773/nationalfamilyhealthfsurvey3/411384/stats.aspx indicators. Yet it ranks eighteenth among all states and union territories on wealth; Gujarat ranks second.

To contextualize the debate, it is appropriate to present a brief sketch of what the Kerala model is. Kerala is the southwestern state of India on the coast of the Arabian Sea. It is considered to be a tourist haven; the state tourist ministry's slogan claims that it is "the gods' own country." Its lush green tropical vegetation, clean white sandy beaches for hundreds of miles washed by the deepest blue ocean, the soothing cool breeze from the Arabian Sea, and the most gorgeous sunsets that only van Gogh would dare to paint, conjure magic. But Kerala is famous for something else: Dr. Mahbub ul Haq, the pioneer of the HDI system, was among the first to notice it. Kerala is not among the richest states in India, but in spite of its lower economic achievement, Kerala ranks at the top of the nation on several important measures including the HDI, life expectancy at birth, literacy, gender parity, low infant mortality, and proactive social organization and participation. Haq and Sen advocated Kerala as the model for other poor nations and states to follow. Others, including Bhagwati and Panagariya, strongly argue that poor states and nations should follow Gujarat, a state also on the west coast of India, which achieved significantly higher economic growth than Kerala. The government of Gujarat, led by Narendra Modi, the leader of the conservative Hindu nationalist Bharatiya Janata Party (BJP), emphasized more private initiatives, and entrepreneurships; the state spent less public funds on education, health, and human development; and invested less governmental effort in social welfare. (Modi is the BJP leader who won the prime ministership of India in the April–May 2014 national election by a landslide victory. He will no doubt push for the Gujarat model.) A brief review of how Kerala could accomplish so much with less money would be relevant to the debate between Sen and Bhagwati on the relative merit of Kerala versus Gujarat. Table 11.1 presents comparative data on key indicators of development of these two states on the HDI.

On measures of gender parity, empowerment, literacy, and social participation, Kerala is at par or better than several economically advanced nations. The gender ratio is a measure of gender empowerment; Kerala has 1,084 women per 1,000 men alive; indeed, Kerala is the only state in India that has more women than men alive. Gujarat has 82 women missing for every 1,000 men. Life expectancy at birth for Kerala is more than ten years longer than that in Gujarat. The adult literacy rate in Kerala is very high (96% for men and 92% for women); although a slightly lower percentage of women are literate than men in Kerala, nearly 20% more women in Kerala are educated than in Gujarat (92% versus 70%). The IMR, a key measure of the health status of a population, is very low in Kerala; it is almost one-fifth of the IMR in Gujarat (11 per 1,000 live births in Kerala, compared to 51 for Gujarat). TFR for Kerala is 1.8 births per woman, much lower than that in Gujarat (2.3 per woman); and lower than that in the United States (2.1). The coverage of recommended vaccinations for Kerala and Gujarat are 79% and 44% respectively; for India as a whole it is 51.2%. Finally, the number of homes without sanitary latrines is a measure of health risk; in Kerala, less than 5% (4.8%) of homes are without latrines; in Gujarat, over 40% (42.7%) of homes are without latrines. In spite of higher GDP and per capita income, the poverty level in Gujarat is more than twice as high as in Kerala (16.3% and 7.5% respectively). These statistics and other evidence show that on several measures of human development, health, and gender empowerment, Kerala has made notable progress.

We need to understand why and how Kerala achieved these developments. Several historical and social developments have paved the way for Kerala's progress; it is appropriate to identify these developmental processes that stood Kerala in good stead.

Two other recent studies confirm the Kerala experience; these are measurements of happiness and social progress. Earlier we discussed the results of a recent *World Happiness Survey* (2013) that showed that five small Scandinavian countries topped the list of the happiest nations in the world (the happiest children in the world are in Denmark) on measures of subjective happiness; these five nations are not among the richest nations in the world. On the other hand, the richest nations of the world ranked much lower than the five Scandinavian nations on the happiness index (e.g., the U.S. ranked 17, the U.K. 22, France 25, Germany 26, Kuwait 32, Saudi Arabia 33, Taiwan 42, Russia 68, Bahrain 79, China 93, and South Africa 96). Benin, the Central African Republic, and Togo ranked at the very bottom of the list. These results confirmed what most of us know intuitively; that money alone does not buy happiness (WHR, 2013).

The second study, by Michael Porter and Scott Stern of Harvard University, measures a Social Progress Index or SPI (Porter & Stern, 2014) based on the premise that:

> A broader and more inclusive model of development requires new metrics with which policymakers and citizens can evaluate national performance. We must move beyond simply measuring Gross Domestic Product (GDP) per capita, and make social and environmental measurement integral to national performance measurement. (Porter & Stern, 2014, p. 3)

They used four principles for developing their SPI: that the indicators must be

1. exclusive social and environmental indicators,
2. measures of outcomes not of inputs,
3. actionable indicators for policy development, and
4. relevant to all cultures.

They defined "social progress" as the capacity of a society to meet the basic human needs of its citizens, establish the building blocks that allow citizens and communities to enhance and sustain the quality of their lives, and create the conditions for all individuals to reach their full potential. Their SPI includes three domains: *basic human needs, foundations of well-being,* and *opportunities.* They used this SPI to rank 132 countries across the world. New Zealand, Switzerland, Iceland, the Netherlands, and Norway rank at the top in that order. The United Kingdom ranks 13, Japan 14, Iceland 15, and the United States 16. Chad, the Central African Republic, and Burundi rank at the bottom of the list (Porter & Stern, 2014). Both measurements (happiness and SPI) confirm one conclusion: that the level of income or economic growth (PPP GDP per capita) alone is not a good predictor of either happiness or social progress.

These two studies (happiness and social progress) confirmed what the Kerala model found through its emphasis on human development initiatives.

How Kerala Achieved Higher HDI with Lower Wealth

Various hypotheses or explanations of how Kerala accomplished higher levels of human development with a lower level of economic growth include:

1. the tradition of enlightened rulers' emphasis on universal education;
2. investments in public education and health care;
3. high female education and gender parity in social participation;
4. strong political activism, grassroots movements, and strong pro-poor policies and programs by Kerala's Communist Party and leftist governments;
5. redistribution of agricultural lands and resources to reduce the extreme disparities between the wealthy minority of high-caste landowners and the tenant farmers and landless peasants; and
6. collective actions by an ethnically diverse population for promoting social reforms that benefit all (e.g., education, health, land distribution, gender parity, and absence of social segregation based on the traditional caste system).

Historically, the rulers of the three kingdoms that were combined to form the state of Kerala in 1956 (Kochi, Malabar, and Travancore) demonstrated strong records in investment in universal education, especially women's education, and welfare reforms including health care for their people. These enlightened rulers believed that better-educated subjects are easier to rule, are a more productive workforce, and are better able to enhance the reputation of the state and its rulers. These rulers also believed that it is the primary responsibility of the rulers to provide essential welfare services to their subjects. This philosophy of governance was prevalent in Buddhist rulers as early as the fourth century BCE during the reign of Emperor Ashoka of the Mauryan dynasty.

Under Ashoka's patronage, Buddhism spread from India to south India (where Kerala is located), and then to the south in Sri Lanka and the Far East; to Nepal, Tibet, China, and Japan in South-East Asia; to Pakistan, Afghanistan, and to the Indo-Greek kingdoms in the northwest. The extent of deaths and sufferings inflicted on millions of people by Ashoka's triumphant wars and the expansion of his empire caused him great repentance, and he converted to Buddhism. As a true Buddhist ruler, Ashoka dedicated himself to serving his subjects according to Buddha's teachings of compassion and *Dharma* (in Sanskrit; or *Dhamma* in Pali/Buddhist texts), which means "education," "discipline," or proper conduct" according to Buddha's teachings. Ashoka left behind 23 major edicts carved on stone pillars that spelled out his moral principles and public pronouncements of his vows that he considered essential for a just ruler. Ashoka's edicts proclaimed that there are two types of morality in a just society: public and private. "Public morality" refers to the moral duties of a ruler to his subjects, and "private morality" is the duties of a citizen toward the family and society.

Ashoka's public edicts clearly emphasized that it is the ruler's responsibility to ensure the well-being of all citizens, including education and health care for all. His edicts further stipulated that health care is a basic right of all citizens, and it should be available to all humans and animals, and furthermore it is the responsibility of the ruler to procure and distribute herbs, minerals, and medicines to all medical practitioners in the kingdom so that the citizen will have access to proper health care. To the best of our knowledge, Ashoka's edicts spell out the very first public declaration of universal health care and the state's responsibility for guaranteeing citizens' basic rights for health care; 2,500 years later, numerous countries in the world, including the world's wealthiest nation, the United States, still does not have universal health care funded by the State and available to all (several Scandinavian nations have). The Buddhist teachings also valued egalitarianism, opposed the caste hierarchy, and promoted higher status for women than did non-Buddhist Indian societies.

Buddhist influence in Kerala began during Ashoka's rule; he sent numerous Buddhist monks and scholars to South India who established many monasteries and engaged in education and social reforms, including the elimination of the caste system in the region. It is not surprising to find the influence of Buddhist teachings and values (or *Dhamma/Dharma*) on the rulers in their pronouncements, policies, emphasis on women's education and social participation for centuries in the South Indian kingdoms that were later combined to establish the modern state of Kerala in 1956.

In a recent assessment of Kerala's past, Rigzin (2014) reminds us that Kerala also has the longest history of European colonization in India.

The Portuguese explorer, Vasco da Gama landed in Kozhikode in 1498 A. D. and this marked the beginning of European Colonization in India.

Dutch and British followed the Portuguese colonization in Kerala. By the end of 18th Century, the whole of Kerala fell under the control of British colonist. However, ruler of Cochin and Travancore, two of three-major Malayalam speaking region, signed treaty of subsidiary alliance with British and become princely state of British India. This treaty allows the ruler of those two princely states a regional autonomy in return for fixed annual tribute to the British.

It was during this period that Kerala witness several social and educational reforms directed toward eradication of social evils such as practices of 'untouchability' and Sati system. The role-played by rulers of princely state, Christian missionaries and other social reformers have made significant contribution in creating welfare system in Kerala in general and progress of education in particular. (Rigzin, 2014)

The beginning of the monarch's responsibility for universal education and health care in Travancore can be traced back to the Royal Rescript by Rani (Queen) Gouri Parvati Bai in 1817. She introduced free and universal education for all her citizens. It is important to note that universal education at the State's cost was not practiced in most countries in the West at that time. The Queen's Rescript of 1817 says:

> The state should defray the entire cost of the education of its people in order that there might be no backwardness in the spread of enlightenment among them, that by diffusion of education they might become better subjects and public servants and that the reputation of the state might be advanced thereby. The Queen's proclamation of 1817 is hailed by all educational historians as "the Magna Carta of education" in Travancore. Through this Rescript the State was proclaiming its entire responsibility to provide budgetary accommodation for costs involved. A rule was also enforced that every school run on systematic lines was to have two teachers paid by the State. This may be regarded as the first formal recognition by the State to the right of education from public revenue (Aiya, 1906).

Commenting on the queen's progressive social reforms, historian V. Nagam Aiya, the author of the *Travancore State Manual*, in 1906 wrote:

> Her Highness was an enlightened and thoughtful ruler who illumined her reign by many humane acts of good government, the memory of which gladdened her last days ... she used to refer with pride and satisfaction to her various acts of administration for the amelioration of her people for many acts of redress of public wrongs had been either carried out or inaugurated during her reign. This was no small achievement for a Travancore queen when we remember that in the early years of the reign

of Queen Victoria of England, the condition of women in England was far worse than in Travancore.

In addition to education of the general people, women's education was especially emphasized in Kerala. The historical tradition of emphasizing State-funded universal education for both genders and health care became the norm of the former kingdoms of southern India that later became the state of Kerala. Table 11.1 shows that more than 92% of women in Kerala were educated in 2001; that is significantly higher than female literacy rates in Gujarat and India as a whole (65%) and also much higher than that of Indian men (82%). The estimated literacy rate in Kerala in 2013 was 97%. In addition to education, some authors speculated that Kerala's historical matrilineal tradition empowered the women; while it is true that Kerala's Nairs practice matrilineal inheritance of property, Nairs constitute less than 20% of the state's population. Consequently, the matrilineal tradition of the Nairs is not likely to be a dominant cause of the higher status of women and overall prosperity in Kerala.

In addition to high literacy, especially female literacy, Kerala's strong tradition of social activism and more recently its Communist Party and governments had significant roles to play. Major social reforms in Kerala that were sponsored or strongly supported by the Communist regimes for more than four decades included: (a) social reforms that eliminated crippling caste barriers, (b) redistribution of land and property that benefited the poor, and (c) democratization of governance by diminishing the monopoly of political and financial power by the high-caste Brahmins and Nairs. When the state Communist Party was in power, it forcefully led these reforms, and when not in power, it put strong pressure on the ruling coalition governments for these reforms. Franke and Chasin (1989) concluded:

> Land reform has redistributed wealth and political power from a rich elite to small holders and landless laborers. Public food distribution at controlled prices, large-scale public health actions, accessible medical facilities, and widespread literacy combine with and reinforce each other to maintain and expand Kerala's achievements. Serious unemployment threatens the Kerala experiment, but Kerala nonetheless offers important lessons to development planners, policymakers, and Third World activists.

In a subsequent letter to the editor and an exchange with Sen, Chasin and Franke (1991) further added:

> He (Sen) minimizes Kerala's radical political traditions in improving the lives of all of its people, including women. Though he does credit recent "left-wing governments," he gives far too much weight to Kerala's pre-independence rulers' stress on public education, and to a tradition of inheritance through the female line in much of Kerala that he says gives

women more material means for survival. He also fails to account for the availability of the medical care that he correctly points out is one of the major factors accounting for the better health of women in Kerala. (Chasin & Franke, 1991)

Chasin and Franke place more emphasis than Sen does on the importance of political activism and the impact of modern Communist rule in Kerala on its remarkable human development records. This author believes that, had Chasin and Franke appreciated more Kerala's unique cultural and historical heritage (including the influence of Buddhist, European, and progressive Rulers' legacies), their conclusion would have been different. Yes, Leftist/ Communist parties and governments played important roles and fought for the poor, but the sound foundation of universal education, women's literacy and status, healthcare services, various social reforms against caste-based exclusion, and strong social activism by peasant and landless laborers that led to Kerala's achievements were in motion for centuries before Kerala's Communist Party came to power in 1957. Sen concedes that Leftist governments and political activism of the masses had significant effects, but he traces the roots of these historical and unique developments to Kerala's traditional emphasis on education, especially women's education, health care, emancipation, and empowerment aided by matrilineal tradition and the status of women in Kerala. Sen concludes with this:

> Its (Kerala's) contemporary female–male ratio of 1.04 is indeed close to the values that obtain in modern Europe and North America (1.05 or so), and is totally different from that in India as a whole (0.93), and also from those in many other countries in Asia (such as, China's 0.94, Bangladesh's 0.94, Pakistan's 0.90). Modern Kerala does deserve credit for consolidating and building on past achievements. But the background to these developments has to be traced, to a considerable extent, back to Kerala's remarkable past, and we have to take note, among other things, of its old policy of educational expansion. These issues are important since the role of education, and in particular of female education, may well be central to many problems of the contemporary world. (Sen, 1991)

One important point to add is that Kerala, in spite of its ethnic diversity, worked together for common causes that affected all. According to the 2001 Indian census, Kerala's population was divided as follows—Hindus 56%; Muslim 24%; Christians 19%. The Hindus were subdivided into Brahmins, Nairs (families are matriarchal groups of decedents of common female ancestors) and other caste case-Hindus are those in four castes above the Dalits Hindus (four castes that are all above the subaltern underclass or the *Dalits* it literally means the "oppressed"), who were formerly called the "Untouchables." In spite of these serious class, caste, and religious differences and social cleavages, the fact that Kerala as a whole has been able to come together for the social reforms that affected all positively is not a small matter. The important lesson we may learn from Kerala's example is that universal education, especially women's education, gender parity, and empowerment; social activism for reforms, including land redistribution among landless farmers; and political activism inspired by Leftist ideologies/governments, enabled Kerala to confront disastrous disparities and caste segregation effectively. This combination empowered the powerless in Kerala and uplifted the entire state.

Lessons Learned from an Application of the EMPOWER Model

To recapitulate: The EMPOWER model was constructed to identify various categories of empowerment dimensions (or categories of empowerment methods), to extract qualitative and quantitative data from case studies, and to compare the quantitative data from 80 case studies. The model identifies seven EMPOWER *dimensions* used by these movements to promote one or more domains of life. The model includes four *domains* of life that affect our overall sense of QOL. These four domains are: human rights, equal rights, health, and economic self-reliance. (Several movements referred to the importance of the spiritual domain, but the definition and indicators of spiritual empowerment were not well articulated; for that reason, this fifth domain is not included in the domains of empowerment). The EMPOWER framework was also used to compare whether the seven dimensions or methods of empowerment used varied in economically more and less advanced societies. Chapter 5 presented the theoretical and conceptual framework of the EMPOWER model for the meta-analysis. Chapter 6 presented the results of the comparative quantitative data on seven empowerment dimensions/methods by the four empowerment domains.

This section reviews the lessons learned from the meta-analysis of empowerment movements and the implications of the EMPOWER model for future research and interventions.

SIX RESEARCH QUESTIONS

The key lessons learned from the qualitative findings of our meta-analysis project as they relate to the six research questions are presented below.

Can and Do Ordinary Women Lead Effective Empowerment Movements?

The answer is a resounding "Yes." However, it is impossible to enumerate all movements because there is no reliable databank or network that identifies and lists all women's self-organized movements. Consequently, we can never know how many self-organized movements actually occurred, succeeded, or failed during a given time period. These grassroots movements are mostly organized by the victims themselves and/or by persons and organizations who care for them. These people are not always scholars or journalists; they are activists dedicated to seeking justice and remedying problems through citizens' collective actions. As a result, they do not usually write about their work or publish it. Until Internet browsing became popular, it was not possible to search for news about most movements online; and even after the Internet became widely accessible, grassroots movements that were not posted online could not be accessed. In addition, Internet searches can be problematic for three reasons. First, unlike peer-reviewed journals and articles, Internet entries are not always edited or curated by experts in the subject area; anyone can post just about anything. So the credibility of the items is always questionable and needs to be corroborated and verified from independent credible sources. Second, the sheer volume of information generated by an Internet search makes it impossible to verify the authenticity of the items detected. For instance, a Google search using "women's empowerment movements" as a search term on April 28, 2014, generated 28 million items; a Google Scholar search with the same keywords generated more than 300,500 items. Many items are repeated countless times, and not all items have sufficient information to allow anyone to evaluate the veracity of the items posted. Third, unless a case study or report contains sufficient information on all six research questions of our meta-analysis, that case study cannot be used for quantitative content analysis and it does not meet our criteria of inclusion. Our extensive multiple search methods identified 426 case studies that appeared to meet our criteria of inclusion for content analysis, but only 80 (or 18.7%) of these case studies provided necessary information on all six dimensions and met our criteria of inclusion. This winnowing was a highly labor-intensive process, and less than one out of five case studies could be used for our meta-analysis. Yet, to the best of our knowledge, as of now this study includes the largest number of case studies on women's self-organized empowerment movements. All of these case studies, except one, were initiated, led, and organized by women who were victims of abuse or were closely related to victims. The exceptional case is the Grameen Bank's microfinance movement in Bangladesh; it was originated by Mohammad Yunus, a male economist. We included this case because the movement was for poor village women, and it was collectively implemented by the women: more than 97% of the beneficiaries of this movement were women, and the movement was organized and implemented by small work-groups of women who were collectively responsible for managing their loans, performing the activities that generated the income needed to repay their loans, and collectively taking responsibility for repaying their loans on time (the timely loan repayment rate was astoundingly more than 97%!).

Our case studies are from both rich and poor countries in all continents, from rural and urban areas, and represent all major religious groups. For these reasons, we conclude that ordinary women can and do lead grassroots movements that significantly improve the HRQOL of their families and communities.

What Are the Characteristics of Women Who Organize These Movements?

We excluded women who are in a position of power through inheritance, marriage, or membership of a powerful elite group; for instance, we excluded the likes of India's Prime Minister Indira Gandhi (daughter of India's first prime minister); or Benazir Bhutto of Pakistan (the world's first Muslim woman to be head of state, and the daughter of Pakistan's prime minister); or Sirimavo Bandaranaike, world's first woman Prime Minister, of Sri Lanka (her wealthy husband was the Prime Minister of Sri Lanka); or Queen Elizabeth II of England. They are powerful women to start with, and we expect them to do exceptionally good deeds, but often they do not. These women do not need empowerment. It was refreshing to discover that the women who led and organized movements came from all sorts of backgrounds; there is no special characteristic that separates them from most ordinary women. They include the likes of:

1. Then-15-year-old Malala Yousafzai, considered to be the bravest girl in the world, from the Taliban-infested Swat Valley in Pakistan—she was shot in her face by an extremist Talib because she advocated for girls' rights for school education;
2. The uneducated Rigoberta Menchu (a Nobel Peace Prize laureate at the young age of 33), a Quiche Indian woman from a poor peasant family in Guatemala who struggled against ruthless land owners who brutalized indigenous Indians and the poor peasants;
3. The 14 middle-aged, simple, semiliterate women of the Madres de Playa Mayo in Buenos Aires, Argentina, who bravely challenged the brutal military junta to reveal where their loved ones had "disappeared" to after the junta dragged them out of their homes in the dark of night; and who helped bring a regime change in that nation;
4. The ordinary mother from California, Candice (Candy) Lightner, who was outraged when her 13-year-old daughter was killed by a drunk driver, who led a movement against drunk driving and went on to become the co-founding president of Mothers Against Drunk Driving (MADD), which now has more than 600 chapters in the United States and abroad, and has made our roads much safer;
5. A registered nurse, Margaret Sanger, who was imprisoned because she asserted women's right to have reproductive and contraceptive information and her right to distribute such information to other women publicly; who later went on to found the International

Planned Parenthood Federation (IPPF) that now serves women in almost all nations;

6. The uneducated, stigmatized, and pariah sex-workers who organized the Sonagachi Mahila Darbar movement in Kolkata (India) to protect themselves and their children from HIV/AIDS, police brutality, abusive pimps, and sex-traffickers;

7. The grandmothers in Argentina and Chile (Abuelas de Plaza de Mayo) who are still active in finding their grandchildren who were taken away from the children's "disappeared" and tortured mothers by the military junta and given for adoption in secret to unidentified military families;

8. The illiterate Indian peasant women who tied themselves to trees to prevent cutting of trees and deforestation, and to reclaim their land from unscrupulous logging and mining industries who obtained contracts to occupy the ancestral lands of the villagers (the Chipko movement);

9. The poor, overworked, and helpless women in textile industries in Ahmedabad, India, who organized the SEWA, which has become a model for human development movements globally;

10. An ordinary woman, Wangari Maathai, who organized a movement of peasant women in rural Kenya, known as the "Greenbelt movement," to plant trees to stop soil erosion from their lands, which later expanded to other income-generating enterprises that subsequently elevated her to international fame and a Nobel Peace Prize in 2004;

11. Those involved in the "Apne Aap" (On Your Own) movement in India to protect the members of the "Third Sex" (a broad umbrella group of marginalized and stigmatized persons who do not identify with or fit in the traditional two-gender system, including the lesbians, gays, bisexuals and transgendered, and the *Hinjras* of India, Pakistan, and Bangladesh who dress like women and entertain others with songs and dance) who struggle for their basic rights as human beings;

12. The band of housewives in rural Andhra Pradesh in India, who famously mobbed and raided liquor shops in their villages and destroyed wine bottles and launched the now-famous "Arrak Ban" movement that prohibits liquor shops in rural villages (*Arrak* means liquor); they were outraged that their husbands would spend all their money at the liquor shops, then come home drunk and abuse their wives and children, the women refused to cook, clean, or have sex with their drunken husbands;

13. A single young Christian woman, Angela Gomes, a social worker and the founder of Banchte Shekha ("Survival Learning" NGO), who traveled from village to village to help desperate Muslim women in

rural Bangladesh, and led a successful movement in spite of the fact that Muslim men slandered, defamed, and labeled her as a woman of bad moral character who was corrupting young Muslim girls, converting girls to Christianity, and worse still, luring poor girls to human trafficking. The stigma of a young unmarried woman going against the cultural norms was so deep that she had to "invent" a husband (who is not with her because he is "studying abroad") and a couple of children (who "live with their grandparents so that they can go to better schools") to manufacture a sense of protection from insults and threats of violence. The fact that Gomes was internationally honored by the Ramon Magsaysay Award (some consider this the poor people's Nobel Prize) did not protect her fully from serious threats, abuse, and insults dispensed by her antagonists.

The list goes on.

Four chapters (7–10) of this book presented summaries of these 80 movements, which would constitute an inspiring and instructive volume even without any further narratives or analysis. In essence, they are ordinary women doing extraordinary things for their families and communities.

It is important to point out that, unlike academic researchers or business entrepreneurs, these women did not begin with a research design, or a business plan, or a well-developed strategy or a concept paper; they often did not even have a written statement of a problem and what they intended to do about it. They usually began with a just cause and were driven by a parental motivation to protection their loved ones, or by moral outrage; but they were never alone. Initially they may have been obscured by a spiral of silence (defined as a condition when some powerless people feel that they are a small minority of persons unable to do anything to solve their problems and therefore they are not vocal about asserting their rights).

Two additional characteristics of these women are worth noting. First, their gender seems to offer them some protection in many situations; all societies, including gangs and military juntas, treat mothers and women with some degree of deference. These women were not perceived as a threat or as confrontational; they were not seen as people trying to grab political power or seeking a regime change. A violent confrontation against such mothers was likely to generate community outrage against the perpetrators of the violence (ironically, most of the violence against women is perpetrated by their family members, someone they know, or their intimate partners; that is another matter that deserves separate discussion). For these reasons their gender often acts as a protective shield. For instance, when the mothers of the Madres de Playa Mayor in Argentina began their weekly demonstrations demanding news about their "disappeared" sons, husbands, and relatives, the military junta in power faced a dilemma. The junta did not dare to arrest these women, fearing public outrage; the military instead tried to discredit them by branding them as the "crazy women" of the Playa Mayor. Some of the women received anonymous death threats, and two of them were abducted, tortured, and murdered by unidentified assailants. But the junta did not use force against these mothers openly. Several mothers' organizations, in the United States and abroad, including the MADD and mothers against gun and drug violence, have found some protection from direct violence from gangs and pro-gun groups because they are perceived as caring and apolitical mothers concerned about the safety of their children. Above all, they give and receive strong support from other victims like them with whom they form inseparable bonds that empower and embolden them. Finally, these women demonstrate an immeasurable degree of resilience, courage, and patience while facing their ordeal and abuse. Given the opportunity, they learn marketable skills very quickly, keep their promises (e.g., 98% of the Grameen or SEWA women repay their loans on time), and "get by with a little help from their friends." The moral imperative of professionals is to discover such movements and offer help.

What Motivates These Women?

According to Maslow's five-step hierarchy of needs, these women are motivated primarily by the needs at the bottom two levels; physical survival and protection from imminent danger (safety), and a little bit of opportunity necessary to live like human beings. Although their sustained struggles always have profoundly empowering effects on them, and many women actually gain social status and enhanced self-esteem, these movements do not begin with a motivation for self-enhancement or personal growth like the people in the middle or highest levels of the need hierarchy. While motivation theorist David McClelland may argue that their struggles enable them to develop some level of affiliation with their network of peers (need for affiliation) and some position of influence over others who are less fortunate than they (need for power), they believe their struggle is effective if they are able to overcome the survival and safety threats that drive them to act. Most of them are struggling for very basic survival and safety needs: a roof over their head, steady income, food security, welfare and education for their children, access to health care, and a chance to live in peace like ordinary human beings. Their needs are so basic and the cause of struggle is so fair that no one, except their unscrupulous abusers who stand to gain by exploiting them, opposes them. A just cause is a powerful force that motivates them to act and wins supporters for their cause. No fair and decent person would oppose them. We find evidence of external support for their struggle from altruistic, compassionate, or idealistic citizens, community leaders, and human service professionals in every successful movement.

A small initial success (or gain) in their struggle has an enormously rewarding effect on them. Two important findings about the motivations of the women in our case studies deserve our attention. First, while their struggle begins with simple survival and protection needs, all involvement empowers them at different ways and levels. The second is the deep concern for the well-being of their children which unite them for a common cause across ethnic, linguistic, religious, and other social groups. Prevention of "harms" to their children is a great unifying force.

Rising Aspirations and Capabilities

One of the most refreshing findings is that the aspirations and capacities (skills) of the women rise as they become more involved and empowered. The illiterate village women of the Grameen Bank, the part-time women workers in SEWA projects, and the Rescatando Salud *promotoras* illustrate the steps of progressive empowerment. Initially they are passive, unsure of themselves, avoid eye contact, and never speak unless spoken to. As they become involved in various group activities, the women become more communicative, cultivate social skills and a network of peers, and become optimistic. Their group network provides them with protection and emotional and instrumental support. They no longer believe that they are alone in their struggle, and believe that as a group they can achieve goals that were not possible before. Their work experience allows them to develop marketable skills and find jobs that generate income and elevate their sense of self-efficacy and status within their families and communities. In many instances, they surprise themselves and the sponsors of these projects by setting goals that were beyond their initial expectations.

The work experience of the *promotoras* combined with their on-the-job English classes enabled them to speak and write enough English and made them more employable than before. After a decade in the life of this project, *promotoras* were sending their children to better schools and finding better-paid full-time jobs for themselves. Four of them became homeowners through the low-income housing projects. These secondary but higher goals (e.g., college education for children, home ownership) were not in the original project goals; neither the organizers nor the *promotoras* ever imagined that these goals were attainable by them.

Similar phenomena were discovered by the SEWA and Grameen projects; some 20 years after these projects began, some children of the women beneficiaries are studying in colleges and getting professional jobs. The illiterate poor women could not even have dreamt of such goals. From these secondary gains, we conclude that successful empowerment interventions have moving targets; over time they seek and accomplish goals that are higher and beyond the initial goals that drove them to action.

What Unifies a Diverse Community? Protecting Children from Harm Is a Unifying Force

Chapter 4 discussed the realities of multicultural communities that consist of different ethnic groups with different immigration histories and experiences. Consequently, based upon ethnicity and the length of acculturation experiences in this country, different groups rank their priorities differently. For instance, the recent first-generation immigrants assign higher priorities to immigration assistance, language competency, employment, and housing; the second-generation emigrants often assign higher priorities to intra-family and gender role conflicts, equality in employment and wages, and ethnic identity–related issues; more established (third or subsequent) generations assign higher priorities to social equality, quality of education, and better QOL. This difference in priorities by different groups in a community poses a problem when a participatory needs-assessment and planning process is trying to identify common problem/s for unifying the community for action. The key issue in this situation is to answer: what unifies an ethnically diverse community? The answer from our multiethnic community organization involvement in Los Angeles is: "Prevention of harm to their children." We discovered that, regardless of ethnic and other differences, almost all parents want to protect their children from harm, and that when resources are limited and they must choose only one program for external assistance, they are willing to compromise on other priorities. We hardly require scientific evidence to conclude that the overwhelming majority of parents make sacrifices for their children; it is true that some parents abuse or neglect their children, but we conclude that these cases are aberrations. Perhaps our own beliefs, experience, and observations are enough to accept that parental sacrifices and caring for our children are products of natural law (i.e., even animals take care of and fight to protect their offspring). Biologists may suggest that these are behavioral expressions of our nurturing instincts; sociobiologists and the advocates of parental investment theories (PIT) argue that parental sacrifice is due to evolutionary traits designed to promote our self-perpetuation needs; utilitarians and economists may suggest that this is driven by our need to maximize our own old-age security; social scientists (anthropologists, psychologists, and sociologists) may claim that this is due to internalized and universal values learned through our socialization processes; philosophers may present theories of altruism or moral obligations; and some may argue that this is due to our unconditional love for our children. But hardly anyone would argue that parental motivation to protect their dependent children is not universal.

Personal Sacrifice

When the rich spend astronomical amounts of money for their children's education or health, it may not be considered a personal sacrifice. But parents who cut their own comfort, take on heavy loans for children's education or work a second job, or single mothers who pull double duty as mothers at home and as breadwinners or a poor mother who would go hungry so that her children may have food, are clear examples of parental sacrifices. Is this due to a sense of parental obligation or unconditional love? The question is not easy to answer; it would require a separate volume to review the range of moral, ethical, psychological, and empirical justifications to do it the justice it deserves.

For a good discussion of the type of psychology that goes into the human sense of obligation and may motivate some of these activities in real life, see Robin Bradley Kar, *The Deep Structure of Law and Morality* (RB Kar, 2006). This work draws on a broad range of natural and social sciences to suggest that humans are

> motivated by a sense of obligation, which is not reducible to instrumental reasoning—though it may employ instrumental reason to produce actions. This sense of obligation gives rise to characteristic patterns in our social lives and structures a number of our interpersonal actions and reactions to one another. (p. 880)

These motivations can be quite powerful, but they also have complex properties, which structure a complex form of human social life. For example, they incline ordinary people to take certain duties to have intrinsic authority as parents, teachers, etc., but they also incline ordinary people to have a strong sense of reciprocity, which causes them to react to deviations with criticism and other forms of serious social pressure (RB Kar, 2006, pp. 909–919). Psychological attitudes like these play a large role in many aspects of human social life, and have undoubtedly contributed to the types of norms and values that have promoted public health and human flourishing in many different cultures and societies for millennia (RB Kar, 2014, personal communication).

For this volume it is sufficient to accept the axiom that parental sacrifice is a universal phenomenon, not an exception. The last, and perhaps the most important, characteristic that the women in our case studies share is the level of extreme personal sacrifice they made for their cause. Beyond the persistent investment of time and effort, they were willing to risk their own lives for what they believed in. Even after several threats against their lives, and often after fatal attacks on the originators of the movements, their struggles prevailed, and they showed the courage to continue. Sometimes, the attack on them may not have been fatal, but may have destroyed their careers or reputations and subjected them to inhuman treatments, torture, and violence. Others were publicly humiliated to persuade them to quit.

Who Supports and Opposes Them

All movements have their supporters and detractors; some are selfless patrons, and others are ruthless killers and criminals who exploit the poor and powerless. The case studies show that all successful movements for a just cause attracted supporters and mentors who offered their struggle the credibility they needed, and offered material resources including funds, professional expertise, mentoring, and training for developing necessary skills for the members of the movement. Examples include:

1. The plight and inhumane sufferings of the poor and powerless drove Rabindranath Tagore to initiate, with his personal funds, Asia's first microcredit enterprise and farmers' cooperative in India in 1905;
2. Ila Bhatt, a famous social reformer and effective lawyer for the textile workers' union in Ahmedabad, took up the case of their wives who had to seek part-time jobs without health benefits and with insecure income to help them organize the SEWA cooperative in 1972;
3. Economics professor Yunus started the Grameen Bank in Bangladesh in 1976, initially with his own funds;
4. Indian author Arundhati Roy (named by *Time* Magazine in 2014 as one of the 100 most influential people in the world) who donated the money from her Booker Prize award and royalties from her books and joined Medha Patkar, an eminent social reformer, to support the Sardar Sarovar Dam movement (that threated to uproot and literally drown millions of poor villagers in India);
5. Famous author and feminist Gloria Steinem joined Ruchira Gupta, the founder of the NGO Apne Aap (On Your Own) to battle human trafficking for the sex-trade across the world;
6. America's First Lady Eleanor Roosevelt dedicated her later life to helping the poor, women, and children;
7. Dr. Bina Lakshmi Nepram was also named by AOVC (Action On Armed Violence) among the 100 most important people in 2014 for her dedicated work to prevent gun violence; she was the recipient of many international and national awards;
8. Bill and Melinda Gates invested hundreds of millions of dollars to eradicate HIV/AIDs and deadly diseases in poor communities.
9. Media: both printed and electronic media (including public sector media, commercial and social media) often played a critical role in raising public awareness and support for grassroots movements. The role played by the world press in publicizing the plights of the Madres des Playa Mayor in Argentina (one of the case studies in this book) and ubiquitous use of social media during the recent Arab Spring movements are powerful examples.
10. Donors: both public and non-profit donors provide critical support to empowerment movements in two important ways: (a) funding empowerment movement activities including incentives or boosting legitimacy, and (b) offering global recognition to the leaders of movements

498 Global Health and Quality of Life

and thus enhancing their credibility and effectiveness. The Nobel
Peace Prize and other prestigious international and national awards
for humanitarian causes significantly enhance personal leadership and
empower their movements.

The opponents of women's movements and progress fall in these overlap-
ping categories:

1. Conservatives who oppose ethnic and gender equality in general;
   they often defend their positions on the ground of the preservation of
   cultural gender roles and traditions;
2. Misogynists who oppose any policy that promotes gender equality
   including women's right to choose an education, independent career,
   abortion, divorce, birth control, or single-parenthood;
3. Unscrupulous exploiters of human rights of the poor and powerless
   for their own selfish greed; more than 70% of the world's poor and
   powerless are women and consequently the exploiters harm women
   more often; they also include those who violate existing laws against
   human trafficking of women and children;
4. Sociopaths who inflict immeasurable sufferings on others, especially
   women through the use of violence, rape, trafficking, torture, ethnic
   strifes, and genocides. Most frequently women and children are the
   victims of these crimes.
5. Oppressive regimes that extract and exploit their people's resources
   (e.g., labor, talents, freedom, and dignity) and constitute crimes against
   humanity; helpless women and children suffer more in these conditions.
6. Cultural crimes perpetuated by extremist groups or organizations
   who commit despicable crimes in the name of preserving their anti-
   gender and anti-ethnic cultural heritage.

It is important to note that most of the violations of women's rights
that are rooted in social and cultural traditions are not often considered as
"criminal" acts by the perpetrators and their peers. A recent UN-sponsored
multi-country study on violence against women in six Asian nations
discovered that:

1. The prevalence of sexual violence, including rape, varies from 26% to
   as high as 80%;
2. The majority of the violence against women is perpetrated by intimate partners and men known to the victims;
3. Most men when they force sex on women do not consider that as rape;
4. A prevalent "culture of rape" allows men to perpetrate the crime and
   go unpunished; and

5. The culture of violence also includes the lack of appropriate societal actions to prevent the crimes in the first place. (UN Women, 2013)

Sometimes a brutal attack on a powerless woman can trigger global outrage and support for a just cause; the worldwide support and attention that Malala Yousafzai (another of the 100 most influential persons in the world named by *Time* magazine) received for her movement to educate Pakistani girls was one example. Finally, politicians driven by ideologies and theories (e.g., growth versus development models discussed before) adopt policies that favor the rich and cut investments in human development; these policies adversely affect hundreds of millions of women and their families. The summaries of case studies (Chapters 7–10) included in this book provide illustrations of the important roles that women, their supporters, as well as their adversaries play in these struggles.

WHAT EMPOWERMENT METHODS ARE USED?

Chapter 6 presented the quantitative and comparative results of various empowerment methods used by the 80 movements. This section presents some qualitative observations on the methods that empowered these movements.

Modernization theorists (including Inglehart et al., Hoftstader, Weber, Durkheim, Lipset, Lerner, Rostow, and others) have argued that poor agrarian and pre-industrial societies must achieve a threshold of economic growth, literacy, and industrialization before they can accomplish the preconditions for modernization, specifically in terms of transforming traditional and survival values to self-expressive and emancipative values (e.g., economic prosperity, freedom, empowerment, and egalitarian values). The pro-poor position represented by the UNDP's HDA holds that human development cannot be achieved and measured by economic growth alone; that expansion of choice, freedom, education, good health, and equality of opportunity are the preconditions for human development. At the micro-level, where the self-organized movements originate and mature, a confluence of forces enables them to succeed. These are:

1. a deeply compelling survival motivation of the women,
2. the opportunity to form peer groups to work together to improve their condition,
3. external support including instrumental or tangible help from dedicated mentors, professionals, or local leaders; and
4. the capacity for building profitable skills through empowerment initiatives (e.g., including training), microenterprise, and legal reforms.

These were elaborated on in Chapter 6. However, one factor is worth reemphasizing: the synergy between the group process and the communication media (available to them).

Innovations may originate from the least likely sources and cash-poor situations. A few examples will illustrate these lessons.

Triesman's Merit Immersion for Students and Teachers (MIST) model, which demonstrated that collaborative learning and group-based problem-solving assignments, supported by competent mentors and social media access, while deemphasizing lectures in classrooms by experienced teachers and tests, dramatically improved math and science performance among minority students at UC Berkeley and elsewhere who could not afford private lessons and tutors.

Sugata Mitra's pioneering "Hole in the Wall" experiments showed that poor slum children can self-teach computer competencies without having a computer teacher or owning a personal computer.

Salman Khan's "Khan Academy" showed that children and adults alike can learn math, science, and other technical subjects on their own, from free online lessons that Khan initially designed and uploaded on the Internet to help his cousin struggling with these subjects, and later made available online to everyone.

Each of these highly successful projects used a social medium, but the central lesson is that they began with a bold new idea *supported* by a creative use of social media in peer-group interactions (not simply pressing a button on a cell phone or a personal computer). Before the social media era, Tagore (the pioneer of the "microcredit" project in India), Bhatt (of the SEWA), and Yunus (of the Grameen Bank in Bangladesh) showed that "microcredit" combined with efficient cooperatives, group-based assignments and performance, and effective mentorship can significantly enhance education, income, and HRQOL of the poorest villagers, while investments of hundreds of billions of dollars of foreign assistance per year over the last several decades failed to benefit the poorest in both rich and poor countries.

Jody Heymann (2010) discovered that when companies pay higher wages and provide health care and other employment benefits to their workers at the BOL, the industry itself benefits more; at the same time, appreciative workers become more productive, loyal, and satisfied. Based on her in-depth international case study analysis, Heymann stated:

> This book shows how profit sharing increased the productivity of a box manufacturer in British Columbia and a cookie manufacturer in Roxbury, Massachusetts. It tells the story of how investments in health care provisions at a scrap metal company in AIDS-ridden South Africa and at a cement manufacturer in rural India made these companies more profitable in the long run. (Heymann, 2010, p. 13)

The meta-analysis presented in this book has shown that poor and ordinary women across the world can and do lead self-organized movements that fundamentally transform themselves and promote the health and QOL of their families and communities. These and other innovations show that the inherent power of positive human relations, effective management of groups, and "self-organized" and "collaborative" learning, when supported by competent mentors and trusted professionals, can significantly enhance the performance of groups and empower them as well. Vicarious learning from these and similar movements is a rich source of information about how to empower the poor and powerless.

Four thinkers who have significantly influenced this author's philosophy of empowerment are Rabindranath Tagore, Mahatma Gandhi, Amartya Sen, and Paulo Freire.

1. The philosopher-poet Tagore nearly a century ago emphasized the importance of establishing *bonds of relations* with disparate groups and communities, and of *atma-shakti* or self-strength akin to self-efficacy (Tagore, 1925).
2. Freire's axiomatic book title emphasizes the importance of *Education for Critical Consciousness*; this book taught me the value of a praxis or a two-way interaction between the teacher and the student for collaborative problem-solving tasks from which both can learn (Freire, 2013).
3. Gandhi demonstrated the power of seeking truth, nonviolence and passive resistance as important tools for confronting brutal colonial and military force (Erickson, 1993).
4. Sen has argued that maximizing freedom and capabilities are the ultimate goals of human development, and that the argumentative nature or critical dialogue enriched cultures in general and India in particular and that served them well (Sen, 1999, 2006b).

As our communities are becoming more multicultural, professionals working in these communities must learn what divides and unites people from different cultures, and how some communities effectively cope with the problems unique to multicultural communities. I am not satisfied if I do not learn something myself from teaching a graduate course or working in the field. Public health education should combine these insights to better educate our professionals to become both competent specialists and effective mentors in multicultural communities.

This book is guided by the philosophy of self-organization, vicarious learning, and critical analysis of exemplary case studies as important sources of empowerment education. Hopefully, the summaries of the case studies presented in this book will serve as a powerful source of learning about the empowerment of women for GPH.

An Application of the EMPOWER Model: The Rescatando Salud Project

This chapter concludes with the lessons learned from an application of the EMPOWER model for our *Rescatando Salud* ("Save Health") project in poor and under-served Latino communities in Los Angeles. This project was based on the results of our meta-analysis of women's empowerment movements and the EMPOWER framework for needs assessment, program development, implementation, and evaluation. It exemplifies what a truly participatory study and intervention looks like. The project won the national award in the category of "Excellence in Reducing Ethnic Diversity in Immunization" in 2001 from the National Coalition for Minority Health and Immunization. This award was an external validation of the effectiveness of the model.

Those interested in more details may wish to see a 14-minute video available on the Rescatando Salud Project on YouTube: http://www.youtube.com/watch?v=OXRp7LzuKdE (accessed January 26, 2016).

THE RESCATANDO SALUD (SAVE HEALTH) PROJECT

This project was a four-way innovative and collaborative project among the UCLA Office of Public Health Practice, the Los Angeles County Immunization Program, La Esperanza Community Housing Project, and the South Central Community Health Center (all located in Los Angeles). The health objective of this project (initially funded by the Health Resources and Services Administration [HRSA] and the State of California) was to promote the level of age-appropriate full-immunization coverage of children under three years of age in under-served Latino communities in Los Angeles. For various reasons, including the fear that the police and Immigration and Naturalization Service (INS) staff could be disguised as immunization workers searching for undocumented immigrants, the mothers were unwilling to allow vaccinators to come into their homes or visit local community clinics to have their children immunized in a timely manner.

Methods

The project recruited local women from the poor and under-served Latino communities as *promotoras* (promoters) to increase childhood immunization rates in Latino communities. Unlike other *promotora* projects in the country, which paid their promoters a poor salary as community health aides or assistants to outreach health workers, we did not hire them as poorly paid staff who cost less. Instead, we used the funds available on their training and the development of marketable skills so that when our short-term immunization project fund expired, they would have lifelong marketable skills to earn a living.

The choice of empowerment methods and outreach methods was informed by the EMPOWER model. For instance, instead of paying them a poor salary, we paid their tuition and costs to become a certified phlebotomist, word processor, secretarial assistant, hairdresser, or video recorder; or provided funds needed to start their own microenterprise (one aspiring videographer produced the 14-minute video on this project mentioned above). The *promotoras* received training and a certificate as a *promotora* in a chosen service profession, and they had to do immunization outreach work and education among their peers in their own communities.

Outreach strategies and implementation were planned through regular participatory meetings; indeed, the name of the project was chosen by the *promotoras*. They always worked as a team for planning and executing the outreach work. The *promotoras* kept diaries to record what they did, what worked or did not, the difficulties they faced, and their own evaluation of the program, and their personal efficacy. Weekly meetings were held with their project supervisors to review operational and tactical planning. Monthly meetings including the project co-directors, field supervisors, and *promotoras* were held to review the program's process (including their diaries) and operational decisions.

The Project Team

The project was jointly directed by four co-directors representing the four partner organizations: Cheri Todoroff, director of the L.A. County Department of Health (Chief of Immunization); Nancy Ibrahim, the director and chief of La Esperanza Community Housing Program; myself (Prof. Snehendu Kar, director of public health practice at UCLA); and John Kotick, the director of the South Central Community Health Center, which was serving the population of the project area. Laticia Iberra served as the overall project coordinator and project manager, and Kirstin Chickering served as the program manager at the Public Health Practice office at UCLA. In less than two years, we exceeded our initial target. In 2001, the third year, we received the national award for "Excellence in Reducing Ethnic Disparities" in immunization from the National Coalition for Immunization and the Office of Minority Health at the HRSA. All *promotoras* gained valuable English-language skills; significant professional experience in outreach health care; certified competencies in several service occupations (several of them found full-time paid employment); and enhanced self-efficacy. By the fifth year, several *promotoras* proposed that Rescatando Salud establish a *promotora* training program for training outreach workers from other community-based organizations, and they were eager to serve as field supervisors in the proposed training. This proposal represented a high level of self-efficacy and aspiration among the *promotoras*. This unexpected outcome was beyond the scope of the original project goals. It established that empowerment process results in shifting of expectations and goals; and an effective empowerment evaluation should be able to measure shifting aspirations and moving targets.

REFLECTIONS ON WHY THE PROJECT SUCCEEDED

First: All six key members (the four co-directors and the two program managers) and the field coordinator were members of the UCLA School of Public Health family who subsequently occupied key positions in our partner organizations. Both Nancy Ibrahim and Cheri Todoroff were alumnae of our Masters in Public Health (MPH) program at UCLA; they were both elected to the UCLA Public Health Hall of Fame. Kirstin Chickering and Laticia Iberra were also graduates from the same program. John Kotick, the director of South Central Community Health Center, did not have an MPH from UCLA (he had a law degree), but he had worked closely with me as the program manager of the Public Health Practice office, which I directed. Consequently, all six key persons had a common professional perspective, conceptual framework (empowerment), outcome priorities, and core public health leadership competencies, but each brought additional expertise that complemented others' strengths. There was mutual respect and trust.

Second: The project had clear, specific, and measurable goals that were highly important (complete and timely childhood immunization coverage and the empowerment of the *promotoras*).

Third: In addition to the common project objectives, the team members had respective institutional goals that were better served by the partnership; and these goals were not in conflict. For instance, UCLA students could gain practical field experience, and faculty members could conduct applied research; the Esperanza program could offer added public health experience to their *promotora* training programs; and our collective outreach health-education efforts produced higher immunization coverages that both the L.A. County Health Department and the South Central Family Health Center strove to achieve. There were no conflicts of interest; the six key professionals complemented one another's roles and goals.

Fourth: The *promotoras* were Latinas from the same neighborhoods where they lived and worked for the project; they shared a culture and language and were indeed part of the same community. As a result, the Latina mothers trusted the *promotoras* and were not afraid of them. The *promotoras* began to gain some tangible benefits (albeit psychological); their status as opinion leaders in health was enhanced, and they were learning a new language (English) and new professional skills. As program directors and university professors appreciated their input, their involvement in planning sessions boosted their self-esteem and self-efficacy. There was palpable hope and optimism in them. The project directors invited four *promotoras* to attend an annual American Public Health Association (APHA) conference in Washington, D.C., where Rescatando Salud was presented at a panel discussion session. For the first time in their lives, the *promotoras* had the opportunity to fly to a professional meeting and answer questions from public health professionals, including how they did what they did and how the project helped them. We could only be impressed by their poise, confidence, and pride. They heard more than some kind words; they got respect. One could only guess how profoundly this experience affected them. When something good happened, the credit legitimately belonged to them; and if something did not work, there were no individual failures because all decisions were collective. The national award was the jewel on our crown. That confirmed that our project and the EMPOWER model worked.

Clearly, all events like these have multiple causes of success and failure. In this case it clearly succeeded because there was a confluence of several positive forces: a just cause of protecting children, empowering poor Latina women as *promotoras*, group-work for a project that all members wanted to succeed; bottom-up participatory planning; public health professional competencies of the key members of the team; the EMPOWER framework that was based on lessons learned from 80 self-organized empowerment movements; and above all, mutual trust and respect among the key members of the project team.

Postscript

As a postscript, six points are highlighted to emphasize their significance for empowerment theories and interventions. Some of these were mentioned earlier in various contexts; but it would be unfortunate if they were lost in the substantive texts of the earlier chapters of this book.

FIRST: EMPOWERMENT LEVELS

Some widely cited empowerment theories/models include only three levels of empowerment (i.e. individual, community, and organization); these need to be expanded to include two essential but missing *levels* of empowerment from an ecological perspective. These missing levels are *family* and *cultural and social conditions*. Family has an indisputable influence on our socialization process and behavior, from conception through death. Research on social determinants of health also confirms the importance of these missing levels (e.g., WHO, 2008: WHO Commission on Social Determinants of Health). The ecological model proposed by the IOM and the CDC also identifies five levels, including family and society (macro level determinants of health). Finally the UN HDA justly emphasizes the importance of including culture, gender, and societal norms in studying and enhancing HQOL. A meaningful and ecological empowerment theory/model would be incomplete without these two missing levels.

In addition, a sound empowerment theory/model should also emphasize *gender* and *culture* (cultural values distinct from social class) as major *determinants* of behavior and health status by gender and ethnicity. Gender equality is recognized by scholars and health-related global organizations (e.g.,

UN, UNDP, WHO) as one of the most important determinants and goals of human development; gender equality/development is considered so important that these and other global health agencies have included this as one of the eight MDGs (MDG #3). Many of the health disparities between and within nations are deeply rooted in our cultures (e.g., inequality, violence against women, and gender role segregation); they have direct effects on HRQOL.

Consequently, gender and cultural differences should be included as important causal (independent determinants) variables. In a world where cultural diversities, gender inequalities, and the powerlessness of poor families cause the major share of our problems, family and culture as causal forces cannot be relegated to the status of "background" or exogenous factors. Theories should "explain" and "predict" causal and interaction effects of these causal variables. The scholars who, in the pursuit of an abstract and universal theory of empowerment, ignore family and culture/society as determinants or levels of empowerment, will only produce inadequate theories at best, and irrelevant ones at worst.

SECOND: ECOLOGICAL OR MULTILEVEL INTERVENTION (MLI) APPROACH

Over the past few decades, a consensus has emerged among health related researchers that health behavior and outcomes are determined by causal factors at multiple levels; consequently, several major health research institutions (e.g., IOM, National Institutes of Health [NIH], CDC, National Cancer Institute [NCI]) have insisted that we need to adopt an "ecological" or multilevel intervention (MLI) model in our health promotion research and interventions. These bodies have proposed ecological models with five to six levels. But in practice, most social research and interventions still address the "individual" level. In a meta-analysis of 157 peer-reviewed publications related to health behavior over a period of 20 years, it was discovered that 95% of these studies dealt with individual-level activities; 67% with interpersonal behaviors; 20% with the community level; and only 6% with health policy (Golden & Earp, 2012). Similarly, in 2012, the NCI sponsored a meeting to review and promote MLI research related to tobacco use and cancer prevention. A review of the papers and proceedings of that MLI meeting concluded that MLI studies were highly under represented, and one of the problems is that the field lacks a single unifying theory to guide MLI research (Clauser et al., 2012). More recently, the Office of Behavioral and Social Science Research (OBSSR) of the NIH sponsored several initiatives to promote "Systems Science Research" (SSR) and published a special issue of the *Health Education and Behavior* (March 2013) dealing with this model. The advantage of the SSR model is that "it can examine non-linear relationships, bidirectional feedback loops, and how time-delayed effects work within a complex system that a standard linear model using a cross-sectional survey is unable to do. Adding up individual survey responses does not give us an ecological understanding of how a dynamic and MLI system works. However, while the SSR is widely used in systems and engineering sciences, this method is not a component of standard social science research curricula in the health sciences. The OBSSR plans to offer training and technical support to promote SSR; but it would be important for the academic social sciences and research institutions to promote SSR and use this model more often.

THIRD: EMPOWERMENT EVALUATION

Standard research and evaluation textbooks and courses offer basic competencies in evaluation, and the CDC and NIH have websites that present the basic concepts, evaluation types, and designs that address empowerment evaluation needs and challenges. In addition, there are specialized programs on leadership development programs and evaluation and books on empowerment evaluation (e.g., David M. Fetterman and Abraham Wandersman, Editors). If the program has a tangible health goal (e.g., childhood immunization coverage), and empowerment (e.g., empowered *promotoras*) is used as a means toward that goal, then the evaluation design would have to include both process and impact evaluations in two dimensions or tracks: health outcomes (increase in immunization level) and empowerment goal. The empowerment outcomes would be further measured at two levels: (1) empowerment of the individuals involved, and (2) the empowerment of the program/organization as a whole.

Finally, empowerment is a dynamic and multidimensional process, and its outcome or impact can be moving targets. A standard evaluation design that is designed to measure objective and measurable goals (e.g., competent job performance) that were set at the onset of an intervention is not adequate to measure the full impacts of empowerment over time. For instance, in our Rescatando Salud project, after several months, some of our *promotoras* began to leave for full-time jobs with better prospects. One may consider a resignation as a negative outcome, but from the *promotoras'* empowerment perspective they were leaving for a better job because they were more qualified than before. So this is an empowerment success story. In our original evaluation design, we did not identify an early resignation by a *promotora* as an indicator of empowerment or "success" (we began to track every *promotora* when she left, to determine her career advancement).

In addition, empowerment evaluation must include organizational capacities beyond individual empowerment outcomes (as a unit); for instance the organizational capacities and work environment for planning and implementing culturally appropriate and participatory prevention interventions in multicultural communities. Simply hiring bilingual outreach workers is a far cry from having organizations with multicultural capabilities. Standard research and evaluation methods book, do address this problem.

We also discovered that one intrinsic incentive for the *promotoras* was that their prestige and reputation were enhanced among their peers in the community. Once again, in our original evaluation plan, we did not select their reputation in the community as an indicator of their empowerment. Empowerment evaluation design would have to be flexible enough to accommodate emerging needs and goals like this. As an empowerment program matures and succeeds, the program becomes more empowered. The indicators or external measures of successful empowerment, in our case, were: (a) the national award we received (which we never set as a goal), and (b) replication/adoption of a successful model by others in geographical areas beyond the original program. Emerging goals of the *promotoras* and external recognition or validations (awards and replication) are the two empowerment impacts we had not included in our original program evaluation design.

Finally, empowerment includes both subjective (e.g., self-efficacy, self-esteem) and objective (e.g., objective indicators) dimensions; therefore, empowerment evaluation would have to include valid and sensitive individual and program level indicators. There are several frameworks and methods for developing appropriate evaluation designs and indicators (Abelin et al., 1987; Fetterman et al., 2004; Kar, 1989). Interim gains in empowerments are legitimate "process" indicators, and a sound evaluation plan should have a feedback loop to detect such process indicators.

FOURTH: LESSONS FROM EXEMPLARY MOVEMENTS

Lessons from exemplary empowerment movements dealing with various problems and sociocultural settings are a major source of inspiration as well as teaching us what works and when. Meta-analyses are a better source for this type of learning because they tend to reveal clusters of factors and effective methods across sociocultural divides that individual case studies, however successful, do not reveal.

In our case, the EMPOWER framework, based on our meta-analysis, provided us with findings on determinants and methods that were effective in empowerment movements in diverse problems and situations. As we were planning to launch our Rescatando Salud project, we had already gained considerable empirical knowledge about empowerment processes and methods that had worked in diverse situations across the world.

To the best of our knowledge, this is the first meta-analysis of case studies on women's self-organized empowerment movements across the world, and naturally, we were wondering whether other studies would support or challenge our findings. We are grateful for the positive feedback from credible sources involved in global health and empowerment. Two examples are cited here to illustrate this process of external corroboration. The WHO's South-East Asia Regional Office (SEARO) produced a monograph on the internationally famous SEWA empowerment project in India, in which they cited our EMPOWER paper and confirmed that our results are consistent with SEWA's experiences. This WHO/SEARO monograph states:

> A case is now being made for using empowerment, together with economic development and health sector reforms, as a strategy for reducing persistent disparities in health and quality of life across gender and ethnic groups (Kar et al). It is believed that in the process of empowering itself, a group or community would tackle the underlying social, structural and economic conditions that impact on its health. As a result, it would gain more control over the social determinants of health. (Aggrawal, 2005)

The second example is the "Safer Motherhood" project that was involved in maternal and child health initiatives globally for more than two decades. Author Moore in 2000, in an extensive review of innovative models for community empowerment and saving mothers, summed up our EMPOWER model first presented in 1999, in these words:

> A powerful meta-analysis of forty successful case studies of community development and empowerment model utilizes some interesting acronyms as part of its evaluation framework The paper identifies common characteristics of effective women-led empowerment movements, despite cultural geographic political and socioeconomic differences, and integrates key findings into an empowerment model for social action and health promotion movements centered around "WAM"—Women And Mothers. Some basic theoretical constructs of empowerment are discussed and a six-dimensional evaluation framework is utilized. The analysis identified seven empowerment methods most frequently used, with significant differences in frequency of use among successful programs. In descending order the interventions are enabling services, rights protection/promotion, public education, media use/advocacy, organizing associations/unions, empowerment education and work training, and microenterprise.

Moore (2000) further reviews the key components of our EMPOWER model:

> The EMPOWER model consists of five stages: 1) motivation for action; 2) empowerment support; 3) initial individual action; 4) empowerment program; and 5) institutionalization and replication. Although the article itself makes no mention of the stages of change behavioral model, obvious parallels and overlaps can be identified. The EMPOWER analysis categorizes the dimensions of support—CORE support and media support. CORE is another acronym for Community support, Organizational

support from community based organizations, Resource support, and Empowerment support. The category of enabling services and assistance, though not described as such, falls within the parameters of social support defined previously for safe motherhood community interventions. The author also discusses the use of media in empowerment, dividing media use into two complementary objectives: 1) media support or 2) media advocacy. A clear distinction is made between the role of media support for advocacy and program objectives and public education and participation, which is more face-to-face, at both interpersonal and community network levels.

Empowerment of women for human development and health is an emerging field; many established authors have yet to get seriously involved in this area. Theories and models of empowerment for health promotion are also in their formative stages; we need more evidence to develop a better grasp of how empowerment processes work across genders, social class, and cultures. Cumulative empirical knowledge from multicultural empowerment movements, systematic analyses and applications of the lessons learned, and Participatory Action Research (PAR) (which Kurt Lewin and his colleagues promoted) are essential steps in these processes. Meta-analysis would serve as an indispensable empirical foundation for progress in this endeavor.

FIFTH: SOCIAL SETTINGS

Independent of our perceived reality, the social setting determines our behavior to the extent that a sound prevention strategy in one social setting may not be effective in another. A personal experience of this author illustrates this point.

I was invited to serve as a consultant to São Paulo (Brazil) to help develop indicators of health promotion program evaluation. Our immediate objective was to prioritize top health risks and identify behavioral indicators to prevent these risks. São Paulo is a major industrial city with a population of more than 14 million; local epidemiologists reported that injury to industrial workers was a major health risk and financial loss to industries. Injuries caused by automobile accidents emerged as one of the top health risks. My first question to the local public health epidemiologists was: "What proportion of automobile drivers in São Paulo use seat belts?" Loud laughter was their response. Naturally, I asked why they laughed. There was strong evidence from other industrialized nations that seat-belt use reduced the severity of automobile accidents; so why would that be a laughable question? Their response was: "Dear Professor— seat-belt use may be a good preventive measure against automobile accidents in the USA, but in Brazil the drivers are well protected inside their cars. It is the pedestrians who are getting hit by the cars." In this situation, obviously, seat belts were not the best preventive measure. São Paulo needed alternative measures such as busing the workers to and from the factories, building more underground pedestrian walkways and overpasses in busy intersections, and instituting harsher punishment for reckless driving, etc. This incident shows that an indicator that is valid in one context may not be so in another.

Behavioral expression of one empowerment measure may not be socially acceptable in another. There are anecdotal reports that, in many societies and situations, if a woman acts like an "independent" person, she invites hostility from some men, and even women may consider her a tactless or unwise person. In other words, the "social costs" for behaving like a successful and autonomous woman may be too high; so she acts submissively ("learned helplessness": Martin Seligman). Empowerment research and intervention cannot be oblivious to social contexts in which people live and act. According to a recent news report, girls' enrollment in secondary grades sharply dropped in Afghanistan because most secondary schools there do not have running water and toilets for girls (this is true for many poor countries). Until this reality is changed for the better, we are not going to meet the MDG of gender equality in education, and subsequently, gender equality in employment and income. Empowerment, especially of women and girls, depends significantly on the social realities of poor and traditional societies; consequently, any empowerment theory or model that ignores these realities would be ineffective in designing proper interventions and evaluations.

SIXTH: CULTURE AND EMPOWERMENT

Finally, empowerment is a multidimensional and multilevel process that is affected by dominant cultural values and the social context in which one lives and acts. Relationships among cultural values, modernization, and human development are well established by sociologists, and more recently by several iterations of the World Values Survey (WVS; Inglehart & Norris, 2003). These studies show that two factors determine modernization and gender equality attitudes: (1) Survival versus Self-Expression values, and (2) Traditional versus Secular/Rational values. The WVSs show that the intersections of these two factors have strong relationship with levels of modernization and gender equality values across the world. Higher Self-Expression values and Secular-Rational values correlate strongly with higher levels of modernization and gender equality attitudes. This means that a society that is more modernized would provide better opportunities for women's empowerment. In conservative societies, where women do not have the opportunities necessary for higher education and professional careers outside homes, they endure greater gender inequality. A program that makes a small gain in women's empowerment in a traditional society would deserve more credit than a similar small gain in a modernized society. Empowerment goals and evaluations would have to consider the level of cultural support for women's education and empowerment and give weight to the program outcome accordingly.

There is also a rich literature on how situations, including the subjective perception of social situations, affect human behavior. In a spectacular psychological experiment known as the Stanford Prison Experiment, Philip Zimbardo demonstrated the powerful effects of role expectations and social setting on people's behavior toward one another. His research question was: "What happens when you put good people in an evil place? Does humanity win over evil, or does evil triumph?" (Zimbardo, 2007).

Zimbardo randomly divided his students in two groups: "prisoners" and prison "guards." They were then asked to behave (role-play) as if they were prisoners or guards in real life. It soon became clear that the students assigned to play "guards" became aggressive and abusive toward the "prisoners"; and those who played the role of "prisoners" became more tolerant of the abusive behaviors of the "guards." The interactions between these two groups soon became so hostile that the experiment had to be abandoned after a couple of weeks. Zimbardo concluded that the students' **beliefs** about how prisoners and guards actually behave in a prison, their **perception** of how they are expected to behave (subjective role) in the actual situation (prison), and the **value** they attached to the experiment affected their behavior towards one another.

Zimbardo was recently invited to study and advise how to deal with offensive treatment of Iraqi prisoners in the infamous Abu Ghraib prison. In his book titled *The Lucifer Effect* he explained how a good angel, Lucifer, would behave offensively and violently if he were banished to a bad situation—in hell.

Major threats to women's empowerment are culturally rooted practices that cause/tolerate violence against and sexual abuse of women and girls. Women's rights activists claim that cultural undervaluation of women, lack of appropriate education, absence of effective alternatives to escape from abuse, poor prevention measures, and ineffective deterrence and punishment of the perpetrators create a "rape culture." It is defined as:

> an environment in which rape is prevalent and in which sexual violence against women is normalized and excused in the media and popular culture. Rape culture is perpetuated through the use of misogynistic language, the objectification of women's bodies, and the glamorization of sexual violence, thereby creating a society that disregards women's rights and safety. (UN/WHO, 2013)

One of the largest studies so far on sexual violence against women is sponsored by the UN/WHO in South Asia and the Pacific. In Chapter 1, we briefly referred to this major six-nation survey of violence against women in South-East Asia. Several important findings are worth special attention (Jewkes et al., 2013). The study conducted in-depth interviews of 10,178 men in six nations to determine the prevalence of rapes and the reasons for these crimes. The prevalence ranged between 4% in urban Bangladesh and 41% in Papua New Guinea. The prevalence of intimate partner rape ranged between 13% in Bangladesh and 59% in Papua New Guinea. When asked about the reason for the most recent (non-partner) rape, 73% of the men said because they "felt entitled to have sex"; the next most frequent reason was "seeking entertainment" at 59%; "anger or punishment" at 38%; and "alcohol or substance use" was 27%.

Another major study, the WHO Study on Women's Health and Domestic Violence against Women, analyzed data collected from more than 24,000 women in ten countries. Key objectives of this study were to: estimate the prevalence of "intimate partner violence" (IPV), also called "domestic violence"; explore health outcomes of IPV; identify factors associated with IPV; and document the strategies and services the victims used to cope with the violence (Garcia-Moreno et al., 2005a). This cross-cultural/national study demonstrated that: prevalence of IPV vary across nations, meanings of perceptions of IPV differ significantly, victims are often blamed for inviting IPV, and social and cultural systems treat the perpetrators very differently.

These findings are consistent with the UN study cited above. The major conclusions that arise from these findings are that violence against women is universal, the underlying reasons extend much beyond economic development, and culture and traditional practices significantly affect violence against women, blaming the victims, and letting the perpetrators go unpunished.

In two recent incidents of gang rape of two young women in India (in Delhi and Mumbai), one of the victims later died, and these crimes caused nationwide anger and demand for the punishment of the perpetrators, as well as mass anger regarding the lack of adequate protection of women in public spaces, and ineffective societal response against violence against women. Often the victims are blamed and the perpetrators are set free. In the United States there is a widespread demand and movement for protecting young college students (women) on campus. Because most of the crimes are not reported or are covered up, this is a cause of anger and concern. The situation of sexual abuse of women in the military is also a major issue for concern. According to several press accounts (no accurate estimates are available), tens of thousands of women in the military may be sexually abused annually. Prevalent sexual abuse, inadequate protection and prevention, and ineffective implementation of justice constitute what some activists term a "rape culture." The term "rape culture" may not sound pleasant, but that does not make the crimes less serious. Activist Ruchira Gupta, the founder and president of Apne Aap, an international movement against violence against women including human trafficking, insists that the problem is much deeper and more widespread and needs global action (see http://apneaap.org/).

These crimes against women are committed primarily because of devaluation of women and traditional cultural practices that allow or ignore these violations. Given these findings, it is imperative that these and other repulsive barriers to women's empowerment rooted in cultural values and practices be proactively reformed and removed. Critics might ask: What right does a reformer have to confront or change traditional cultural practice in another culture? The answer is: When a brutal traditional practice violates the basic human rights of powerless victims against their wishes, and such violation contradicts multiple global consensuses on *universal human declarations* that their own nations have ratified, then fighting against these cruel and criminal acts is not only justified, but it is our moral rightful obligation.

CASE STUDIES IN FOUR DOMAINS

The case studies in this volume are in four domains: Human Rights (HR; Nos. 1–13); Equal Rights (ER); Economic Development (ED; Nos. 28–42); and Health Promotion and Disease Prevention (HPDP). Each case has an identity number for tracking it for additional information.

Serial#	ID#	Case Study Title	Page#
1	3	*Agrupación de los Familiares de Detenidos-Desaparecidos* ("Association of the Relatives of the Detained and Disappeared"), Chile, 1974 (HR)	227–229
2	7	Prevention of Dowry-Death Movement, India (HR)	229–232
3	2	Black Sash, Cape Town, South Africa, 1955 (HR)	232–235
4	5	CoMadres of El Salvador (Committee of Mothers and Relatives of Political Prisoners, Disappeared, and Assassinated of El Salvador Monseñor Romero, 1977 (HR)	235–238
5	10	Equality Now, United States, 1992 (HR)	239–240
6	6	FORWARD International (Foundation for Women's Health Research and Development), London, England, 1980 (HR)	241–243
7	8	*Grupo de Apoyo Mutuo* ("Mutual Support Group") for the Reappearance of Our Sons, Fathers, Husbands, and Brothers (GAM), Guatemala, 1984 (HR)	243–246
8	4	Madres de Plaza de Mayo, Argentina, 1977 (HR)	246–250
9	9	Mothers of East Los Angeles (MELA), United States, 1985 (HR)	250–254
10	11	Okinawan Women Act Against Military Violence, Okinawa, 1995 (HR)	254–256
11	85	Apne Aap, p. 267: Sex-Workers' Human Rights and International Anti-Trafficking Movement, India (Ruchira Gupta and Gloria Steinem) 2015 (HR)	256–257
12	24	Asian Immigrant Women Advocates (AIWA), California, 1993 (EQRT)	259–264
13	20	ATABAL Collective and La Esperanza, Mexico City, 1986 (EQRT)	265–267
14	17	Baltimore Working Women (BWW), Maryland, 1978 (EQRT)	268–270

15	15	COYOTE, United States, 1973 (EQRT)	270–273
16	18	Export Processing Zone (EPZ), Sri Lanka, 1979 (EQRT)	273–275
17	19	GABRIELA, Philippines, 1984 (EQRT)	275–278
18	23	Innabuyog, Philippines, 1990 (EQRT)	278–280
19	25	National Asian Pacific American Women's Forum (NAPAWF), California, 1996 (EQRT)	281–284
20	13	NOW (National Organization for Women), United States, 1966 (EQRT)	284–287
21	22	Rural Workers' Organizations (RWOs), India, Philippines, Sri Lanka, 1987 (EQRT)	287–290
22	14	Union of Women Domestic Employees (UWDE), Recife, Brazil, 1970 (EQRT)	290–294
23	21	Women Living Under Muslim Laws (WLUML), Muslim Countries, 1986 (EQRT)	294–299
24	12	YWCA (Young Women's Christian Association), International, 1849 (EQRT)	299–303
25	28	Working Women's Forum (WWF), India, 1978 (ED)	304–307
26	30	Bankura Women's Samities (Societies), West Bengal, India, 1980 (ED)	308–312
27	29	Barrio Indio Guayas Guayaquil, Ecuador, 1979 (HPDP)	312–315
28	67	Chipko Movement, India, 1973 (ED)	315–319
29	69	"Chipko" Movement for Water, Doon Valley, India, 1986 (ED)	319–321
30	31	Community Kitchens in *Pueblos Jovenes*, Peru, 1980s (ED)	321–325
31	27	Grameen Bank, Bangladesh, 1976 (ED)	325–329
32	26	SEWA (Self-Employed Women's Association), Ahmedabad, India, 1972 (ED)	329–335
33	81	The Chatra Lokahita Project, West Bengal, India (ED)	335–336
34	86	Banchte Shekha ("Learning to Survive"), Jessore, Bangladesh	336–338
35	82	Karma Kutir (Handicraft Hut), Kolkata, India (ED)	338
36	41	Asian and Pacific Islanders for Reproductive Health (APIRH), California, 1989 (HPDP)	339–342
37	46	The Boston Women's Health Book Collective, United States, 1969 (HPDP)	342–344
38	40	Centro de Informacíon y Desarrollo de la Mujer (CIDEM) Kumar Warmi, El Alto, Bolivia, 1985 (HPDP)	345–347
39	68	Comite Por Rescate de Nuestra Salud (CPRNS), Mayagüez, Puerto Rico, 1983 (HPDP)	347–350
40	44	Girls' Power Initiative (GPI), Nigeria, 1993 (HPDP)	350–353
41	59	The International Network of Women Against Tobacco (INWAT), 1990 (HPDP)	353–355

42	34	International Planned Parenthood Federation (IPPF), 1952 (HPDP)	355–358
43	42	La Casa de la Mujer, Santa Cruz, Bolivia, 1990 (HPDP)	358–361
44	35	La Leche League International, 1956, United States (HPDP)	361–363
46	57	MADD (Mothers Against Drunk Driving), United States, 1980 (HPDP)	363–366
47	36	Family Planning Mothers' Clubs, South Korea, 1968 (HPDP)	367–369
48	74	Mothers' Voices United to End AIDS (Georgia)	369–372
49	78	National Alliance for the Mentally Ill (NAMI), United States, 1979 (HPDP)	372–375
50	64	Narika, Berkeley, California, 1992	375–377
51	48	National Black Women's Health Project, United States, 1981 (HPDP)	377–380
52	51	National Latina Health Organization (NLHO; Organizacion Nacional de la Salud de la Mujer Latina), Oakland, California, 1986 (HPDP)	380–383
53	52	Native American Women's Health Education Resource Center, Lake Andes, South Dakota, 1988 (HPDP)	384–388
54	45	De Madres a Madres, Houston, Texas, 1990s (HPDP)	388–390
55	53	National Asian Women's Health Organization (NAWHO), San Francisco, California, 1993 (HPDP)	390–393
56	77	National Eating Disorders Associations (NEDA), United States, 1977	394–396
57	47	Over Sixty Health Center (OSHC), California, 1976 (HPDP)	396–398
58	54	Pacific Institute for Women's Health (PIWH), Los Angeles, California (HPDP)	398–401
59	38	Women's Center of Jamaica Foundation (WCJF) Program for Adolescent Mothers, Jamaica, 1978 (HPDP)	401–403
60	58	Prototypes: A Center for Innovation in Health, Mental Health, and Social Services, California, 1986 (HPDP)	403–405
61	62	Rape Crisis, Cape Town, South Africa, 1975 (HPDP)	405–407
62	63	Sakhi, New York, 1989 (HPDP)	407–410
63	71	The SALTA Project, San Diego, California, 1995 (HPDP)	410–412
64	72	South Carolina AIDS Education Network (SCAEN), South Carolina, 1987 (HPDP)	412–414
65	55	Sisters Network, Inc., Houston, Texas, 1994 (HPDP)	414–417
66	49	Supportive Older Women's Network (SOWN), Philadelphia, Pennsylvania, 1982	417–418
67	79	Step Up on Second: A Center for Recovering Mentally Ill Adults, Santa Monica, California, 1984 (HPDP)	418–420

68	37	Traditional Childbearing Group, Boston, Massachusetts, 1978 (HPDP)	420–423
69	70	Tri-Valley Citizens Against a Radioactive Environment (CAREs), California, 1980s (HPDP)	423–424
70	66	Women Against Gun Violence (WAGV), California, 1994 (HPDP)	425–428
71	56	Women For Sobriety (WFS), United States, 1975 (HPDP)	428–431
72	39	Women's Health Care Foundation, Quezon City, Philippines, 1980	431–434
73	60	Women in New Recovery (WINR), United States, 1994 (HPDP)	434–436
74	75	Women Alive Coalition, Inc., Los Angeles, California, 1991 (HPDP)	436–439
75	76	Women at Risk, California, 1991 (HPDP)	439–440
76	65	Mothers Against Violence in America (MAVIA), United States, 1993	440–442
77	43	Women's Reproductive Health and Development Program (WRHDP), Yunnan, China, 1991 (HPDP)	442–444
78	61	Arrak Ban (Anti-Alcohol Campaign), India, 1996 (HPDP)	444–446
79	1	The Rescata ndo Salud: Promotora EMPOWER Model (See Discussion of this Case in the Text in pp. 150–151 in Chapter 5 and Chapter 11)	447
80	33	Mahila Milan, Bombay, India, 1988 (D)	447–449
81	50	DisAbled Women's Network (DAWN) Canada, 1985 (HPDP)	449–452
82	73	WORLD (Women Organized to Respond to Life-threatening Diseases): Oakland, California, USA, 1990 (HPDP)	452–454

EPILOGUE

Since the manuscript of this book was first submitted, several major events have reinforced its central theme: that self-organized women's empowerment movements are a *third path* for human progress (the first two are economic growth and human development initiatives by the United Nations). These major events include (a) the award of the 2014 Nobel Peace Prize to 16-year-old Malala Yousefzai of Pakistan for her bold advocacy for girls' education in spite of deadly Taliban threats to her life; (b) the award of the 2015 Nobel Prize for Economics to Angus Deaton for his pioneering research on household/family-level variations in consumption and governmental incompetency as powerful forces that affect the health, wealth, and well-being of nations; (c) the emergence of a terrorist state (ISIS/ISIL) that sponsors mass destructions that disempower millions globally. The purpose of this postscript is not to summarize these events nor to recapitulate the content of this volume, but rather to highlight the significant implications of these recent events and to present an integral and analytical framework of social determinants of empowerment that has emerged from our meta-analysis presented in this book (see Figure E1).

Figure E1 presents a framework for examining the social determinants of empowerment with several components and dimensions within each component. The major components of an empowerment system are sources of powerlessness, levels of empowerment, domains of empowerment, and the seven EMPOWER methods. This volume has shown that women's powerlessness is a function of the combined effects of five social determinants (5Ps): poverty, prejudice, patriarchy, political exclusion, and psycho-physical disabilities. This book has also shown that self-organized movements by ordinary women used seven EMPOWER methods that have significantly empowered them and accomplished extraordinary benefits to their families and communities. In addition, the figure identifies six "exogenous" forces; they are "macro level" forces that effect a local empowerment movement, but they are not affected by isolated local empowerment movements (our focus is on social determinants of empowerment; hence genetics and genomes are not included). Each component includes several dimensions or subsets of entities that combine to constitute it; for instance, the level of empowerment includes five levels (dimensions) of empowerment. The figure includes a "Spiritual" dimension as a part of the empowerment domain; this point is further elaborated below. The figure also identifies serendipities and disasters as exogenous **519**

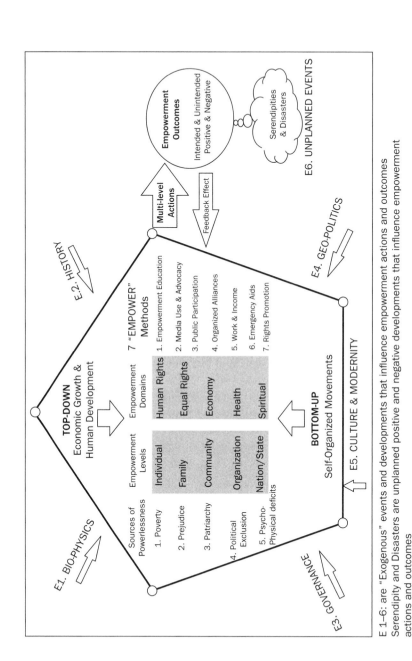

E 1–6: are "Exogenous" events and developments that influence empowerment actions and outcomes
Serendipity and Disasters are unplanned positive and negative developments that influence empowerment
actions and outcomes

FIGURE E1   A Framework of Social Determinants of Empowerment.

determinants (positive and negative) because these are not parts of planned movements, but they have significant effects on a movement. These two items present serious challenges to empowerment research and policy. This framework presents a holistic view of an empowerment process for research and policy analysis. It is integral because it integrates different sets of conceptual and empirical knowledge from previous chapters; it is analytical because it critically reviews the ideas and information presented in this book.

The Malala event has shown that a courageous voice for a just cause, even from a powerless teenage girl in a male-dominated traditional society, can create a major movement; she did not have a project grant, a business plan, nor a planned strategy for change. Ironically a destructive force (Taliban) that threatened her life emboldened her and outraged the world to take actions for her cause. Deaton's research shows that variations in consumption patterns within household/families can have serious effects on our well-being; therefore, neglecting family as a unit of analysis is a major flaw in a theory of social determinants empowerment. Deaton further presents evidence which shows that when a government is corrupt or incompetent, massive foreign aids, however well intentioned, do not solve any problem; aids may even be counterproductive. They can promote destructive corruption and sectarian violence. Deaton advocates effective interventions to enhance governmental capacities and to empower local organizations and community initiatives (Deaton, 2013). While he does not single out self-organized women's movements as the panacea, he certainly includes women's movements as a part of the overall capacity building at the community level. The rise of ISIS/ISIL poses an unprecedented and complex threat that requires global actions on two fronts simultaneously: addressing the distal causes of extremism over a very long period and offering effective relief services to disempowered victims who are mostly women and children. While local actions may not prevent extremist threats, our case studies repeatedly show that ordinary women are especially effective in helping powerless victims of violence who are most often women and children. Incidentally, critics often argue that localized empowerment movements, even when successful, serve a number of people too small to make any difference nationally. If this is true, then the answer is to multiply the number of empowerment movements to cover most of the needy population, not to reject an option that has been proven to be successful (e.g., SEWA, Grameen, and cases included in this volume). A major obligation of human service professionals is to learn from effective movements and develop professional competencies to better support these movements.

For a consequentialist, success is the primary justification for an action. For a reformist, the will to sustain right actions for a just cause, even in the absence of a decisive victory or quick success, is in itself, a valid outcome of empowerment. We find it in every case study; the will to right action for a just cause is a major driving force. The group of women who began the Las Madres de Plaza de Mayo (Case study No. 4) movement in the late 1970s in Argentina by now have grown very old and many among them have died, but the movement has attracted others to sustain their collective struggle as the "Grandmothers of the Disappeared" (Abuelas de Plaza de Mayo). We also discovered that violent action by antagonists can empower victims and embolden a movement; direct action by the victims may not be the only force for change. Several women in our case studies were murdered and/or raped. Their tragedy enraged others to act. Malala, the teenage girl in Pakistan, enraged the extremist Taliban; a savage Talib shot her almost to death. While this act of unforgivable violence shocked the world, it also emboldened her and she was awarded the Nobel Peace Prize in 2014. She fully deserved the Nobel, but one wonders where her movement would be today had she not been shot? On the positive side, several case studies have shown that serendipities (unexpected positive events) have a significant empowerment effect. For instance, the world press came to Buenos Aires to cover the 1978 World Cup soccer games and perchance observed a demonstration of the Madres de Plaza de Mayo movement (Case Study No. 4). The moral shock felt by the journalists drove them to broadcast the mothers' plight globally through printed and electronic media. Even before that, the media blitz emboldened the mothers, and global support for their cause swelled. We cannot evaluate the direct effect of this media blitz, but it drew global attention on the atrocities committed by the Junta and played a major role in the subsequent downfall of that brutal regime. These and other case studies show that sustained right action for a just cause is a dimension common to all successful empowerment movements, yet we know very little about how to define and measure it.

Spirituality and Empowerment

One of the key lessons we have learned from this project is that empowerment includes an important spiritual dimension that cannot be measured by standard experimental designs using randomized clinical trials. By definition, spirituality is something that is not made of material entities. Within the context of empowerment, spirituality is a core component that is shared by several spiritual traditions; this core component *is* a quest to answer several fundamental questions including What is the true reality? Who am I? What is the purpose of my life? How best may I achieve the purpose of my life? and What happens to the soul after I die? A spiritual quest seeks to answer these related questions. From this perspective, spiritual empowerment is a sustained quest for seeking the truth and liberation through right actions. That is why Gandhi named his nonviolent struggle for India's freedom as *Satyagraha* or "seeking for truth." One can be highly spiritual without believing in an anthropomorphic God; at least two major world religions do not require the existence of God. Buddhism is an agnostic religion, and the Jains are atheists. At a more pragmatic level, spiritual beliefs and practices have tangible health benefits especially in managing chronic illnesses, dying and deaths, and bereavements.

Readers interested in the spiritual dimension related to empowerment may read Huston Smith's (1991) excellent volume *The World's Religions: Our Great Wisdom Traditions* and Philip Goldberg's (2010) book *American Veda* that describes the upsurge of interest in Vedic/Vedantic wisdom in America. Goldberg presents a fascinating history of spiritual empowerment in America that is based on the wisdoms of Hinduism/Vedanta philosophy and Buddhism. It describes the roles played by major luminaries including Swami Vivekananda, Sri Aurobindo, Aldous Huxley, H. G. Wells, Alan Watts, Allen Ginsberg, Joseph Campbell, Huston Smith, Sri Ramakrishna, Abraham Maslow, Michael Murphy, Paramahansa Yogananda, Ralph Emerson, Ram Das, Christopher Isherwood, Juddu Krishnamurthi, Maharshi Mahesh Yogi, Timothy Leary, Amma (the Mother), founders of the Esalen Personal Growth movement (including Richard Price, Steve Jobs, Steve Wozniak, Michael Murphy, Andrew Weil), the founder of Self-Realization Centers, and numerous spiritual and yoga centers. The excerpts below from three spiritual leaders give us an idea of what spirituality means for empowerment.

Smith (1991) justly includes the phrase "Our Great Wisdom Traditions" in the title of his book because it reviews the spiritual edicts that transcend specific religions. A distinction between spirituality and organized religion is very important for our understanding of empowerment because persons and groups can be highly spiritual without being religious. In the name of religion, countless wars, persecutions, and genocides have been committed by dogmatic believers who pervert or misinterpret their religious scriptures. The spiritualists, on the other hand, believe in unity diversity in, tolerance, and universal peace; they are dedicated to right action for just cause. The excerpts below from three great spiritual leaders give us an idea of what spirituality means to them. Swami Vivekananda, in his famous speech that introduced the Vedanta philosophy at the Parliament of World Religions meetings in Chicago in 1893, quoted from the Gita to emphasize the concept of unity in diversity of religions. In his quote, the Supreme God Krishna tells his disciple Arjuna, the mighty warrior/prince:

> Whosoever comes to Me, through whatsoever form, I reach him; all men are struggling through paths which in the end lead to Me. (Vivekananda, 1893/2013, p. 64)

Another important ascetic, Sri Ramakrishna, the spiritual Guru of Swami Vivekananda, asserted that one divine includes all diverse religions in this metaphor. He once said to his followers:

> Imagine that there are several Ghats (docks) around a lake. The Hindus who drink water from a Ghat call it "jal"; the Muslims at another Ghat call it "pani"; and the Christians at a third Ghat call it "water." They all drink the same water but call it by different names. (Ramakrishna, cited in Goldberg, 2010, p. 69).

A third spiritual master, Sri Aurobindo, the spiritual innovator of *Integral Yoga*, who inspired millions including Aldous Huxley, Abraham Maslow, Michael Murphy (the founder of Esalen Institute), and others, stressed that the goal of human existence is a higher level of evolution of human consciousness. The goal of his Integral Yoga is to achieve the highest level of consciousness possible for humans. The excerpt below sums up his basic philosophy. Sri Aurobindo, who led the personal human growth movement, began his youth as an armed revolutionary and ended his life as a great sage. He held that the human race is by no means at the final stage of evolution; humans are at an intermediate stage halfway between animals and the divine consciousness. The first stage of evolution developed life from matters in lower forms (without mind/cognition); the second stage gave rise to humans with a mind and cognition; and the final stage would be the evolution of a "supermind" in humans dominated by divine consciousness. Integral Yoga integrates the strengths of various forms of yoga and Western science and is dedicated to developing the "super-mind"; unlike the more popular *Hata-Yoga* that depends heavily on various yoga postures, Integral Yoga is solely a method for spiritual growth. Aurobindo held that through Integral Yoga, individuals can not only advance their own evolution, but also that of the universe (Aurobindo, 1934/ 2016).

To Sri Aurobindo, spirituality is a quest for reaching the maximum human potential. A spiritual person does not divide and rank groups of people (prejudice) or treat them differently (discrimination) in a way that disempowers people. A spiritual quest is not driven by greed or a desire to win battles, gain more wealth or assets, power, or pleasure. Smith (1991) summarized three sets of universal ethical edicts that guide spiritual quests. These are actions to (a) *avoid vices*: murder, stealing, lying, and adultery; (b) *promote virtues*: humility, charity, and veracity (capacity to see things as they are); and (c) *seek a vision* of the ultimate character of things or comprehend the full picture of the true reality (Smith, 1991, pp. 386–389). In sum, spirituality requires actions that are very different from those who are materialistic. Spiritualism requires firm beliefs and sustained actions that promote unity in diversity, secularism, equality, nonviolence, and personal growth. It promotes societies where people are dedicated to peace and harmony that empower all. For these reasons, spirituality is a strong antidote of prejudice, injustice, greed, and actions by those in power that disempowers others.

Recently, several highly credible health-related research institutions (e.g., US National Institutes of Health) have acknowledged the importance of spiritual dimensions of health; this spiritual dimension has not yet been explored adequately. A Google search on February 4, 2016, using "spiritual research teaching centers" as keywords, listed more than 2.1 million items. This book concludes with a plea to better integrate spirituality as a unique component of global health and empowerment research and action. We may call this spiritual component "the will to sustain right actions for just cause" or Will for Action (WFA). The WFA belongs to a higher level of consciousness that is not preoccupied with what psychologist McClelland identified as human motivations: that is, need for achievement, need for affiliation, or need for power (McClleland, 1953). This WFA is much more than a desire to promote four freedoms (defined by former U.S. President Franklin Roosevelt as freedom of speech, freedom of worship, freedom from want, and freedom from fear); it is also more than actions for achieving the eight UN millennial development goals (MDGs); these are goals for our society as a whole. These initiatives do not address the issue of the spiritual dimension of empowerment. The WFA is also beyond what social psychologists call a "Behavioral Intention"; that is, the intention to perform a specific action (Fishbein & Ajzen, 1975). The WFA is more akin to what Maslow (1962) called a striving for self-actualization and closer to what Tagore defined as *Atma-Shakti* (or Self-Power). Joan of Arc, Gandhi, Martin Luther King Jr., Nelson Mandela, and Aung San Suu Kyi, among many visionaries have shown this sustained WFA that transcends individual self-interest; it is a commitment to sustain right actions for a just cause regardless of personal pain and sufferings resulting from their actions. In case after case we discovered ordinary women doing extraordinary things for long periods of time, not for personal power, wealth, or glory, but to protect and promote the survival and quality of life of their loved ones at great personal suffering and even facing real threats to their own lives. Their courage and WFA have inspired many to follow their footsteps.

Conventional empowerment evaluation is often guided by a research paradigm which depends on applying established theories and models of social determinants, testing hypotheses based on empirical evidence, and using standardized research tools. Empowerment activists, on the other hand, are driven by a quest for justice, concerns for loved ones, and a willingness to pay a heavy personal price for a just cause; conviction in their cause and endurance of pain in the pursuit of that cause are their main tools. Rather than relying on replicating past success, the innovative movements often use audacious and untested methods. For instance, no social science theory or experiment ever predicted that the Gandhian nonviolent freedom movement would succeed in defeating the mighty imperialist military power, Great Britain, in India's freedom fight. In addition, the basic values of open societies would not permit double-blind social experiments. Unlike standard research projects, the movements in this book did not start with a measurable baseline, did not use a standard research design or a business plan. Their empowerment approach was not experimental but evolutionary; their methods and goals changed over time. There are important differences between these two approaches: social experiments and empowerments. This means that methods that are effective for the former are not adequate for the latter approach.

Finally, some empowerment efforts may not lead to predefined goals, but from an empowerment perspective, this may not be a measure of total failure. Success is often overrated as a teacher; one may also learn from failures and become more efficient. Nietzsche is credited for saying: "That which does not kill us, makes us stronger." In addition, some outcomes may be invisible but have a direct effect by inspiring others to act. We shall never know how many people were inspired by the Buddhist monks who self-immolated for religious freedom that they never lived to relish. The basic difference between these monks and the suicide bombers is that the monks kill themselves, not others, and for a basic religious right denied them. To them, the absence of a visible success is not a proof of failure. One who believes this truth is truly empowered. Efforts well executed may enhance self-efficacy, competency, or resilience, even when a material goal is not reached due to external conditions. A freedom fighter does not consider her/his personal sufferings or death to be futile. Tagore describes this concept saying an unfinished struggle is not really a futile effort in these words:

> *The prayers of my life that remain undone,*
> *I know that they are not in vain.*
> *The buds that dropped on the ground*
> *before they could bloom,*
> *the streams that dried on desert sands,*
> *on their way to a distant ocean,*
> *I know deep in my heart,*
> *that they were not in vain.*

(Kar, 2015, p. 19, Tagore's *The Unfinished Prayers*)

The ancient Indian wisdom captured in the *Bhagavad Gita* is relevant to our understanding of the importance of right action as a spiritual dimension of empowerment. In the Gita, Krishna (the Supreme God in human form) serves as the spiritual guide and the chariot-driver of the greatest warrior Arjuna. Arjuna, a consequentialist, loses his desire to fight his enemy when he finds out that the enemy includes his relatives, teachers, and childhood playmates. Still, Krishna urges Arjuna to fight. The Gita spells out in detail Krishna's reasoning as to why Arjuna should fight for the sake of moral obligations and preservation of justice. Unfortunately, the scope of this book and the space available would not permit us a deeper discussion of the Gita; however, Krishna's mantra and advice to Arjuna would be instructive. Krishna tells Arjuna:

> *You have the right to perform your duty*
> *But never expect the fruits of your action*

> *(Krishna uses the term* Karma *for moral duties and obligations).*
> *(*The Bhagavad Gita, *2009, Chapter 2: Verse 2.47, p. 49)*

Scholars will no doubt continue to debate and interpret this central thesis of the Gita on our moral obligations and imperatives for doing what is right even if it does not produce the expected result. A consequentialist may be quick to abandon a mission if it does not produce the desired results; however, gender equality and empowerment of the powerless are our moral imperatives. Also, there is a global consensus on these imperatives. We cannot expect to build a healthy and just society unless we act tirelessly on our moral obligations to promote equity and empowerment of the powerless. Nor can we show our due respect and admiration for the intrinsic value of that ideal or those who are committed to it. Hopefully this volume will help us to learn from those who have struggled for these goals and have made a difference.

REFERENCES

Abelin T, Brzezinski ZJ, & Carstairs VDL (1987). *Measurement in Health Promotion and Protection.* Copenhagen: WHO Regional Office for Europe.

Abraído-Lanza AF, Dohrenwend BP, Ng-Mak DS, & Turner JB (1999). The Latino mortality paradox: A test of the "salmon bias" and healthy migrant hypotheses. *American J Public Health,* 89(10), 1543–1548.

Abrams G (1986, October 2). Program gives a step up to the mentally ill. *Los Angeles Times,* V-3–4.

Acemoglu D & Robinson J (2012). *Why Nations Fail: The Origins of Power, Prosperity, and Poverty.* New York: Crown Business.

Acosta M (1993). The CoMadres of El Salvador: A case study. In: *Surviving Beyond Fear: Women, Children and Human Rights in Latin America.* Fredonia, NY: White Wine Press.

Africa Check (2014). *Institute for Security Studies and Africa Check (2014).* Available at https://africacheck.org/factsheets/factsheet-south-africas-official-crime-statistics-for-201314/. Accessed July 19, 2015.

Afshar H (1991). *Women, Development and Survival in the Third World.* New York: Longman.

Afshar H (1998). *Women and Empowerment: Illustrations from the Third World.* London: Macmillan.

Aggrawal S (2005). Tackling Social and Economic Determinants of Health through Women Empowerment: The SEWA Case Study, WHO/SEARO: 8. Available at http://www.who.int/social_determinants/resources/isa_sewa_ind.pdf. Accessed July 30, 2015.

Agosin M (2002). *Women, Gender, and Human Rights: A Global Perspective.* New Brunswick, NJ: Rutgers University Press:115–127.

Agosin M (Ed.) (1993). *Surviving Beyond Fear: Women, Children and Human Rights in Latin America.* Fredonia, NY: White Wine Press.

Aiya VN (1906). *Travancore State Manual.* Available at http://en.wikipedia.org/wiki/Gowri_Parvati_Bayi). Accessed July 30, 2015.

Alam F & Chakravarty R (Eds) (2011). *Essential Tagore.* Cambridge, MA: Harvard University Press.

Albrecht GL, Fitzpatrick R, & Scrimshaw SC (Eds) (1999). *The Handbook of Social Studies in Health and Medicine.* Thousand Oaks, CA: Sage.

Alinsky S (1962). *Citizen Participation and Community Organization in Planning and Urban Renewal.* Chicago, IL: Industrial Area Foundation.

Alinsky S (1971). *Rules for Radicals.* New York: Vintage.

Alleyne GAO (1986). Preface. *Health Promotion: An Anthology.* Washington, DC: PAHO/WHO, Scientific Publication No. 557:vi.

529

Allport G & Postman L (1947). *The Psychology of Rumor.* Oxford, England: Henry Holt.

Allport GW (1935). Attitudes. In: Murchison C (Ed.), *Handbook of Social Psychology.* Worcester, MA: Clark University Press:798–844.

Almadovar NJ (2013, July 18). Web site of the executive director. Available at https://jasmineanddora.wordpress.com/media/press-releases/joint-press-release-from-coyote-la-and-iswface/.

American Anthropological Association (AAA) (2015). Available at http://www.aaanet.org/about/WhatisAnthropology.cfm p.1. Accessed May 26, 2015.

American Peace Caravan (1996). *Okinawan Women Act Against Military Violence.* Available at http://www.walrus.com/~dawei/articles/apc-e.html. Accessed July 3, 2015.

Americas Watch (1985). *Guatemala: The Group for Mutual Support 1984–1985.* Washington, DC: Americas Watch:37–63.

Americas Watch (1988). *Closing the Space: Human Rights in Guatemala May 1987 - October 1988.* Washington, DC: The Americas Watch Committee:23–60.

Amnesty International (AI) (2013). *Violation Against Women Information.* Available at http://www.amnestyusa.org/our-work/issues/women-s-rights/violence-against-women/violence-against-women-information. Accessed December 26, 2015.

Anand A (Ed.) & Women's Feature Service (WFS) (1992). *The Power to Change: Women in Third World Redefine Their Environment.* London, UK: Zed Books.

Anand S & Ravallion M (1993). Human development in poor countries: On the role of private incomes and public services. *J Econ Perspect.,* 7(1), 133–150.

Anderfuhren M (1994). The union of women domestic employees, Recife, Brazil. In: Martens M & Mitter S (Eds), *Women in Trade Unions: Organizing the Unorganized.* Geneva: International Labour Office:17–32, 147–164.

Anderson NB (2015). Training Institute for Dissemination and Implementation Research in Health (TIDIRHI). Available at http://obssr.od.nih.gov/about_obssr/BSSR_CC/BSSR_definition/definition.aspx. Accessed May 26, 2015.

Andrews FM (1989). The evolution of a movement. *J Public Policy,* 9(4), 401–405.

Andrews FM & Robinson JP (1991). Measures of subjective well-being. In: Robinson JP, Shaver PR, Wrightsman LS (Eds), *Measures of Personality and Social Psychological Attitudes, Volume 1 of Measures of Social Psychological Attitudes.* New York: Academic Press:61–114.

Andrews P (1996). *Sisters Listening to Sisters: Women of the World Share Stories of Personal Empowerment.* Westport, CT: Bergin & Garvey.

Anti-Arrack Movement (AAM) (1991). Available at http://www.ukessays.com/essays/history/anti-arrack-movement-in-andhra-pradesh-history-essay.php#ixzz3Ryrlem9l. Accessed July 20, 2015.

Apne Aap (2015a) ("On Your Own"). Available from http://apneaap.org/blog-6/. Accessed June 12, 2014.

Apne Aap (2015b). *Red Light Dispatch Delhi, Kolkata, and Forbesganj (Bihar)* (vol. VIII, issue 9). Available at http://apneaap.org/wp-content/uploads/2012/11/RLD_September-2015.pdf.

Archive for Research on Women and Gender (ARWG) (2009). *Archive for Research on Women and Gender Feminist Studies.* San Antonio: University of Texas. Available at http://www.smith.edu/libraries/libs/ssc/links.html. Accessed January 4, 2016.

Arditti R & Lykes MB (1993). The disappeared children of Argentina: The work of the grandmothers of Plaza de Mayo. In: Agosin M (Ed.), *Surviving Beyond Fear: Women, Children and Human Rights in Latin America*. Fredonia, NY: White Wine Press.

Argyris C (1970). *Intervention Theory and Method: A Behavioral Science View*. Reading, MA: Addison-Wesley.

Arunachalam J (1978). Our Founder WWF. Available at http://www.workingwomensforum.org/wwf_ourfounder.htm. Accessed July 13, 2015.

Arunachalam J (2004). *Hundred Years of Co-operative Development in India (1904–2004)*. Women Workers: WWF Experiment in Indian Cities. Available at http://www.mixmarket.org/sites/default/files/medialibrary/20501.1846/ICNW_Case_Study_04.doc. Accessed August 1, 2014.

Ashworth G & Bonnerjea L (Eds) (1985). *The Invisible Decade: UK Women and the UN Decade for Women*. Hants, UK: Gower.

Ashworth G (1982). The United Nations "Women's Conference" and International Linkages in the Women's Movement. In: Willetts P (Ed.) *Pressure Groups in the Global System. The Transnational Relations of Issue-Orientated Non-Governmental Organisations*. London: Frances Pinter.

Ashworth G (Ed.) (1995). *A Diplomacy of the Oppressed: New Directions in International Feminism*. Atlantic Heights, NJ: Zed Books.

Asian and Pacific Islanders for Reproductive Health (APIRH) (2015). Available at http://strongfamiliesmovement.org/assets/docs/ACRJ-A-New-Vision.pdf. Accessed July 7, 2015.

Asian Immigrant Women Advocate (AIWA) (2015). *AIWA History*. Available at http://www.aiwa.org/history/. Accessed July 6, 2015.

Asians and Pacific Islanders for Reproductive Health (APIRH) (2010). Available at http://www.apair.at/conferences/past-conferences/asia-conference-2010/en/. Accessed July 16, 2015.

Asia-Pacific Report (APR) (2015). Available at http://thediplomat.com/2015/06/asia-pacific-population-growth-and-the-un-post-2015-development-agenda/. Accessed July 16, 2015.

Asiaweek (2000, November). Excerpt from Announcement of Magsaysay Award. Available http://edition.cnn.com/ASIANOW/asiaweek/99/0806/sr2.html. Accessed July 14, 2015.

Associated Press (2006, November 17). *Brazil City Ready to Introduce Women-Only Buses*. Available at http://www.nbcnews.com/id/15772398/#.VaCJV_IVhBc. Accessed July 10, 2015.

Association of Schools of Public Health in the European Region (ASPHER) (2011). *Annual Forum*. ASPHER, Copenhagen, Available at http://aspher.org/annual-forum.html. Accessed January 6, 2016.

Association for Voluntary Surgical Contraception (AVSC). Available at http://www.xyonline.net/category/authors/avsc-international-and-international-planned-parenthood-foundation/-western-hemisph. Accessed February 5, 2015.

Association of Schools and Programs in Public Health (ASPPH) (2014, July 25). *Friday Letters from ASPPH*.

Aurobindo, Sri (1934/2016). *The Life Divine:* Book 1, Chapter 1. *Writings by Sri Aurobindo.* Pondicherry, India: Sri Aurobindo Ashram, Auroville. Available at http://saccs.org. in/texts/sriaurobindo/-sa-humanaspiration.php. Accessed January 3, 2016.

Azad Foundation (2001). *Women Empowerment—A Reality or Myth?*Available at http:// www.icrw.org/what-we-do/economic-empowerment. Accessed January 10, 2016.

Azad N (1986). *CEDAW: Empowering Women Workers: The WWF Experiment in Indian Cities.* Madras, India: Working Women's Forum. Available at http://www.worldcat. org/title/empowering-women-workers-the-wwf-experiment-in-indian-cities/oclc/ 15906140. Accessed January 8, 2016.

Azad N (1988). *Creating Bases for Women's Solidarity: A Study of Grassroots of the Working Women's Forum.* Ann Arbor, MI: University of Michigan Press.

Azad N (2011). *A Model for Social Performance.* Available at http://microcreditwom-enindia.com/articles/nandini-azad-a-model-for-social-performance1. Accessed January 10, 2016.

Bair B & Cayleff SE (1993). Historical context. In: *Wings of Gauze: Women of Color and the Experience of Health and Illness.* Detroit, MI: Wayne State University Press:202–225.

Ball P, Konrak O, & Spirer AA (1999). *A State Violence in Guatemala, 1960–1996: A Quantitative Reflection.* New York: American Association for the Advancement of Science. Available at https://hrdag.org/wp-content/uploads/2013/ 01/state-violence-guate-1999.pdf.

Bandura A (1986). *Social Foundation of Thought and Action: A Social Cognitive Theory.* New Jersey: Prentice-Hall.

Banerjee NK (1984). *Women, Participation and Development: A Case Study from West Bengal.* Availableatfile:///C:/Users/Kar/Downloads/WomenParticipationandDevelopment%20 (2).pdf. Accessed July 13, 2015.

Bangassar CL (1994). The working women's forum: A case study of leadership develop-ment in India. In: Martens M & Mitter S (Eds), *Women in Trade Unions: Organizing the Unorganized.* Geneva; International Labour Office:131–214.

Barnaby F (Ed.) (1988). *The Gaia Peace Atlas.* London: Pan Books:98.

Barnett B, Eggleston E, Jackson J, & Hardee K (1999). Sexual attitudes and behavior among young adolescents in Jamaica. *Int Fam Plan Perspect.,* 25(2),78–84, 91.

Barraza-Roppe B, Moya M, & Takvorian D (1998, January/February). San Diego's answer to environmental racism: The SALTA Project. *Poverty and Race Research Action Council (PRRAC) Newsletter*, 7(1).

Basu A (1995). *The Challenge of Local Feminisms: Women's Movements in Global Perspective.* Boulder, CO: Westview Press.

Basu RL (2005). Why the Human Development Index does not measure up to ancient Indian standards. *Culture Mandela: Bull Centre East-West Cult Econ Stud.,* 2(1), 1–7.

Basu RL (2009a). *Rabindranath Tagore on Ecology and Sustainable Development.* Washington: WBRi.

Basu RL (2009b, December). The eco-ethical views of Tagore and Amartya Sen. Culture Mandala: Bull Centre East-West Cult Econ Stud., 8(2), 56–61. Available at http://www.international-relations.com/CM8-2/Eco-Ethical-Views.pdf. Accessed January 8, 2016.

Batis Center for Women/Aid Philippines (2011). Available at http://www.aidphilippines. com/2011/08/21/batis-center-for-women/. Accessed July 2, 2015.

Batis/Association of Women in Action for Rights and Empowerment (AWARE) (2015). Available at http://www.batiscenterforwomen.org/about.php. Accessed July 3, 2015.

BBC (2014). Available at www.bbc.co.uk/ethics/war/against/nonviolence.shtm. Accessed January 8, 2016.

Bearak B (1996, December 12). The battle against the bottle. *Los Angeles Times*.

Beck AT (1976). *Cognitive Therapy and Emotional Disorder*. Madison, CT: International University Press.

Beckels M (1988). Strange bedfellows: Women and gender stereotypes in Argentine politics. Master's thesis. Los Angeles: UCLA Latin American Studies Center.

Bedi K (2012). *A Police Chief with a Difference* (TED Talk). Available at https://www. ted.com/talks/kiran_bedi_a_police_chief_with_a_difference. Accessed January 4, 2016.

Bell D (1973). *The Coming of Post-Industrial Society: A Venture in Social Forecasting*. New York: Basic Books.

Berelson B (1966). KAP studies on fertility. In Berelson B, Anderson RK, Harkavy O, Maier J, Mauldin WP, & Segal SJ (Ed.), *Family Planning and Population Programs: A Review of World Developments*. Chicago: University of Chicago Press:655–668.

Berelson B (1969). Beyond family planning. *Studies Fam Plan*, 1(38), 1–16.

Berelson B (1974). World population: Status report 1974. *Reports on Population/Family Planning*. The Population Council:197.

Berelson B, Anderson RK, Harkavy O, Maier J, Mauldin WP, & Segal SJ (Eds) (1966). *Family Planning and Population Programs: A Review of World Developments*. Chicago: University of Chicago Press.

Bhagavad Gita, The (2009). A view by Swami Vivekananda (compiled by Swami Madhuranda). Kolkata, India: Advaita Ashrama:49.

Bhatt I (2007). *Organizing Working Poor Women: The SEWA Experience*. University of Chicago Law School. Available at https://soundcloud.com/uchicagolaw. Accessed December 24, 2015.

Bhatt I (2010, May 17). *A Discussion with Ela Bhatt*. Berkeley Center for Religion, Peace & World Affairs, Georgetown University. Available at http://berkleycenter.george-town.edu/interviews/a-discussion-with-ela-bhatt-founder-self-employed-women-s-association-sewa. Accessed December 30, 2015.

Bhattacharya P (2013, July 20). Everything You Wanted to Know about the Sen-Bhagwati Debate. *Live Mint*. Available at http://www.livemint.com/Politics/zvxkjvP9KNfar-GagLd5wmK/Everything-you-wanted-to-know-about-SenBhagwati-debate.html. Accessed August 4, 2015.

Bishop D (1991). The Black Sash: White women confront apartheid. In: Russell DEH (Ed.), *Lives of Courage: Women for a New South Africa*. New York: Basic Books:213–226.

Bisnath SE (2000). *Women's Empowerment Revisited*. Available at www.unifem.undp. org.

Black Sash (2015). Homepage, "Our History." Available at http://www.blacksash.org.za/ index.php/our-legacy/our-history. Accessed July 2, 2015.

Black Women's Health (BWH) (2012). Available at http://www.blackwomenshealth.com/. Accessed July 17, 2015.

Black Women's Health Initiative (BWHI) (n.d.). Available at http://www.bwhi.org/about-us/our-story/. Accessed July 18, 2015.

Blackburn E (2008). *Work Life Balance—Nobel Winner Elizabeth Blackburn's Work Life Balance Story.* Available at http://womensissues.about.com/od/intheworkplace/a/WorkLifeBalanceElizabethBlackburn.htm. Accessed December 30, 2015.

Blow the Whistle (2014). Available at https://africacheck.org/factsheets/factsheet-south-africas-official-crime-statistics-for-201314/. Accessed July 19, 2015.

Bogardus ES (1922). *A History of Social Thought.* Los Angeles: University of Southern California Press.

Bogardus ES (1933). A social distance scale. *Sociol Soc Res.,* 17, 265–271.

Bollyky TJ (2014, January 21). *L.A. Times,* A-11. Available at http://www.cfr.org/experts/global-health-economics-international-law-trade/thomas-bollyky/b11198).

Bongaarts J, Mauldin WP, & Phillips JF (1990, November–December). The demographic impact of family planning programs. *Stud Fam Plan.,* 21(6), 299–310.

Bornstein D (1996). *The Price of a Dream—The Story of the Grameen Bank and the Idea that Is Helping the Poor to Change Their Lives.* New York: Simon & Schuster.

Bornstein D (2013, April 17). *Beyond Profit: A Talk With Muhammad Yunus.* Available at http://opinionator.blogs.nytimes.com/2013/04/17/beyond-profit-a-talk-with-muhammad-yunus/. Accessed August 4, 2015.

Boserup E (1970/2007). *Women's Role in Economic Development.* London: Allen & Unwin.

Boserup E (1981). *Population and Technological Change: A Study of Long-Term Trends.* Chicago: University of Chicago Press.

Boston Women's Health Book Collective (BWHBC) (2000). Black Women's Health Book Collective, Available at http://guides.library.harvard.edu/schlesinger_bwhbc. Accessed December 10, 2014.

Boston Women's Health Book Collective (BWHBC) (2015). Available at http://www.our-bodiesourselves.org/history/. Accessed July 16, 2015.

Bourne PA, Eldemire-Shearer D, McGrowder D, & Crawford T (2009, October). Examining health status of women in rural, peri-urban and urban areas in Jamaica. *N Am J Med Sci.,* 1(5), 256–271.

Bouvard MG (1996). *Women Reshaping Human Rights: How Extraordinary Activists Are Changing the World.* Wilmington, DE: Scholarly Resources.

Boxer B (2011). Available at http://www.freerepublic.com/focus/news/2666841/posts?page=1. Accessed July 18, 2015.

Boxer B (2015, March 11). Available at https://www.boxer.senate.gov/press/release/boxer-colleagues-urge-hhs-secretary-sylvia-burwell-to-improve-access-to-emergency-contraception-at-indian-health-services-facilities/. Accessed December 27, 2015.

Bradburn NM (1969). *The Structure of Psychological Well-Being.* Chicago: Aldine.

Braveman P, Egerter S, & Williams DR (2011). The social determinants of health: Coming of age. *Annu Rev Public Health,* 132, 381–398.

Breslow B (2012, April 15). Lester Breslow, Who Linked Healthy Habits and Long Life, Dies at 97 (Obituary). *New York Times,* A-20.

Broad WJ (2012). *The Science of Yoga: The Risks and Rewards.* New York: Simon & Schuster.

Bronfenbrenner U (1977). Toward an experimental ecology of human development. *Am Psychologist,* 32(7), 513–524.

Brown TT (2014). How effective are public health departments at preventing mortality? Evidence from California County Departments of Public Health. *Econ Hum Biol.,* 13, 34–45.

Brownson RC, Fielding JE, & Maylahn CM (2009). Table constructed from data. In: Fielding J, et al. (Eds), *Mortality in LA County: 2009.* Available at http://publichealth.lacounty.gov/dca/dcareportspubs.htm.

Buchanan, R. (1975): Breast-feeding: Aid to infant health and fertility control. *Popul Rep.,* J(4), 503–510.

Buenafe M (1998). *Health Related Quality of Life (HRQOL).* WHOCenter.

Burgos-Debray E (1996). *I, Rigoberta Menchu: An Indian Woman in Guatemala.* New York: Verso.

Buvinic ML (1983). Women's issues in Third World poverty: A policy analysis. In: Buvinic ML & McReevey W (Eds), *Women and Poverty in the Third World.* Baltimore, MD: Johns Hopkins University Press.

BUZZ (2013, July 13). Bhagwati vs Sen Updated. *Outlook.* Available at http://www.outlookindia.com/blogs/post/bhagwati-vs-sen-updated/3009/31. Accessed August 4, 2015.

Cantril H (1965). *The Pattern of Human Concerns.* New Brunswick, NJ: Rutgers University Press.

Caplan NS, Choy MH, & Whitmore JK (1991). *Children of the Boat People: A Study of Educational Success.* Ann Arbor, MI: University of Michigan Press.

Carabillo T (1993). *Feminist Chronicles 1953–1993.* Los Angeles: Women's Graphics.

Carr W & Kemmis S (1986). *Becoming Critical: Education, Knowledge, and Action Research.* London: Falmer.

Castillo A (1988, May 15). Advocate for East L.A., in Obituary Section by Myrna Oliver. *Los Angeles Times* Staff Writer. Available at http://articles.latimes.com/1998/may/15/local/me-50072. Accessed December 28, 2015.

Center for Elementary Mathematics and Science Education (CEMSE). Available at cemse.uchicago.edu/staff. Accessed July 16, 2015.

Center for Health and Gender Equity (CHANGE): JHU (2000). *Violence Against Women Report.* Baltimore, MD: Johns Hopkins University.

Center for Inherited Disorders of Energy Metabolism (CIDEM) (2004). Available at http://www.case.edu/med/CIDEM/cidem.htm. Accessed July 16, 2015.

Center for Inherited Disorders of Energy Metabolism (CIDEM). Available at http://www.case.edu/med/CIDEM/cidem.htm. Accessed July 16, 2015.

Center for Integrated Services for Families and Neighborhoods (CISFAN) (2007, March). On Angela Gomes. Available at http://word.world-citizenship.org/wp-archive/1118. Accessed August 1, 2015.

Center for Integrated Services for Families and Neighborhoods (CISFAN) (1994). *Strategies for Distressed Neighborhoods.* Sacramento, CA: Center for Integrated Services for Families and Neighborhoods. Available at http://word.world-citizenship.org/wp-archive/1118.

Center for Women's Development Studies (CWDS) (2014). *Center for Women's Development Studies, Partnership with Peasant Women (and Men) in West Bengal—Bankura.* Available at http://www.cwds.ac.in/bankura.htm. Accessed July 13, 2015.

Center for Women's Development Studies (CWDS) (2014). *Partnership with Peasant Women (and Men) in West Bengal—Bankura*. Available at http://www.cwds.ac.in/bankura.htm. Accessed July 13, 2015.

Centers for Disease Control and Prevention (CDC) (1981). *BRFSS: The Behavioral Risk Factor Surveillance System*. Atlanta, GA: Centers for Disease Control and Prevention. Available at http://www.cdc.gov/brfss/about/.

Centers for Disease Control and Prevention (CDC) (2015). *CDC Study of Hispanic Health*. Available at http://www.hispanichealth.org/its-about-time.html. Accessed July 18, 2015.

Centers for Disease Control and Prevention (CDC) (2015). *Ross and the Discovery that Mosquitoes Transmit Malaria Parasites*. Available at http://www.cdc.gov/malaria/about/history/ross.html. Accessed July 13, 2015.

Chamorro-Premuzic (2014). *Does Having More Money Make People Happier?* Available at http://www.theguardian.com/profile/tomas-chamorro-premuzic. Accessed July 29, 2015.

Chan M (2008). Director General of WHO, Speech at an International Conference on Complementary and Alternative Medicine (CAM), China. Available at http://www.who.int/dg/speeches/2008/20081107/en/. Accessed July 28, 2015.

Charaka Samhita (200–300 BCE). Indian medical text, *Encyclopedia Britannica*, http://www.britannica.com/topic/Charaka-samhita; *Susruta Samhita*, http://medical-dictionary.thefreedictionary.com/Sushruta%2BSamhita. Accessed July 28, 2015.

Chasin BH & Franke RW (1991, October 24). The Kerala Difference. *New York Review of Books*. Available at http://www.nybooks.com/articles/archives/1991/oct/24/the-kerala-difference/. Accessed July 29, 2015.

Chatterjee M (1993). The Self Employed Women's Association (SEWA): A case study from India. In: Young G, Samarsinghe V, & Kusterer K (Eds), *Women at the Center: Development Issues and Practices in the 1990s*. Hartford, CT; Kumarian Press:81–93.

Chipko (2015a). Available at https://www.iisd.org/50comm/commdb/desc/d07.htm. Accessed July 13, 2015.

Chipko (2015b). *The Legend*. Available at https://en.wikipedia.org/wiki/Chipko_movement.

Chipko (2015c). *Today's Heroes: The Chipko Movement: India's Call to Save Their Forests*. Available at http://www.womeninworldhistory.com/contemporary-04.html. Accessed July 14, 2015.

Chipko Movement, The: 1996–2013 (2015). Available at http://www.womeninworldhistory.com/contemporary-04.html. Accessed January 9, 2016.

Christian Science Monitor (2008, July 29). Peru's women unite in kitchen—and beyond. Available at http://www.csmonitor.com/World/Americas/2008/0729/p01s01-woam.html. Accessed July 15, 2015.

Christian Science Monitor (2015). Available at http://www.csmonitor.com/World/Making-a-difference/Change-Agent/2015/0409/How-SEWA-brings-access-to-energy-across-India. Accessed July 14, 2015.

Chuchryk PM (1993). Feminist anti-authoritarian politics: The role of women's organizations in the Chilean transition to democracy. In: Jaquette J (Ed.), *The Women's Movement in Latin America: Feminism and the Transition to Democracy*. Boston, MA: Unwin Hyman:149–184.

Citizens Against a Radioactive Environment (CARE) (2015). Available at http://www. trivalleycares.org/new/aboutus.html. Accessed July 20, 2015.

Clark H (2010). *UNDP: Human Development Report*, Foreword, p. iv. Available at http:// hdr.undp.org/sites/default/files/reports/270/hdr_2010_en_complete_reprint.pdf. Accessed July 30, 2015.

Clark H (2013). *UNDP Human Development Report*. Available at http://hdr.undp.org/en/ humandev.

Clark KB & Clark MK (1940). Skin color as a factor in racial identification of Negro preschool children. *J Soc Psychol.*, S.P.S.S.I. Bulletin, 11, 159–169.

Clark KB & Clark MP (1947). Racial identification and preference among negro children. In: E. L. Hartley (Ed.) *Readings in Social Psychology*. New York: Holt, Rinehart and Winston.

Clark KB (1955). *Prejudice and Your Child*. Boston: Beacon Press.

Clark KB (1989). *Dark Ghetto: Dilemmas of Social Power*, Wesleyan Edition. Middletown, CT: Wesleyan University Press.

Clauser SB, Tapin CH, Foster MK, Fagan P, & Kaluzny AD (2012, May). Multilevel intervention research: Lessons learned and pathways forward. *J Natl Cancer Inst.* (44), 127–133.

CNN Report (2014). Available at http://edition.cnn.com/2013/09/09/business/earth-institute-world-happiness-rankings/index.html.

Cochran WG (1950). The comparison of percentages in matched samples. *Biometrika*, 37, 256–266.

Coleman J (1956, December). Social capital in the creation of human capital. *Am J Sociol.* (Suppl) 94, S95–S120.

Coleman J, Katz E, & Menzel H (1957). The diffusion of an innovation among physicians. *Sociometry*, 20(4), 253–270.

Collier P (2007). *The Bottom Billion: Why the Poorest Countries Are Failing and What Can Be Done About It*. London: Oxford University Press.

CoMadres (2015). Available at https://en.wikipedia.org/wiki/COMADRES. Accessed July 2, 2015.

Convention on the Elimination of Discrimination Against Women (CEDAW) (1979). *International Convention on the Elimination of Discrimination Against Women, Women Workers: The WWF Experiment in Indian Cities*. Mylapur, India: WWF. Available at www.un.org/womenwatch/daw/cedaw. Accessed January 8, 2016.

Convention on the Elimination of Discrimination Against Women (CEDAW) (2008). Short History of the CEDAW Convention, UN Department of Public Information, Commission on the Status of Women, Geneva, Switzerland, WHO.

Cordillera Women's Education Action Research (CWEARC) (2014). Part 1. Available at http://www.cwearc.org/main/kali/101-cordillera-indigenous-women-pursuing-indigenous-knowledge-for-food-sovereignty. Accessed July 8, 2015.

Cordillera Women's Education Action Research (CWEARC) (2015). Part 2. Available at http://www.cwearc.org/main/kali/103-cordillera-women-pursuing-indigenous-knowledge-for-food-sovereignty-part-2. Accessed July 8, 2015.

Corey S (1949a). Action Research, Fundamental Research, and Educational Processes. *Teachers College Rec.*, 50, 509–514.

Corey S (1949b, December). Curriculum development through action research. *Educ Leadership*, 7, 147–153.

Cornell ILR Program and UC Berkeley Labor Center (2010). *New Approaches to Organizing Women and Young Workers, Social Media and Work Family Issues.* Available at http://www.bergermarks.org/resources/NewApproachestoOrganizingWomenandYoung Workers.pdf

Corporate Watch website. Available at http://www.corpwatch.org/article.php?list=class t&class=11&all=1. Accessed July 11, 2015.

Corsa L & Oakley D (1979). *Population Planning.* Ann Arbor, MI: University of Michigan Press.

Council for Accreditation in Public Health (CEPH) (2015). Council on Education for Public Health. Available at http://ceph.org/. Accessed January 8, 2016.

COYOTE (Founder NJ Almodovar), telephone interview, November 12, 1996. Augmented with information from Coyote web site. Available at http://www.wal-net.org/csis/groups/coyote.html. Accessed July 31, 2015.

COYOTE (Founder: NJ Almodovar) website (2013). Call off Your Old Tired Ethics. Available at http://www.coyotela.org. Accessed January 10, 2016.

Credit Suisse (2013). *Global Wealth Report*, p.10. Available at https://publications.credit-suisse.com/tasks/render/file/?fileID=BCDB1364-A105-0560-1332EC9100FF5C83. Accessed July 28, 2015.

Cusk R (2010). The female eunuch, 40 years on. *The Guardian.* Available at http://www.theguardian.com/books/2010/nov/20/rachel-cusk-the-female-eunuch. Accessed December 26, 2015.

Dasgupta P (2015). Zoom Infopost. Available at http://www.zoominfo.com/p/Partha-Dasgupta/276599208. Accessed July 29, 2015.

Dasgupta RK (2004). *Gandhi's Political Philosophy*, p. 1. Available at http://www.mkgandhi.org/articles/dasgupta.htm. Accessed June 10, 2015.

Dasgupta S (2007, March 21). Philosophical Assumptions for Training in Non-violence, vol. 2. Shri Jamnalal Bajaj Institute of Studies in Ahimsa Monograph. University of California.

Davis F (1991). *Moving the Mountain: The Women's Movement in America Since 1960.* New York; Simon & Schuster:15–25, 52–68.

De Beauvoir S (2004). *Stanford Encyclopedia of Philosophy.* Available at http://plato.stanford.edu/entries/beauvoir/. Accessed December 28, 2014.

De Bruyn M (1995). *In Advancing Women's Status.* Amsterdam: Royal Tropical Institute (KIT).

Deaton A (2008). Income, aging, health and wellbeing around the world: Evidence from the Gallup World Poll. *J Econ Perspect.,* 22, 53–72.

Deaton A (2013). *The Great Escape: Health, Wealth, and the Origins of Inequality.* Princeton, NJ: Princeton University Press:ch. 7, p. 312.

Denison R (1995). Call us survivors! Women Organized to Respond to Life-threatening Diseases (WORLD). In: Schneider BE & Stoller NE (Eds), *Women Resisting AIDS: Feminist Strategies of Empowerment.* Philadelphia: Temple University Press:195–207.

Department of Health and Human Services (DHHS) (1991). *Healthy People 2000: National Health Promotion and Disease Prevention Objectives.* Washington, DC: PHS Publication No. 91-50-212.

Dhammacaro (2013). *Female Monks in Buddhism.* Available at http://www.buddhapadipa.org/buddhism/female-monks-in-buddhism/. Accessed December 17, 2015.

Dhammika SV (1993). *The Edicts of King Ashoka.* Available at http://www.cs.colostate. edu/~malaiya/ashoka.html. Accessed May 26, 2015.

Dhillon HS & Kar SB (1965). Malaria eradication: An investigation of cultural patterns and belief among tribal populations in India. *J Health Edu.*, 1, 31–40.

Diamonds J (2005). *Collapse: How Societies Choose to Fail or Succeed.* New York: Penguin.

DiAna D (1990). Talking the talk. In: *The ACT UP/NY Women and AIDS Book Group: Women, AIDS, and Activism.* Boston, MA: South End Press:219–222.

Diener E, Kahneman D, Tov W, & Arora R (2009). Income's differential influence on judgements of life versus affective well-being. In: Diener E (Ed.), *Assessing Well-being: The Collected Works of Ed Diener.* Oxford, UK: Springer:20–21.

Doktor P (1996, March 7). Okinawa is a global issue. *Golden Gater Online.*

Dorkenoo E (1994). *Cutting the Rose, Female Genital Mutilation: The Practice and Its Prevention.* London: Minority Rights.

Doula (2011). Available at http://ictcmidwives.org/about-ictc/ictc-history/. Accessed July 20, 2015.

Dovidio JF, Glick P, & Rudman L (Eds) (2005). *On Nature of Prejudice: Fifty Years After Allport.* Somerset, NJ: Wiley-Blackwell

Duncan S (1991). Forced removals mean genocide. In: Russell DEH (Ed.), *Lives of Courage: Women for a New South Africa.* New York: Basic Books:227–240.

Duncan S (2015). SAHO (South African History online posted in 2010). Available at http://www.sahistory.org.za/people/sheena-duncan#content-top. Accessed July 2, 2015.

Dunlop DD, Hughes SL, & Manheim LM (1997, March). Disability in activities of daily living: Patterns of change and a hierarchy of disability. *Am J Public Health,* 87(3), 378–383.

Dunst CJ, Trivette CM, & Hamby DW (2007). Meta-analysis of family-centered help giving practices research. *Mental Retard Dev Disabil Res Rev.*, 13(4), 370–378. Available at http://www.ncbi.nlm.nih.gov/pubmed/17979208.

Eating Disorder Education (2015). Available at http://www.edcatalogue.com/eating-disorders-parenting-2015/. Accessed July 18, 2015.

Economic and Social Survey of Asia and the Pacific (ESCAP) (2015). *Asia Pacific Report.* Available at http://www.unescap.org/sites/default/files/Economic%20and%20Social%20 Survey%20of%20Asia%20and%20the%20Pacific%202015.pdf. Accessed July 16, 2015.

Economist (2012, November 3). Bangladesh and development, References. Available at http://www.economist.com/news/briefing/21565617-bangladesh-has-dysfunctional-politics-and-stunted-private-sector-yet-it-has-been-surprisingly?zid=300&ah=e7b 9370e170850b88ef129fa625b13c4. Accessed July 14, 2015.

Egenes KJ (n.d.). *History of Nursing.* Sudbury, MA: Jones & Bartlett.

Eidelson RJ & Eidelson JI (2003). Dangerous ideas: Five beliefs that propel groups toward conflict. *Am Psychologist,* 58(3), 182–192.

Ember C & Ember M (2003). Breast-feeding practices in the west. *Encyclopedia of Medical Anthropology: Health and Illness in the World's Cultures.* New York: Springer:234. ISBN 9780306477546.

Encuesta Nacional sobre Discriminación en México (Enadis) (2010). *National Survey on Discrimination.* Available at http://www.academia.edu/931652/National_Survey_ on_discrimination_in_Mexico_ENADIS_2010_. Accessed July 7, 2015.

Engle L (2002, January/February). Listening to mothers' voices. Helping parents talk to their kids about sex, choices and HIV/AIDS. *Body Positive.* Available at http://www. thebody.com/content/art30929.html. Accessed February 14, 2015.

Environmental Health Coalition (2015, December 17). Available at https://www.facebook.com/EHCSanDiego. Accessed July 19, 2015.

Equality Now web site. Available at http://www.equalitynow.org.

Erickson E (1993). *Gandhi's Truth: On the Origins of Militant Nonviolence*. New York: W.W. Norton.

Euromonitor (2013). Available at http://blog.euromonitor.com/2012/03/special-report-income-inequality-rising-across-the-globe.html#sthash.Cu3v7rQ3.dpuf) (Accessed July 29,2015)

European Public Health Association (EUPHA) (2014). Available at http://www.eupha.org/site/history.php. Accessed July 13, 2015.

Family Health International (FHI) (1997, November 6). *Case Study of the Women's Health Care Foundation*. Quezon City, Philippines: UP Center for Women's Studies.

Family Health International (FHI) (2007a). *Family Corporate Report*. Available at http://www.fhi360.org/sites/default/files/media/documents/FHICorporateReport2007.pdf. Accessed July 20, 2015.

Family Health International (FHI) (2007b). *Program Report*. Available at http://www.fhi360.org/about-us/annual-report. Accessed June 18, 2015.

Farquhar JW, Fortmann SP, Maccoby N, Haskell WL, Williams PT, Flora JA, et al. (1985, August). The Stanford Five-City Project: Design and methods. *Am J Epidemiol.*, 122(2), 323–334.

Fawcett JT (Ed.) (1973). *Psychological Perspectives on Population*. New York: Basic Books.

Feldman S & Beneria L (Eds) (1992). *Unequal Burden: Economic Crises, Persistent Poverty, and Women's Work*. Boulder, CO: Westview Press.

Fenner RM & Gifford MH (2012). Women for Sobriety: Thirty-five years of challenges, changes and continuity. *J Group Addict & Recov.*, 7(2–4), 142–170. Posted at www.williamwhitepapers.com/ with permission of the authors and Taylor & Francis.

Fetterman DM, Kaftarian SJ, & Wandersman A (Eds) (2014). *Empowerment Evaluation: Knowledge and Tools for Self-Assessment, Evaluation Capacity Building, and Accountability*. Thousand Oaks, CA: Sage.

Fielding J (2009). Key Indicators of Health, Los Angeles County Department of Health (LACDH). Available at http://publichealth.lacounty.gov/ha/docs/kir_2013_finals.pdf Accessed August 1, 2015.

Fielding J et al. (2009). Leading Causes of Death and Premature Death. Los Angeles County Department of Health (LACDH). Available at http://publichealth.lacounty.gov/wwwfiles/ph/hae/dca/MortalityReport2009.pdf. Accessed August 1, 2015.

Fielding JE (2009). Health in all policies: Lessons learned by L.A. County DPH. *CDC Leaders to Leaders Conference*, July 8, 2008, L.A. County Department of Public Health. Available at file:///G:/Fielding%20CDC%20L2L%207.8.08%20-%20FINAL.pdf.

Fillenbaum, GG (1987). Activities of daily living. In: Maddox GL et al. (Eds), *The Encyclopedia of Aging: A Comprehensive Resource in Gerontology and Geriatrics* (2 vols, 3rd edn). New York: Springer.

Fishbein M & Ajzen I (1975). *Belief, Attitude, Intention, and Behavior: An Introduction to Theory and Research*. Reading, MA: Addison-Wesley.

Fletecher MA (1998, April 7). Melting Pot: America's Racial and Ethnic Divides. Available at http://www.washingtonpost.com/wp-srv/national/longterm/meltingpot/melt2.htm

Foreign Relations (0000). US Library of Congress, Country Studies: Peru. Available at http://countrystudies.us/peru/96.htm. Accessed July 15, 2015.

Fortmann SP & Varady AN (1999). Effects of a Community-wide Health Education Program on Cardiovascular Disease Morbidity and Mortality: The Stanford Five-City Project. *Am J Epidemiol.*, 152(4), 316–323.

Fox Business News (2011). Eight Cities Where Minorities Are Now in the Majority. Available at http://www.foxbusiness.com/industries/2011/09/06/eight-cities-where-minorities-are-now-in-majority/. Accessed August 3, 2015.

Franke RW & Chasin BH (1989). *Kerala: Radical Reform as Development in an Indian State* (2nd edn). San Francisco, CA: Institute for Food and Development Policy.

Free Burma Coalition (1995, August 31). Beijing '95 website. Opening Keynote Address by Aung San Suu Kyi. Available at http://danenet.wicip.org/fbc/beijing.html.

Freedman R & Berelson B (1976). The records of family planning programs. *Studies Fam Plan.*, 7(1), 1–40.

Freeman RC, Collier K, & Parillo KM (2015, April 9). Early life sexual abuse as a risk factor for crack cocaine use in a sample of community-recruited women at high risk for illicit drug use. *Am J Drug Alcohol Abuse*, 28, 109–131. Available at www.ncbi.nlm.nih.gov/pmc/articles/PMC2096682. Accessed December 16, 2015.

Freire P (1968). *Pedagogy of the Oppressed*. New York: Seabury Press.

Freire P (1973). *Education for Critical Consciousness*. New York: Seabury Press.

Freire P (1974). *Education: Practice of Freedom*. London: Writers and Readers Publishing Cooperative.

Freire P (2015). *Concepts Used by Paulo Freire*. Freire Institute:1. Available at http://www.freire.org/paulo-freire/concepts-used-by-paulo-freire/. Accessed August 10, 2015.

French JRPJr. & Raven BH (1959). The bases of social power. In: Cartwright D (Ed.), *Studies in Social Power*. Ann Arbor, MI: Institute for Social Research:150–167.

Frerichs RR (2015). Competing Theories of Cholera. Available at http://www.ph.ucla.edu/epi/snow/choleratheories.html. Accessed May 24, 2015.

Frese H (2012, February). Women's power: The Anti-Arrack Movement in Andhra Pradesh. *South Asia Chronicle* 2(2012), S.219–S.234. Available at http://edoc.hu-berlin.de/suedasien/band-2/219/PDF/219.pdf. Accessed July 20, 2015.

Friedan B (1963). *The Feminine Mystique*. New York: W.W. Norton.

Friends of CoMadres (2014). Available at http://www.foco-madres.org/patricia-garcia-president-co-madres-dies-47/. Accessed July 2, 2015.

Fulu E, Jewkes R, Roselli T, Garcia-Moreno C, & on behalf of the UN Multi-country Cross-sectional Study on Men and Violence Research Team (2013). Prevalence of and factors associated with male perpetration of intimate partner violence: Findings from the UN Multi-country Cross-sectional Study on Men and Violence in Asia and the Pacific. *Lancet Glob Health*, 1, e187–e207.

GABRIELA (2015). Available at http://www.gabrielaph.com/. Accessed January 7, 2016.

GABRIELLA Philippines (2008). Available at https://gabrielaphilippines.wordpress.com/2008/02/. Accessed July 2015.

Gahlot D (1993). A SPARC of hope for slum-dwellers. In: Women's Feature Service, *The Power to Change: Women in the Third World Redefine their Environment*. London: Zed Books:138–143.

Gallup (2009). World Poll Methodology. Technical report. Washington, DC: Gallup World Headquarters. Available at scale.aspxhttp://www.gallup.com/poll/122453/understanding-gallup-uses-cantril-scale.aspx. Accessed December 28, 2015.

Gandhi M (1916). From "On Civil Disobedience," by Mohandas Gandhi. Available at http://powpak.dl.noacsc.org/powpak/data/csiebeneck/articles/document_ar65.pdf. Accessed January 12, 2016.

Garcia-Moreno C, Jansen H, Ellsberg M, et al. (2005b). *WHO Multi-country Study on Women's Health and Domestic Violence against Women: Initial Results on Prevalence, Health Outcomes, and Women's Responses.* Geneva: World Health Organization. Available at http://www.who.int/gender/violence/who_multicountry_study/Introduction-Chapter1-Chapter2.pdf. Accessed July 31, 2015.

Garcia-Moreno C, Jansen H, Ellsberg M, et al. (2006, October 7). Prevalence of intimate partner violence: Findings from the WHO multi-country study on women's health and domestic violence. *Lancet*, 368(9543), 1260–1269.

Garcia-Moreno C, Jansen H, Ellsberg M, et al. (2005a). Violence against women: An urgent public health priority. 89(1), 1–80. Available at www.who.int.

Gill TM & Feinstein AR (1994). A critical appraisal of the quality of quality-of-life measurements. *JAMA,* 272(8), 619–626.

Gimmell M (1990). *The Supply and Education of Public Health Professionals.* Washington, DC: Association of Schools of Public Health.

Girl's Power Initiative (GPI) (1996). Nigeria. Available at http://www.gpinigeria.org/pages/article/about-us. Accessed January 10, 2016.

Glanz K, Rimer B, & Viswanath K (2008). *Health Behavior and Health Education: Theory, Research, and Practice* (4th edn). San Francisco: Jossey Bass.

Glazer N (1988). *We Are All Multiculturalists Now.* Cambridge, MA: Harvard University Press.

Gleick J (1987). *Chaos: Making a New Science.* New York: Viking.

Global Survival Network (1999). Available at http://www.globalsn.net/.

Goda T (2013, May). Changes in income inequality from a global perspective: An overview. Post Keynesian Study Group (PKSG). Working Paper 1303. Available at www.postkeynesian.net/downloads/wpaper/PKWP1305.pdf. Accessed July 29, 2015.

Goldberg R (1993). *Organizing Women Office Workers: Dissatisfaction, Consciousness and Action.* New York: Praeger.

Goldberg RA (1991). *Grassroots Resistance: Social Movements in Twentieth Century America.* Belmont, CA: Wadsworth:193–217.

Goldberg P (2010). *Aurobindo, American Veda.* New York: Harmony Books:69, 136.

Golden SD & Earp JA (2012). Social ecological approaches to individuals and their contexts: Twenty years of *Health Education & Behavior* health promotion interventions. *Health Edu Behav*, 39(3), 364–372.

Gomes A (2007). *Banchte Sekha (Learn to Live).* Available at http://blog.worldcitizenship.org/wp-archive/677. Accessed January 8, 2016.

Goodenough P (2010, October 22). Statistics Show Women Fare Badly in Muslim Countries, but U.N. Official Says Critics Are "Stereotyping" Islam. *CNNews.* Available at http://www.cnsnews.com/news/article/statistics-show-women-fare-badly-muslim-countries-un-official-says-critics-are. Accessed January 9, 2016.

Goodenough P (2014). *World's Women Report: 2010.* UN.

GPI Alumna Association (GAA) (2015). Available at http://gpinigeria.org/pages/article/gaa. Accessed February 13, 2015.

Graham C (1991). The APRA government and the urban poor: The PAIT program in Lima's pueblos jovenes. *J Lat Am Stud.*, 23, 91–130.

Grameen Bank. Mohammad Yunus, founder. Bangladesh. Available at http://www.grameenfoundation.org/.

Green LW & Kreuter M (2004). *Health Promotion Planning: An Educational and Ecological Approach.* New York: McGraw-Hill.

Greer G (1970). *The Female Eunuch.* New York: Harper-Collins.

Group for Mutual Support (GAM) (1985). *Guatemala: Group for Mutual Support 1984–85.* Washington, DC: Americas Watch.

Gupta R & Steinem G (2015). *Gloria Steinem on Combating Sex Trafficking*, Apne Ap ("On Your Own"). Available at http://apneaap.org/?s=gloria+steinem+. Accessed July 9, 2015.

Gutiérrez G (1994). Mothers of East Los Angeles strike back. In: Bullard RD (Ed.), *Unequal Protection, Environmental Justice and Communities of Color.* San Francisco: Sierra Club Books.

Hamburg D, Eliott GR, & Parron DL (1982). *Health Behavior: Frontiers of Research in the Biobehavioral Sciences: A Report of the Institute of Medicine.* Washington, DC: National Academies Press.

Hari-Correa N (1994). Workers' education for women members of rural workers' organizations in Asia. In: Martens M & Mitter S (Eds), *Women in Trade Unions: Organizing the Unorganized.* Geneva: International Labour Office:107–114.

Harter JK & Arora R (2008, June 5). *Social Time Crucial to Daily Emotional Well-being in U.S. Gallup Polls.* Available at http://www.gallup.com/poll/107692/Social-Time-Crucial-Daily-Emotional-Wellbeing.aspx. Accessed August 10, 2009.

Harter JK & Gurley VF (2008). Measuring health in the United States, Association for Psychological Science (APS). *Observer*, 21(8), 23–26.

Harvard University (2010). *The Harvard Conference on Sustaining Momentum: Ten Years into the Asian Century.* Available at http://www.apair.at/conferences/past-conferences/asia-conference-2010/en/. Accessed July 16, 2015.

Hayes-Bautista D (2010, November 14). The Latino Paradox. Editorial. *Los Angeles Times.*

Hayes-Bautista D (2011, December 8). Latino Health Paradox: Latinos Boast Low Infant Mortality, Long Lives Despite Risk Factors. Posted by Janell Ross, *Huffington Post.* Available at http://www.huffingtonpost.com/2011/08/11/latino-health-a-mystery_n_924820.html. Accessed August 2, 2015.

Health Alert Network (HAN) (2015). *Emergency Preparedness Response.* Available at http://emergency.cdc.gov/HAN/index.asp. Accessed January 7, 2016.

Health-related Quality of Life (HRQOL) (2000). *Measuring Healthy Days Population Assessment of Health-Related Quality of Life.* Available at http://www.cdc.gov/hrqol/pdfs/mhd.pdf. Accessed January 6, 2016.

Heckler M (1985). *Report of the Secretary's Task Force on Black and Minority Health.* Washington, DC: U.S. Department of Health and Human Services.

Hélie-Lucas MA (1993). Women living under Muslim laws. In: Kerr J (Ed.), *Ours By Right: Women's Rights as Human Rights.* London: Zed Books:52–64.

Henry J. Kiser Family Foundation (2013, March 13). *Health Coverage by Race and Ethnicity: The Potential Impact of the Affordable Care Act*, figure 6. Available at http://kff.org/disparities-policy/issue-brief/health-coverage-by-race-and-ethnicity-the-potential-impact-of-the-affordable-care-act/. Accessed July 18, 2015.

Herdman M, Fox-Rushby J, & Badia X (1997). "Equivalence" and the translation and adaption of health-related quality of life questionnaires. *Qual Life Res.*, 6, 237–247.

Heymann J (2010). *Profit at the Bottom of the Ladder: Creating Value by Investing in Your Workforce.* Boston: Harvard Business Press.

Hills MD (2002, August). Kluckhohn and Strodtbeck's Values Orientation Theory. *Online Readings in Psychology and Culture*, 4(4). Available at http://dx.doi.org/10.9707/2307-0919.1040.

Hipp JR (2010). Micro-structure in micro-neighborhoods: A new social distance measure, and its effect on individual and aggregated perceptions of crime and disorder. *Soc Net.*, 32(2), 148–159.

Hobbs T (1909). *Leviathan.* London: Oxford University Press:66–67.

Hofstede G (1980). *Culture's Consequences.* Beverly Hills, CA: Sage.

Hofstede G, Hofstede GJ, & Minkov M (2010). *Cultures and Organizations, Software of the Mind: Intercultural Cooperation and Its Importance for Survival* (3rd edn). New York: McGraw-Hill Professional.

Holwell JZ (1767). *An Account of the Manner of Inoculating for the Smallpox in the East Indies.* Available at http://www.reformation.org/holwell.html.

https://en.wikipedia.org/wiki/Sioux >. Accessed July 18, 2015

Huntington S (1993, Summer). Clash of civilizations. *Foreign Affairs,* 2(3), 22–49.

Indian National Trust for Art and Cultural Heritage (INTACH) (1986) *India's Civilisational Response to the Forest Crisis.* New Delhi, India: INTACH.

Indians for Collective Action (ICA) (2015). Available at http://icaonline.org/. Accessed February 15, 2015.

Inglehart I & Norris P (2003). *The Rising Tide: Gender Equality and Cultural Change Around the World.* Cambridge, UK: Cambridge University Press.

Inglehart R & Welzel C (2005). *Modernization, Cultural Change, and Democracy: The Human Development Sequence.* Cambridge, UK: Cambridge University Press.

Inglehart R & Welzel C (2010). *World Values Survey (WVS).* Available at www.worldvaluessurvey.org. Accessed January 6, 2016.

Inkeles A & Smith DH (1974). *Becoming Modern: Individual Change in Six Developing Countries.* Cambridge, MA: Harvard University Press.

Institute of Medicine (IOM) (1988). *Institute of Medicine's Report on the Future of Public Health.* Washington, DC: National Academies Press.

Institute of Medicine (IOM) (2002). *The Future of the Public's Health in the 21st Century.* Washington, DC: National Committee on Assuring the Health of the Public in the 21st Century.

Institute of Medicine (IOM) (2009). *Race, Ethnicity, and Language Data: Standardization for Health Care Quality Improvement.* Washington, DC: National Academies Press. Available at http://www.ahrq.gov/research/findings/final-reports/iomracereport/iomracereport.pdf. Accessed August 2, 2015.

Intermon (1997). Translated from Spanish by L Macera & T Oyola. Available at www.intermon.org.

Intermon (2008). Lima's Community Kitchens: Combating Hunger and Loneliness (a Report by Zibechi R). Available at http://upsidedownworld.org/main/

peru-archives-76/1088-limas-community-kitchens-combating-hunger-and-loneliness. Accessed August 2015.

International Center for Traditional Childbearing (ICTC) (1991). Available at http://ictc-midwives.org/about-ictc/ictc-history/. Accessed July 20, 2015.

International Conference on Population and Development (ICPD) (2014c). *Global Review Report*. Available at http://icpdbeyond2014.org/uploads/browser/files/icpd_global_review_report.pdf. Accessed August 2, 2015.

International Institute for Sustainable Development (IISD) (1997). Available at http://iisd1.iisd.ca/50comm/commdb/desc/d07.htm. Accessed July 14, 2015.

International Labor Organization (ILO) (2002). *Promoting Gender Equality: A Resource Kit for Trade Unions*. Booklet No. 6. Geneva, Switzerland. Available at http://www.workinfo.com/free/links/Gender/cha_7.htm. Accessed July 10, 2015.

International Labor Organization (ILO) (2015). *Gender Equality in the World of Work, and R165–Workers with Family Responsibilities Recommendation, 1981* (No. 165). ILO Gender Equality web site. Available at http://www.ilo.org/inform/online-information-resources/research-guides/gender-equality/lang--en/index.htm. Accessed July 10, 2015.

International Labour Organization (ILO) (2015). Available at http://www.ilo.org/public//english/region/asro/bangkok/arm/ind.htm. Accessed July 10, 2015.

International Labour Organization (ILO). *World Employment Report 1998–1999*. Available at http://www.ilo.org/global/about-the-ilo/media-centre/press releases/WCMS_007996/lang--en/index.htm. Accessed August 2, 2015.

International Nutrition Foundation (INF) (1991). *World Food Prize*. Available at http://www.inffoundation.org/about/founder.htm. Accessed November 15, 2014.

International Planned Parenthood Federation (IPPF) (2014–2015). *Annual Performance Report*. Available at http://www.ippf.org/resource/Annual-Performance-Report-2014-15-0. Accessed July 16, 2015.

International Planned Parenthood Federation (IPPF) (2015). *Our Work*. Available at http://www.ippf.org/our-work. Accessed July 2015.

International Planned Parenthood Federation (IPPF) (2015a). Available at http://www.ippf.org/. Accessed July 2015.

International Planned Parenthood Federation (IPPF) (2015b). Available at http://www.ippf.firmwareservice.com/login.php. Accessed February 13, 2015.

International Planned Parenthood Federation (IPPF) Western Hemisphere Region. (1994). *Forty Years of Saving Lives with Family Planning*. An Anniversary Publication. New York: IPPF.

International Planned Parenthood Federations (IPPF) (2015c). Available at http://www.ippf.org/about-us. Accessed May 25, 2015.

International Seminar Workshop on Indigenous Studies (ISWIS) (2013). *Synthesis, Conference Report, International Seminar Workshop on Indigenous Studies*. Philippines: University of Philippines, Baguio, Cordillera Studies Center:21. Available at http://www.up.edu.ph/tag/indigenous/. Accessed January 6, 2016.

International Women's Health Coalition (IWHC) (1993). *Advancing Gender Equality in Nigeria Through Girls' Empowerment*. Available at https://iwhc.org/event/advancing-gender-equality-in-nigeria-through-girls-empowerment/. Accessed December 28, 2015.

International Women's Health Coalition (IWHC) (2010). *Annual Gala 2010*. The MacArthur Foundation. Available at https://www.macfound.org/grantees/453/. Accessed January 12, 2016.

International Network of Women Against Tobacco (INWAT) (1990). Available at http://inwat.org/content/. Accessed July 16, 2015.

International Network of Women Against Tobacco (INWAT) (2014). Available at http://inwat.org/content/about/our-work/. Accessed July 16, 2015.

International Network of Women Against Tobacco (INWAT) (2015). Available at https://www.facebook.com/pages/INWAT-Europe-International-Network-of-Women-Against-Tobacco/254091551276926. Accessed February 13, 2015.

Israel BA, Checkoway B, Schulz A, Zimmerman M (1994, Summer). Health education and community empowerment: Conceptualizing and measuring perceptions of individual, organizational, and community control. *Health Educ Q.*, 21(2), 149–170.

Jackson KE (2015). Available at http://www.sistersnetworkinc.org/founder.html. Accessed February 15, 2015.

Jamaica Observer (JO) (2014). Available at http://www.jamaicaobserver.com/columns/Abortion-----let-s-get-rid-of-those-ancient-laws_16773601.

James GS (1995). Yet women's development is still regarded as a separate issue. In: Thin N (Ed.), *Advancing Women's Status: Gender, Society, and Development: Women and Men Together*. Amsterdam: Royal Tropical Institute (KIT):24.

Jameson KR (1999). *Night Falls Fast*. New York: Alfred Knopf:48–52.

Jamison JT, Summers LH, Alleyne G, Arrow KJ, et al (2013). Global Health 2035: Grand convergence. *Lancet* (special issue). Available at http://www.thelancet.com/commissions/global-health-2035. Accessed July 30, 2015.

Japan Times News (2015, June 23). Okinawa reflects on battle's end 70 years later. Available at http://www.japantimes.co.jp/news/2015/06/23/national/history/japan-marks-70th-anniversary-since-guns-fell-silent-battle-okinawa/#.Vo7fBvkrJD9. Accessed January 6, 2016.

Jasper K (1958). The future of mankind. *Stanford Encyclopedia of Philosophy*. Available at http://plato.stanford.edu/entries/jaspers/. Accessed January 14, 2016.

Jenness V (1991). From Sex as Sin to Sex as Work: COYOTE, Organizational Legitimation and the Contemporary Prostitutes' Rights Movement. Doctoral dissertation. Santa Barbara, CA: University of California.

Jethmalani R & Women's Action Research and Legal Action for Women (WARLAW) (1995). *Kali's Yug: Empowerment, Law, and Dowry Deaths: Women's Action Research and Legal Action for Women (WARLAW)*. New Delhi, India: Har-Anand.

Jewkes R, Fulu E, Roselli T, and Garcia-Moreno C (2013). A six nation surveys in South Asia on men's attitudes towards sexual partner. *Lancet Global Health*, 1(4). Available at http://www.thelancet.com/journals/lancet/article/PIIS2214-109X(13)70069-X/abstract. Accessed July 31, 2015.

Johnson C (2002). *Okinawa Between United States and Japan, JPRI*. Available at http://www.jpri.org/publications/occasionalpapers/op24.html. Accessed July 2, 2015.

Judge TA, Piccolo RF, Podsakoff NP, Shaw JC, & Riche BL (2010). The relationship between pay and job satisfaction: A meta-analysis of the literature. *J Vocat Behav.*, 77, 157–167.

Kabeer N (2010a). *Can the MDGs Provide a Pathway to Social Justice?* New York: UNDP.

Kabeer N (2010b). Women's empowerment, development interventions and the management of information flows. *IDS Bull.,* 41(6), 105–113.

Kabilsingh C (1991). *Thai Women in Buddhism.* Foreword, p. xiii. Berkeley, CA: Parallax Press.

Kabilsingh C (1998). *Women in Buddhism: Questions and Answers.* Bangkok: Thammasat University.

KABOO (2015). Available at http://kboo.fm/program. Accessed July 20, 2015.

Kagawa-Singer M, Dadia AV, Yu MC, & Surbone A (2010, January–February). Cancer, culture, and health disparities: Time to chart a new course? *CA Cancer J Clin.,* 60(1), 12–39, doi: 10.3322/caac.2005.

Kahneman D (2011). *Thinking. Fast and Slow.* New York: Farrar, Straus, & Giroux.

Kahneman D & Deaton A (2010). High income improves evaluation of life but not emotional well-being. *Proc Natl Acad Sci USA.,* 107(38), 16489–16493. doi: 10.1073/pnas.1011492107. Available at http://www.pnas.org/content/107/38/16489.full. Accessed January 6, 2016.

KALFOU (2010). *Immigrant Women Workers at the Center of Social Change: AIWA Takes Stock of Itself.* Available at http://www.aiwa.org/wp-content/uploads/2014/08/KalfouArticle_SocialChange.pdf. Accessed January 6, 2016.

Kalisch PA & Kalisch BJ (1995). *American Nursing: A History* (4th edn). New York: Lippincott Williams & Wilkins.

Kang KC (1998, October 7). Okinawans Bring Drive to L.A. *Los Angeles Times*, Metro Section B, B1, B4.

Kar RB (2006). The deep structure of law and morality. *Texas Law Rev.,* 84(4), 877–942.

Kar RB (2012a, August 4). On the Proto-Indo-European Language of the Indus Valley Civilization (and Its Implications for Western Prehistory). The Sindhu-Sarasvati Civilization: New Perspectives (Essays in Honor of Dr. S.R. Rao) (2014). Available at SSRN: http://ssrn.com/abstract=2124180. Accessed August 10, 2015.

Kar RB (2012b). Western legal prehistory: Reconstructing the hidden origins of western law and western civilization. *Univ Illinois Law Rev.,* 5, 1499–1702.

Kar SB & Alex S (1999). Public health approaches to substance abuse prevention: A multicultural perspective. In: Kar SB (Ed.), *Substance Abuse Prevention in Multicultural Communities.* Amityville, NY: Baywood.

Kar SB (1978). Consistency between fertility attitudes and behavior: A conceptual model. *Popul Stud.,* 32(1), 173–185.

Kar SB (1990). Primary health care: Implications for medical profession and education. *Acad Med.,* 65(5), 291–297.

Kar SB (1994). Health promotion in the Asian Pacific Region. Commissioned paper, World Health Organization, Western Pacific Regional Office, Manila, Philippines (WHO/WPRO Conference 1992).

Kar SB (1999). *Substance Abuse Prevention: A Multicultural Perspective.* New York: Baywood.

Kar SB (2000a, March 6–8). Acculturation and quality of life among Asian immigrants: A cross-national study. Paper presented at the Second International Conference of Quality of Life, International Society of Quality of Life Studies, Singapore.

Kar SB (2000b, April 5–7). Better health and welfare systems. Background paper for the International Meeting on Women and Health. WHO Kobe Centre, Awaji, Japan.

Kar SB (2001). *Women's Health Development: Imperatives for Health and Welfare Systems.* Background paper for International Meeting on Women and Health. Kobe Center, Japan: World Health Organization.

Kar S (2015). *Coming and Going: Poems and Songs of Rabindranath Tagore* (translations and photos by Snehendu B. Kar). Kolkata, India: Bee Books/Patra Bharati:19. Available at http://beebooks.in/portfolio/coming-and-going-poems-and-songs-of-rabindranath-tagore/. Accessed January 20, 2016.

Kar SB (Ed.) (1989). *Health Promotion Indicators and Actions.* New York: Springer.

Kar SB, Afifi AA, Scrimshaw S, & Evans C (1993, November 2). Community-based public health practice. Paper presented at the Annual Convention of the APHA.

Kar SB, Alcalay R, & Alex S (Eds) (2001). *Health Communication: A Multicultural Perspective.* Thousand Oaks, CA: Sage.

Kar SB, Campbell K, Jimenez A, & Gupta S (1995/1996). Invisible Americans: An exploration of Indo-American quality of life. *Amerasia J.,* 21(3), 25–52.

Kar SB, Campbell K, Jimenez A, & Sze F (1998a). Acculturation and quality of life: A comparative study of Japanese Americans and Indo-Americans. *Amerasia J.,* 24(1), 129–142.

Kar SB, Chickering C, & Pascual C (1998b). Public health practice in a multicultural and under-served Los Angeles Community: A case-study. Revised version of paper presented at American Public Health Association (APHA) in 1997, UCLA Office of Public Health Practice.

Kar SB, Gill J, Jimenez A, Wong L, & Sze F (2002). Acculturation and quality of life: A comparative study of Asian Indians, Japanese Americans, and Korean Americans. *Asian Am Policy Rev (Harvard).,* 11, 37–55.

Kar SB, Pascual C, & Chickering K (1999). Empowerment for health promotion: A meta-analysis. *Soc Sci Med.,* 49(11), 1431–1460.

Kar SB & Srivastava VP (1968). Impact of mass communication in a smallpox vaccination campaign. *Health Edu J.,* XXVII(4), 205–2l4.

Karma Kutir (2013). Available at https://www.facebook.com/Karmakutirkolkata. Accessed July 14, 2015.

Kaskutas LA (1994). What do women get out of self-help? Their reasons for attending Women for Sobriety and Alcoholics Anonymous. *JSAT.,* 11(3), 185–195.

Kaskutas LA (1996). A road less traveled: Choosing the "Women for Sobriety" program. *J Drug Issues.,* 26(1), 77–94.

Kaye LW (1997). *Self-Help Support Groups for Older Women: Rebuilding Elder Networks Through Personal Empowerment.* Washington, DC: Taylor & Francis.

Kelman HC (1997). Group processes in the resolution of international conflicts: Experiences from the Isreli-Palestenian case. *Am Psychol.,* 52(3), 212–220.

Kelman HC (1987). The political psychology of the Israeli-Palestinian conflict: How can we overcome the barriers to a negotiated solution. *Polit Psychol.,* 8, 347–363.

Kennedy P (1989). *The Rise and Fall of the Great Powers.* New York: Vintage.

Khan Academy (2015). *Personalized Learning Resources.* Available at https://www.khanacademy.org/about. Accessed August 3, 2015.

Khan M (1964). Pakistan: The rural pilot family planning action project at Comilla. *Stud Fam Plan.,* 3, 9–11.

Kickbush I (1996). Health promotion: A global perspective. In: *Pan American Health Organization Health Promotion.* An Anthology Scientific Publication No. 557. Washington, DC: Pan American Health Organization:14–22.

King Jr. (1963). *I Have a Dream* (text). Available at https://www.archives.gov/press/exhibits/dream-speech.pdf. Accessed January 8, 2016.

King Jr. ML & Nelson K (2012). *I Have a Dream* (book/CD). New York: Schwartz & Wade.

Kluckhohn FR & Strodtbeck FL (1961). *Variations in Value Orientations.* Evanston, IL: Row, Peterson.

Koh H (2014). Available at http://www.surgeongeneral.gov/library/reports/50-years-of-progress/sgr50-chap-1.pdf. Accessed July 30, 2015.

Kohli A (1989). *Democracy and Development in India: From Socialism to Pro-Business.* New Delhi, India: Oxford University Press.

Korbin JE & Coulton CJ (1996). The role of neighbors and the government in neighborhood-based child protection. *J Soc Issues,* 52(3), 163–176.

Kumar H (2013, August 22). Sen-Bhagwati debate: Rival economists in public battle over cure for India's poverty. *New York Times,* p. A-10.

Kusterer K (1993). Women-oriented NGOs in Latin America: democratization's decisive wave. In: Young G, Samarsinghe V, & Kusterer K (Eds), *Women at the Center: Development Issues and Practices in the 1990s.* Hartford, CT; Kumarian Press:182–192.

L.A. County Department of Public Health (2008). *CDC Leaders to Leaders Conference,* July 8. Available at http://www.utsandiego.com/news/2009/Apr/14/1m14kessler234037-lois-kessler-sdsu-womens-studies/. Accessed September 4, 2014.

L.A. Department of Health (2012). *Key Indicators of Health.* Available at http://publichealth.lacounty.gov/ha/docs/kir_2013_finals.pdf.

LA Almanac (2005). Lack of Health Insurance in LA County: Ethnicity data. Available at http://www.laalmanac.com/health/he05.htm. Accessed August 4, 2015.

La Leche League International (LLLI) (0000). *A Brief History of La Leche League International.* Available at https://www.llli.org/lllihistory.html. Accessed February 14, 2015.

La Leche League International (LLLI) (2012). Available at http://www.llli.org/thewomanlyartofbreastfeeding. Accessed February 14, 2015.

La Leche League International (LLLI) (2015). Available at https://en.wikipedia.org/wiki/La_Leche_League_International#History. Accessed July 16, 2015.

Labor/Community Strategy Center (2015). Available at http://www.thestrategycenter.org/transformative-organizing. Accessed February 8, 2016.

Lakota Law Project (2005, August 11). Available at http://lakotalaw.org/about-us/our-team. Accessed July 18, 2015.

Lancet Editorial (1991). Quality of life. *Lancet,* 338, 350–351.

Land KC & Spilerman S (Eds) (1975). *Social Indicator Models.* New York: Russell Sage Foundation.

Large J (1997, June). Disintegration conflicts and the restoring of masculinity. *Gender Dev,* 5(2), 23–32.

Lashuay N, Burgel BJ, Harrison R, et al (2002). *A Report on Workplace Injuries, Asian Immigrant Women Advocate (AIWA).* Oakland, CA: AIWA. Available at aiwa@igc.org and http://www.aiwa.org/wp-content/uploads/2015/02/working-in-pain-clinic-report-2002.rev_.pdf. Accessed July 12, 2015.

Law Center to Prevent Gun Violence (LCTPGV) (2014). Available at http://gunlawscorecard.org/. Accessed February 16, 2015.

Laxmi CS (2000, May 21, Sunday). Lessons from the Mountains. *The Hindu.* Available at http://www.thehindu.com/2000/05/21/stories/13210414.htm. Accessed February 9, 2015.

Lazarini RJ & Martinez O (2001). Unions and domestic workers in Mexico City. In: Martens M & Mitter S (Eds), *Women in Trade Unions: Organizing the Unorganized*. Geneva: International Labour Office:83–88.

Lenten R (1993). *Cooking Under the Volcanoes—Communal Kitchens in the Southern Peruvian City of Arequipa*. Amsterdam, the Netherlands: Centro de Estudios y Documentación Latinoamericanos. Available at http://www.worldcat.org/title/cooking-under-the-volcanoes-communal-kitchens-in-the-southern-peruvian-city-of-arequipa/oclc/659394314. Accessed December 16, 2015.

Lewin K (1939). Field theory and experiment in social psychology. *Am J Sociol.*, 44(6), 868–896.

Lewin K (1951). *Field Theory in Social Science: Selected Theoretical Papers*. In: D. Cartwright (Ed.). New York: Harper & Row.

Lewin K (1997). *Resolving Social Conflicts: Field Theory in Social Science*. Washington, DC: American Psychological Association.

Lewin K, Dembo T, Festinger L, & Sears PS (1944). Level of aspiration. In: Hunt JMcV (Ed.), *Personality and the Behavior Disorders*, Vol. 1. New York: Ronald Press:333–378.

Liburd LC & Sniezek JE (2007). Changing times: New possibilities for community health and well-being. *Prevent Chronic Dis* [serial online], 4(3). Available at http://www.cdc.gov/pcd/issues/2007/jul/07_0048.htm. Accessed January 2016.

Li V & Wang S (Eds) (1998). *Collaboration and Participation: Women's Reproductive Health of Yunnan, China*. Beijing: Beijing Medical University.

LifeLong Medical Care (LLMC) (2015). Available at http://www.lifelongmedical.org/. Accessed February 15, 2015.

Lifelong over 60 Medical Care (n.d.) Available at http://www.lifelongmedical.org/locations/our-locations/over-60-health-center.html. Accessed December 27, 2015.

Lindow M (2009, June 20, Saturday). South Africa's Rape Crisis: "1 in 4 Men Say They've Done It." Time Magazine, Cape Town.

Lipset SM (1959, March). Some social requisites of democracy: Economic development and political legitimacy. *Am Polit Sci Rev.*, 53, 69–105, doi:10.2307/1951731.

Lopez A (2005). *Global Burden of Disease Project*. Cambridge, MA: Harvard University Press.

Lord JH (1990). MADD: The heart of America's anti-drunk driving movement. *J Traffic Med.*, 18(4), 191–197.

Los Angeles Department of Health Services (2012). Annual Report 2010–2011. Available at http://file.lacounty.gov/dhs/cms1_205090.pdf

Luepker RV, Murray DM, Jacobs Jr DR, Maurice B, Mittelmark MB, et al. (1994). Community education for cardiovascular disease prevention: Risk factor changes in the Minnesota Heart Health Program. *AJPH*, 84(9), 1383–1393. Available at http://www.ncbi.nlm.nih.gov/pmc/articles/PMC1615184/pdf/amjph00460-

Macera L & Oyola T (1997, Winter). Empowering women: A critical analysis of community kitchens in Peru. Unpublished paper. UCLA/SPH.

MADD35 (Mothers Against Drunk Driving) (2015). Available at http://www.madd.org/about-us/history/. Accessed July 17, 2015.

Madres del Este de Los Angeles—Santa Isabel (1999). Available at http://clnet.ucr.edu/community/intercambios/melasi/.

Madunagu (1993). Girls' Power Initiative (GPI), Nigeria. Available at http://www.gpinigeria.org/pages/article/about-us. Accessed July 16, 2005.

Maheshwari K (2015). Ahimsha Paramo Dharma. Hindupedia. Available at http://www.hindupedia.com/en/Ahimsa_Paramo_Dharma. Accessed June 20, 2015.

Majumder S (2009). Education as empowerment. *Indian J Educ.,* XXXV(3), 5–17.

Manekshaw S (2014). Quoted in *Deusche Welle, Made for Minds.* Available at http://www.dw.com/en/gurkhas-nepalese-warriors-in-world-war-i/a-17632181. Accessed January 6, 2016.

Mann V, Eble A, & Frost C (2010). Retrospective comparative evaluation of the lasting impact of a community-based primary health care programme on under-5 mortality in villages around Jamkhed, India. *Bull WHO,* 88, 727–736.

Marguerite R (2002, April). Moving forward: Addressing the health of Asian American and Pacific Islander women. *Am J Public Health,* 92(4), 516–519.

Markides K (2011). Latino Health Paradox: Latinos Boast Low Infant Mortality, Long Lives Despite Risk Factors. Available at http://www.huffingtonpost.com/2011/08/11/latino-health-a-mystery_n_924820.html.

Martens H & Mitter S (Ed.) (1994). *Women in Trade Unions: Organizing the Unorganized.* Geneva: International Labour Office.

Martens MH (1994). Organizing experiences in export processing zones in other countries. In: Martens M & Mitter S (Eds), *Women in Trade Unions: Organizing the Unorganized.* Geneva: International Labour Office:1–57.

Martin LR (1991). *A Survey of Agricultural Economics Literature: Agriculture in Economic Development 1940s to 1990s.* Minneapolis: University of Minnesota Press.

Martinez M (1995, September 7). Legacy of a mother's dedication: Juana Gutierrez, a beacon for East L.A., wins national award. *Los Angeles Times,* Metro Part B, p. 1.

Maslow (1943). A theory of human motivation. *Psychol Rev.,* 50, 370–396.

Maslow A (1962). *Toward a Psychology of Being.* Reprint. Eastford, CT: Martino Fine Books.

Mason MA (2002). *The Equality Trap.* New Brunswick, NJ: Transaction:180.

Matsumoto V & Allmendinger B (1999). *Over the Edge: Remapping the American West.* Oakland, CA: University of California Press:323–335.

Mauldin WP (1967, March). Measurement and evaluation of national family planning programs. *Demography,* 4(1), 71–80.

Mauldin WP, Watson WB, & Noe LF (1971). *KAP Surveys and Evaluation of Family Planning Programs.* New York: Population Council.

MAVIA (n.d.). Annual Report. Mothers Against Violence. Available at http://www.mav4life.org/. Accessed January 4, 2016. Also see https://www.youtube.com/watch?v=oZvcqI_iVMg. Uploaded August 11, 2011. Accessed January 4, 2016.

Mayne A (1989). Feminism and the anti-rape movement. *Fem Psychol.,* 6(2), 176–180.

Maza Coin (2014). Available at https://en.wikipedia.org/wiki/MazaCoin. Accessed July 18, 2015.

Mazumdar V (1989). Peasant Women Organize for Empowerment: The Bankura Experiment. Occasional Paper No. 13. New Delhi: Center for Women's Development Studies.

McCaffey (1999, February 24). Available at http://www.csdp.org/publicservice/troubled.htm. Accessed July 17, 2015.

McClelland DC (1953). *The Achievement Motive*. New York: Appleton.

McClelland A (1961). *The Achieving Society*. Princeton, NJ: D. Van Nostrand.

McClelland DC & Winter DG (1969). *Motivating Economic Achievement*. New York: Free Press.

McClelland DC (1953). *The Achievement Motive*. New York: Appleton.

McClelland DC (1988). *Human Motivation*. London: Cambridge University Press.

McFarlane J & Fehir J (1994). De Madres a Madres: A community, primary health care program based on empowerment. *Health Educ Q., 21*(3), 381–394.

McGinnis JM & Foege WH (1993). Actual causes of death in the United States. *JAMA, 270*(18), 2207–2212.

McKnight JL (1978). Community health in a Chicago slum. *Dev Dialogue, 1*, 62–68.

McKnight JL (1997). *Keynote address on resource-based community development. Conference on Community Campus Partnerships for Health (CCPH)*. San Francisco, CA: CCPH: UCSF.

McLeroy KR, Bibeau D, Steckler A, & Glanz K (1988, Winter). An ecological perspective on health promotion programs. *Health Educ Q.*, 1988, 15(4), 351–377. Available at http://www.ncbi.nlm.nih.gov/pubmed/3068205)

MDG Funds (2008). *Winning Rights for Brazil's Domestic Workers*. Available at http://www.mdgfund.org/node/3693. Accessed July10, 2015.

Medicinenet (2013). Available at http://www.medicinenet.com/script/main/art.asp?articlekey=169013. Accessed July 20, 2015.

MELA (2015). The Goldman Environmental Foundation. Available at http://www.goldmanprize.org/recipient/aurora-castillo/. Accessed December 29, 2015.

Menchú R (1983). *I Rigoberta Menchu: An Indian Woman in Guatemala*. London: Verso.

Michel A (1995). Militarisation of contemporary societies and feminism in the north. In: Ashworth G (Ed.), *A Diplomacy of the Oppressed: New Directions in International Feminism*. Atlantic Heights, NJ: Zed Books:49.

Millennium Development Goals Achievement Fund (MDG-F) (2012). *Advancing Gender Equality: Promising Practices*. Available at http://www.unwomen.org/mdgf/downloads/MDG-F_Case-Studies.pdf. Accessed July 16, 2015.

Minkler M & Roe KM (2004, November). Grandmothers as care givers: Raising children of the crack cocaine epidemic. *J Fam Iss., 25*, 1005–1025.

Minkler M (1992). Community organizing with elderly poor in San Francisco's Tenderloin District. In: M Minkler (Ed.), *Community Organizing and Community Building for Health* (2nd edn). New Brunswick, NJ: Rutgers University Press:272–287.

Mitra S (1982). Hole in the Wall Beginnings. Available at http://www.hole-in-the-wall.com/Beginnings.html. Accessed August 3, 2015.

Mitra S (2007). TED award talk (video). Available at http://www.ted.com/talks/sugata_mitra_shows_how_kids_teach_themselves?language=en. Accessed August 3, 2015.

Mittal S (2013, April 27–28). The Role of CBO in Social Protection—Some Experiences of the Self-Employed Women's Association (SEWA), India. Paper presented at the Rethinking Economy: Social/Solidarity Economy in China and the World conference, Beijing, China. Available at http://wiego.org/sites/wiego.org/files/publications/files/Shah_Mittal_SEWA_2013.pdf. Accessed July 14, 2015.

Mittlemark M, Akerman M, GillisD, et al. (2001). Health Promotion and Chronic Disease: Building on the Ottawa Charter, Not Betraying It? *Mexico Conference on*

Health Promotion, 16(1). Oxford University Press:3–4. Available at heapro.oxford-journals.org/content/16/3/215.full.pdf. Accessed January 9, 2016.

Mizan AN (1994). *In Quest of Empowerment: The Grameen Bank's Impact on Women's Power and Status.* Dhaka: University Press.

Moghadam VM (1994). *Identity, Politics, and Women: Cultural Reassessment and Feminism in International Perspective.* Boulder, CO: Westview Press

Mondal WI & Peters MR (2012, April–June). Microcredit at a crossroads: A question of principled leadership. (Story of Patisar and Kaligram Krishi Bank.) *Integral Leadersh Rev.* Available at http://integralleadershipreview.com/author/wali-i-mondal-and-mark-r-peters/. Accessed August 4, 2015.

Monte T & the Editors of East West Natural Health (1993). *World Medicine—The East West Guide to Healing Your Body.* Los Angeles: Jeremy P. Tarcher/Perigee Books.

Moon B (2014, March 26). International Women's Day: Equality for Women is Progress for All. *Harare.* Available at http://www.zw.one.un.org/newsroom/news/international-women%E2%80%99s-day-equality-women-progress-all. Accessed June 10, 2015.

Moore M (2000). *Safer Motherhood 2000,Convening the Communication and Media for Development Community.* The Communication Initiative Network. Available at http://www.comminit.com/global/content/safer-motherhood-2000. Accessed July 31, 2015.

Moser C (1987). Women, human settlements, and housing: A conceptual framework for analysis and policy-analysis. In: Moser C & Peake L (Eds), *Women, Human Settlements, and Housing.* London: Tavistock:481–482.

Moser C (1991). Barrio Indio Guayas, Guayaquil, Ecuador. In: Sontheimer S (Ed.), *Women and the Environment: A Reader. Crisis Development in the Third World.* New York: Monthly Review Press:146.

Moser C (1993). *Gender Planning and Development: Theory, Practice and Training.* London: Routledge.

Mothers Against Drunk Driving (MADD) (2015). Available at http://www.madd.org. Accessed February 14, 2014.

Mothers Against Violence (MAV). *MAV: UK.* Available at http://mavuk.org/ and https://www.youtube.com/watch?v=oZvcqI_iVMg. Accessed July 21, 2015.

Mothers' Voices (2015). Available at http://www.mvgeorgia.org/. Accessed July 17, 2015.

MSNBC (2013). Available at http://www.msnbc.com/all/california-did-tough-gun-control-laws-cut. Accessed July 20, 2015.

Muñoz-Vázquez M (1996). Gender and politics: Grassroots leadership among Puerto Rican women in a health struggle. In: Ortiz A (Ed.), *Puerto Rican Women and Work: Bridges in Transnational Labor.* Philadelphia, PA: Temple University Press:56–71.

Murthi M, Guio A, & Drèze J (1995). Fertility and gender bias in India: A district-level analysis. *Popul Dev Rev.,* 21(4), 745–782.

Nair GB & Narain JP (2010). From endotoxin to exotoxin: De's rich legacy to cholera. *Bull WHO,*88, 237–240, doi: 10.2471/BLT.09.0725.

Narayana P (1675/2005). *Hitopedesha* ("Beneficial Advice"), originally in Sanskrit. Translated by Chandramoni GL (Ed.) (2005). Mumbai, India: Jaico:35.

Narika (2009). Available at http://2009.artsinsociety.com/index.html.

Narika (n.d.). Available at http://www.narika.org/. Accessed January 6, 2016.

National Alliance for Hispanic Health (NAHH). Available at http://www.hispani-chealth.org/. Accessed July 18, 2015.

National Alliance on Mental Illness (NAMI) (2012). *Program Evaluation Report.* Available at https://www.nami.org/About-NAMI. Accessed July 17, 2015.

National Asian Pacific American Women's Forum (2015). Available at https://napawf.org/about/contact/.

National Asian Pacific American Women's Forum (NAPAWF) (2015). Available at http://www.napawf.org/. Accessed July 10, 2015.

National Asian Women's Health Organization (NAWHO) (2013). Available at http://www.nawho.org/. Accessed February 14, 2015.

National Black Women's Health Project (NBWHP) (2009). *National Latina Health Organization. 1998–1999 Annual Report.* Oakland, CA.

National Black Women's Health Project (NBWHP) (2015). Available at https://en.wikipedia.org/wiki/National_Black_Women%27s_Health_Project. Accessed July 18, 2015.

National Center for Complementary and Alternative Medicine (NCCAM) (2015). NCCIH Pub No.: D347. Available at https://nccih.nih.gov/health/integrative-health.

National Center for Educational Research and Technology (NCERT) (n.d.). Memorial Lecture Series. New Delhi, India: NCERT.

National Council of Women's Organizations (NCWO) (2015). Available at http://www.womensorganizations.org/index.php?option=com_content&view=article&id=2&Itemid=3. Accessed July 18, 2015.

National Eating Disorders Associations (NEDA) (2015). Available at http://www.nationaleatingdisorders.org/. Accessed July 18, 2015.

National Institutes of Health (NIH) (2012). Available at https://www.nlm.nih.gov/exhibition/survivingandthriving/digitalgallery/detail-A027784.html. Accessed July 20, 2015.

National Institutes of Health (NIH)/National Cancer Institute (NCI) (2005). *Theories at a Glance: A Guide for Health Promotion Practice* (2nd edn). Washington, DC: U.S. Department of Health and Human Services.

National Institutes of Health (NIH)/OBSSR (2015). *Ecological Models.* Available at http://www.sfu.ca/uploads/page/26/GERO820_2012_ECOLOGICAL_MODELS.pdf. Accessed December 28, 2015.

National Latino Health Organization (NLHO) (2015). Available at http://www.migrant-clinician.org/toolsource/resource/national-latino-health-organization-nlho.html. Accessed July 18, 2015.

National Organization of Women (NOW) (1966). *Statement of Purpose.* Available at http://now.org/about/history/statement-of-purpose/. Accessed July 2015.

National Organization of Women (NOW) web site (2012). Available at http://www.now.org. Accessed August 4, 2015.

Native American Community Board (NACB) (1993, November). Health Survey for Yankton Sioux Reservation Community, Health Order #409. Posted on December 7, 2010. Available at http://www.cbc.ca/news/canada/north/yukon-health-care-survey-worked-official-1.958030. Accessed January 2016.

Native Shop home page (2008, December 21). Available at http://www.nativeshop.org/index.html.

New York Times (2012, April 15). Lester Breslow, Who Linked Healthy Habits and Long Life, Dies at 97, p. A20.

Nguyen TUN, Kagawa-Singer M, & Kar S (2003). *Multicultural Health Evaluation: Literature Review and Critique*. Los Angeles, CA: California Endowment.

Noer M (2012). One Man, One Computer, 10 Million Students: How Khan Academy Is Reinventing Education. *Forbes*. Available at http://www.forbes.com/sites/michael-noer/2012/11/02/one-man-one-computer-10-million-students-how-khan-academy-is-reinventing-education/. Accessed August 3, 2015.

Norsigian J, Diskin V, Doress-Worters P, Pincus J, Sanford W, & Swenson N (1999, Winter). The Boston Women's Health Book Collective and Our Bodies, Ourselves: A brief history and reflection. *J Am Med Women Assoc.*, Special Issue, 54(1):35–38.

Nozick R (1974). *Anarchy, State, and Utopia*. Oxford, UK: Blackwell.

Nuyen T, Kagawa-Singer M, & Kar SB (2003). *Multicultural health evaluation*. Oakland, CA: California Endowment.

Nyswander D (1966). Open Society August 2013—Society for Public Health. Available at www.sophe.org/APPL_Open_Society_August_2013.pdf.

Nzo A (1994). *South Africa's Post-Apartheid Foreign Policy. Alfred Nzo has been Minister of Foreign Affairs between 1994 and 1998. For Post-Apartheid Foreign Policy, see Obituary of Alfred Nzo by African National Congress*. Available at http://www.anc.org.za/show.php?id=7301.

O'Connell K (2010). Rabindranath Tagore: Envisioning Humanistic Education at Santiniketan (1902–1922). *Int J Humanistic Ideology*, 2, 15–42.

O'Connell KM (2002). *Rabindranath Tagore: The Poet as Educator*. Kolkata: Visva Bharati.

O'Connell KM (2003). Rabindranath Tagore on education. In: *The Encyclopaedia of Informal Education*. Available at http://infed.org/mobi/rabindranath-tagore-on-education/. Accessed August 4, 2015.

Oakland Tribune (1992, May 12). The Gray Crusader: Lillian Rabinowitz Forces the Needs of the Elderly into the Public Light.

Occupational Safety and Health Administration (OSHA) (1994). Program Narrative (PHS-5151-1). Building Health and Independence: A New Geriatric Facility for Lifelong Medical Care. Available at https://www.osha.gov/html/Feed_Back.html and https://www.whitehouse.gov/the-press-office/2015/07/13/fact-sheet-white-house-conference-aging. Accessed August 4, 2015.

OHSC (1994–1995, Fall//Winter). *Health and Aging*.

Organismo Nacional del Menor, Mujer y Familia (ONAMFA; National Organization of Minors, Women and Family). Available at https://books.google.com.bo/books/about/ONAMFA_Regional_Santa_Cruz.html?id=aaIutwAACAAJ. Accessed July 16, 2015.

Orley J & Kuyken W (Eds) (1994). *Quality of Life Assessment: International Perspectives WHOQOL Group. The Development of the WHO Quality of Life Assessment Instruments (the WHOQOL)*. Berlin: Springer-Verlag:41–57.

Ortiz A (Ed.) (1996). *Puerto Rican Women and Work: Bridges in Transnational Labor*. Philadelphia: Temple University Press:161–180.

Ortiz I & Cummings M (2011). Global Inequality: Beyond the Bottom Billion—A Rapid Review of Income Distribution in 141 Countries. UNICEF working paper.

Available at www.unicef.org/socialpolicy/files/Global_Inequality.pdf. Accessed January 9, 2016.

OSHC Program Narrative (PHS-5151-1) (n.d.). *Building Health and Independence: A New Geriatric Facility for Lifelong Medical Care.* Available at http://www.lifelongmedical.org/services/senior-independence. Accessed January 9, 2016.

Oteri M (2015). Available at https://evanstoncommunitykitchen.wordpress.com/about/. Accessed July 15, 2015.

Ottawa Charter for Health Promotion (1986). *An International Conference on Health Promotion, Ottawa, Canada.* Geneva: WHO.

Our Bodies, Ourselves (OBOS) (1972). Boston Women's Health Book Collective (BWHBC). Preface. New York: Simon & Schuster. Available at http://www.ourbodiesourselves.org/global-projects/usa-latin-america-collaboration/preface-nuestros-cuerpos-nuestras-vidas/. Accessed July 16, 2015.

Our Bodies, Ourselves (OBOS) (2015). Our bodies ourselves. Available at http://www.ourbodiesourselves.org/2015/10/a-message-from-gloria-lena-obos/. Accessed January 6, 2016.

Over 60 Health Center (OSHC) (2014). Available at http://www.berkeleyside.com/2014/03/04/years-of-work-culminate-in-new-berkeley-medical-clinic/. Accessed July 19, 2015.

Over 60 Health Center (OSHC) (2015). Available at http://gis.oshpd.ca.gov/atlas/places/facility/306014161. Accessed February 6, 2015.

Over 60 Health Center (OSHC) (n.d.) Available at http://www.berkeleyside.com/tag/the-over-60-health-center/. Accessed July 19, 2015.

Pardo M (1997). Mexican American women grassroots community activists: Mothers of East Los Angeles. In: Jameson E & Armitage S (Eds), *Writing the Range: Race, Class, and Culture in the Women's West.* Norman: University of Oklahoma Press:553–568.

Park HJ et al. (1974). *Mothers' Club and Family Planning in Korea.* Seoul: Seoul National University.

Park HJ, Kincaid DL, Chung KK, Han DS, & Lee SB (1976, October). The Korean Mothers' Club Program. *Stud Fam Plan.,* 7(10), 275–283.

Parker D (1999). *Health, Civilization, and the State: A History of Public Health from Ancient to Modern Times.* New York: Routledge.

Parrillo VN & Donoghue C (2005). Updating the Bogardus social distance studies: A new national survey. *Soc Sci J.,* 42(2), 257–271.

Parsons T, Tolman E, & Sills E (1935). *The Structure of Social Action.* New York: Free Press.

Parsons T, Shils E, & Tolman C (1951). *Toward a General Theory of Action.* Cambridge, MA: Harvard University Press.

Paulson S & Bailey P (2003). Culturally constructed relationships shape sexual and reproductive health and health care in Bolivia. *Culture Health Sexual.,* 5(6), 483–498.

Paulson S (2000, April). Cultural bodies in Bolivia's gendered environment. *Int J Sexual Gender Stud.,* 5(2), 125–140.

Paulson S, Gisbert ME, & Quinton M (1996). *Case Studies of Two Women's Health Projects in Bolivia.* International Women's Study Project No. 96-04. Triangle Park, NC: Family Health International. Available at http://www.fhi.org/en/RH/Pubs/wsp/caseSTudies/BoliviaCS.htm. Accessed December 28, 2015.

Paulson S, Gisbert ME, & Quiton M (1996, December). Triangle Park, North Carolina, Family Health International. Family Health International Women's Studies Project No. 96-04. Available at http://www.popline.org/node/306664. Accessed July 16, 2015.

Pearson NK (1993). The story of two self-help organizations: Women for the survival of agriculture and farmworkers Self-Help, Inc. In: Young G, Samarsinghe V, & Kusterer K (Eds), *Women at the Center: Development Issues and Practices in the 1990s*. Hartford, CT: Kumarian Press:94–103.

Penn N, Kar SB, Kramer J, Skinner J, & Zambrana R (1995). Ethnic minorities, health care systems, and behavior. *Health Psychol.*, 14(7), 641–646.

People Assisting the Homeless (PATH). Available at http://www.epath.org/site/main. html. Accessed February 15, 2015.

Periera I (2013, August 6). Rising number of dowry deaths in India: NCRB. *The Hindu*, front page headline.

Perkins DD & Zimmerman MA (1995). Empowerment theory, research, and application. *Am J Commun Psychol.*, 23(5), 569–579.

PEW Research Center (1993, February). *Health Professions Education for the Future: Schools in the Service to the Nation*. San Francisco, CA: Report of the PEW Health Professions Commission.

PEW Research Center (2013). *The World's Muslims: Religion, Politics and Society*. Available at http://www.pewforum.org/2013/04/30/the-worlds-muslims-religion-politics-society-women-in-society/. Accessed 2015.

PEW Research Center (2014). PEW Research Internet Project. Available at http://www. pewInternet.org/2013/12/30/social-media-update-2013/.

PEW Research Center (PRC) (2015, January 9). *Growing Public Support for Gun Rights*. Available at http://www.pewresearch.org/fact-tank/2015/01/09/a-public-opinion-trend-that-matters-priorities-for-gun-policy/ Accessed July 20, 2015.

Piero A, Raven B, Amato C, & Belanger JJ (2013). Bases of social power, leadership styles, and organizational commitment. *Int J Psychol.*, 48(6), 1122–1134.

Piketty T (2014). *Capital in the Twenty-First Century*. Cambridge, MA: Belknap Press.

Pilisuk M, McAllister J, & Rothman J (1996). Coming together for action: The challenge of contemporary grassroots community organizing. *J Soc Iss.*, 52(1), 15–37.

Pillsbury B & Andina M (1998). Trust: An approach to women's empowerment. "Let women's organizations just do it." Los Angeles: Pacific Institute for Women's Health Working Paper Series.

Pineo RF (1996). *Social and Economic Reform in Ecuador: Life and Work in Guayaquil*. Gainesville: University Press of Florida.

PIWH (0000). Available at http://www.piwh.org/. Accessed July 19, 2015.

Planned Parenthood vs Casey (1992). Available at https://en.wikipedia.org/wiki/Planned_Parenthood_v._Casey. Accessed July 16,2015 and http://en.wikipedia.org/wiki/Webster_v._Reproductive_Health_Services. Accessed February 13, 2015.

Population Reference Bureau (PRB) (2012). *The Decline in U.S. Fertility*. Available at www.prb.org/Publications/Articles/2012/us-fertility.aspx.Accessed July 28, 2015.

Porter M & Stern S (2014). *Social Progress Index, Executive Summary*. Washington, DC: Social Progress Imperatives.

Prahalad CK (2006). *The Fortune at the Bottom of the Pyramid: Eradicating Poverty Through Profits*. Upper Saddle River, NJ: Wharton School.

Prigogine I & Stengers I (1984). Foreword by Alvin Toffler. *Order Out of Chaos: Man's New Dialogue with Nature*. New York: Bantam Books.

Prototype (2015). Available at https://www.prototypes.org/treatment-programs/success-stories/. Accessed July 19, 2015.

Puska P, Nissinen AA, Toumilehto J, et al. (1996). Community-based strategy to prevent heart disease: Conclusions from the 10 years of the North Karelia Project. *Health Promotion Anthology*, Scientific Publication No. 557. Washington, DC: PAHO/WHO:97.

Ramakrishna, S (2010). Parable of lake and water, cited by Goldberg P (2010). *American Veda*. New York: Harmony Books:69.

Randall M (1994). *Sandino's Daughters Revisited: Feminism in Nicaragua*. New Brunswick, NJ: Rutgers University Press.

Randall M (1997). *Hunger's Table: Women, Food and Politics*. London: Papier-Mache Press.

Rao MM (2004). The battle of the bottle in Andhra Pradesh. *Hindu: The Online Edition*, posted on March 27, 2004. Available at http://www.thehindu.com/2004/03/27/stories/2004032707371200.htm. Accessed January 4, 2016.

Rao R (1990). Doon Valley: A significant ecological triumph. *Ambio.*, 19(5), 274–275.

Rao SB & Parthasarathy G (Eds) (1997). *Anti-Arrack Movement of Women in Andhra Pradesh and Prohibition Policy*. New Delhi: Har-Anand.

Rappaport J (1981). In praise of paradox: A social policy of empowerment over prevention. *Amer J Commun Psychol.*, 9(1), 1P25.

Rappaport J (1984). Studies in empowerment: Introduction to the issue. *Prev Hum Serv.*, 3(2), 1–7.

Rappaport J (1987). Terms of empowerment/exemplars of prevention: Toward a theory for community psychology. *Am J Commun Psychol.*, 15(2), 121–148.

Raturi G (2015). *The Chipko Movement*. Available at http://edugreen.teri.res.in/explore/forestry/chipko.htm. Accessed July 14, 2015.

Raven B (1992). A power interaction model on interpersonal influence: French and Raven thirty years later. *J Soc Behav Personal.*, 7(2), 217–244.

Raven B (2008). The bases of power and the power/interaction model of interpersonal influence. *Analyses Soc Issue Public Policy*, 8(1), 1–22.

Raven BH (2012). Power, Six Bases of. *Encyclopedia of Leadership*. Thousand Oaks, CA: Sage:1242–1249.

Rawls J (1971). Social unity and primary goods. In: Rawls J (Ed.), *A Theory of Justice*. Cambridge, MA: Harvard University Press.

Rawls J (1999). *A Theory of Justice* (rev edn). Cambridge, MA: Harvard University Press. Available at http://plato.stanford.edu/entries/rawls/. Accessed August 4, 2015.

Reddy DN & Patnaik A (1993). Anti-Arrak Movement in Andhra Pradesh. *Econ Polit Weekly*, 28(21), 1059–1066.

Reichenbach BR (1988, October). The Law of Karma and the principle of causation. *Philos E W.*, 38(4), 399–410.

Renaud S & De Lorgeril M (1992). Wine, alcohol, platelets, and the French paradox for coronary heart disease. *Lancet,* 339, 1523–1526. Available at http://www.ncbi.nlm.nih.gov/pmc/articles/PMC1768013/.

Reynolds J (1972, February). Evaluation of family planning program performance: A critical review. *Demography*, 9(1), 69–86.

Rice AL, Sacco L, Hyder A, & Black RE (2000). Malnutrition as an underlying cause of childhood deaths associated with infectious diseases in developing countries. *Bull World Health Organ.*, 78(10), 1207–1221. Available at http://www.ncbi.nlm.nih.gov/pmc/articles/PMC2560622/. Accessed July 30, 2015.

Rice AV (1947). *A History of the World's Young Women's Christian Association.* New York: Woman's Press.

Rigzin T (2014). Kerala: An anomalous case of development. *Int J Peace Educ Dev.*, 2(2 and 3), 107–110.

Rogers EM (1973). *Communication Strategies for Family Planning.* New York: Free Press.

Rojas M (1997, January 31 to February 13). Mental wellness. *LA Weekly*, W-6.

Rose K (1992). *Where Women Are Leaders: The SEWA Movement in India.* London: Zed Books.

Rose K (1993). *Where Women Are Leaders: The Story of SEWA (Self-Employed Women's Association).*Trenton, NJ: Humanities Press.

Rosen G (1993/1958). *A History of Public Health.* Baltimore, MD: Johns Hopkins University Press.

Ross LJ (2006). *Voices of Feminism, Oral History Project.* Sophia Smith Collection. Northampton, MA: Smith College.

Rossi PH, Berk RA, & Lenihan KJ (1980) *Experimental Evidence.* Available at https://www.ncjrs.gov/App/publications/abstract.aspx?ID=81280.

Rostow WW (1960). *The Stages of Economic Growth.* Cambridge, UK: Cambridge University Press.

Rothman J & Tropman JE (1987). Models of community organization and macro practice perspectives: Their mixing and phasing. In: Cox FM, et al. (Eds), *Strategies of Community Organization* (4th edn). Itasca, IL; Peacock:3–26.

Roy A (1999). *Greater Common Goods.* Bombay, India: India Book Distributor.

Roy A (2001). *Power Politics.* Cambridge: MA: South End Press.

Roy A (2014). Is India on a Totalitarian Path? Available at http://www.democracynow.org/2014/4/9/is_india_on_a_totalitarian_path. Accessed December 27, 2015.

Rushdie S (1981). *Midnight's Children.* London: Jonathon Cape.

Russell, DEH (1991). *Lives of Courage, Women for a New South Africa.* New York: Basic Books.

Ryukyu Shinpou (local newspaper) (1995, October 22). 80,000 at anti-base rally.

Saavedra L (2013). *ILO and FAO 2013 (International Labor Organization and Food and Agricultural Organizations), Food, Agriculture, and Decent Work , ILO and FAO Working Together.* Available at http://www.fao-ilo.org/more/fao-ilo-ruralworkers/en/. Accessed July 10, 2015.

Saighal V (2008, June 29, Sunday). Field Marshall Sam Manekshaw. *The Guardian*, India. Available at http://www.theguardian.com/world/2008/jun/30/india. Accessed December 20, 2015.

Sakhi (1989). Available at http://www.sakhi.org/about-sakhi/mission-and-history/. Accessed July 19, 2015.

Sakhi (2015). Impact Report 2015. Available at http://sakhiimpactreport2015.tumblr.com/. Accessed January 4, 2015.

Salud Ambiental Lideres Tomando Accion (SALTA) (2015). Available at http://www.environmentalhealth.org/index.php/en/what-we-do/leadership-development/salta. Accessed February 15, 2015.

Sanjek R (2009). *Gray Panthers*. Philadelphia, PA: University of Pennsylvania Press.

Sarveswara Rao B & Parthasarathy G (Eds) (1997). *Anti-Arrack Movement of Women in Andhra Pradesh and Prohibition Policy*. New Delhi: Har-Anand.

Schofield JW (1995). Review of research on school desegregation's impact on elementary and secondary school students. In Banks JA & Banks CAM (Eds), *Handbook of Research on Multicultural Education*. New York: Macmillan:597–616.

Scrimshaw N (2013, February). *Nevin S. Scrimshaw, Pioneer Nutritionist, Dies at 95.* Available at http://www.nytimes.com/2013/02/13/us/nevin-s-scrimshaw-pioneer-nutritionist-dies-at-95.html.

Scrimshaw S & Hurtado E (1987). *Rapid Assessment Procedures for Nutrition and Primary Health Care: Anthropological Approaches to Improving Program Effectiveness (RAP)*. UCLA, CA: Latin American Studies Center, University of California.

Scrimshaw S (2006). Culture, behavior, and health. In: Merson MH, Black R, & Mills AJ (Eds), *International Public Health* (2nd edn). London: Jones & Bartlett:43–70.

Scrimshaw SM & Hurtado E (1987). *Rapid Assessment Procedures for Nutrition and Primary Health Care*. Los Angeles: University of California Press.

Self-Employed Women's Association (SEWA) & Selliah S (1989). *The Self-Employed Women's Association*. Ahmedabad, India: Geneva, ILO.

Self-Employed Women's Association (SEWA) (1995). *Self-Employed Women's Association: Annual Report 1995*. Ahmedabad, India: SEWA.

Self-Employed Women's Association (SEWA) (2009) web site. Available at http://www.sewa.org. Accessed August 4, 2015.

Self-Employed Women's Association (SEWA) (2015). Home page. Available at http://www.sewa.org/. Accessed July 14, 2015.

Selliah S (1989). *The Self-Employed Women's Association*. Ahmedabad, India. Geneva: International Labour Office.

Selliah S (1989). *The Self-Employed Women's Association*. Geneva: ILO.

Sen A (1983). *Poverty and Famines: An Essay on Entitlement and Deprivation*. Oxford, UK: Oxford Scholarship Online.

Sen A (1990). Gender and cooperative conflicts. In: Tinker I (Ed.), *Persistent Inequalities: Women and World Development*. New York: Oxford University Press:123–149.

Sen A (1991). *The Kerala Difference, The* New York Review of Books. Response to Chasin and Frankie. Available at http://www.nybooks.com/articles/archives/1991/oct/24/the-kerala. Accessed July 30, 2015.

Sen A (1992). Missing women. *BMJ*, 304, 586–587.

Sen A (1998). *The Possibility of a Social Choice*. Nobel Award lecture. Available at http://www.nobelprize.org/nobel_prizes/economic-sciences/laureates/1998/sen-lecture.pdf. Accessed December 20, 2015.

Sen A (1999). *Development as Freedom*. New York: Alfred A. Knopf.

Sen A (2001, November 19). Many faces of gender inequality. *Frontline*, 2001, 18, 4–14. Available at www.hinduonnet.com/fline/fl1822/18220040.htm. Accessed September 15, 2003.

Sen A (2003, December). Missing women—revisited: Reduction in female mortality has been counterbalanced by sex selective abortions. *BMJ*, 6, 327(7427), 1297–1298, doi:10.1136/bmj.327.7427.1297.

Sen A (2006a). *The Argumentative Indian.* New York: Picador.

Sen A (2006b). *Identity and Violence: The Illusion of Destiny.* London: Allen Lane.

Senge P (2006). *The Fifth Discipline: The Art and Practice of the Learning Organizations.* New York: DoubleDay.

SG (2014). *The Health Consequences of Smoking—50 Years of Progress: A Report of the Surgeon General, 2014* (The Second Surgeon General's Report on Smoking). Rockville, MD: U.S. Department of Health and Human Services, Office of the Surgeon General. Available at http://www.surgeongeneral.gov/library/reports/50-years-of-progress/. Accessed May 22, 2015.

Shah S (2014, November 28). Gloria Steinem versus prostitution in India, The World Post. *The Huffington Post* (US edition). Available at http://www.huffingtonpost.com/american-anthropological-association/gloria-steinem-vs-prostit_b_6198614.html. Accessed December 29, 2015.

Sharma K & Zodpey S (2011). Public health in India: Need and demand paradox. *Indian J Commun Med., 36*(3), doi: 10.4103/0970-0218.86516. Available at http://www.frontiersin.org/profile/publications/22090669.

Shiva V (2002). *Staying Alive: Women, Ecology, and Development* (8th edn). New Delhi, India: Zed.

Shiva V (1993, December 9). Diversity and Freedom. Acceptance Speech of the Right Livelihood Award. Available at www.rightlivelihood.org/v-shiva.html. Accessed August 4, 2015.

Shiva V (2011). Organic Solutions to Hunger and Malnutrition. Acceptance Speech of Honorary Doctorate Degree from University of Oslow. Available at http://www.uio.no/english/research/interfaculty-research-areas/leve/newsevents/events/2011/0901-vandana-shiva-honorary-speach.html. Accessed August 4, 2015.

Shiva V (2013a). A Conversation with Vandana Shiva—Question 3—Treehugging and the Chipko Movement. Video available at https://www.youtube.com/watch?v=i3EDEqr7haU

Shiva V (2013b). Common Dreams. Available at http://www.commondreams.org/author/vandana-shiva. Accessed August 4, 2015.

Short D (2014, September 25). Happiness revisited: A Household Income of $75K? *Advisor Perspective.* Available at http://www.advisorperspectives.com/dshort/commentaries/Happiness-Benchmark.php. Accessed July 25, 2015.

Shumaker SK & Berzon R (Eds) (1995). *The International Assessment of Health-Related Quality of Life: Theory, Translation, Measurement and Analysis.* London: Oxford Rapid Communications.

Sibelius K (2014). *Smoking—50 Years of Progress: A Report of the Surgeon General, Executive Summary.* Rockville, MD: U.S. Department of Health and Human Services, Public Health Service Office of the Surgeon General:1.

Simon JM (1984). *Guatemala: The Group for Mutual Support.* Available at http://ssrn.com/abstract=2329201 or http://dx.doi.org/10.2139/ssrn.2329201.

Simon JM (1987). *Guatemala: Eternal Spring—Eternal Tyranny.* New York: W.W. Norton:159, 161.

Simon JM (graduate of Harvard Law School) (May 25, 2014). *Was There Genocide in Guatemala?* (May 25, 2014). Available at http://hablaguate.com/recordings/133-was-there-genocide-in-guatemala. Accessed January 9, 2016.

Singh N (1991). The Bankura story: Rural women organize for change. In: Sontheimer S (Ed.), *Women and the Environment: A Reader. Crisis and Development in the Third World*. New York: Monthly Review Press:179–205. Available at http://www.popline.org/node/342685. Accessed July 14, 2015.

Sinha K (2014, August 18). UK researchers unravel reasons behind India's farmer suicides (reported in the *Times of India*). Available at http://timesofindia.indiatimes.com/world/uk/UK-researchers-unravel-reasons-behind-Indias-farmer-suicides/articleshow/33878275.cms. Accessed December 28, 2015.

Sisters Network (1994). Available at www.sistersnetworkinc.org. Accessed July 20, 2015.

Skinner BF (1953). *Science and Human Behavior*. New York: Free Press.

Smith H (1991). *The World's Religions: Our Great Wisdom Traditions*. New York: Harper Collins.

Smith MK (2010). *Kurt Lewin: Groups, Experiential Learning and Action Research*. Available at http://www.infed.org/thinkers/et-lewin.htm/. Accessed August 4, 2015.

Solomon BB (1977). *Black Empowerment: Social Work in Oppressed Communities*. New York: Columbia University Press.

Sontheimer S (Ed.) (1991). *Women and the Environment: A Reader. Crisis and Development in the Third World*. New York: Monthly Review Press.

SOS CORPO ("Safe city for Women") (2015). Available at http://www.palgrave-journals.com/development/journal/v54/n3/full/dev201161a.html. Accessed July 10, 2015.

South Carolina AIDS Education Network (SCAEN) (2015). Available at https://en.wikipedia.org/wiki/DiAna_DiAna. Accessed July 20, 2015.

Squatriglia C (1995, May 31). Health Center Chief Leads Way in Caring for the Elderly Poor. *West County Times*.

SRS: Government of India (2012). *SRS Statistical Report 2012*. New Delhi, India. Available at http://www.censusindia.gov.in/vital_statistics/SRS_Reports_2012.html. Accessed January 21, 2014.

States E (2014). A Discussion of the Impact of Political and Economic Forces on Equitable Access to Potable Water in Ecuador and Recommendations for Improvement through Better Watershed Management. Pitzer Senior Theses, Paper 52. Available at http://scholarship.claremont.edu/pitzer_theses/52. Accessed July 13, 2015.

Stead M (1991). Women, war and underdevelopment in Nicaragua. In: Afshar H (Ed.), *Women, Development, and Survival in the Third World*. New York: Longman:53–87.

Steinem G (1992). *Revolution from Within: A Book of Self-Esteem*. Boston: Little, Brown.

Steinem G (2012). Speeches: Gloria Steinem on combating sex trafficking. Posted by Apne Ap. Available at http://apneaap.org/speeches-gloria-steinem-on-combating-sex-trafficking. Accessed December 26, 2015.

Step Up on 2nd (2014). Newsletter, 7(2). Permanent Supportive Housing, Santa Monica, CA:1–2. Available at http://www.stepuponsecond.org/services/home/. Accessed December 28, 2015.

Stephen L (1997). *Women and Social Movement in Latin America: Power from Below*. Austin, TX: University of Texas Press.

Stephenson H & Zeldes K (2008, October). Write a chapter and change the world. How the Boston Women's Health Book Collective transformed women's health then—and now. *Am J Public Health*, 98(10), 1741–1745 (Abstract).

Stolen KA & Vaa M (Eds) (1991). *Gender and Change in Developing Countries.* Oslo: Norwegian University Press.

Stone AA, Schwartz J, Broderick, & Deaton A (2010). A snapshot of the age distribution of psychological well-being in the United States. *Proc Natl Acad Sci USA*, 107(22), 9985–9990, doi: 10.1073/pnas.1003744107.

Stringer ET (1999). *Action Research* (2nd ed.). Thousand Oaks, CA: Sage.

Stromquist N (1990). Women's education in development: From welfare to empowerment. *INNOTECH J.*, 14(1), 78–84.

Summers L (2014a, Spring). The Inequality Puzzle: Piketty book review. *Democracy*, 32, 1. Available at http://larrysummers.com/2014/05/14/piketty-book-review-the-inequality-puzzle/#sthash.aeWkF6vZ.dpuf. Accessed December 28, 2015.

Summers L (2014b, Summer). Review of Thomas Piketty's book: Capital in the twenty-first century. *Democracy*, 33.

Summers LH (1992). Investing in all the people: Educating women in developing countries. Paper presented at the Development Economics Seminar, 1992 Annual Meeting of the World Bank:2–7. Available at http://faculty.ucr.edu/~jorgea/econ181/summers_women94.pdf. Accessed August 4, 2015.

Sumpter B (1990). We have a job to do. In: *The ACT UP/NY Women and AIDS Book Group Women, AIDS, and Activism.* Boston, MA: South End Press:223–224.

Swendeman D, Basu I, Das S, Jana S, and Rotheram-Borusa (2009), Empowering sex workers in India to reduce vulnerability to HIV and sexually transmitted diseases Soc Sci Med. 2009 Oct; 69(8): 1157–1166.

Tagore R (1905). Micro Finance Initiative: Kaligram Krishi Bank. Available at http://www.rediff.com/business/report/was-tagore-the-founder-of-microfinance-schemes/20130519.htm.

Tagore R (1913). The Nobel Prize acceptance speech. In: Alam F & Chakravarty R (2011) (Eds). *The Essential Tagore.* Cambridge, MA: Belknap Press:183–186.

Tagore R (1925). On Education. In: *Talks in China.* New Delhi, India: Rupa.

Tagore R (1928). Sriniketan: The Institute of Rural Reconstruction. *Visva Bharati Bull.*, 4:8.

Tagore R (1929, April–July). Ideals of education. *Visva-Bharati Q.*, 73–74.

Tagore R (1966). Visva-Bharati. In: Chakravorti A (Ed.), *Talks in China: A Tagore Reader.* Boston: Beacon.

Tapin-Chinoy S (2015). *Muslim Women's Fund.* Available at http://www.wisemuslimwomen.org/muslimwomen/bio/shahnaz_taplin-chinoy/. Accessed July 11, 2015.

Tennyson RD (1999). *Instruction Development Methodology.* Available at Wiley Online Library, http://onlinelibrary.wiley.com/doi/10.1002/pfi.4140380607/abstract. Accessed January 9, 2016.

Terris M (1996). Concepts of health promotion. In: *Health Promotion: An Anthology,* Scientific Publication No. 557. Washington DC: PAHO: World Health Organization.

Terry L (1964). *Surgeon General's Report on Health Consequences of Smoking.* Rockville, MD: U.S. Department of Health and Human Services, Office of the Surgeon General.

The Goldman Environmental Foundation (2015). Available at http://www.goldmanprize.org/recipient/aurora-castillo/. Accessed December 29, 2015.

The Ottawa Charter (1986). Available at http://www.who.int/healthpromotion/conferences/previous/ottawa/en/. Accessed August 4, 2015.

The Pioneer (2014, July 16). State Edition. Available at http://www.dailypioneer.com/state-editions/dehradun/green-leader-chandi-gets-gandhi-peace-prize.html. Accessed July 13, 2015.

The World Facts (2015). Peru. Available at http://worldfacts.us/Peru.htm. Accessed July 15, 2015.

Thin N (1995). *Advancing Women's Status: Gender, Society, and Development: Women and Men Together*. Amsterdam: Royal Tropical Institute (KIT):22–36.

Tickner JA (1992). *Gender in International Relations: Feminist Perspective on Achieving Global Security*. New York: Columbia University Press.

Tinker I (1990a). *Persistent Inequalities: Women and World Development*. New York: Oxford University Press.

Tinker I (1990b). *Towards a Strategy for Full Participation in All Phases of the United Nations Global Strategy for Shelter to the Year 2000*. Nairobi: United Nations Economic Commission for Africa.

Tinker I (1993). Women and shelter: Combining women's roles. In: Young G, Samarsinghe V, & Kusterer K (Eds), *Women at the Center: Development Issues and Practices in the 1990s*. Hartford, CT: Kumarian Press:63–77.

Toubia N (1995). *Female Genital Mutilation: A Call for Global Action*. New York: Rainbow.

Triesman U (1992). Studying students studying calculus: A look at the lives of minority mathematics students in college. *College Math J.*, 23(5), 362–372.

Triesman U (2007). Merit Immersion for Students and Teachers (MIST). Available at http://merit.illinois.edu/educators_treisman.html. Accessed August 4, 2015.

Triandis HC (1993). Collectivism and individualism as cultural syndromes. *Cross Cultural Res.*, 27, 155–180.

Tri-Valley (2015, December 19). Available at http://www.trivalleycares.org/new/. Accessed December 28, 2015.

Tuchman B (1984). *The March of Folly: From Troy to Vietnam*. New York: Random House.

Tula MT (2015). *Disappeared*. RFK Center for Justice and Human Rights. Available at http://rfkcenter.org/maria-teresa-tula-2. Accessed July 2, 2015.

U.S. Department of Commerce (USDC) (2011). *Exploring the Digital Nation: Computer and Internet Use at Home*. Washington, DC: Economics and Statistics Administration and National Telecommunications and Information Administration. Available at https://www.ntia.doc.gov/report/2011/exploring-digital-nation-computer-and-internet-use-home. Accessed January 10, 2016.

UK Essay (1991). Anti-Arrak Movement in Andhra Pradesh. Available at http://www.ukessays.com/essays/history/anti-arrack-movement-in-andhra-pradesh-history-essay.php. Accessed August 4, 2015.

UN Women (2013). *Productive Patrimonial Assets Building and Citizenship Programme for Women in Extreme Poverty*. New York:73–76. Available at http://www.unwomen.org/mdgf/downloads/MDG-F_Case-Studies.pdf. Accessed July 16, 2015..

UN Women (2015). *World's Women Report: Progress of the World's Women: 2014–2015*. Available at http://progress.unwomen.org/en/2015/. Accessed January 7, 2016.

UN:MDG (2015). *Progress Report*. Available at http://progress.unwomen.org/en/2015/pdf/SUMMARY.pdf. Accessed July 29, 2015.

UNDHR (1948). *Universal Declaration of Human Rights, the United Nations*. New York. Available at http://www.un.org/en/universal-declaration-human-rights/index.html. Accessed December 28, 2015.

UNDP (2015). *The Millennium Development Final Report*, New York, Available at United Nations.

UNFPA (2012). *MDG Targets.* Available at http://www.unfpa.org/webdav/site/global/shared/documents/publications/2012/Trends_in_maternal_mortality_A4-1.pdf. Accessed July 28, 2015.

UNFPA (2013). Available at https://www.unfpa.org/gender/docs/Sex_Ratio_by_Country_in_2013.pdf. Accessed February 20, 2015.

UNFPA (2014a). *Adding it Up: Executive Summary.* Available at http://www.unfpa.org/sites/default/files/resource-pdf/AIU3%20Exec%20Summary-ENG-12.2.14.pdf. Accessed July 29, 2014.

UNFPA (2014b). *ICPD Global Report (2014).* Available at http://www.unfpa.org/public/home/sitemap/ICPDReport.

UNICEF (2013). Female Genital Mutilation/Cutting: A statistical overview and exploration of the dynamics of change by UNICEF. Available at http://www.unicef.org/protection/57929_58002.html. Accessed January 10, 2016.

UNICEF(2015). Goal: Reduce child mortality. New York Plaza: UNICEF. Available at http://www.unicef.org/mdg/childmortality.html. Accessed November 4, 2015.

United Nations (2014). *Millennium Development Goals: Gender Charts.* Available at http://mdgs.un.org/unsd/mdg/Resources/Static/Products/Progress2014/GenderChart201'4.pdf.

United Nations (UN) (1948). *Universal Declaration of Human Rights.* Available at http://www.ohchr.org/en/udhr/pages/introduction.aspx. Accessed August 4, 2015.

United Nations (UN) (1995). *Beijing Declaration.* Available at http://www.un.org/geninfo/bp/women.html.

United Nations (UN) (1996). *Beijing Declaration: 1995.* New York: United Nations.

United Nations (UN) (2013). *MDGs—Millennial Development Goals and Beyond 2015.* Available at http://www.un.org/millenniumgoals/. Accessed August 20, 2015.

United Nations (UN) (2014). *Millennium Development Goals and beyond 2015.* Available at http://www.un.org/millenniumgoals/education.shtml. Accessed July 29, 2015.

United Nations (UN) (2015). *The World's Women Report 2010: Trends and Statistics.* Available at http://unstats.un.org/unsd/demographic/products/Worldswomen/WW2010pub.htm. Accessed August 4, 2015.

United Nations (UN) (2016). *World's Women Report: Progress of the World's Women- 2014–2015.* Available at http://progress.unwomen.org/en/2015/. Accessed January 7, 2016.

United Nations (UN) (n.d.) (2000–2009). Committee on the Elimination of Discrimination, the CEDAW Convention. Available at http://www.un.org/women-watch/daw/cedaw/history.htm. Accessed January 4, 2016.

United Nations (UN) Committee on the Elimination of Discrimination Against Women (CEDAW) (1979). *International Convention on the Elimination of Discrimination Against Women.* Available at http://www.un.org/womenwatch/daw/cedaw/. Accessed August 3, 2015.

UN: Conference on Population and Development Report (2014). *World Population Situation in 2014: A Concise Report.* Department of Economic and Social Affairs Population Division ST/ESA/SER.A/354, New York.

United Nations (UN) Human Rights Watch (2015, June). *Report.* Available at https://www.hrw.org/world-report/2015. Accessed January 6, 2016.

United Nations (UN) International Conference on Population and Development (ICPD) (2014a). *Beyond 2014 Global Report.* Available at http://icpdbeyond2014.org/about/view/29-global-review-report. Accessed July 30, 2015.

United Nations (UN) International Conference on Population and Development (ICPD) (2014b). *Global Report, UN Review of ICPD Progress.* Available at http://www.unfpa.org/public/home/sitemap/ICPDReport.

UN: International Conference on Population and Development (ICPD) (2014c). *International Conference on Population and Development (ICPD). Beyond 2014, Report of the UN Secretary-General*, E/CN.9/2014/4.

United Nations (UN) Women (2014). *Commission on the Status of Women.* Available at http://www.unwomen.org/en/csw/csw58-2014.

United Nations (UN): United Nations Development Programme (UNDP) (2013). *Human Development Report, 2013: The Rise of the South*, New York. Available at http://www.undp.org/content/undp/en/home/librarypage/hdr/human-development-report-2013/. Accessed January 10, 2016.

United Nations Development Programme (UNDP) (1999). *Human Development Report.* Available at http://hdr.undp.org/en/content/human-development-report-1999, Accessed November 15, 2000.

United Nations Development Programme (UNDP) (1999). *Human Development Report.* New York: UNDP.

United Nations Development Programme (UNDP) (2000). *The Millennium Development (MDGs) for 2015.* Available at http://www.undp.org/content/undp/en/home/mdgoverview/mdg_goals.html. Accessed August 4, 2015.

United Nations Development Programme (UNDP) (2013). *Annual Human Development Reports.* Available at http://hdr.undp.org/en/reports. Accessed January 4, 2016.

United Nations Development Programme (UNDP) (2014). *Annual Report.* Available at http://icpdbeyond2014.org/uploads/browser/files/icpd_global_review_report.pdf. Accessed December 2014.

United Nations Development Programme (UNDP) (2014a). *Beyond 2015 MDGs.* Available at http://www.er.undp.org/content/eritrea/en/home/presscenter/articles/2014/un-day-2014-eritrea-looking-beyond-20150.html. Accessed August 5, 2015.

United Nations Development Programme (UNDP) (2014b). *Human Development Report, HDR 2014.* Available at http://hdr.undp.org/en/content/human-development-report-2014. Accessed August 3, 2015.

United Nations Development Programme (UNDP) (2014c). *The Millennium Development Goals Report* 2014. Available at www.un.org/millenniumgoals/2014%20MDG%20report/MDG...

United Nations Development Programme (UNDP) (2014d). *Sustainable Development Goals (SDGs).* Available at http://www.undp.org/content/undp/en/home/sdgoverview.html. Accessed January 2016.

United Nations Development Programme (UNDP) (2015). *Human Development Approach (HDA).* Available at http://hdr.undp.org/en/2015-report. Accessed December 28, 2015.

United Nations Development Programme (UNDP) HDR (2014, July 24). *Report.* Available at http://hdr.undp.org/en/content/human-development-report-2014. Accessed July 30, 2015.

United Nations Development Programme (UNDP) HDR (2015). *Gender Inequality Index (GII)*. Available at http://hdr.undp.org/en/content/gender-inequality-index-gii. Accessed July 30, 2015.

United Nations Statistical Division (UNSTATS) (2010). *The World's Women 2010: Trends and Statistics*. Available at http://unstats.un.org/unsd/demographic/products/Worldswomen/WW2010pub.html. Accessed July 2015.

United Nations Statistics Division (2014, March 10–21). *Millennium Development Goals*. Special Edition for the 58th Session of the Commission on the Status of Women. New York: Gender Chart. Available at http://mdgs.un.org/unsd/mdg/Resources/Static/Products/Progress2014/Gender%20Chart%202014.pdf.)

United Nations/United Nations Development Programme (UNDP) (2015a). *The Millennium Development Goals Report*. Available at http://www.un.org/millenniumgoals/2015_MDG_Report/pdf/MDG%202015%20rev%20%28July%201%29.pdf. Accessed January 10, 2016.

United Nations/United Nations Development Programme (UNDP) (2015b). *The Future of Human Development*. Available at https://www.project-syndicate.org/focalpoints/the-future-of-human-development. Accessed January 10, 2016.

United Way (1994). *Los Angeles 1994: State of the County Report. Los Angeles: United Way of Greater Los Angeles*. Available at http://www.unitedwayla.org/. Accessed January 8, 2016.

University of Chicago (2015). *Family Planning and Population Programs*. Chicago. Available at http://familyplanning.uchicago.edu/ Accessed March 16, 2015.

US Census (2011). *Census Bureau Releases 2011 American Community Survey Estimates*. Available at https://www.census.gov/newsroom/releases/archives/american_community_survey_acs/cb12-175.html. Accessed January 9, 2016.

US Institute of Peace (USIP) (2011). *Gender, War and Peacebuilding*. Washington, DC: United States Institute of Peace:10–11. Available at http://www.usip.org/sites/default/files/files/NPECSG12.pdf. Accessed August 3, 2015.

US Surgeon General (2014). *The Health Consequences of Smoking—50 Years of Progress.*. Available at http://www.surgeongeneral.gov/library/reports/50-years-of-progress/full-report.pdf. Accessed January 9, 2016.

Varkey P, Kureshi S, & Lesnick T (2010, January). Empowerment of women and its association with the health of the community. *J Women Health (Larchmt).*, 19(1), 71–6, doi: 10.1089/jwh.2009.1444.

Vedanta Philosophy (2015). Available at http://www.ramakrishnavivekananda.info/vivekananda/volume_1/lectures_and_discourses/the_vedanta_philosophy.htm. Accessed May 25, 2015.

Visaria L, Jeejebhoy S, & Merrick T (1999, January). From Family Planning to Reproductive Health: Challenges Facing India. *Fam Plan Perspect.*, 25(Suppl), 1.

Vivekananda Swami (1893/2013). *A Short Life Of Vivekananda*. Edited by Swami Tejasananda. Kolkata, India: Advaita Ashrama:64.

Vivekananda Swami (1983, September 11). *Lecture on Vedanta Philosophy at At the World's Parliament of Religions*. Chicago. Available at http://www.ramakrishnavivekananda.info/vivekananda/volume_1/addresses_at_the_parliament/v1_c1_response_to_welcome.htm. Accessed January 9, 2016.

Vivekananda Swami (2010, March). *The Vedanta Philosophy: An Address Before the Graduate Philosophical Society of Harvard University, March 25, 1896*. Available at http://www.vivekananda.net/PDFBooks/The_Vedanta_Philosophy.pdf. Accessed May 25, 2015.

Vroom V (1964). Vroom's expectancy models and work-related criteria: A meta-analysis. *J Appl Psychol.*, 81(5), 575–586.

Waite G (1993). Childbirth, lay institution building, and health policy, the Traditional Childbearing Group, Inc., of Boston in a historical sense. In: Bair B & Cayleff SE (Eds), *Wings of Gauze: Women of Color and the Experience of Health and Illness*. Detroit, MI: Wayne State University Press:202–225.

Waldrop MM (1992). *Complexity: The Emerging Science at the Edge of Order and Chaos*. New York: Simon & Schuster.

Walker A & Parmar P (1993). *Warrior Marks: Female Genital Mutilation and the Sexual Blinding of Women*. New York: Harcourt Brace.

Wallack L (1993). *Media Advocacy and Public Health: Power for Prevention*. Newbury Park, CA: Sage.

Wallerstein N (2006). *The Effectiveness of Empowerment Strategies to Improve Health*. Copenhagen: Health Evidence Network, World Health Organization.

Wallerstein N & Bernstein E (1994). Health education and community empowerment: Conceptualizing and measuring perceptions of individual, organizational and community control. *Health Educ Q.*, 21(2), 141–148.

WebMD (2015). Available at http://www.webmd.com/fitness-exercise/walking-for-wellness.

Webster v. Reproductive Health (1989). Available at https://www.law.cornell.edu/supremecourt/text/492/490. Accessed November 26, 2014.

Weeks vs Bell (1967). Court Listener. Available at https://www.courtlistener.com/opinion/1868780/weeks-v-southern-bell-telephone-telegraph-company/. Accessed July 10, 2015.

Weldon W (2011, January). Fix the health care crisis, one employee at a time. *Harvard Business Review,* 4/5. Available at https://hbr.org/2011/01/web-exclusive-fix-the-health-care-crisis-one-employee-at-a-time. Accessed February 20, 2015.

Wells HG (1922). *A Short History of the World*. XXIX. King Asoka. Available at http://www.bartleby.com/86/29.html. Accessed August 3, 2015.

Wheeler CC (1991). *Peace and Power: A Handbook of Feminist Process*. New York: NY National League for Nursing Press.

Willetts P (1981). *Pressure Groups in the Global System*. London: Frances Pinter.

Winslow CE (1920). The untilled fields of public health. *Science,* 51(1306), 23–33.

Wollstonecraft M (1792). *A Vindication of the Rights of Women*. Available at http://www.britannica.com/biography/Mary-Wollstonecraft. Accessed August 4, 2015.

Women Against Gun Violence (WAGV) (2013). Available at http://wagv.org/about-wagv/. Accessed July 20, 2015.

Women Alive (2015). Available at http://women-alive.org/services.html. Accessed February 16, 2015.

Women at Risk International (2005). Available at http://warinternational.org/about-us/our-history/. Accessed January 14, 2016.

Women for Sobriety (WFS) (2011). Available at www.womenforsobriety.org and http://womenforsobriety.org/beta2/about-wfs/. Accessed July 20, 2015.

Women in New Recovery (WINR) (2014). Available at http://www.winr.org/. Accessed July 20, 2015.

Women Living Under Muslim Laws (WLUML) (2015). Available at https://www. myphilanthropedia.org/top-nonprofits/international/violence-against-women/ 2011/women-living-under-muslim-laws-wluml. Accessed July 11, 2015.

Women's Centre of Jamaica Foundation (WCJF) (n.d.). Programme for Adolescent Mothers. Available at http://www.advocatesforyouth.org/publications/1330-womens-centre-of-jamaica-foundation-programme-for-adolescent-mothers and http://www.jamaica-kidz.com/womenscentre/. Accessed July 19, 2015.

Women's Feature Service (WFS) (1992). *The Power to Change: Women in Third World Redefine Their Environment.* New Jersey: Zed Books.

Women's Health Gov (2015, August 13). *Substance Abuse.* Available at http://www. womenshealth.gov/statistics/statistics-by-topic/substance-abuse.html. Accessed January 9, 2016.

Working Women's Forum (India) (WWF) (2015). Available at http://wiego.org/content/ working-womens-forum-india. Accessed July 13, 2015.

Working Women's Forum (WWF) (2009). Available at http://www.workingwomensforum.org/pdf/Awards_final.pdf. Accessed July 13, 2015.

Working Women's Forum (WWF) (2010). Available at http://wiego.org/content/working-womens-forum-india. Accessed July 13, 2015.

World Bank (1999, 2014). *World Development Report.* Washington, DC: World Bank.

World Bank (2012). *World Development Report 2012: Gender Equality and Development (By Topics).* Available at https://openknowledge.worldbank.org/browse?value=Gender+%3A%3A+Gender+and+Development&type=topic.

World Bank (2014). *Maternal Mortality Ratio Table.* Available at http://data.worldbank. org/indicator/SH.STA.MMRT)

World Bank (2015). *Gini Indicators.* Available at http://data.worldbank.org/indicator/ SI.POV.GINI. Accessed December 24, 2015.

World Development Report (WDR) (2014). *The World's Women Report: Gender at Work.* Available at https://www.worldbank.org/en/topic/gender/publication/gender-at-work-companion-report-to-world-development-report-2013-jobs. Accessed July 30, 2015.

World Happiness Report (WHR) (2013). Available at http://unsdsn.org/wp-content/ uploads/2014/02/WorldHappinessReport2013_online.pdf. Accessed July 29, 2015.

World Health Organization (WHO) (1948). *The Constitution of the World Health Organization.* Geneva: WHO. Available at http://www.who.int/governance/eb/who_constitution_en.pdf. Accessed January 2014.

World Health Organization (WHO) (1966). *Annual Report.* Geneva, Switzerland: WHO. Available at http://www.worldcat.org/title/second-ten-years-of-the-world-health-organization-1958-1967/oclc/467865&referer=brief_results. Accessed December 12, 2015.

World Health Organization (WHO) (1986). *Ottawa Charter for Health Promotion. An International Conference on Health Promotion*, PAHO Scientific Publications No. 557. Ottawa, Canada: WHO.

World Health Organization (WHO) (1996). Investing in Health Research and Development. *Report of the Ad Hoc Committee on Health Research Relating to Future Intervention Options.* Geneva: World Health Organization.

World Health Organization (WHO) (1997a). *The Jakarta Declaration.* Available at http://www.who.int/healthpromotion/conferences/previous/jakarta/declaration/en. Accessed August 3, 2015.

World Health Organization (WHO) (1997b). Measuring Quality of Life. Available at http://www.who.int/mental_health/media/68.pdf. Accessed August 2, 2015.

World Health Organization (WHO) (1997c). WHOQOL—Measuring Quality of Life and The World Health Organization Quality of Life Instrument. WHO/MSA/MNH PSF 197-4. Geneva: Division of Mental Health and Prevention of Substance Abuse, WHO.

World Health Organization (WHO) (1998). CHOICE (Choosing Interventions that are Cost-effective). Available at http://www.who.int/choice/cost-effectiveness/en/. Accessed July 28, 2015.

World Health Organization (WHO) (1998). *CHOICE (CHOosing Interventions that are Cost-Effective).* Available at http://www.who.int/choice/cost-effectiveness/en/. Accessed August 4, 2015.

World Health Organization (WHO) (1999a). *Health and Development in the 20th Century.* Geneva: WHO. Available at http://www.who.int/whr/1999/en/. Accessed August 4, 2015.

World Health Organization (WHO) (1999b). *The World Health Report 1999.* Geneva: WHO.

World Health Organization (WHO) (2000). *Global Health Estimates (GHE).* Available at http://www.who.int/healthinfo/global_burden_disease/en/

World Health Organization (WHO) (2002). *The World Health Report 2002—Reducing Risks, Promoting Healthy Life.* Available at http://www.who.int/whr/2002/en/. Accessed November 16, 2014.

World Health Organization (WHO) (2004). *The Global Burden of Disease: 2004 Update.* Geneva, Switzerland: WHO. Available at http://www.who.int/healthinfo/global_burden_disease/GBD_report_2004update_full.pdf. Accessed November 16, 2014.

World Health Organization (WHO) (2008). *Commission on Social Determinants of Health (CSDH), Final Report.* Geneva, Switzerland. Available at http://apps.who.int/iris/bitstream/10665/43943/1/9789241563703_eng.pdf. Accessed January 26, 2012.

World Health Organization (WHO) (2013). *World Health Report 2013: Research for Universal Health Coverage.* Available at http://www.who.int/whr/en/.

World Health Organization (WHO) (2015). *Call to Involve, Mobilize and Empower Health-Workers to End Female Genital Mutilation.* Available at http://www.who.int/reproductivehealth/topics/fgm/zero-tolerance-day/en/. Accessed December 29, 2015.

World Health Organization (WHO) (n.d.). *Health-Related Quality of Life (HRQOL).* Available at http://www.who.int/substance_abuse/research_tools/whoqolbref/en/.

World Health Organization (WHO)/EURO (1986). *The Ottawa Charter.* Available at http://www.who.int/healthpromotion/conferences/previous/ottawa/en/. Accessed August 4, 2015.

World Health Organization (WHO)/European Regional Office (EURO) (1986). The Ottawa Charter for Health Promotion. In: *Health Promotion: An Anthology. Proceedings of the International Conference on Health Promotion*, Ottawa, Canada. Washington, DC: Pan American Health Organization. Available at http://www.euro.who.int/__data/assets/pdf_file/0004/129532/Ottawa_Charter.pdf. Accessed January 10, 2016.

World Health Organization (WHO)/Female Genital Mutilation (FGM) (2014). *Fact Sheet 241*. Available at http://www.who.int/mediacentre/factsheets/fs241/en/. Accessed November 25, 2015.

World Health Organization (WHO)/FGM/C (2015). Female Genital Mutilation and Other Harmful Practices. Available at http://www.who.int/reproductivehealth/topics/fgm/prevalence/en/. Accessed July 2, 2015.

World Health Organization (WHO)/HRQOL (2004). *WHO Health Related Quality of Life*. Available at http://www.who.int/substance_abuse/research_tools/whoqolbref/en/. Accessed August 4, 2015.

World Health Organization (WHO)/Pan American Health Organization (PAHO) (1986). *Health Promotion Anthology*. Scientific Publication No. 557. Washington, DC: PAHO.

World Health Organization (WHO)/ Pan American Health Organization (PAHO) (1996). *Health and Human Development in the New Global Economy: The Contribution and Perspectives of Civil Society in the Americas*. Available at http://publications.paho.org/pdf/HealthHumanDev.pdf. Accessed January 26, 2014.

World Health Organization (WHO)/SEARO (1995). *SEWA Case Study*. Available at http://www.who.int/social_determinants/resources/isa_sewa_ind.pdf. Accessed July 14, 2015.

World Health Organization (WHO)/SEARO (1995). The SEWA Case Study. Available at http://www.who.int/social_determinants/resources/isa_sewa_ind.pdf. Accessed August 4, 2015.

World Health Organization (WHO)/SEARO (1999). *The Kolkata Declaration*. New Delhi, India: WHO/SEARO.

World Health Organization (WHO)/SEARO (2000). The Calcutta declaration on public health. *J Health Popul Dev Ctries.*, 3(1).

World Health Organization (WHO)/UNICEF (1978a). *The Alma-Ata Declaration, Primary Health Care: Report of the International Conference on Primary Health Care, Alma-Ata, USSR*. Geneva, Switzerland: WHO. Available at http://www.who.int/publications/almaata_declaration_en.pdf. Accessed November 15, 2015.

World Health Organization (WHO)/UNICEF (1978b). *Declaration of Alma-Ata: International Conference on Primary Health Care*. Geneva: WHO.

World Health Organization (WHO)/Western Pacific Regional Office (WPRO) (1997). *Renewing the Strategy for Health for All: Report of the Sub-Committee of the Regional Committee on Programmes and Technical Cooperation*, Part II. Manila, Philippines: WHO/WPRO.

Worlds Women/UN (2015). *Progress of the Worlds Women: 2015–2016*. Available at http://progress.unwomen.org/en/2015/. Accessed January 9, 2016.

World-YWCA (2015). *YWCA: Our History*. Available at http://www.worldywca.org/About-us/Our-History. Accessed January 8, 2016.

Yates WB (1913). *An Introduction to Gitanjali (Offerings of Singa) by Rabindranath Tagore*. Available at http://www.sacred-texts.com/hin/tagore/gitnjali.htm/. Accessed January 6, 2016.

Young G, Samarasinghe V, & Kusterer K (1993). *Women at the Center: Development Issues and Practices for the 1990s*. West Hartford, CT: Kumarian Press.

Yunus M (2003). *Banker to the Poor: Micro-Lending and the Battle Against World Poverty*. US: Public Affairs.

Yunus M (2006). *Woman Are Better with Money.* Available at http://www.spiegel.de/international/spiegel/0,1518,453234,00.html. Accessed February 10, 2015.

Yunus M (2010, May 4). *Building Social Business, Public Affairs* (reprint edn). Available at http://muhammadyunus.org/index.php/for-test-only/580-building-social-business-the-new-kind-of-capitalism-that-serves-humanitys-most-pressing-needs. Accessed June 1, 2015.

Yunus M (2015a). *Management Study Guide (MSG), Seven Principles of Social Business.* Available at http://www.managementstudyguide.com/social-business-principles.htm. Accessed July 14, 2015.

Yunus M (2015b). *Social Business Is a Cause-Driven Business.* Dhaka, Bangladesh: Yunus Centre. Available at http://muhammadyunus.org/www.muhammadyunus.org/index.php/social-business/social. Accessed August 4, 2015.

YWCA (2007, May). *Advocacy Kit.* Available at http://intranet.ywca.org/atf/cf/%7B38f90928-ee78-4ce9-a81e-7298da01493e%7D/YWCA_ADVOCACY_TOOLKIT.PDF. Accessed July 12, 2015.

YWCA (2014). *Strategic Framework.* Available at http://www.worldywca.org/About-us/Strategic-Framework-2012-2015. Accessed July 11, 2015.

Z News (2014, July 15). Available at http://zeenews.india.com/news/nation/president-presents-gandhi-peace-prize-to-chandi-prasad-bhatt_947473.html

Zahidi S (2014). *Women in the Muslim World Taking the Fast Track to Change.* Available at http://www.mckinsey.com/insights/social_sector/women_in_the_muslim_world_taking_the_fast_track_to_change. Accessed July 11, 2015.

Zimbardo P (2007). *The Lucifer Effect: How Good People Turn Evil.* New York: Random House.

Zimmerman M (1989). Empowerment theory: Psychological, organizational and community levels of analysis. In: Rappaport J & Seidman E (Eds), *Handbook of Community Psychology.* New York: Kluwer Academic/Plenum:43–63.

Zimmerman M (1995). Psychological empowerment: Issues and illustrations. *Am J Commun Psychol.,* 23(5), 581–599.

Zimmerman M, Israel BA, Schultz A, & Checkoway B (1992). Further explorations in empowerment theory: An empirical analysis of psychological empowerment. *Am J Commun Psychol.,* 20(6), 707–727.

ADDITIONAL READING

Gomes (2015). Banchte Sekha web site. Available at http://word.world-citizenship.org/wp-archive/1118 and http://www.mixmarket.org/mfi/banchte-shekha.

KABOO (2015). Available at http://kboo.fm/program. Accessed July 20, 2015.

Large J (1995). Feminist conflict resolution. In: Ashworth G (Ed.), :23–32.

Mothers' Voices United to End AIDS (0000). Available at http://www.mvgeorgia.org/ and http://www.mvgeorgia.org/programs/hisstd-public-advocacy/. Accessed July 17, 2015.

Perry L (1964a). The First Surgeon General's Report—Smoking and Tobacco Use, CDC. Available at http://archive.tobacco.org/resources/history/1964_01_11_1st_sgr.html. Accessed May 22, 2015.

Perry L (1964b). The Reports of the Surgeon General: The 1964 Report on Smoking and Health. Bethesda, MD: National Library of Medicine. Available at http://profiles.nlm.nih.gov/ps/retrieve/Narrative/NN/p-nid/60. Accessed July 28, 2015.

Stanford Encyclopedia of Philosophy (0000). "Justice is Fairness." Available at http://plato.stanford.edu/entries/rawls/. Accessed August 4, 2015.

United Nations Development Programme (0000). What Is Human Development? Available at http://www.undp.org/hdro/hd.htm.

United Nations Statistical Division (UNSTATS) (2015). Available at http://unstats.un.org/unsd/demographic/products/Worldswomen/WW_full%20report_color.pdf and http://unstats.un.org/unsd/demographic/products/Worldswomen/WWreports.htm. Accessed July 12, 2015.

Women and Substance Abuse (0000). Available at http://alcoholism.about.com/od/women/ Accessed July 20, 2015.

Women in New Recovery (WINR) (0000). Available at http://treatment-facilities.healthgrove.com/l/245/Women-in-New-Recovery. Accessed July 20, 2015.

INDEX